# HANDBOOK OF MEDICINE
# OF THE FETUS & MOTHER

# HANDBOOK OF MEDICINE
# OF THE FETUS & MOTHER

## E. ALBERT REECE, MD
The Abraham Roth Professor and Chairman,
Professor of Obstetrics, Gynecology,
Reproductive Sciences, and Internal Medicine
Director, Division of Maternal Fetal Medicine
Temple University School of Medicine
Philadelphia, Pennsylvania

## JOHN C. HOBBINS, MD
Professor and Chief of Obstetrics
Director of Prenatal Diagnosis and Genetics
University of Colorado, School of Medicine
Denver, Colorado

## MAURICE J. MAHONEY, MD
Professor of Genetics, Pediatrics and Obstetrics and Gynecology
Director of The Prenatal Diagnosis Unit
Director of Clinical Affairs
Yale University School of Medicine
New Haven, Connecticut

## ROY H. PETRIE, MD, ScD
Professor and Chairman of Obstetrics and Gynecology
Division of Maternal-Fetal Medicine
Department of Obstetrics and Gynecology
St. Louis University School of Medicine
St. Louis, Missouri

**129 contributors**

**J.B. LIPPINCOTT COMPANY**
Philadelphia

Acquisitions Editor: Lisa McAllister
Developmental Editor: Paula Callaghan
Indexer: Michael Loo
Production Service: Textbook Writers Associates
Cover Designer: Tom Jackson
Production Manager: Janet Greenwood
Production Editor: Mary Kinsella
Compositor: Circle Graphics
Printer/Binder: RR Donnelley & Sons, Crawfordsville

6  5  4  3  2  1

Library of Congress Cataloging-in-Publication Data

Handbook of medicine of the fetus & mother / E. Albert Reece . . .
    [et al.] ; 129 contributors.
        p.      cm.
    Includes index.
    Condensed version of: Medicine of the fetus & mother. c1992.
    ISBN 0-397-51347-X
    1. Pregnancy.  2. Obstetrics.  I. Reece, E. Albert.  II. Medicine
of the fetus & mother.
    [DNLM:  1. Pregnancy Complications.  2. Pregnancy.  3. Fetal
Development. WQ 240 H236 1995]
RG551.H36      1995
618.3-dc20
DNLM/DLC
For Library of Congress                                        94-30432
                                                                    CIP

The authors and publisher have exerted every effort to ensure that drug selection and dosage set forth in this text are in accord with current recommendations and practice at the time of publication. However, in view of ongoing research, changes in government regulations, and the constant flow of information relating to drug therapy and drug reactions, the reader is urged to check the package insert for each drug for any change in indications and dosage and for added warnings and precautions. This is particularly important when the recommended agent is a new or infrequently employed drug.

# PREFACE

The field of maternal–fetal medicine has been recognized as the academic arm of obstetrics since the 1970s. In recent years, the specialty has flourished and now encompasses many other allied fields, including genetics, teratology, diagnostic imaging, endocrinology, fetal physiology and pathology. Various technological advances now permit in utero diagnosis, as well as both medical and surgical treatment of the fetus.

This handbook has been designed to complement the textbook *Medicine of the Fetus & Mother*. It is our hope that clinicians will turn to this handbook for assistance and guidance as they encounter the complex and often perplexing issues involving care of the fetus and mother. This handbook is intended to provide the practicing obstetrician with succinct, clinically focused and easily retrievable information regarding both the maternal and fetal complications of pregnancy. Each chapter focuses on a specific aspect of maternal–fetal medicine and highlights current modalities for diagnosis, evaluation, and treatment.

E. Albert Reece, MD
John C. Hobbins, MD
Maurice J. Mahoney, MD
Roy H. Petrie, MD, ScD

# CONTRIBUTING AUTHORS

Diana M. Adams
N. Scott Adzick
Erol Amon
Frederick C. Battaglia
David A. Beckman
Richard L. Berkowitz
Pravit Bisalbutra
John M. Bowman
D. Ware Branch
Robert L. Brent
G. N. Burrow
Tim Chard
Frank A. Chervenak
Cecilia Y. Cheung
David A. Clark
Steven L. Clark
Mark J. Clinton
Wayne R. Cohen
Joshua A. Copel
David B. Cotton
Donald R. Coustan
Joe Craft
Robert K. Creasy
F. Daffos
Alan H. DeCherney
Gary A. Dildy
James O. Donaldson
Jennifer I. Downey
Mark I. Evans
Fiona M. Fairlie
Ann M. Ferris
Mieczyslaw Finster
John C. Fletcher
F. Forestier
Axel Forman
Harold Fox
Sandro Gabrielli
A. B. Galway
Alessandro Ghidini
Ronald S. Gibbs
J. S. Ginsberg
Mitchell S. Golbus

James D. Goldberg
Ian Gross
John H. Grossman III
James E. Haddow
Zion J. Hagay
Michael R. Harrison
Jean C. Hay
John P. Hayslett
Washington Clark Hill
J. Hirsh
John C. Hobbins
Angela R. Holder
Lillian Y. F. Hsu
Alan J. Hill
Frederick R. Jelovsek
Mark Paul Johnson
Ervin E. Jones
Russell K. Laros, Jr.
Nicholas Kadar
Ruben Kier
Charles S. Kleinman
William Ledger
Jean M. Lien
Charles J. Lockwood
Barbara Luke
Lauren Lynch
Maurice J. Mahoney
Frank A. Manning
Linda J. Van Marter
Richard A. Matthay
Donald R. Mattison
Laurence B. McCullough
James G. McNamara
Philip B. Mead
Aubrey Milunsky
Fernando R. Moya
Katherine V. Nichols
Jennifer R. Niebyl
Michael S. Niederman
Barbara M. Nies
Carl A. Nimrod
Jose Nores

Glenn E. Palomaki
Valerie M. Parisi
Richard Paul
Hilda Pedersen
David B. Peisner
T. V. N. Persaud
Lone K. Petersen
Roy H. Petrie
Jeffrey P. Phelan
Gianluigi Pilu
Edward Quilligan
C. W. G. Redman
E. Albert Reece
Deborah L. Reid
Caroline A. Riely
Roberto Romero
Mortimer G. Rosen
Benjamin P. Sachs
Alan C. Santos
I. L. Sargent
Philip M. Sarrel
Peter E. Schwartz
James R. Scott
Ulla M. Sellgren

John L. Sever
Kathryn Shaw
Jaye M. Shyken
Baha M. Sibai
Joe Leigh Simpson
Ray Bahado-Singh
Susan L. Sipes
Kristjar Skajaa
Danny Svane
Richard L. Sweet
Michael de Swiet
Samuel S. Thatcher III
David Trock
Brian J. Trudinger
Niels Uldbjerg
Richard R. Viscarello
Joseph J. Volpe
Cheryl K. Walker
Carl P. Weiner
Selman I. Welt
Agnes H. Whitaker
Karen A. Hutchinson-Williams
Kim B. Yancey

# CONTENTS

# HANDBOOK OF MEDICINE OF THE FETUS & MOTHER

# PART I. PREGNANCY AND THE FETOPLACENTAL UNIT

## 1. NORMAL PLACENTATION AND DEVELOPMENT

### NORMAL PLACENTATION

The placenta as expelled from the uterus is generally regarded as a complete organ. The fetal placenta, is not, however, the total structure; there is also a vitally important maternal component of the placenta, which comprises the placental bed and the uteroplacental vessels.

### DEVELOPMENT OF THE FETAL PLACENTA

The fertilized ovum enters the uterine cavity as a morula that rapidly converts into a blastocyst and loses its surrounding zona pellucida. The outer cell layer of the blastocyst proliferates to form the primary trophoblastic cell mass, from which cells infiltrate between those of the endometrial epithelium. The latter degenerates and the trophoblast thus comes into contact with the endometrial stroma. This process of implantation is complete by the 10th or 11th postovulatory day. In the 7-day conceptus, the trophoblast forms a peripheral circumferential plaque, which rapidly differentiates into two layers, an inner layer of large, mononuclear cytotrophoblastic cells with well-defined, limiting membranes, and an outer layer of multinucleated syncytiotrophoblast, which is a true syncytium. That the syncytiotrophoblast is derived from the cytotrophoblast, not only at this early stage but throughout gestation, is now well established.

Between the 10th and 13th postovulatory days, a series of intercommunicating clefts, or lacunae, appear in the rapidly enlarging trophoblastic cell mass (Fig. 1-1). These are probably formed as a result of engulfment within the trophoblast of endometrial capillaries. These lacunae soon become confluent to form the precursor of the intervillous space and, as maternal vessels are progressively eroded, this becomes filled with maternal blood. At this stage the lacunae are incompletely separated from each other by trabecular columns of syncytiotrophoblast which, between the 14th and 21st postovulatory days, tend to become radially orientated and come to possess a central cellular core that is produced by proliferation of the cytotrophoblastic cells at the chorionic base. These trabeculae are not true villi but serve as the framework, or scaffolding, from which the villous tree will later

E. Albert Reece, John C. Hobbins, Maurice, J. Mahoney and Roy H. Petrie (Eds).
*Handbook of Medicine of the Fetus & Mother.* Copyright © 1995 by J.B. Lippincott Company

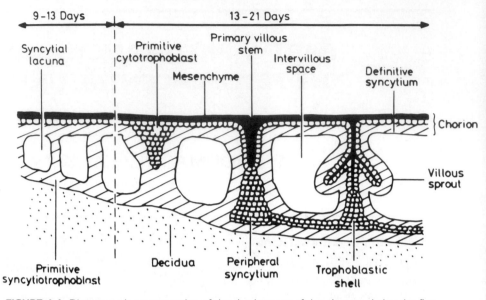

**FIGURE 1-1.** Diagrammatic representation of the development of the placenta during the first 21 days of gestation.

develop. The placenta at this time is a labyrinthine rather than a villous organ and the trabeculae act as "primary villous stems."

Between the 21st postovulatory day and the end of the fourth month of gestation, there is not only continuing growth but also considerable remodelling of the placenta. The villi orientated toward the uterine cavity degenerate and form the chorion laeve, while the thin rim of decidua covering this area gradually disappears to allow the chorion laeve to come into contact with the parietal decidua of the opposite wall of the uterus. The villi on the side of the chorion orientated toward the decidual plate proliferate and progressively arborize to form the chorion frondosum, which develops into the definitive fetal placenta.

The placental septa appear during the third month of gestation: they protrude into the intervillous space from the basal plate and divide the maternal surface of the placenta into 15 to 20 lobes. These septa are simply folds of the basal plate, formed partly as a result of regional variability in placental growth and partly by the pulling up of the basal plate by the anchoring columns, which have a poor growth rate. Because the basal plate is formed principally by the remnants of the trophoblastic shell embedded in fibrinoid material, it follows that the septa are similarly constituted, although some decidual cells may also be carried up into the folds. The septa are simply an incidental by-product of the architectural remodelling of the placenta, and have no physiological or morphological role to play.

By the end of the fourth month of gestation, the fetal placenta has achieved its definitive form and undergoes no further anatomical modification. Growth continues, however, until term and is due principally to the continuing branching of the villous tree and formation of fresh villi.

## DEVELOPMENT OF THE MATERNAL PLACENTA

During the early weeks of gestation, cytotrophoblastic cells stream out from the tips of the anchoring villi, penetrate the trophoblastic shell, and extensively colonize the decidua and adjacent myometrium of the placental bed. These cells are known as the "interstitial extravillous cytotrophoblast"; in addition, trophoblastic cells stream into the lumens of the intradecidual portions of the spiral arteries of the placental bed, where they form intralumenal plugs and constitute the "intravascular extravillous cytotrophoblast." These endovascular trophoblastic cells destroy and replace the endothelium of the maternal vessels and then invade the media, with resulting destruction of the medial elastic and muscular tissue: the arterial wall becomes replaced by fibrinoid material that appears to be derived partly from fibrin in the maternal blood and partly from proteins secreted by the invading trophoblastic cells. This process is complete by the end of the first trimester, at which time these "physiological" changes within the spiral arteries of the placental bed extend to the myometriodecidual junction. There then appears to be a pause in this process, but between the 14th and 16th week of gestation there is a resurgence of endovascular trophoblastic migration, with a second wave of cells moving down into the intramyometrial segments of the spiral arteries, extending as far as the origin of these vessels from the radial arteries. Within the intramyometrial portion of the spiral arteries the same process that occurs in their intradecidual portion is repeated (i.e., replacement of the endothelium, invasion and destruction of the medial musculo-elastic tissue, and fibrinoid change in the vessel wall). The end result of this trophoblastic invasion of, and attack on, the vessels is that the thick-walled muscular spiral arteries are converted into flaccid, sac-like uteroplacental vessels (Fig. 1-2) that can passively dilate in order to accommodate the greatly augmented blood flow through this vascular system, which is required as pregnancy progresses.

It will be apparent that the extravillous intravascular population of trophoblastic cells plays a key role in placentation, and that via these cells the placenta estab-

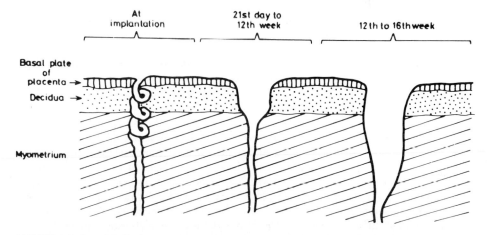

**FIGURE 1-2.** Diagrammatic representation of the conversion of the spiral arteries in the placental bed into uteroplacental vessels.

lishes its own low-pressure, high-conductance vascular system, thus ensuring an adequate maternal blood flow to itself and an ample supply of oxygen and nutrients to the fetus.

## ANATOMY OF THE FETAL PLACENTA

The fetal placenta is made up of a number of subunits that are now generally known as lobules. The primary stem villi break up just below the chorial plate into a number of secondary stem villi that, after running parallel to the chorionic plate for a short distance, divide into a series of tertiary stem villi. The lobules are derived from these tertiary stem villi, which sweep down through the intervillous space to anchor onto the basal plate; during the course through the intervillous space they give off multiple branches that ramify into the terminal villous network. As the tertiary stem villi pass down toward the basal plate, they are arranged in a circular fashion around the periphery of an empty cylindrical space; the lobule thus forms a hollow globule, with the bulk of the terminal villi mainly in the outer shell of this globular structure and the center of the lobule relatively empty and free of villi. The lobules are separated from each other by interlobular areas that are in continuity with the subchorial space.

## THE MATERNAL UTEROPLACENTAL CIRCULATORY SYSTEM

Maternal blood enters the intervillous space via arterial inlets in the basal plate and is then driven by the head of maternal pressure toward the chorionic plate as a funnel-shaped stream. The driving head of maternal pressure is gradually dissipated, a process aided by the baffling effect of the villi, and lateral dispersion of the blood occurs. This forces the blood already present in the intervillous space out through basally sited wide venous outlets, into the endometrial venous network. The maternal blood enters the space "much as water from an actively flowing brook penetrates a reed-filled marsh."

The physiological basis for this circulatory system is a series of pressure differentials. The pressure in the maternal arterioles is higher than the mean intervillous space pressure which, in turn, exceeds that in the maternal veins during a myometrial diastole. This entire system is, however, a low-pressure one, for whereas in most organs there is a progressive decrease in the diameter of the arteries as they approach their target tissues, the reverse is true for the placenta. The uteroplacental vessels assume an increasing diameter as they approach their entry into the intervillous space. There is, therefore, a considerable drop in pressure from the proximal to the distal portion of these vessels, and the full arterial pressure is not transmitted to the intervillous space. The placenta itself offers little flow resistance to maternal blood and has a high vascular conductance; there is thus very little fall in pressure across the intervillous space, and the main factor governing the rate of maternal blood flow in a normal pregnancy is the vascular resistance within the radial arteries. Despite the fact that the pressure difference between arterial and venous sides of the intervillous space is small, it is apparently sufficient to drive arterial blood toward the chorionic plate, to stop short-cutting of the stream into adjacent venous outlets, and to prevent mixing of neighboring arterial inflows.

Cineangiography has shown that the individual uteroplacental arteries act independently of each other. They are not all patent and do not discharge blood simultaneously into the intervillous space. Furthermore, during myometrial contractions, the afferent blood flow through the intervillous space may be markedly reduced or can even cease. This is probably due to compression and occlusion of the veins draining the intervillous space, but ultrasonic studies have shown that during a myometrial contraction the intervillous space distends, so the fetus is not severely deprived of an oxygen supply during myometrial systole.

## RELATIONSHIP OF MATERNAL CIRCULATORY SYSTEM TO FETAL LOBULE

A definite relationship exists between the maternal vessels and the fetal lobules. This is not coincidental, because it is probable that the lobules tend to develop preferentially around the flow from eroded maternal vessels. The exact nature of this relationship is still not fully determined, and two contrasting schemes have been proposed. Some have thought that arterial inlets into the intervillous space are so situated that the inflow from each uteroplacental vessel is into the central, villous-free space of a fetal lobule, and that the maternal blood then flows laterally through the lobule into the interlobular area, from which it is drained by basal venous outlets (Fig. 1-3). Others consider that the maternal vessels open, not into the central space of a lobule, but into the interlobular spaces, and that the maternal blood then encircles the lobule in streams to form a shell around them, entering and leaving the lobule while doing this and before draining through the basal outlets.

Whichever of these two concepts is correct, it is clear that maternal–fetal exchange takes place principally in those villi that form the shell of the lobule, and that it is only here that a true functional intervillous space, which is probably only

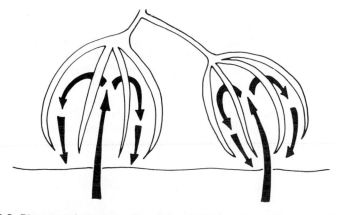

**FIGURE 1-3.** Diagrammatic representation of the relationship between the maternal blood flow (*black arrows*) and the fetal lobule as envisaged by Wigglesworth. (Wigglesworth, JS. Vascular organization of the human placenta. Nature 1976;216:1120.)

of capillary caliber, exists; elsewhere, in the subchorial lake, the interlobular spaces, and the central intralobular spaces, villi are either sparse or absent, and these areas are, in functional terms, "physiological dead spaces."

## HISTOLOGY OF THE PLACENTAL VILLI

In the first 2 months of pregnancy, the villi are relatively few in number, have a homogenous pattern, and measure approximately 170 μm in diameter. Their outer surface is covered by a trophoblastic mantle, which has two layers: an outer layer of syncytiotrophoblast, and an inner layer of cytotrophoblastic cells (Langhans' cells).

The villous stroma is, at this stage, formed by loose mesenchymal tissue: by the end of the second month of gestation, small, centrally placed vessels, lined by large, immature endothelial cells, are present. Hofbauer cells are a prominent feature of the villous stroma: these cells may be round, ovoid, or reniform, measure about 25 μm in diameter, and have an eccentrically placed nucleus. There is now overwhelming evidence that the Hofbauer cells are fetal tissue macrophages; their origin is, however, obscure, for they are present in the villi before they are vascularized by fetal vessels and before hematopoiesis begins in the fetus.

Between the 8th and 30th weeks of gestation, the villi become more numerous, and the predominant form of villus has an average diameter of about 40 μm. In these villi the cytotrophoblastic cells are less prominent, while the syncytiotrophoblast is thinner and somewhat irregular: the syncytial nuclei are less evenly distributed than in the first trimester, and often show a degree of clustering. A distinct, but thin, trophoblastic basement membrane is present, separating the trophoblast from the stroma.

From about the 30th week of gestation, small terminal villi, measuring about 40 μm in diameter, begin to appear; these are the predominant form of villi seen in the term placenta. Their trophoblastic-covering layer is irregularly thinned, and cytotrophoblastic cells are few and inconspicuous.

In the terminal villi, there are usually between two and six fetal capillary vessels, which are characteristically situated toward the villous periphery in close approximation to the covering trophoblast. These vessels are commonly sinusoidally dilated and occupy most of the cross-sectional area of the villus. Some have thought that the dilatation of the fetal villous vessels was a mechanism for crowding flow lines, and hence increasing concentration gradients, for substances crossing from maternal to fetal blood, and was thus a mechanism for augmenting the efficiency of placental transfer mechanisms. By contrast, others have considered that the sinusoidal dilatation of these vessels was a means of decreasing blood flow resistance, for allowing an evenness of blood flow throughout the placenta, and for facilitating fetal placental perfusion.

# 2. PLACENTAL HORMONES AND METABOLISM

Pregnancy is a time of major physiological and metabolic changes in the mother. These changes are assumed to be adjustments of maternal physiology to ensure optimal survival of the fetus.

There are four mechanisms by which the fetoplacental unit* can influence maternal physiology and metabolism:

1. The uteroplacental circulation is a massive arteriovenous shunt that demands major adaptations in the maternal cardiovascular system.
2. The fetoplacental unit consumes large quantities of nutrients to support its normal metabolism and growth, and at the same time excretes a range of waste products.
3. The conceptus and uterus have major mechanical effects on surrounding organs and vessels.
4. The fetoplacental unit secretes a number of "specific" products that may have hormonal activity in the mother.

## PRODUCTS OF THE HUMAN FETOPLACENTAL UNIT

Fetal products (e.g., alphafetoprotein) are not considered to play any role in maternal physiology, and will not be discussed further here.

The placenta secretes a wide range of materials that are considered to be specific to that organ (Table 2-1). The specificity may be either quantitative or qualitative. Quantitative specificity refers to estrogens and progesterone that are secreted by the ovary but are secreted in much greater quantities by the placenta. Qualitative specificity refers to those placental proteins that are associated almost exclusively with pregnancy. However, small quantities of the placental proteins are found in sites such as seminal plasma and ovarian follicular fluid.

The tissue of origin of the "placental" proteins (see Table 2-1) is either the placental syncytiotrophoblast (Groups 1 and 2) or the maternal decidua (Group 3).† The secretion of the major pregnancy estrogen, estriol ($E_3$), is dependent on precursors from the fetal adrenal and liver. The trophoblast proteins (Groups 1 and 2) are secreted almost exclusively into the mother; the levels in the fetal circulation are 100-fold less.

---

* "Fetoplacental unit" is used here as a convenient term for the ensemble of the conceptus, although to some extent fetus and placenta may behave as independent organisms.

† The decidual proteins (PP12 and PP14) were originally isolated from the placenta, and were only subsequently recognized as being of maternal origin (endometrium/decidua). As a result, the terminology is confused; until a final agreement is reached, most of the reproductive literature will probably prefer the original "PP" terminology, and this convention is followed here.

E. Albert Reece, John C. Hobbins, Maurice, J. Mahoney and Roy H. Petrie (Eds).
*Handbook of Medicine of the Fetus & Mother.* Copyright © 1995 by J.B. Lippincott Company

**TABLE 2-1.** A Classification of Human Placental Products
Based on a Variety of Biological and Clinical Characteristics

| Group 1 | Group 2 | Group 3* |
|---|---|---|
| Heat stable alkaline phosphatase (HSAP) | Placental protein 5 (PP5) Pregnancy-associated plasma protein A (PAPP-A) | Placental protein 12† (PP12) Placental protein 14† (PP14) |
| Cystine aminopeptidase (CAP; oxytocinase) | | |
| Estrogens (E) | | |
| Progesterone (P) | | |
| Human chorionic gonadotropin (hCG) | | |
| Human placental lactogen (hPL) | | |
| Schwangerschaftsprotein 1 (SP1) | | |
| Releasing hormones | | |

* Group 3 products, although originally isolated from placental extracts, are synthesized by the maternal endometrium/decidua.
† There are many synonyms for these materials.

The functional characteristics of the placental proteins are summarized in Table 2-2. These characteristics are derived from experimental observations that cannot necessarily be extrapolated to a function in a normal pregnant woman.

## SOME PROBLEMS WITH THE ATTRIBUTION OF METABOLIC EFFECTS TO PLACENTAL PRODUCTS

It is difficult to specify the precise functional role of any one of the placental products. The reasons for this problem are:

1. The hormonal effects of placental products are only one of a number of mechanisms that can alter maternal physiology.
2. There is a multiplicity of placental products, and some of these might have very similar effects.
3. Most of the proposed functions of placental products (see Table 2-2) are based on experiments in animals, in nonpregnant humans, or in tissue culture. None of these can provide a satisfactory emulation of the complete pregnant woman.
4. There are rare pregnancies in which one or another of the placental products is completely absent. This has been described many times for hPL and estriol. The pregnancy itself is usually entirely normal. This may exclude an essential function for these materials.
5. Some of the most dramatic alterations in maternal physiology occur during the first trimester, when the synthesis of placental products is relatively limited.
6. There is a notable absence of the feedback control mechanisms that characterize most classical endocrine systems.
7. Although there are random time-to-time fluctuations in the levels of placental products, there is no systematic change in circulating levels over a 24-hour period.

TABLE 2-2. A Summary of the Main Functional Characteristics
of the Three Groups of Placental Products

| Material | Functional Characteristics |
|---|---|
| **Group 1** | |
| Heat stable alkaline phosphatase (HSAP) | Unknown |
| Cystine aminopeptidase (CAP) | Proteolysis of oxytocin |
| Estrogens and progesterone | Various physiological and metabolic adjustments in the mother (see Tables 2-3 and 2-4) |
| Human chorionic gonadotropin (hCG) | Maintenance of corpus luteum |
| Human placental lactogen (hPL) | Mammotrophic. Various metabolic effects |
| Placental growth hormone (pGH) | Control of IGF-I levels |
| Schwangerschaftsprotein 1 (SP1) | Unknown |
| **Group 2** | |
| PAPP-A | Antiproteolytic; anticomplementary |
| PP5 | Antithrombin |
| **Group 3** | |
| PP12 | IGF-binding protein |
| PP14 | Beta lactoglobulin |

## MATERNAL METABOLIC EFFECTS OF PLACENTAL PRODUCTS

### PRODUCTS THAT ARE NOT CONSIDERED TO HAVE SIGNIFICANT METABOLIC EFFECTS

Of the materials listed in Table 2-1, the following are not generally considered to have significant metabolic functions: HSAP, CAP, hCG, SP1, PAPP-A, and PP14.

### EFFECTS OF ESTROGENS AND PROGESTERONE

All of the maternal metabolic changes in pregnancy could be attributed to either or both of estrogens and progesterone secreted by the placenta (Tables 2-3 and 2-4). However, a large part of the literature consists of observations of the effects of oral contraceptive agents on nonpregnant woman. The spectrum of estrogenic and progestogenic steroids in these is not necessarily representative of endogenous materials. Furthermore, orally administered estrogens have a far greater effect on metabolic functions than do parenterally administered steroids. Of the various metabolic changes listed in Tables 2-3 and 2-4, the least ambiguous in terms of attribution are the substantial gestational increases in various circulating binding proteins (thyroxine-binding globulin, cortisol-binding globulin, sex hormone-binding globulin).

### BIOLOGICAL EFFECTS OF HUMAN PLACENTAL LACTOGEN (HPL)

A great variety of biological activities has been proposed for hPL, including growth promotion, lactogenesis, an effect on carbohydrate and lipid metabolism,

**TABLE 2-3.** Metabolic Changes in Pregnancy That Have Been Attributed to Estrogens

| Effects |
| --- |
| Immunosuppression |
| Increased insulin response and glucose intolerance |
| Increase in sex hormone binding globulin (SHBG) |
| Increase in renin substrate and angiotensin II |
| Sodium diuresis and potassium retention |
| Inhibition of lymphocyte transformation |
| Overbreathing and reduction of $pCO_2$ |
| Increase of thyroxine binding globulin |
| Decrease in pulmonary gas transfer |
| Ureteral dilatation |
| Increased urinary excretion of phosphate |
| Increase in serum cholesterol |
| Liver phagocytosis increased (Kupffer cells) |
| Dilatation of small vessels |
| Increase in triglycerides |

**TABLE 2-4.** Metabolic Changes in Pregnancy That Have Been Attributed to Progesterone

| Effects |
| --- |
| Increase in renin substrate and angiotensin II |
| Overbreathing and reduction of $pCO_2$ |
| Reduction of potassium secretion |
| Change in appetite leading to fat accumulation |
| Vasodilation |
| Ureteral dilatation |
| Immunosuppression |

stimulation of the corpus luteum, erythropoiesis, inhibition of fibrinolysis, and immunosuppression.

Human placental lactogen has only weak somatotrophic activity, variously estimated at 0.1% to 10% of that of pituitary prolactin. However, the growth-promoting activity of hPL may be greater than that of hGH for some fetal tissues.

The lactogenic activity of hPL has been estimated as 20% to 100% of that of prolactin. Administration of hPL in animals leads to a rise in blood sugar and free fatty acids due to increased peripheral resistance to insulin. In rhesus monkeys hPL can decrease the hypoglycemic response to exogenous insulin, without affecting glucose tolerance or the insulin response to glucose.

In the mouse, hPL can stimulate erythropoietin secretion. Both hPL and hCG can suppress phytohemagglutinin-induced lymphocyte transformation. However, the suggestion that either of these compounds plays a role in the immune survival of a pregnancy is now discredited.

Administration of releasing hormones and steroid hormones has no effect on circulating hPL levels. Blood levels of hPL decrease following intravenous administration of glucose, although the change is small and inconsistent.

Increases of blood hPL levels have been shown during insulin-induced hypoglycemia, prolonged starvation, and intravenous arginine, but changes are small when compared with those of pituitary growth hormone under similar circumstances. There is no change in hPL levels after oral administration of glucose. Experimentally induced changes in circulating levels of free fatty acids do not produce any consistent change in hPL concentrations. There is no direct relationship between circulating hPL levels and standard parameters of glucose metabolism, such as the fasting blood glucose and the response to intravenous glucose. Pregnancies in which there is a partial or total deletion of the hPL gene have been widely documented.

## BIOLOGICAL EFFECTS OF PLACENTAL GROWTH HORMONE

Placental growth hormone (GH) is the product of the hPL-V gene. The fact that a "normal" pregnancy has been described in which there was a total deletion of the hPL-V gene clearly does not support a vital role for this hormone in the mother.

## BIOLOGICAL EFFECTS OF PLACENTAL PROTEIN 5

Placental protein 5 (PP5) is biologically analogous to antithrombin III. A sharp increase in maternal blood levels is seen following administration of small doses of heparin, and substantial increases may also occur in severe preeclampsia and placental abruption. It has been suggested that PP5 is a natural defense of the placenta against coagulation in the intervillous space.

## BIOLOGICAL EFFECTS OF PLACENTAL PROTEIN 12

Placental protein 12 (PP12) was originally isolated from placental extracts, then shown to be synthesized by the endometrium/decidua, and finally demonstrated to be identical to the small molecular weight IGF-I binding protein (IGFBP-I).

The function of IGFBP-I (PP12) is binding of IGF-I in the circulation and an important but not yet completely specified role in the action of IGF-I and its cell surface receptors. The latter may be significant in the control of fetal growth, there being an *inverse* relationship between maternal PP12 levels and the size of the fetus. At the metabolic level, there is an inverse relationship between the levels of IGFBP-I and insulin, and IGFBP-I is probably an important part of the insulin-glucose homeostasis system.

## THE CLINICAL SIGNIFICANCE OF PLACENTAL PRODUCTS IN RELATION TO MATERNAL METABOLISM

At one time, measurement of hPL and estriol was widely used in the assessment of fetal well-being in late pregnancy. These "placental function tests" have now been superseded by biophysical procedures. The main parameter to which the maternal circulating levels of Group 1 products relate is the weight of the fetus, but there is no evidence for a functional relationship between some of these products and fetal growth.

An association between elevated levels of hPL and maternal diabetes was described by virtually all of the earlier workers. No such changes are seen in well-controlled diabetic pregnancies. The phenomenon is a secondary consequence of the overgrowth of the trophoblast that is (or was) characteristic of maternal diabetes.

## CONCLUSION

The dramatic changes in maternal physiology and metabolism during normal pregnancy may be attributed to four factors: the uteroplacental unit as an arterio-venous shunt, the nutrient and excretory demands of the fetus and placenta, the mechanical obstructive effects of the pregnancy, and the secretion of hormonal products by the placenta. Despite the emphasis often given to the last of these, the placental products may in reality make only a small contribution to maternal changes during pregnancy.

# PART II. FETAL DEVELOPMENTAL BIOLOGY

# 3. FETAL LUNG DEVELOPMENT AND AMNIOTIC FLUID ANALYSIS

## FETAL LUNG DEVELOPMENT

Respiratory distress syndrome (RDS) is a developmental disorder of prematurely born infants characterized by progressive atelectasis and respiratory insufficiency. It is caused, in part, by a developmental deficiency of pulmonary surfactant, a mixture of phospholipids and proteins that acts to reduce the surface tension at the air-alveolar interface and prevent alveolar collapse (Tables 3-1, 3-2, 3-3). The overall incidence of RDS is 1% to 15% in infants with birth weight less than 2500 g. The incidence varies inversely with gestational age, with a 35% to 60% incidence in infants less than 30 weeks and a 10% to 25% incidence in infants 30 to 33 weeks gestational age.

## EVALUATION OF FETAL LUNG MATURITY

### THE LECITHIN/SPHINGOMYELIN (L/S) RATIO

Assessment of fetal lung maturity by analysis of phospholipids in amniotic fluid began in 1971, when Gluck reported gestational changes in amniotic fluid phos-

**TABLE 3-1.** Phases of Lung Development

| Phase | Gestation | Characteristics |
|---|---|---|
| Glandular | 28 days–16 weeks | Branching of bronchial tree; large distance between terminal airways and pulmonary capillaries |
| Canalicular | 13–25 weeks | Airways end in alveolar ducts; much interstitial tissue between terminal airway and capillaries, limiting potential for gas exchange |
| Terminal sac | 24 weeks–birth | Primitive alveoli; Type II alveolar cells and surfactant production |

True alveolarization begins at 34–36 weeks.

At birth, one-eighth to one-sixth of the adult number of alveoli are present. The number of alveoli increases until adult members are reached in the eighth year.

**TABLE 3-2.** Surfactant Composition

| | % Total Weight |
|---|---|
| Protein | 10–15* |
| Phospholipid | 85–90 |

| | % Total Phospholipid |
|---|---|
| Phosphatidylcholine (lecithin) | 80–85 |
| (Disaturated phosphatidylcholine (DSPC) | (45–50) |
| Phosphatidylglycerol (PG) | 6–11 |
| Phosphatidylethanolamine | 3–5 |
| Phosphatidylinositol | 2 |
| Sphingomyelin | 2 |

Surfactant Proteins

SP-A (28–36 kd)
Surfactant recycling and formation of tubular myelin
SP-B, SP-C (4–8kd)
Important for surface activity
SP-D
Lectin-like, function unknown

*Ninety percent of the protein in surfactant obtained by lung lavage represents serum proteins.

**TABLE 3-3.** Influences on Lung Development and Surfactant Secretion

| Labor | Increases the rate of surfactant secretion; lower incidence of RDS after labor regardless of mode of delivery |
|---|---|
| Fetal sex | Biochemical maturity of females precedes males by about 1 week |
| Maternal diabetes | Greater incidence of RDS at each gestational age |
| Glucocorticoids | Accelerated maturity and increased surfactant production |
| Thyroid hormone | Increased surfactant production |
| β-adrenergic agents | Increased surfactant secretion |
| Adenosine/ATP | Increased surfactant secretion |

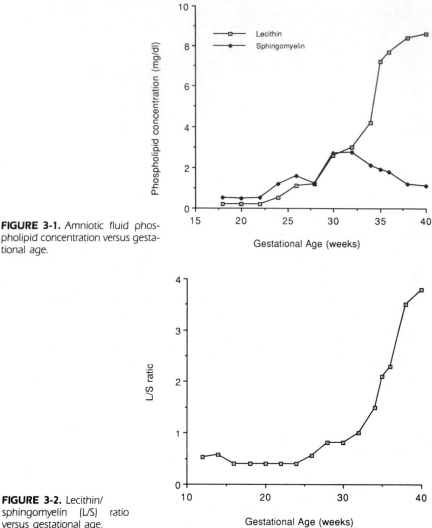

**FIGURE 3-1.** Amniotic fluid phospholipid concentration versus gestational age.

**FIGURE 3-2.** Lecithin/sphingomyelin (L/S) ratio versus gestational age.

pholipid concentrations.* Total phospholipids in amniotic fluid increase throughout gestation, with a sharp increase at about 35 weeks, when there is a sharp increase in the lecithin concentration. Thereafter, lecithin continues to increase while sphingomyelin declines slightly (Fig. 3-1). Because sphingomyelin remains fairly constant while lecithin increases, a ratio between the two is used to correct for changes in amniotic fluid volume. The L/S ratio reaches 2:1 at about 35 weeks (Fig. 3-2, Table 3-4).

---

* Gluck L, Kulovich MV, Borer RC, et al. Diagnosis of the respiratory distress syndrome by amniocentosis. Am J Obstet Gynecol 1971;109:440.

**TABLE 3-4.** Conditions Associated With Accelerated or Delayed Lung Maturation by L/S Ratio

| Accelerated Maturation | Delayed Maturation |
|---|---|
| Pregnancy-induced hypertension | Diabetes, Class A, B, C |
| Hypertensive renal disease | Nonhypertensive renal disease |
| Hypertensive cardiovascular disease | Hydrops fetalis |
| Sickle cell disease | |
| Narcotics addiction | |
| Diabetes, Class D, F, R | |
| Premature rupture of membranes >24 hr | |
| Placental insufficiency | |
| Chronic retroplacental bleeding | |

## PHOSPHATIDYLGLYCEROL (PG)

PG appears at 34 to 35 weeks and increases thereafter. The appearance of PG as 3% or more of total phospholipids is predictive of lung maturity. In Class A, B, and C diabetes, appearance of PG is delayed until 37 to 39 weeks.

The positive predictive value of L/S-PG (immature test = RDS) is about 70%. The negative predictive value (mature test = no RDS) is close to 100%. A variety of other tests using simpler methodologies have been developed in an attempt to improve the predictive value (Table 3-5).

The phospoholipids in blood and meconium interfere with the L/S ratio, making it an invalid test in the presence of these contaminants.

**TABLE 3-5.** Predictive Value of Prenatal Tests for Lung Maturity

| Test | Positive Accuracy | Negative Accuracy |
|---|---|---|
| L/S | 0.541 | 0.982 |
| L/S-PG | 0.470 | 0.993 |
| Shake test | 0.120 | 1.0 |
| OD 650 | 0.128 | 0.987 |
| 35 kD protein | 0.315 | 1.0 |
| 35 kD + L/S + PG | 0.714 | 1.0 |
| FELMA | 0.330 | 1.0 |
| TDX-FLM | 0.307 | 0.996 |

Positive accuracy: Immature test = RDS
Negative accuracy: Mature test = no RDS
FELMA = microviscosity by fluorescence polarization
TDX-FLM = fluorescence polarization, Abott Laboratories

Reduction of RDS Incidence with Optimum Antenatal Steroid Therapy

| Gestational Age | Without Steroids | With Optimum Steroids |
|---|---|---|
| <30 weeks | 60% | 35% |
| >30–33 weeks | 25% | 10% |

## USE OF ANTENATAL STEROIDS

Glucocorticoids accelerate anatomical, biochemical, and physiological maturation of the lung. Accumulation of phospholipid and protein components of surfactant is enhanced by steroids. Maximum benefit of steroids is realized if

1. they are used before 32 weeks.
2. two doses of betamethasone are given over 48 hours.
3. delivery is at least 2 to 3 days but less than 7 to 10 days after starting treatment.

---

# 4.   RECURRENT PREGNANCY LOSS

Human reproduction is an inefficient process, with losses possibly following 70% to 80% of fertilizations. Please see Chapter 15, in Reece EA, Hobbins JC, Mahoney MJ, and Petrie RH, eds. *Medicine of the fetus & mother*. J.B. Lippincott, 1992.) A significant proportion (28%) of fertilized ova appear to be lost before implantation. A number of investigators have reported losses in 39% (217/560) of confirmed postimplantation pregnancies. Two-thirds of these postimplantation losses could not be detected clinically, consistent with the generally observed 10% to 15% clinical spontaneous abortion rate.

Recent data derived from early gestational sonography and aggressive karyotype analysis have demonstrated a 77% chromosomal abnormality rate in very early losses, although not all investigators have confirmed this high correlation between early losses and chromosomal aberrations. The high spontaneous loss rate observed in older women (>45% over age 40 years) supports the etiologic role of chromosomal abnormalities in early pregnancy loss. However, it is uncertain whether aneuploidy alone is responsible for this maternal age-related increase in early pregnancy loss.

Given the high rate of pregnancy wastage inherent in normal human reproduction, it would not be unusual for successive early losses to occur by chance. Indeed, the risk of a spontaneous abortion following one prior loss may not be appreciably different from the risk following four prior losses (23.7% versus 25.9%). Therefore, any evaluation of possible causes for recurrent pregnancy loss or its treatment must take into account both the high background rate of pregnancy loss and the inherently high "spontaneous remission" rate. Furthermore, most studies of recurrent pregnancy loss inappropriately use patients' prior loss rates as statistical support for a given cause or as "controls" to document therapeutic efficacy. Ascertainment biases distort the relative frequencies of possible causes for recurrent pregnancy loss.

### GENETIC ETIOLOGIES

As noted previously, chromosomal abnormalities may be associated with the majority of first trimester spontaneous abortions. Approximately 50% of these abnormalities are autosomal trisomies, most frequently trisomy 16. Monosomy X and polyploidy each account for an additional 20% to 25% of cases. Although cytogenetic abnormalities may account for most sporadic losses, chromosomal aberrations may also account for at least half of recurrent losses.

## CHROMOSOMAL CAUSES: RECURRENT ANEUPLOIDY

Parental factors that increase the likelihood of a chromosomally abnormal conceptus should increase the likelihood of recurrent pregnancy losses.

### Parental Chromosomal Abnormalities

About 3% to 6% of couples experiencing two or more losses have identifiable chromosomal abnormalities. This compares with a 0.2% prevalence in the general population. Most (75% to 83%) abnormalities are balanced translocations, with two thirds reciprocal and one third Robertsonian. An additional 12% to 36% are low-grade chromosomal mosaicisms, usually involving the X chromosome. Couples with balanced translocations have spontaneous loss rates ranging from 50% for reciprocal translocations to 25% for Robertsonian translocations. Minor chromosomal variants (1qh, 9qh, 16qh, Yqh, and satellites—p+) do not appear to be associated with increased rates of pregnancy loss. Peri- and paracentric inversions are of uncertain significance, but could theoretically increase the risk of lethal chromosomal recombinants.

It appears prudent to assess couples having two or more spontaneous losses with parental karyotype analysis before their next conception. High-resolution banding techniques, if available, should be employed in these karyotypic assessments. Couples with documented chromosomal abnormalities should be offered fetal karyotype analysis in subsequent ongoing pregnancies.

Affected couples may wish to attempt repetitive conceptions, understanding that their success rate will be at least 50% per conception. Alternatively, adoption, artificial insemination, or ova donations from in vitro fertilization programs may be opted for.

### Parental Predispositions to Meiotic Nondisjunction

A number of investigators have demonstrated an increased incidence of hypermodal chromosomal spreads (meiotic nondisjunction) in lymphocyte cultures derived from recurrent aborters. These involve both autosomes and the X chromosome. Meiotic nondisjunctional events might also occur more frequently in these patients, accounting for their increased pregnancy loss rates. However, caution must be exercised because not all investigators have confirmed this phenomenon.

Our ability to detect increased risks for meiotic nondisjunction in couples with normal parental karyotypes is limited. Therefore, it is essential to evaluate the karyotypes of each abortus in couples suffering recurrent pregnancy loss. Detailed vaginal sonography early in pregnancy may also be of value in recurrent aborters. The presence of only a yolk sac-like structure within the gestational sac may be a marker for an abnormal karyotype. Such a sonographic finding in a recurrent loss patient should prompt karyotype analysis of the products of conception or, possibly, chorionic villus sampling (CVS).

Therapy in cases of recurrent aneuploidy of unknown cause is not possible beyond the use of donor gametes. Moreover, the couple's prognosis is difficult to make because there is no a priori reason to believe that defects in germ cell chromosomal segregation will universally occur. Karyotype assessment by amniocentesis may be indicated in pregnancies progressing past 8 weeks if recurrent aneuploid losses have been previously documented.

### Hyperspermia

Higher sperm counts and superior sperm motility and morphology have been associated with recurrent pregnancy loss. One proposed explanation for this phenomenon is polyspermia resulting in zygotic polyploidy. However, these data have not been further evaluated, and the clinical utility of semen analysis in the partners of recurrent loss patients is unknown.

## SINGLE-GENE CAUSES AND LETHAL GENE INTERACTIONS

Mutations critical to cell function or tissue morphogenesis can lead to early embryonic loss. Such mutations inherited in an autosomal recessive fashion are presumably quite rare and should only result in a 25% loss rate (e.g., α-thalassemia) unless affected gametes are selected for. In contrast, a parental germ line lethal mutation would lead to a 50% loss rate or higher, if the mutation conferred a conceptive advantage. Certain disorders appear to be lethal in the hemizygous or heterozygous male, causing an increased spontaneous loss rate. Examples include focal dermal hypoplasia, incontinentia pigmenti, and oral-facial-digital syndrome (Type I). These disorders may have a X-linked recessive inheritance or are caused by an autosomal dominant mutation lethal in males. They should be suspected when the ratio of females to males in affected families is 2:1, when one-half of female sibs are affected, and when all male sibs are unaffected. Lethal multiple pterygium syndrome (LMPS) appears to be an X-linked cause of recurrent midgestational loss without affected female heterozygotes.

There appears to be an increased spontaneous loss rate in couples with a family history of either neural tube defects or cleft lip with or without cleft palate. Because these polygenic anomalies may result in part from unfavorable gene interactions, the associated pregnancy losses may have an analogous cause.

The potential for single-gene disorders or complex gene interactions to cause recurrent euploid pregnancy loss is substantial. However, our ability to identify their frequencies or potential causes is rudimentary. This underscores the importance of a detailed genetic history in the assessment of affected couples. Serial high-resolution vaginal sonography may be of use in the detection of lethal single-gene abnormalities (e.g., LMPS), because postmortem evaluation of macerated tissue is often inadequate for phenotype ascertainment.

## MÜLLERIAN ANOMALIES AND OTHER
## UTERINE ABNORMALITIES

Abnormalities of müllerian duct fusion most commonly result in symmetric defects, including didelphic uterus, bicornuate uterus, and septate uterus, less commonly in unicornuate uterus with or without a rudimentary horn (Table 4-1). Müllerian anomalies reportedly occur in 0.25% (0.1% to 0.5%) of patients; however, prevalence statistics are undoubtedly underestimated, because only in pa-

**TABLE 4-1.** Müllerian and Other Uterine Abnormalities

| Etiology | Diagnosis | Therapy |
|---|---|---|
| **Müllerian Anomalies** | | |
| Septate uterus | HSG/hysteroscopy with laparoscopy | Hysteroscopic resection |
| Didelphic and bicornuate uteri | HSG/hysteroscopy with laparoscopy | Strassman procedure |
| Unicornuate uterus | HSG/hysteroscopy with laparoscopy | None |
| **Other Uterine Abnormalities** | | |
| Submucous myomas | HSG/hysteroscopy with laparoscopy | Myomectomy |
| Asherman's syndrome | HSG/hysteroscopy | Hysteroscopic resection or D & C |
| DES-Hypoplasia | HSG/hysteroscopy | ? Cerclage |

tients with pregnancy complications are these anomalies likely to be ascertained. Conversely, in patients with recurrent pregnancy loss, the prevalence of müllerian anomalies is reportedly 15%. This prevalence, however, is likely overestimated secondary to referral population selection biases.

Patients with a history of spontaneous losses associated with preterm labor or abnormal fetal lie are appropriate candidates for diagnostic studies. A family history of uterine myomas, DES use, uterine or renal abnormalities, or a history of multiple prior uterine curettages are indicators of risk. Proper evaluation includes hysterosalpingography (HSG) or hysteroscopy with concomitant laparoscopy. All patients documented to have müllerian anomalies should undergo renal ultrasound and intravenous pyelography. The prevalence of concomitant urinary tract abnormalities in these patients is 20% to 60%; conversely, up to 90% of women with unilateral renal anomalies may have concomitant genital tract abnormalities.

## INFECTIOUS ETIOLOGIES

The role of infectious agents in the genesis of recurrent pregnancy loss, if any, is limited to certain commensal organisms that provoke only a modest host response or chronic infections by organisms of low virulence (Table 4-2). The link between recurrent loss and *Mycoplasma* species, self-replicating prokaryotes that lack a cell wall, has been intensively studied. The two primary genital mycoplasmas with pathogenic potential are *Mycoplasma hominis* and *Ureaplasma urealyticum*. Both are common commensal organisms with a population prevalence of 50% to 70% (greater for *U. urealyticum*).

## ENDOCRINOLOGICAL AND METABOLIC ETIOLOGIES

Maternal endocrinological disorders have been implicated in the genesis of recurrent pregnancy loss, including luteal phase defects and poorly controlled diabetes mellitus (Table 4-3). There is no evidence that mild hyper- or hypothyroidism can

**TABLE 4-2.** Infectious Etiologies: Mycoplasma

| Etiology | Diagnosis | Therapy |
|---|---|---|
| U. urealyticum | Cervical culture | Doxycycline<br>Erythromycin |
| M. Hominis | Cervical culture | ? Need |

**TABLE 4-3.** Endocrinological Etiologies

| Etiology | Diagnosis | Therapy |
|---|---|---|
| Luteal phase defects | Endometrial biopsy<br>Progesterone level | Clomid<br>Progesterone suppositories |
| Poorly controlled diabetes mellitus | Serial blood glucose<br>Hemoglobin A1-c | Insulin |

cause recurrent pregnancy loss. Untreated maternal metabolic disorders can also cause recurrent pregnancy loss, including homocystinuria and Wilson's disease. Fortunately, since these latter disorders are sufficiently rare and generally, although not always, obvious to the obstetrician, they do not pose a significant diagnostic concern.

## LUTEAL PHASE DEFECTS

Luteal phase defects (LPD) should be suspected in patients with short cycles, postovulatory intervals less than 14 days, or the association of secondary infertility with recurrent early losses. The reported prevalence of LPD in recurrent aborters ranges from 20% to 60%, although ascertainment biases undoubtedly inflate these numbers.

Treatment for LPD includes clomiphene citrate or vaginal progesterone suppositories. The latter therapy avoids potential clomiphene-induced embryotoxic effects. Various regimens can be employed: for example, 25 mg of micronized progesterone given intravaginally twice daily until 10 to 12 weeks. Alternatively, the patient can be begun on weekly 17-hydroxyprogesterone caproate (intramuscular) injections. Success rates of up to 90% compared with historical controls have been reported in recurrent aborters; however, other investigators have noted no improvement in outcomes.

## INSULIN-DEPENDENT DIABETES MELLITUS

Poorly controlled diabetes is likely to account for only a fraction of recurrent loss patients. However, one should not ascribe recurrent pregnancy loss in a diabetic to poor metabolic control unless all other potential causes have been ruled out.

**TABLE 4-4.** Autoimmunological Causes

| Etiology | Diagnosis | Therapy |
| --- | --- | --- |
| **Antiphospholipid Antibodies** | | |
| Lupus anticoagulant | aPTT | Aspirin and Heparin |
| | KCT | ? Prednisone |
| | RVVT | ? Plasmaphoresis |
| | TTIT | |
| | PNP | |
| Other antiphospholipid antibodies, including: | ELISA or RIA | Same |
|   Anticardiolipin | | |
|   Antiphosphotidylserine | | |
|   Antiphosphatidic acid | | |

## LUPUS ANTICOAGULANT (ANTIPHOSPHOLIPID ANTIBODIES)

Laurell and Nilsson (1957)* first described the association of a unique circulating anticoagulant and a false-positive Wasserman serology test with recurrent pregnancy wastage. This phenomenon is now termed the lupus anticoagulant (LAC) because of its frequent occurrence in patients with systemic lupus erythematosus (SLE). The term is a misnomer, because its primary clinical effect is thrombosis. Lupus anticoagulants are very closely associated with IgG and IgM class antibodies whose epitopes are negatively charged phospholipids.

Lupus anticoagulants are clearly associated with thromboembolic phenomena, including sundry neurological lesions (cerebral vascular accidents, spinal thrombosis, chorea, and Guillain-Barré syndrome), pulmonary embolism, Budd-Chiari syndrome, renal vein thrombosis, and verrucous endocardial lesions. Approximately 50% of patients with LAC will eventually have a thrombotic event, and the risk of thrombosis in patients with antiphospholipid antibodies may correlate with antibody concentrations.

Recurrent pregnancy loss is common in pregnant patients with LAC. Scott and colleagues† reviewed the literature and described 242 untreated pregnancies in 65 women with lupus anticoagulant. Spontaneous abortions or stillbirths occurred in 220 (91%), with approximately half of the losses occurring before 20 weeks gestation. Indeed, they report that only six untreated patients with LAC have had live births. Additional obstetric complications include preeclampsia and hepatic-splenic rupture. The association of adverse pregnancy outcomes in patients with antiphospholipid antibodies but without LAC appears less certain. Pregnancy wastage, when present, may be mediated by uteroplacental thrombosis and vasoconstriction, although extensive placental infarction has been noted by some, but not all, investigators. Spiral artery vasculopathy, termed "acute atherosis," may also contribute to adverse perinatal outcomes. Additional mechanisms may include immune complex-mediated trophoblast damage or trophoblast-reactive lymphocytotoxic antibody (see Alloimmune section) (Table 4-4).

*Laurell A, Nilsson I. Hypergammaglobulinemia, circulating anticoagulant and biologic false positive Wasserman reaction. J Lab Clin Med 1957;49:694.

†Scott JR, Rote NS, Branch DW. Immunologic aspects of recurrent abortion and fetal death. Obstet Gynecol 1987;70:645.

The diagnosis of recurrent pregnancy loss secondary to LAC/antiphospholipid antibody should be suspected in patients with recurrent abortions or intrauterine fetal growth retardation or demise. The combination of recurrent pregnancy wastage and maternal thromboembolic phenomenon is particularly suggestive. Patients with a history of false-positive syphilis serologies, prolonged PTT, or laboratory evidence of other autoantibody production should be evaluated. All patients with signs, symptoms, or a history of connective tissue disorders should be considered at high risk.

The LAC phenomenon can be detected by functional coagulation assays such as the activated partial thromboplastin time (aPTT). However, assays that employ low phospholipid concentrations appear to be more sensitive. These include the kaolin clotting time (KCT), the Russell's viper venom time (RVVT), the tissue thromboplastin inhibition test (TTIT), and the platelet neutralization procedure. The paradoxical prolongation in coagulation identified by these assays is a consequence of antibody-mediated disruption of the prothrombin complex on phospholipid micelles. Definitive diagnosis requires mixing studies in which normal plasma is added to the patient's sample in a 1:4 ratio without correcting the prolonged coagulation time. This essentially rules out a factor deficiency.

Alternatively, a direct assay for antiphospholipid antibodies can be carried out by either radioimmunoassay (RIA) or enzyme-linked immunoassay (ELISA). There is growing evidence that direct antibody identification by immunoassay is the more sensitive method of determining patients at risk. It is not clear, however, whether the direct identification of antiphospholipid antibodies is as clinically relevant as their indirect detection via a functional coagulation assay because of the former's increased false positives. If an antiphospholipid antibody ELISA or RIA is employed, it is important that each sample serum be assayed for specific and nonspecific binding to a given phospholipid, because generalized immunoglobulin elevations can cause spurious results. Also critical to the interpretation of results is the establishment of clinically rather than just statistically relevant cut-off values.

Treatment of patients with antiphospholipid antibodies has had two aims: reducing the antibody burden with prednisone, azathioprine, or plasmaphoresis with or without immunoglobulin therapy; and reducing the antibody effect with low-dose aspirin (<80 mg) or heparin. The literature suggests a 70% viable pregnancy rate for patients treated with some combination of the above modalities. Such a success rate calls to mind the inherently high "spontaneous remission" rate present in recurrent aborters. Treatment for patients with a history of adverse pregnancy outcomes (or, if primigravid, prior thrombotic events) in whom LAC and high concentrations of antiphospholipid antibody are found should employ combination therapy with aspirin 80 mg per day and either heparin 10,000 U subcutaneously twice a day, or prednisone 60 mg per day. Calcium supplementation is required because of the osteopenic effects of both the prednisone and the heparin. Repeated glucose tolerance testing is also required, given the diabetogenic effects of prednisone.

Additional maternal evaluations include initial echocardiography and serial assessment of renal and liver function. Fetal evaluations include serial sonography to evaluate fetal growth, and Doppler flow analysis, if available. Fetal heart rate testing and biophysical profiles should be initiated at 28 weeks gestation. Delivery is mandated by maternal indications, fetal distress, or the cessation of fetal growth.

The need to treat patients without LAC who have only modest elevations in other antiphospholipid antibodies is unclear. Treatment in this group should be reserved for those patients with documented euploid recurrent pregnancy losses in whom all other causes have been ruled out. Pregnancy should be strongly discouraged in patients with refractory, life-threatening thrombotic disease secondary to LAC/antiphospholipid antibody syndrome.

## SUMMARY

As noted, the sporadic occurrence of early pregnancy loss is so common that recurrent pregnancy loss can be expected to occur frequently by chance. Sporadic losses appear to result most commonly from aneuploidy; however, lethal gene mutations or embryopathic gene interactions may be common. As anticipated, the prognosis for a viable pregnancy in a woman with multiple prior losses is excellent without or despite "therapeutic" interventions. Although this information may provide solace for the perplexed clinician and hope for the anxious couple, it should not take the place of a thorough search for factors that may increase the risk for pregnancy loss. Moreover, because recurrent loss can persist despite a negative evaluation, affected couples should be presented with the limits of our knowledge and not with idle reassurances.

# PART III. VARIATIONS IN EMBRYONAL AND FETAL GROWTH AND DEVELOPMENT

## 5.  ECTOPIC AND HETEROTOPIC PREGNANCIES

Recent research into the epidemiology, etiology, and pathophysiology of ectopic pregnancy (EP) has raised larger issues. The incidence of this disease has increased two- to threefold throughout the industrialized world over the last 25 years. Despite the fact that the risk of dying from an EP has fallen dramatically during the same period, it has not fallen by as much as the risk of dying from other pregnancy-

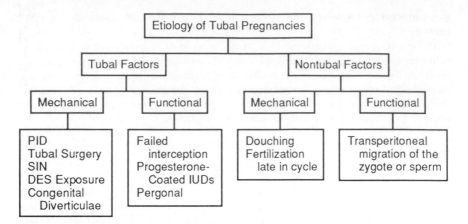

**FIGURE 5-1.** Etiology of tubal pregnancies.

related causes. (Please see Chapter 17, in Reece EA, Hobbins JC, Mahoney MJ, and Petrie RH, eds. Medicine of the fetus & mother. J.B. Lippincott, 1992.)

## ETIOLOGY

Although many theories have been advanced to explain the occurrence of tubal pregnancies, and several recent case-control studies have established an association between EP and a number of factors such as smoking, douching, and spontaneous abortions, the only firmly established, noniatrogenic cause of EP is pelvic inflammatory disease (PID), and the consensus is that the rising incidence of PID probably accounts for much of the recent rise in the incidence of EP.

Some of the mechanisms that have been forwarded to explain the occurrence of tubal pregnancies in humans are listed in Figure 5-1, and a fuller discussion of these is available elsewhere.

## PATHOPHYSIOLOGY

Normal implantation is a process that lasts about a week. Very little is known about how this process operates at the cellular level or how it is regulated in humans. Whether the mechanisms of normal and extrauterine implantations are similar is not known.

Budowick and colleagues (1980)* were the first authors in recent years to describe in detail the behavior of the trophoblast in tubal pregnancies. They stated that after implanting on the surface of the tubal mucosa, the trophoblast rapidly invades the lamina propria and tubal musculature. The pregnancy then grows in the potential space that exists between the outer wall of the fallopian tube and the overlying peritoneum. Growth of the conceptus at this extraperitoneal site occurs both in a direction parallel to the long axis of the tube and circumferentially. Tubal

* Budowick M, Johnson TRB, Genardy R, et al. The histopathology of the developing tubal ectopic pregnancy. Fertil Steril 1980;34:169.

rupture actually entails rupture of the peritoneum overlying the tube. The authors pointed out that the peritoneum was more adherent at the isthmic portion of the tube than at the ampulla, which might explain the propensity of isthmic pregnancies to rupture.

## MANAGEMENT OF SUSPECTED ECTOPIC PREGNANCIES

The cardinal symptoms and signs associated with EP are well known and require no repetition. The clinical presentation of patients with EP falls into two more or less distinct categories. The minority (about 10%) present with a surgical abdomen and symptoms and signs of hypovolemia, if not frank shock. They present no diagnostic problem, require no special investigations, and need immediate laparoscopy or laparotomy. In most patients, however, the diagnosis is far less clear-cut and immediate surgery is not mandatory. In some of these cases, the symptoms and signs will be, of course, much more suggestive of an EP than in others, but the gynecologist must accept that in the absence of shock or symptoms identical to that experienced in a previous pregnancy, EP cannot be reliably distinguished from other disorders on clinical grounds.

## DIAGNOSTIC STUDIES

The literature pertaining to the diagnostic workup of clinically stable women with suspected EP has become very large and to some extent conflicting and continues to grow as new methodologies become available. It is not possible at this time for the clinician to establish an optimal algorithm for the workup of women with suspected EPs. Nonetheless, it is possible to define the principles on which any diagnostic evaluation should be based and those that will serve as a logical framework for any future diagnostic algorithm, regardless of new developments.

## LAPAROSCOPY AND CULDOCENTESIS

Two facts about women with a suspected EP largely govern how these patients should be investigated. First, if a suitably high index of suspicion for the diagnosis is exercised, about 70% to 80% of patients investigated for a suspected EP will not have an EP. It follows immediately that a test that can reliably exclude a diagnosis of EP will be the most cost effective and should be administered first. Second, most women who are suspected of having, but who do not have, an EP are not pregnant at all. Consequently, a sensitive pregnancy test is the most cost effective and useful test in emergency gynecology, because by demonstrating that a pregnancy is not present, a diagnosis of EP can be excluded (in most cases) on the basis of a single test. At the present time, laparoscopy is the only available diagnostic test that enables one to exclude a diagnosis of EP reliably on the basis of a negative result. This is why culdocentesis, for example, is less useful in practice than some of the statistics cited about this procedure might suggest.

## PREGNANCY TESTS

The last remaining obstacles to the routine use of sensitive pregnancy testing in cases of suspected ectopic pregnancy have been removed by the development of enzyme-linked immunosorbent assays (ELISA). In vitro, these assays are as sensitive as rapid RIAs, but no laboratory experience is required to perform them reliably.

A negative result of an RIA or ELISA is reliable, because if an EP is present, the tests will almost always be positive.

## ULTRASOUND

If a patient with a suspected ectopic pregnancy has a positive pregnancy test but does not have an EP, she will have an intrauterine pregnancy (IUP), or a threatened, missed, or complete abortion. In these patients ultrasound has its greatest value. In the absence of a positive pregnancy test, ultrasound is not helpful unless fetal heart activity (FHA) is detected inside or outside the uterus, which is uncommon. Therefore, ultrasound should be reserved for cases in which the pregnancy test is positive, and not used as a primary diagnostic test.

### INTRAUTERINE FINDINGS

The purpose of ultrasound in women with positive pregnancy tests is to try to localize the pregnancy, but usually the diagnosis of EP is still only presumptive, because in at least 80% of cases an ectopic fetus cannot be imaged even with transvaginal (TV) sonography. Because simultaneous IUP and EP (heterotropic pregnancies) are uncommon, the presence of an IUP is taken to exclude an EP, and if an IUP cannot be detected, this is taken as presumptive evidence of an EP. Unfortunately, the situation is not so simple, for two reasons.

First, a pregnancy can be detected by a sensitive pregnancy test up to 2 weeks before it can be imaged by ultrasound. Therefore, failure to detect an IUP when an ultrasound test is positive does not necessarily mean that an early IUP is not present.

Second, sonographically detectable intrauterine "sacs" can be present in EPs (pseudogestational sac). (Blood in the endometrial cavity and a strong decidual reaction presumably give rise to this image.) One cannot automatically equate an intrauterine sac with an IUP. The demonstration of FHA or fetal products within the sac provides conclusive evidence that an IUP is present (Fig. 5-2). An equally reliable, but earlier, indicator of an IUP is the demonstration of the (secondary) yolk sac within an intrauterine sac (Fig. 5-3). In some cases, it is also possible to image the decidua capsularis and parietalis of an IUP, in which case the gestational sac has a double-walled appearance (Fig. 5-4). This so-called double-ring sign can be detected in 30% of pseudogestational sacs and is, therefore, not a reliable indicator of an IUP. With the use of TV sonography, a confident diagnosis of an IUP can be made. Hence EP can be excluded much earlier than by transabdominal (TA) ultrasound, because the yolk sac, fetus, or fetal cardiac activity can frequently be identified prior to their detection by TA ultrasound.

### EXTRAUTERINE FINDINGS

The sonographic features of the adnexa or pouch of Douglas (POD) may also provide strong presumptive evidence for an EP, even if the findings are not specific for that condition. One should look for a mass and fluid but must distin-

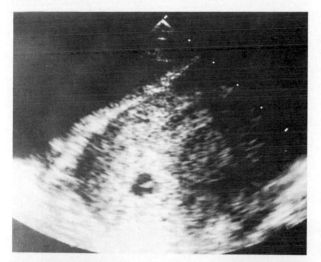

**FIGURE 5-2.** Gestational sac containing fetal parts.

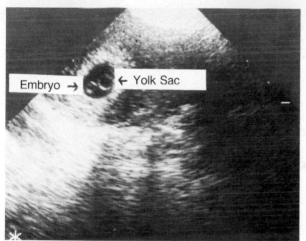

**FIGURE 5-3.** Gestational sac with a demonstrable yolk sac and embryo.

guish between masses that are purely cystic and those that have mixed echogenicity. In the presence of a positive hCG assay, a complex mass in the adnexa or POD is about 80% predictive of an EP, and the figure rises to about 95% if fluid is also present. Up to 50% of women with EP will have these findings, which are an indication for laparoscopy.

## POSITIVE hCG ASSAYS AND NONDIAGNOSTIC SONAR FINDINGS

In approximately 20% of women with a suspected EP and positive pregnancy tests, ultrasound will be nondiagnostic; that is, an IUP cannot be demonstrated, and the extrauterine findings do not provide presumptive evidence of an EP. The management of these patients has reached a high level of sophistication in some

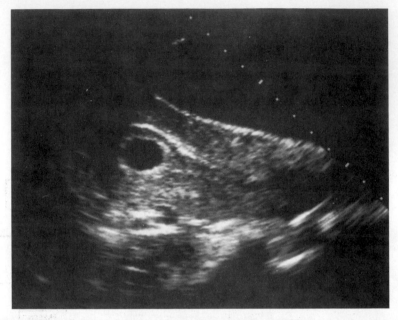

**FIGURE 5-4.** Gestational sac with double-ring image or sign.

centers and involves the use of a quantitative hCG assay and serial hCG testing in some patients, as discussed later in this chapter. The diagnostic approach based on an ELISA and ultrasound is summarized in Figure 5-5.

## PROGESTERONE ASSAYS

An alternative method of evaluating women with nondiagnostic sonar findings (or indeed women with a positive pregnancy test prior to the performance of an ultrasound) may be to measure the serum progesterone with a rapid, direct RIA, or its urinary metabolite (pregnanediol-3-glucuronide) by an immunometric assay.

A possible algorithm that merits further evaluation is shown in Figure 5-6.

The alternative approach to the evaluation of pregnant women with suspected EPs who have nondiagnostic sonar findings starts with a serum hCG determination (blood drawn at the time of the scan). If the serum hCG is found to be above a certain critical value (called the discriminatory zone [DZ]), and an IUP cannot be detected, one can safely assume that the patient has an EP. If the serum hCG is not above this critical value, then the patient may have an EP, a very early normal IUP, or an abortion. Serial hCG measurements are then obtained to try to distinguish between these possibilities.

## THE DISCRIMINATORY HCG ZONE

If the serum hCG is more than 6500 mIU/mL (International Reference Preparation [IRP]; discussed later in this chapter) and an IUP cannot be detected sonographically, the probability is more than 95% that an EP is present.

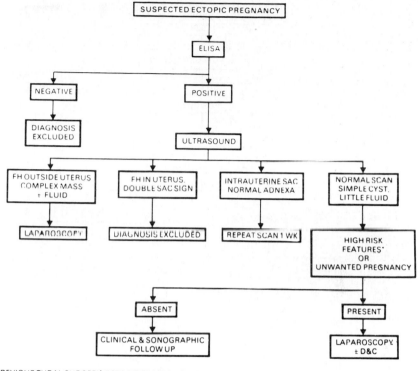

**FIGURE 5-5.** Algorithm for managing cases of suspected FP based on the availability of urinary ELISA and gray-scale sonography.

It is probably safe for the reader to adopt the values shown in Figure 5-7 for the DZ, depending on which type of hCG assay the laboratory is running and which type of sonography is being performed. A fuller discussion of the principles underlying the use of the DZ, and of the correspondence between hCG values obtained in different hCG assays, is available elsewhere.

## SERIAL hCG TESTING

The serum hCG increases exponentially in normal pregnancies at hCG values that are below the original DZ (i.e., the log hCG-time relationship is linear). The 15th percentile of the rate of hCG increase in normal pregnancies corresponds to a doubling time (DT) of 2.7 days, or to a slope of the log hCG-time regression line of 0.25 (or 0.11 if common logarithms [i.e., base 10] are used). In at least 87% of EPs the serum hCG increases at a slower rate, and the levels may in fact be falling. The most suitable and practical way to determine the rate of hCG increase in serum among women with suspected EPs is to measure the hCG again in a blood sample

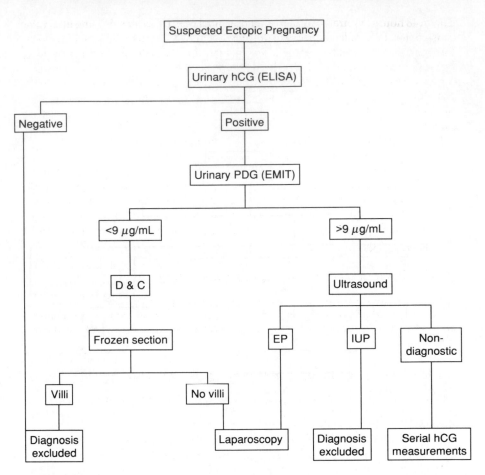

**FIGURE 5-6.** A possible algorithm for managing cases of EP based on a urinary ELISA for hCG and a urinary EMIT for pregnanediol glucuronide (PDG).

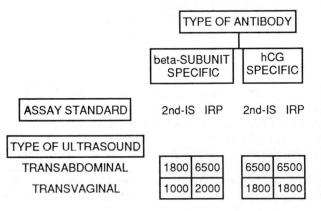

| TYPE OF ANTIBODY | | | |
|---|---|---|---|
| beta-SUBUNIT SPECIFIC | | hCG SPECIFIC | |
| **ASSAY STANDARD** 2nd-IS | IRP | 2nd-IS | IRP |
| **TYPE OF ULTRASOUND** | | | |
| TRANSABDOMINAL 1800 | 6500 | 6500 | 6500 |
| TRANSVAGINAL 1000 | 2000 | 1800 | 1800 |

**FIGURE 5-7.** The hCG level (in mIU/mL) above which failure to detect a gestation should be taken as being indicative of an ectopic pregnancy is a function of both the type of ultrasound and the type of hCG assay being used.

drawn 48 hours (accurately timed) after the initial one. (Shorter sampling intervals cause potential problems, because the increase in hCG expected is less than twice the interassay variability of most assays.) The serum hCG should increase by 66% or more over this time period. Alternatively, one can compute the slope of the increase [log ($hCG_2$/$hCG_1$)-sampling interval], or the doubling time (DT) (log 2/slope). If the rate of increase is subnormal (i.e., percentage of increase is less than 66%, DT is less than 2.7 days, or slope is less than 0.25), laparoscopy is indicated.

If the second hCG value is lower than the first one (i.e., the levels are falling), one can be confident that the pregnancy is not viable, and in most cases it is appropriate to perform a D&C prior to laparoscopy to try to differentiate between an EP and an abortion. One should try to avoid having to give the patient a second anesthetic at a later date, so if there is uncertainty over the nature of the curettings obtained (in most EPs little or no tissue is obtained by gentle curettage), frozen section should be performed if possible. The algorithm incorporating these findings is shown in Figure 5-8.

## THE TREATMENT OF TUBAL PREGNANCIES

The treatment of tubal pregnancies remains primarily surgical, even if no longer exclusively so. The primary goal of surgery is, of course, to remove the pregnancy and thereby arrest or prevent hemorrhage, which can be accomplished in many different ways.

## FACTORS CONFOUNDING TREATMENT COMPARISONS

It is almost axiomatic that several factors besides the operative treatment used can affect both the live birth rate (LBR) and recurrent EP rate (REPR) following treatment of a tubal pregnancy.

The best-established prognostic factor is a history of infertility or evidence of tubal disease at surgery. Some of the other factors that have been found to impair reproductive performance (nulliparity, prior PID, EP or tubal surgery, and increasing age) are probably also linked with infertility. Increasing size of the tubal pregnancy and the presence of tubal rupture may also influence reproductive performance adversely, whereas women with an EP who have an intrauterine device in place may have a more favorable reproductive outcome.

## ABLATIVE OPERATIONS

Salpingectomy remains the standard operation whenever a tubal pregnancy is to be treated by removal of the affected tube. However, it is not the only ablative operation used, since two modifications to Lawson Tait's salpingectomy have been employed for a number of years: concurrent cornual resection and ipsilateral oophorectomy (sometimes called paradoxical oophorectomy).

## CORNUAL RESECTION

Cornual resection appears to have been widely practiced in some centers but has been condemned in recent years. It can be shown by formal "cost-benefit" anal-

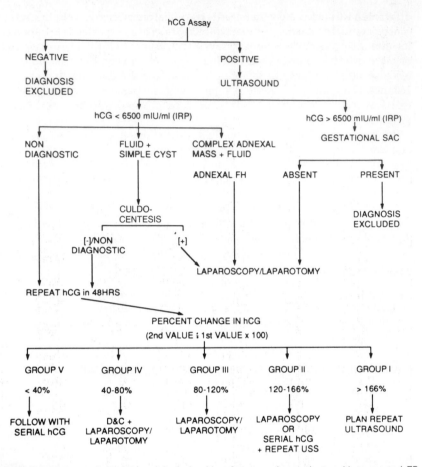

**FIGURE 5-8.** An extension of the original algorithm for managing patients with suspected EP based on transabdominal sonography and a quantitative hCG assay calibrated against the IRP.

ysis that the risk associated with cornual resection in fact outweighs the benefits. This is simply shown by estimating the probability of a homolateral interstitial recurrence (as the probability of a recurrent EP multiplied by the probability of an EP being interstitial) and the probability of a ruptured uterus following cornual resection.

## PARADOXICAL (IPSILATERAL) OOPHORECTOMY

Data justify treating women with a tubal pregnancy by salpingo-oophorectomy if the involved adnexum shows evidence of preexisting tubo-ovarian disease, the contralateral adnexum is normal and patent on intraoperative chromotubation, and the patient admits to a history of infertility of at least a year's duration. However, this set of circumstances will occur in only a small minority of women with EP, perhaps 5%.

Women with a tubal pregnancy should be treated by salpingo-oophorectomy if the involved adnexum shows evidence of preexisting tubo-ovarian disease, the contralateral adnexum is normal and patent on intraoperative chromotubation, and the patient gives a history of antecedent infertility of at least a year's duration.

## CONSERVATIVE OPERATIONS

The operations that are still used today to remove tubal pregnancies without sacrificing the gravid tube are salpingotomy, salpingostomy, segmental tubal resection, and manual expression (ME) of the pregnancy, also referred to as "milking" the tube or fimbrial expression. Of these, salpingotomy and salpingostomy are by far the most commonly performed procedures. For the sake of simplicity, the term *tubotomy* will be used to refer to either or both of these procedures in general terms. A tubotomy that is closed primarily will be referred to as a salpingotomy, and one that is left open to heal by secondary intention will be called a salpingostomy (although, strictly speaking, this is a misnomer, since it is not the surgeon's intention, when performing this operation, to fashion a "stoma").

## SALPINGOTOMY/SALPINGOSTOMY

The reproductive performance of women following tubotomy performed in this setting has been reported by a number of investigators. Women who undergo a tubotomy for an ectopic pregnancy (EP) located in their only fallopian tube can expect to have an LBR of about 40% and a REPR of about 20%. Compared with women who have two fallopian tubes, patients with one oviduct who undergo tubotomy for an EP have a somewhat lower LBR and a somewhat higher REPR. The difference with respect to both outcomes reaches statistical significance when the pooled data are examined by the Mantel Haenszel statistic.

## MANUAL EXPRESSION

The present consensus among tubal surgeons is that ME should be abandoned because it is associated with an inordinately high REPR, regardless of whether the procedure is performed at a laparotomy or through the laparoscope. Delayed hemorrhage from persistent trophoblastic activity also appears to be more common than after salpingostomy (see discussion later in this chapter).

## SEGMENTAL TUBAL RESECTION

Segmental tubal resection is accepted as the procedure of choice whenever a gravid fallopian tube is to be conserved but the tubal wall is ruptured, or there is persistent or uncontrollable bleeding from the tube following a salpingostomy. A few tubal surgeons have advocated that segmental resection with primary or delayed closure should be the primary treatment in all cases of tubal pregnancy. They argue that salpingostomy conserves an abnormal implantation site, because the invading trophoblast is likely to have caused local damage to the tube in addition to any preexisting damage that might have caused the abnormal implan-

**TABLE 5-1.** Live Birth and Recurrent Tubal Pregnancy Rates Following Conservative and Ablative Operations for Tubal Pregnancy

| Type of Operation | Ploman and Wicksall (1960) | | Sherman Langer, Sadovsky, et al (1982) | |
|---|---|---|---|---|
| | Live Birth Rate | Recurrent EP Rate | Live Birth Rate | Recurrent EP Rate |
| Conservative | 16/27 (59%) | 5/27 (18.5%) | 39/47 (83%) | 3/47 (6.4%) |
| Ablative | 29/61 (48%) | 5/61 (8.2%) | 75/104 (72%) | 5/105 (5.8%) |

(Data from Ploman L, Wicksell F. Fertility after conservative surgery in tubal pregnancy. Acta Obstet Gynecol Scand 1960;38:143; and Sherman D, Langer R, Sadovsky G, et al. Improved fertility following ectopic pregnancy. Fertil Steril 1982;37:497.

tation in the first place. Although good results have been obtained from this procedure, there is no evidence that better results are obtained than from salpingostomy. It is obviously a more complicated procedure, and the general consensus is that it is not the primary treatment of choice for most tubal pregnancies for which a conservative procedure is indicated.

## CONSERVATIVE VERSUS ABLATIVE TREATMENT OF TUBAL PREGNANCIES

The most common decision a gynecologist has to make in treating tubal pregnancies is whether to remove the oviduct. From the preceding discussion it is apparent that this decision almost always reduces to a choice between salpingectomy and salpingostomy. Furthermore, the question arises only in women who wish to have children, since tubal conservation serves no purpose in women who have completed their families, and it carries a higher complication rate than salpingectomy.

## SALPINGOSTOMY VERSUS SALPINGECTOMY

Satisfactory comparisons between salpingostomy and salpingectomy are not available. As noted previously, the best available comparative data were reported by DeCherney and Kase (1979),* which showed that the LBR was higher and the REPR lower after salpingectomy (42% and 12%, respectively) than after salpingostomy (39.6% and 18.75%), although the observed differences did not reach statistical significance.

A further comparison between conservative and ablative operations has been made using two papers in which raw data were provided (Table 5-1). It can be seen that the trend toward a higher REPR following tubal conservation persists. In these studies, however, there was also a trend toward a higher LBR following conservative surgery.

*DeCherney AH, Kase N. The conservatie surgical management of unruptured ectopic pregnancy. Obstet Gynecol 1979;54:451.

## THE INFLUENCE OF PATIENT CHARACTERISTICS ON SURGICAL RESULTS

In the only multivariate analysis reported to date, patient characteristics were also found to be a more important determinant of reproductive outcome than the operative treatment used. The type of operation did not affect outcome even after accounting for differences in patient characteristics, although the sample size was rather small and the number of operations considered quite numerous.

## SITE OF RECURRENT TUBAL PREGNANCIES

When both tubes are present, recurrent EPs after salpingostomy are located in the contralateral tube as often as in the conserved tube. This finding has been uniformly interpreted as indicating that in general the conserved tube is at no greater risk of developing an EP than the contralateral one.

## INDICATIONS FOR SALPINGOSTOMY

What, then, are the indications for salpingostomy? Clearly, salpingostomy is indicated whenever the woman wishes to have children and the pregnancy is located in her only remaining oviduct. The procedure is about three times more likely to result in a live birth than in vitro fertilization, and if conception occurs, a term pregnancy is at least twice as likely as an EP. The procedure is also indicated if the contralateral tube is blocked, but the results to be expected in this situation have been less clearly defined.

## LAPAROSCOPIC SALPINGOSTOMY

The laparoscopic treatment of tubal pregnancies has proved to be surprisingly safe, even if not entirely complication-free. Secondary hemorrhage occurs in about 3% of patients, and persistent EP, which is discussed in detail later, also occurs in a significant minority of cases. Conservative laparoscopic procedures also seem to be as effective as their abdominally performed counterparts in terms of tubal patency and subsequent fertility. The results of a recently published randomized clinical trial in which laparoscopic procedures and abdominal salpingostomy were compared are shown in Table 5-2. Interestingly, and for reasons that are unclear, the REPR seems to be higher after abdominal than after

**TABLE 5-2.** Tubal Patency and Fertility Following Laparoscopic and Abdominal Salpingostomy

|  | Tubal Patency on HSG | Intrauterine Pregnancy | Tubal Pregnancy |
|---|---|---|---|
| Laparoscopic salpingostomy (N = 30) | 16/20 (80%) | 9/18 (50%) | 1/18 (6%) |
| Abdominal salpingostomy (N = 30) | 17/19 (89%) | 8/19 (42%) | 3/19 (16%) |

(Data from Vermesh M, Silva PD, Rosen GF, et al. Management of unruptured ectopic gestation by linear salpingostomy's prospective, randomized clinical trial of laparoscopy versus laparotomy. Obstet Gynecol 1989; 73:400.)

laparoscopic salpingostomy. The advantages of laparoscopic surgery are decreased morbidity and lower cost of treatment.

## PERSISTENT ECTOPIC PREGNANCY

In at least 40% of tubal pregnancies the trophoblast penetrates the tubal wall, and some trophoblastic tissue is probably frequently left behind in the oviduct whenever the implantation site is not removed, as is the case with salpingotomy, salpingostomy, or fimbrial expression of the pregnancy. Usually, however, this tissue seems to degenerate, since late postoperative complications after these procedures are uncommon. Occasionally, however, instead of resorbing, the residual trophoblastic tissue persists and resumes growing, until the patient eventually develops symptoms again from intraperitoneal hemorrhage or a pelvic mass. The frequency of persistent ectopic pregnancy after conservative surgery depends on how this entity is defined (i.e., whether seemingly abnormal hCG clearance patterns in asymptomatic women are counted as persistent pregnancies). Several case reports of delayed hemorrhage or pain referable to a pelvic mass have been reported after salpingotomy, salpingostomy, and fimbrial expression, but they give no indication of the frequency of the problem.

In summary, serial hCG monitoring after conservative operations for tubal pregnancy has been recommended by all clinical investigators, even though it is not certain how the results should be interpreted. Much more research is needed in this area to establish the various serial hCG patterns that may herald the development of clinical symptoms and the best way to manage these patients. In the interim it seems reasonable to suggest that in the absence of symptoms intervention should not be undertaken as long as the serum hCG continues to fall, however slowly. Rising values should be considered more ominous but do not inevitably presage continued trophoblastic growth. A reasonable compromise might be to intervene when the doubling time of hCG is in the normal range (less than 2.7 days) or to follow subnormally increasing titers for a few days before intervening to ensure that the pattern is persisting.

## TREATMENT OF PERSISTENT PREGNANCY

The first few reported cases of persistent ectopic pregnancy presented with intraperitoneal hemorrhage or a pelvic mass and were managed by salpingectomy. Since the introduction of postoperative hCG monitoring, patients with rising hCG levels have been treated with chemotherapy on the assumption that rising hCG levels herald the development of the previously mentioned problems. It is clear from the cases reported to date that treatment with chemotherapy has been very effective.

## THE NONOPERATIVE TREATMENT OF TUBAL PREGNANCIES

For years, gynecologists have stressed the need to diagnose and treat EPs as early in their natural history as possible to reduce the mortality and morbidity associated with the disease. Therefore, one might be forgiven for regarding present-day attempts to treat tubal pregnancies nonoperatively as misguided and even as courting disaster. However, it has been known for many years that some ectopic pregnancies resolve without sequelae. Therefore, a number of investigators have managed selected patients with laparoscopically proven tubal pregnancies expectantly, in the hope of identifying those that may not require treatment. The selection criteria used and the results obtained from expectant management by different investigators are summarized briefly in Table 5-3.

## HETEROTOPIC PREGNANCIES

Until now the discussion has centered on ectopically implanted singleton pregnancies, but one or more members of a multiple gestation may also implant outside the endometrial cavity. Ectopic twins are curiosities whose clinical features do not differ from singleton EPs. However, when an EP is combined with an IUP, a potentially disastrous situation exists.

Coexistent intrauterine and extrauterine pregnancies are referred to as combined or heterotopic pregnancies. The extrauterine pregnancy is almost always tubal, although ovarian, interstitial, abdominal, and cervical pregnancies have been described in association with IUPs.

## INCIDENCE

The most recently available estimate of the EP rate across the United States as a whole showed this to be about 1.5% of reported pregnancies for the year 1983, and as high as 2.8% in some segments of the population (black women aged 35 to 44). This translates into a heterotopic pregnancy rate of about 1 out of 2000 to 1 out of 4000 reported pregnancies on the assumption that the rate of fraternal twinning is

**TABLE 5-3.** The Expectant Management of Tubal Pregnancies

| Author/Year | Selection Criteria | Initial HCG (MIU/ML) | Subsequent Surgery | Normal Patient Tube on HSG | Pregnancies |
|---|---|---|---|---|---|
| Carp et al, 1986 | hCG < 250 <2 × 2 CMS | 14, 20, 100, 250, 20,000 | 1/5 | 1/1 | 1 Term 2 Abs 1EP |
| Garcia, Aubert, Sama, Josimovich, 1987 | <4 CMS Falling hCG | All < 4000 10 < 1000 (Stand n/s) | 1/13 | 7/10 | 3 Term 2 ABs |
| Fernandez, Rainhorn, Papianik, Bellet, Frydman, 1988 | Ampullary, <2 CMS, <50 mL Blood | All < 10,000 9 < 1000 (Stand n/s) | 4/14 | 5/6 | 3 IUP |
| Sauer, Vermesh, Anderson et al., 1988 | <3 CMS Falling hCG | 65–1010(IRP) | 0/5 | 3/4 | n/s |

0.8% of conceptions and that the EP rate among singleton and multiple pregnancies is the same.

## CLINICAL FEATURES AND DIAGNOSIS

Inasmuch as the diagnosis of EP has become largely nonsurgical, and in the course of a nonsurgical workup the detection of an IUP is taken as presumptive evidence that an EP is not present, a heterotopic pregnancy can be expected a priori to pose formidable diagnostic problems and to represent a potentially disastrous situation whenever the IUP is diagnosed first. This will be the case if the IUP is aborted electively or spontaneously before the EP becomes symptomatic. However, even if the presenting symptoms are referable to the EP, it is more than likely that the IUP will be detected in the course of the workup, and the possibility of an EP dismissed. The converse situation (i.e., the EP is diagnosed but the IUP is unsuspected) can be equally disastrous, but for the fetus rather than for the mother.

## TREATMENT

Treatment consists of removal of the ectopic pregnancy and avoidance of intrauterine instrumentation if the mother wishes to carry the intrauterine pregnancy. The prognosis for the intrauterine pregnancy is, in fact, excellent, provided that signs and symptoms of abortion are not present, since over 75% are carried to term. Indeed, the intrauterine pregnancy can be carried to term even after a cornual resection for a combined interstitial pregnancy.

---

# 6. MULTIFETAL PREGNANCIES: EPIDEMIOLOGY, CLINICAL CHARACTERISTICS, AND MANAGEMENT

---

## BACKGROUND

### INCIDENCE AND PERINATAL SIGNIFICANCE

The overall incidence of twins worldwide is about 1 in 80 pregnancies (1.13%). The frequency of monozygotic (MZ) twins is relatively constant throughout the world, regardless of maternal age, parity, or race. The incidence is between 3.5 and 4 per 1000 births. The incidence of dizygotic (DZ) twins varies and is affected by a number of factors, including race, maternal age, parity, and ovulation induction agents.

Higher-order gestations are rare except in cases in which fertility medications or IVF have been used. Despite their relative rarity, multiple gestations contribute significantly to perinatal mortality. Overall perinatal mortality for twins in developed countries ranges between 65 and 120 of 1000 births. The perinatal mortality rate for triplets is 148 to 312 of 1000 births.

Prematurity and intrauterine growth retardation (IUGR) leading to the high incidence of low-birth-weight infants in multiple gestations are the main causes of significantly increased mortality and morbidity. Studies reveal that more than 50% of twins weigh less than 2500 g. Approximately 10% of preterm deliveries are twin gestations. Fifty percent of twins are delivered before 37 weeks, which corresponds to a 12-fold increase in incidence compared to singletons. The average length of gestation decreases inversely with the number of fetuses present. (Table 6-1). IUGR contributes to a higher incidence of stillborn babies, and it is estimated that two-thirds of twins show some signs of growth retardation at delivery.

In addition to premature delivery and IUGR, congenital anomalies, placental abnormalities, cord accidents, preeclampsia, and malpresentations all have an increased incidence with twins and contribute to the overall morbidity and mortality.

## DIAGNOSIS OF MULTIPLE GESTATION

Currently more than 90% of twins are diagnosed before delivery because of the widespread availability of diagnostic ultrasound and maternal serum alpha-fetoprotein screening.

### Clinical Indications
Clues which are all suggestive of the diagnosis of multiple gestations include past or family history of twins, report of increased weight gain, increased fetal activity, auscultation of two fetal hearts differing by more than 10 beats per minute heard simultaneously, unexplained anemia, hydramnios of early onset, or early onset of pregnancy-induced hypertension (PIH). The most useful clinical screening tool is the finding of a fundal height greater than dates.

### Maternal Serum Alpha Fetoprotein
Maternal serum alpha fetoprotein elevation (>2.5 MOM) occurs in 20% to 30% of patients with twins. If the elevation is greater than 4 MOM and twins are seen, further evaluation is indicated.

**TABLE 6-1.** Average Length of Pregnancy Relative to the Number of Fetuses (In Pregnancies Beyond 20 Weeks Gestation with Accurate Dates)

| No. of Fetuses | No. of Pregnancies | Days Gestation Completed |
| --- | --- | --- |
| One | 82 | 271 |
| Two | 21 | 246 |
| Three | 5 | 234 |
| Four | 3 | 205 |

From Caspi E, Ronen J, Schreyer P, et al. The outcome of pregnancy after gonadotrophin therapy. Br J Obstet Gynaecol 1976;83:967.

## Ultrasound

Ultrasound is the diagnostic method of choice, since it will confirm both the diagnosis and the number of multiple fetuses. Currently the exact prevalence of the phenomenon of the "vanishing twin" has not been determined and has been reported to range between 13% and 78% of patients scanned before 14 weeks of gestational age, with higher rates in those twins studied before 10 weeks. From another perspective, it is estimated that 5% of patients presenting with first trimester bleeding carry a diagnosis of a vanishing twin. This disappearance phenomenon occurs in multiple gestations of higher order. A definitive diagnosis of multiple fetuses on an early first trimester sonogram should not be made simply on the basis of visualization of more than one cavity, because a blood clot or transducer pressure can mimic a twin gestation, or a "disappearing" twin might be present. A therapeutic D&C in the setting of an "inevitable abortion" should be done only after a sonogram is performed to rule out a potentially viable coexisting fetus.

## EMBRYOLOGY

There are essentially three types of twin placentas—monoamnionic monochorionic, diamnionic monochorionic, and diamnionic dichorionic. All dizygous twins will have dichorionic (diamnionic) placentas. Monozygous gestations, however, can result in any of the three possible configurations, depending on the timing of the "twinning impetus." About 30% of monozygous twins have a diamnionic dichorionic placenta. Most diamnionic dichorionic placentas will be the result of dizygous twinning. To identify the subset that are monozygous, one must look at other parameters. About 70% of monozygous twins have a diamnionic monochorionic placenta. Monoamnionic monochorionic twins are the least common variety of monozygous gestations. They occur in about 1% of twin births.

Examination of the placenta after birth will aid in the determination of zygosity. In approximately 35% of patients, differing sex will establish twins as dizygous. In an additional 20%, careful study of the placenta will lead to the proper diagnosis. In the remaining 45% of like-sex dichorionic twins, most will be dizygotic. Other methods used to determine zygosity after birth in these cases are blood grouping and DNA mapping techniques.

## ABNORMALITIES OF MULTIPLE GESTATION

### Fetal Anomalies

The incidence of fetal anomalies in multiple gestations is one and a half to three times higher than that of singleton gestations. This increase is due to the higher percentage of structural defects found in monozygotic twin gestations. Higher-order multiple gestations have even a greater chance of having an anomaly of one fetus.

More obviously a result of twinning is the anomaly of conjoined twins, which deserves special mention because it is specific to multiple gestations. The incidence ranges from 1 in 50,000 to 1 in 100,000 births, or roughly 1 in 600 twin births. These twins are classified by site of union. Most commonly they are fused at the chest (thoracopagus).

The second category of anomalies to consider are those resulting from the vascular interchange that is a potential complication of any monozygotic gestation. An acardiac twin is believed to arise when arterial-arterial and venous-venous anastomoses exist without any arterial-venous connections. This provides for uncompensated reverse flow, which is then linked to absence of the heart. This anomaly is rare and specific to multiple gestations, affecting approximately 1 in 30,000 infants, or 1 in 100 monozygotic twin births.

Another type of vascular interchange that can lead to abnormalities is the embolization of necrotic material or development of DIC that can happen when one fetus is dead and vascular connections are present. In this setting, the live twin can develop microcephaly, hydranencephaly, intestinal atresia, aplasia cutis, or limb amputation.

The last type of anomaly related to multiple fetuses is that group of problems resulting from intrauterine crowding. Examples are minor foot deformities and skull asymmetry. There also may be an increased frequency of congenital dislocation of the hip.

## Placental Anomalies

Anomalies of the placenta are also much more common among multiple gestations. A bivascular (monoarterial) cord, found in only 1% of pregnancies, is found in closer to 4% of twins. Prolapse of the umbilical cord occurs more frequently. A velamentous cord complicates 1% of singleton pregnancies and 7% of twins. A circummarginate or circumvallate placenta is more frequently seen with twins.

## The Twin-Twin Transfusion Syndrome

The abnormality of vascular connections between placentas has been reported to complicate as many as 85% of monochorial placentas studied. When arterial venous connections are uncompensated and unidirectional flow results, the abnormality of the "twin-twin transfusion syndrome" can occur (Figure 6-1). The diagnosis consists of the three findings of hydramnios, a hemoglobin difference of

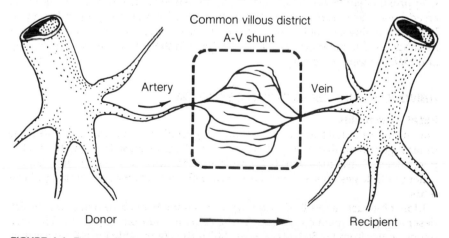

**FIGURE 6-1.** The pathologic arteriovenous connection in the twin transfusion syndrome. (Redrawn from Benirsche K. Twin gestation: incidence, etiology and inheritance. In: Creasy RK, Resnik R, eds. Maternal-fetal medicine: principles and practice, 2nd ed. Philadelphia: WB Saunders, 1989.)

at least 30% (4.4 g/100 mL), and morbid changes of the twins. As many as 30% of monochorial twins have this syndrome to some degree. In its most severe form, the donor fetus is growth retarded, or possibly hydropic due to high-output failure, with anemia and hypotension. The recipient of the transfusion will be more active, it will have increased fluid due to increased urination, and it will have congestive heart failure due to circulatory overload. This recipient twin will have hypovolemia, hypertension, plethora, and thromboses of peripheral vessels. The placenta will reveal pathologic changes in the respective areas. The donor area should be boggy, pale, and edematous, and the receiving area red and congested. The vascular connections should be demonstrable. The degree of morbidity from the syndrome will depend not only on the quality and caliber of the vessels involved, but also on the gestational age of the pregnancy and the presence or absence of any compensatory connections (arterial-arterial or venous-venous). Perinatal mortality in the extreme cases may be as high as 70%. Less affected twins have a much better prognosis. If the smaller twin dies, it is possible for the surviving twin to reach term as the hydramnios resolves.

## PHYSIOLOGY

The physiologic changes of a multiple gestation as compared to the singleton pregnancy are listed in Table 6-2.

## ANTEPARTUM DIAGNOSIS AND MANAGEMENT

### PREVENTION OF PREMATURITY

Premature delivery is the leading cause of morbidity and mortality in this group. The incidence of preterm birth among twins is between 20% and 50%, and even

**TABLE 6-2.** Physiologic Changes of Multiple Gestation as Compared to the Singleton Pregnancy

Increased maternal weight gain
Increased uterine growth
Greater hemodilution
Increased fibrinogen
Greater drop in diastolic blood pressure in the second trimester
Greater rise in diastolic blood pressure before delivery
Increased incidence of pregnancy-induced hypertension
Greater increase in tidal volume
?Higher incidence of gestational diabetes
Increased glomerular filtration rates
Exaggerated ureteral changes, such as dilatation from hormonal changes or compression at the pelvic brim
?Increased incidence of urinary tract infection
?Increased incidence of hyperemesis gravidarum
Increased maternal serum human chorionic gonadotropin
Increased human placental lactogen
Increased levels of estriol, serum estradiol, and progesterone

higher for triplets (75%) and higher-order multiple gestations. Multiple gestations constitute 25% of the perinatal deaths related to prematurity. Most of this mortality (50 to 80%) occurs before 32 weeks. The critical period of gestation appears to be between 26 and 29 weeks, and between 600 and 900 g. Preterm deliveries are the result of premature labor, premature rupture of the membranes, and third trimester bleeding.

## DIAGNOSIS

Patient education, early referral to a specialist, and antepartum care in a special clinic are all measures aimed at earlier identification of the problem of premature labor. Knowledgeable risk assessment, combined with serial cervical examinations, may also help identify patients at highest risk for premature birth (Table 6-3). Home monitoring is a noninvasive modality that can lead to earlier identification and, therefore, treatment of premature uterine activity.

## MANAGEMENT

### Tocolysis

The present consensus of opinion does not support the routine use of prophylactic tocolytics. The use of ritodrine in the treatment of premature labor, on the other hand, has been shown to have beneficial results. The efficacy seen is similar to the benefit of ritodrine therapy for premature labor complicating a singleton pregnancy. Because of the increased maternal blood volume and cardiac output of a multiple pregnancy, the margin of safety with use of tocolytics may be narrowed.

### Bedrest

The value of bedrest in prevention of prematurity is a subject of controversy. It should not be routinely recommended until it has been proven to be beneficial. Of course, certain complications, such as premature cervical dilatation, recurrent contractions, and suspected IUGR, may warrant prolonged hospitalization for rest and closer observation.

**TABLE 6-3.** Risk Factors in Multiple Gestations

Higher-order multiple gestations
Monozygosity
Single fetal death
Polyhydramnios
Anomaly
Growth discordancy
MSAFP > 4 MOM
Premature rupture of the membranes
Antepartum bleeding
Pregnancy-induced hypertension
Premature labor

## Cerclage

The placement of a cerclage to reinforce the cervix under the strain of a multiple gestation has not yet proven to be of benefit for twins, and it is not without significant risks. It is the authors' view that a cerclage should be placed only when suspected cervical incompetence is present in a twin pregnancy. The value of a cerclage for triplets, quadruplets, and greater multiple gestations is not proven at this time.

## Steroid Administration

The use of steroids for the treatment of known or suspected pulmonary immaturity had been shown to be efficacious in certain patients carrying singleton pregnancies. Their use in multifetal pregnancies has remained controversial. A collaborative study did not demonstrate a benefit from dexamethasone for twins or triplets. A recent study using ambraxol found an effectiveness in reducing the incidence of respiratory distress syndrome for twins.

## FETAL ASSESSMENT

### Diagnosis

**Fetal Growth.** It is technically possible to measure multiple parameters with ultrasound. The use of multiple parameters is helpful in assessing fetal growth. Estimated fetal weight is especially useful in this regard. Because growth is a dynamic process, serial scanning is necessary.

**Intrauterine Growth Retardation (IUGR).** To minimize the risks of IUGR, fetal assessment by ultrasound is currently recommended every 3 to 4 weeks, beginning at 26 weeks, and as frequently as every 2 weeks if the diagnosis is suspected. Multiple gestations of higher order may be at risk even sooner. IUGR can be predicted using an estimated fetal weight that is calculated using multiple parameters. Of the individual parameters, abdominal circumference is the most accurate measurement.

**Growth Discordance.** As with IUGR, measurement of abdominal circumference is the most sensitive marker for significant growth discordance. An intrapair difference of 20 mm should be followed with careful estimation of fetal weights based on abdominal circumferences, femur lengths, and BPDs. A difference in fetal weights of greater than 20% will then provide the best predictive value. In the twin-twin transfusion syndrome sonographic findings would include midtrimester hydramnios in the sac of the larger twin that may already have developed hydrops, and a smaller twin with IUGR with diminished fluid volume or frank oligohydramnios. This combination of findings is to be differentiated from a situation in which one twin has simple IUGR and the other twin is growing normally. The least common situation in which a discrepancy is present would involve a normal fetus that is smaller than a twin that is hydropic or macrosomic.

**Amniotic Fluid Volume Assessment.** Assessment of amniotic fluid volume with ultrasound is a mainstay of fetal surveillance for all high-risk singleton pregnancies, including multiple gestations. Increased or decreased fluid may be the first sign of IUGR, discordance from a transfusion syndrome, or hydrops. Abnormal fluid volume may lead to the discovery of an anomaly that had not previously manifested itself. And, certainly, altered fluid volume signals the need for closer surveillance with the other modes of fetal surveillance.

**Fetal Membranes.** Ultrasound is instrumental in making the important diagnosis of a monoamniotic gestation. A monoamniotic sac does not contain an intervening membrane. This finding should be seen on multiple examinations before a definitive diagnosis is made. Monoamniotic twins are rare, occurring in only 1% of twin gestations. Antenatal diagnosis is important because of a mortality rate of 50% to 60% associated with monoamniotic twins.

After excluding a monoamniotic pregnancy, a systematic approach to diagnosing chorionicity may be helpful. This will begin with determination of sex. Discordant sex indicates that the pregnancy is dizygotic and, therefore, the placenta is dichorionic. Likewise, if two separate placental discs are seen, the gestation is dichorionic.

Dichorionic twins carry the lowest perinatal mortality rate, about 9%. This type of placentation does not carry the potential for vascular communications and their associated complications of embolization and transfusion. In addition, most dichorionic placentas are associated with dizygotic twins, which do not have the greatly increased incidence of anomalies found among monozygotic twins

If evaluation of sex and number of placentas identifies twins of like sex and a shared placenta, attention is then turned to the dividing membrane. Two methods of determining chorionicity have been described. The first method determines membrane thickness, which will correctly identify chorionicity in 80% to 90% of patients. A monochorionic membrane should be thin and hairlike. A dichorionic membrane is thick and more easily visualized. The second method involves actual counting the layers in a dividing membrane. When this is possible, the correct diagnosis can be made in almost all cases. Monochorionic dividing membranes should have only two layers; dichorionic membranes should consist of three or four visible layers. Evaluating the dividing membrane to determine chorionicity is optimally performed early in pregnancy.

**Fetal Death In Utero.** The diagnosis of single fetal death complicates 0.5% to 6.8% of multiple gestations. Death of one fetus later in a multiple gestation can be associated with significant morbidity and mortality. The risk of major morbidity or death for the surviving twin has been reported to be as high as 46%. Prognosis will depend on the cause of the initial demise, as well as on the type of placentation—and therefore the degree of shared circulation—and the estimated gestational age or time of delivery. Potential fetal complications include disseminated intravascular coagulation (DIC), thromboembolic phenomena from release of necrotic material into a shared circulation, and anemia from relaxation of the dead twin's vascular bed. With a dead fetus in utero, the mother is also at risk for development of DIC from release of thromboplastic material.

## Fetal Heart Assessment

**Non-Stress Test (NST).** The NST is the screening method of choice for fetal surveillance. This method does not have contraindications and is less time-consuming because it is feasible to test multiple fetuses simultaneously. The NST is reliable and has high predictive value when the results are normal. When the results are abnormal the predictive value is lower, and vibro-acoustic stimulation or another test of fetal well-being should then be used to differentiate the sleeping fetus from the asphyxiated one.

**Contraction Stress Test (CST).** Although a CST may safely be performed in some cases of multiple gestation, this form of fetal surveillance is rarely used.

**Biophysical Profile (BPP).** The fetal BPP is a reliable method of fetal surveillance, and it also can be used as a means of follow-up of a nonreactive NST. Of course, it will be more time-consuming for a multiple gestation, but there are no contraindications to this procedure. It has been found to have as high a sensitivity and specificity for twins as for singletons.

The time to initiate routine screening with these tests of fetal well-being is currently debated. Because they are noninvasive and potentially life-saving, many would begin testing at least weekly at the onset of fetal viability (26 weeks). Certainly they are indicated if a multiple gestation is complicated by other factors that place the fetus at even higher risk for acute hypoxic stresses in utero.

**Doppler Ultrasound.** Doppler velocimetry is an accepted method of evaluating placental impedance in singleton pregnancies, during which it has been shown to predict in utero acid-base status and neonatal morbidity. The role of Doppler in assessment of twins has been outlined by Pardi and Ferrazi.* Their technique uses continuous- and pulsed-wave Doppler coupled in a mechanical sector scanner to ensure proper localization of each twin. They found that for concordant sex pairs without anomalies a significant intrapair pulsatility index (PI) gradient was observed prior to 28 weeks in all pairs that subsequently had birth weight differences of more than 15%. They contend that this finding with Doppler preceded other evidence of growth difference by 4 to 8 weeks. Their recommendation is that doppler assessment of twin fetuses should be initiated at 20 to 22 weeks to help identify pairs at risk for abnormal growth and in need of closer follow-up with the other methods of fetal assessment.

**Percutaneous Umbilical Blood Sampling (PUBS).** PUBS can be performed in a twin gestation for appropriate indications. The exact risks of the procedure, however, are not well defined in multiple gestations.

## MANAGEMENT

### Intrauterine Growth Retardation

When IUGR afflicts one or more fetuses, management is similar to that of IUGR in a singleton. The risks of prematurity must be weighed against the risks of continued stress in utero. In addition, in multiple gestations the gestational age of the normal fetus(es) must be considered. If a decision is made to continue the pregnancy, close fetal surveillance should ensue, with biweekly ultrasound examination to assess fetal growth, frequent heart rate monitoring and BPPs, and possibly Doppler velocimetry. Ideally, delivery of the growth-retarded fetus should await fetal lung maturity of all fetuses. If further evidence of fetal asphyxia becomes evident on the additional testing, delivery may become mandatory prior to documented maturity of all fetuses.

### Growth Discordance

Management consists primarily of tocolysis for the premature labor that results from the progressive polyhydramnios. And, as with IUGR, bedrest and expectant

---

*Ferrazi L, Pardi G. Doppler assessment of multiple gestation. In: Chervenak FA, Isaacson G, Campbell S, eds. Textbook of obstetric and gynecologic ultrasound. Boston: Little, Brown, 1993.

management with close fetal surveillance are indicated. If fetal maturity is reached, delivery should be carried out. In contrast, for severely premature fetuses, allowing one fetus to die in utero in order to avoid severe prematurity for both is recommended. If the smaller twin dies, the hydramnios may resolve. The larger twin may reach a gestation at which survival is much more likely. Between the extremes of fetal lung maturity and severe prematurity, management of cases should be individualized.

## Acute Polyhydramnios

When acute polyhydramnios complicates a multiple gestation, it can be associated with an extremely high rate of fetal mortality from severe prematurity. Some recommend frequent amniocentesis to reduce fluid volume and delay delivery. Others believe that the risks of this procedure, which include abruptio placentae, infection, and premature labor from the tap itself, outweigh the benefits. The authors believe that amniocentesis should be performed to relieve maternal respiratory embarrassment and in some manifestations of intractable premature labor.

## Monoamniotic and Monochorionic Gestations

Monoamnionic pregnancies need intensive fetal surveillance and early delivery in order to reduce their extremely high mortality rates. Monochorionic diamnionic gestations also deserve close monitoring. They are at greater risk for anomalies, and they can have shared circulation with its associated problems. Dichorionic pregnancies progress with the fewest complications. Ultrasound is still indicated to follow fetal growth.

## Single Fetal Death in Utero

After 34 weeks, delivery for all multiple gestations complicated by death of one fetus in utero is recommended after documentation of fetal lung maturity. Before 34 weeks expectant management with close surveillance seems prudent.

## Maternal Complications

**Pregnancy-Induced Hypertension (PIH).** PIH is seen in as many as 37% of multiple gestations. Not only is the incidence of PIH higher than in singleton pregnancies, but the onset is often earlier and the severity greater. PIH is seen even more commonly with multiple gestations with more than two fetuses.

**Hemorrhage.** Maternal hemorrhage is a major concern antepartum, intrapartum, and especially postpartum. Placenta previa and abruptio placentae are both slightly more common with multiple fetuses. There is an increased need for surgical intervention during the intrapartum period and, therefore, an increased risk of blood loss during this period. Overdistention of the uterus, leading to uterine atony, can lead to a significant postpartum hemorrhage.

**Chorionic Villus Sampling (CVS) and Amniocentesis.** CVS is feasible when twins have separate placentas. The transcervical route and transabdominal route, or a combination of approaches, have been used. As with amniocentesis, the risk of fetal loss for twins with this procedure is believed to be approximately equal to the risk of CVS for singletons.

Amniocentesis for analysis of karyotype or AFP analysis requires sampling from both sacs. Tapping the cavities individually should begin with careful sonographic mapping. If there is any uncertainty that separate sacs are being sampled, then the first sac should be identified with contrast. Indigo carmine or Evan's blue dye can be used. Methylene blue should be avoided because it is a chemical reducing agent with the ability to cause fetal hemolysis. Red dyes cannot be used because they might be confused with blood. Ultrasound guidance throughout the procedure is important. The fluid of the second sac should be free of contrast. Amniocentesis for twins in the second trimester, as with singletons, has been found to be a reliable and safe method for prenatal diagnostic testing.

At times, documentation of fetal lung maturity by amniocentesis will aid in clinical management. It is felt that amniocentesis to document fetal lung maturity in most cases can be done by tapping only one sac. Most studies indicate a close correlation between L/S ratios with twins. A ratio above 2.5 is felt to provide a margin of safety even in the setting of intersac variation. Several situations, however, can lead to substantial differences in L/S ratios between twins. In fetuses in which the maturity indices may be altered significantly, the sac of the twin expected to be less mature should be sampled. For example, in the setting of premature rupture of membranes the twin in the unruptured sac should be tapped. After onset of labor, the twin presenting second should be sampled. If a significant discrepancy is present, the larger twin should have the amniocentesis.

**Fetal Anomalies.** Conjoined twins are first suspected when ultrasound evaluation fails to reveal a dividing membrane. Not only are the twins in the same sac, but on repeated examinations their position relative to one another does not change. Hydramnios is present in more than half the cases. Longitudinal scanning of the heads, thoraces, and abdomens will then reveal any sharing of any major organ that is present. A careful search must be made in all cases for other major congenital anomalies, since these often further complicate conjoined twins.

Management of any of the many other anomalies that can be seen with increasing frequency among twins, and management of any karyotype abnormality that is found, will depend upon the severity of the anomaly, as well as the gestational age at which it is diagnosed. The patient herself will have to make the final decision regarding management. One option is selective termination of one fetus.

## INTRAPARTUM MANAGEMENT OF MULTIPLE FETUSES

### LABOR

The patient with a multiple gestation is known to have a greater level of prelabor uterine activity. Therefore, for both multiparas and primiparas the latent phase of labor is shorter, because the patient usually presents with more advanced cervical changes. But the overall duration of labor is not significantly different when compared with singletons, because the active phase is often longer. This prolongation of the active phase may be related to the greater use of anesthetics and analgesics, the much higher incidence of prematurity, or the greater incidence of dysfunctional labor. This in turn is believed to be due to uterine overdistension and the higher incidence of malpresentations. When induction of labor is necessary, it is optimal to use an intrauterine pressure catheter to guide the infusion of oxytocin.

## MONITORING AND THE INTERDELIVERY INTERVAL

The time interval is no longer a critical factor in obtaining a successful outcome. Fetal status can be monitored throughout labor and delivery. Twins should be delivered only in centers with capabilities for real-time ultrasound, electronic fetal heart rate monitoring, and immediate cesarean delivery when necessary. Monitoring of labor with twins usually involves a scalp electrode for twin A, and an external fetal monitor for twin B. After delivery of twin A, electronic or sonographic monitoring of the fetal heart rate of twin B is carried out until its delivery.

## MODE OF DELIVERY

The possible combinations of presentations are varied, but three broad categories provide a working classification to discuss mode of delivery: vertex-vertex, vertex-nonvertex, and nonvertex twin A. The authors' management plan is illustrated in Figure 6-2.

### Twin A Vertex, Twin B Nonvertex

There is no definitive conclusion at this time regarding the optimum management of the vertex-nonvertex twin gestation. Cesarean delivery of all vertex-breech and vertex-transverse twin presentations is an option that is currently accepted. This approach is recommended by some authors because of the possibility of birth

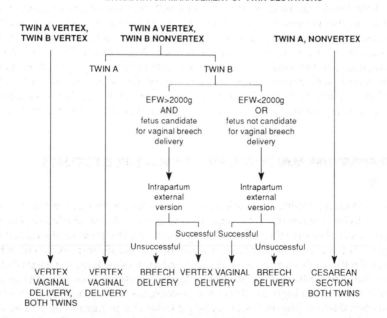

INTRAPARTUM MANAGEMENT OF TWIN GESTATIONS

**FIGURE 6-2.** Outline of proposed intrapartum management of twin gestation. (From Chervenak FA, Johnson RE, Youcha S, et al. Intrapartum management of twin gestation. Obstet Gynecol 1985; 65:119.)

trauma and birth asphyxia to the vaginally delivered nonvertex twin. Two other options exist, however, to avoid routine cesarean section in this setting. Successful version of the second twin has been reported by several investigators. Sonographic assessment of the size of both features should be carried out. If twin B is much larger (i.e., >500 g difference), then version and attempted vaginal delivery are best avoided. Epidural anesthesia to provide abdominal wall relaxation is optimal. Ultrasound guidance facilitates the procedure, and continuous heart rate surveillance is performed. Under these guidelines, version has been found to be a safe and effective procedure to accomplish vaginal vertex delivery.

The specific maneuver is shown in Figure 6-3. Gentle pressure, either with the transducer or one's hands, is used to guide the vertex toward the pelvis. The shortest arc between the vertex and the pelvic inlet should be followed initially. The version can be accomplished as either a forward or a backward roll, but in all patients undue force must be avoided. When the vertex is brought to the pelvic inlet, the membranes are ruptured and delivery accomplished, with oxytocin augmentation as needed. If the version is unsuccessful, vaginal breech delivery or cesarean section is performed. If the fetal heart rate deteriorates, immediate cesarean section is carried out.

Vaginal breech delivery of the second twin is a second option to avoid routine abdominal delivery of vertex-nonvertex twins. This approach will depend upon estimated fetal weights. For twins estimated to be above 2000 g on ultrasound, several studies have not found an excessive risk of asphyxia or birth trauma when these second twins are delivered vaginally as a breech. For breech delivery to be considered, the standard criteria for singleton pregnancy should be met. They are an adequate maternal pelvis, a flexed fetal head, and an estimated fetal weight of 2000 to 3500 g.

For twins estimated to be below 2000 g and therefore potentially in the very-low-birth-weight-group, there is a lack of data demonstrating the safety of vaginal breech delivery. At this time the authors are in agreement with others that these

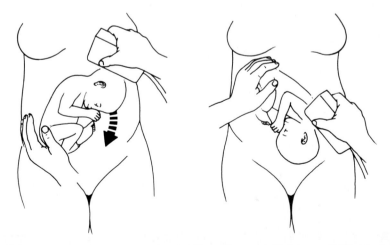

**FIGURE 6-3.** The maneuver of external version (From Chervenak FA, Johnson RE, Youcha S, et al. Intrapartum management of twin gestation. Obstet Gynecol 1983; 62:160.)

infants—whether singleton or breech—should be delivered through an adequate uterine incision.

There are several exceptions to the foregoing management plans. For some patients elective cesarean delivery should follow documentation of fetal lung maturity. For example, monoamniotic twins are optimally delivered by cesarean section at 36 weeks or earlier to minimize their already extremely high perinatal mortality rate and the risks of cord entanglement and fetal interlocking. In most instances of conjoined twins abdominal delivery is indicated as described earlier. Many of the other congenital anomalies seen more frequently among twins can also necessitate abdominal delivery. If one or both of a pair have severe IUGR, the stress of labor and vaginal delivery may be contraindicated. In the authors' opinion, triplets and multiple gestations of higher order warrant cesarean delivery to avoid birth trauma.

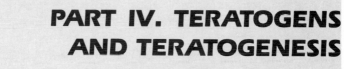

# PART IV. TERATOGENS AND TERATOGENESIS

## 7. PRESCRIBED DRUGS, THERAPEUTIC AGENTS, AND FETAL TERATOGENESIS

### ETIOLOGIES OF CONGENITAL MALFORMATIONS

The etiology of congenital malformations can be divided into three categories: unknown, genetic, and environmental factors (Table 7-1). The etiology of the majority of human malformations, approximately 65% to 75%, is unknown; however, a significant proportion of congenital malformations of unknown etiology are likely to be polygenic (due to two or more genetic loci) or to at least have an important genetic component. Malformations with an increased recurrent risk, such as cleft lip and palate, anencephaly, spina bifida, certain congenital heart diseases, pyloric stenosis, hypospadias, inguinal hernia, talipes equinovarus, and congenital dislocation of the hip, can fit the category of multifactorial disease, as well as the category of polygenic inherited disease. The multifactorial threshold hypothesis involves the modulation of a continuum of genetic characteristics by intrinsic and extrinsic (environmental) factors. Although the modulating factors are not known, they probably include placental blood flow, placental transport, site of implantation, maternal disease states, infections, drugs, chemicals, and spontaneous errors of development.

**TABLE 7-1.** Etiology of Human Malformations Observed During the First Year of Life

| Suspected Cause | Percent of Total |
| --- | --- |
| Unknown | 65–75 |
|   Polygenic | |
|   Multifactorial (gene-environment interactions) | |
|   Spontaneous errors of development | |
|   Synergistic interactions of teratogens | |
| Genetic | 10–25 |
|   Autosomal and sex-linked genetic disease | |
|   New mutations | |
|   Cytogenetic (chromosomal abnormalities) | |
| Environmental | 10 |
|   Maternal conditions: Alcoholism; diabetes; endocrinopathies; phenylketonuria; smoking and nicotine; starvation | 4 |
|   Infectious agents: Rubella, toxoplasmosis, syphilis, herpes, cytomegalic inclusion disease, varicella, Venezuelan equine encephalitis, parvovirus | 3 |
|   Mechanical problems (deformations): Amniotic band constrictions; umbilical cord constraint; disparity in uterine size and uterine contents | 1–2 |
|   Chemicals, prescription drugs, radiation, hyperthermia | <1 |

Adapted from Brent RL. Environmental factors: miscellaneous. In: Brent RL, Harris MI, eds. Prevention of embryonic, fetal, and perinatal disease. DHEW Pub (NIH) 76–853. Bethesda, MD, 1976:211.
Brent RL. The magnitude of the problem of congenital malformations. In: Marois M, ed. Prevention of physical and mental congenital defects, part A: The scope of the problem. New York: Alan R. Liss, 1985:55.
Brent RL, Holmes LB. Clinical and basic science lessons from the thalidomide tragedy: what have we learned about the causes of limb defects? Teratology 1988;38:241.

Spontaneous errors of development may account for some of the malformations that occur without apparent abnormalities of the genome or environmental influence. It has been estimated that up to 50% of all fertilized ova in the human are lost within the first 3 weeks of development. The World Health Organization (1970) has estimated that 15% of all clinically recognizable pregnancies end in a spontaneous abortion, and 50% to 60% of the spontaneously aborted fetuses have chromosomal abnormalities.* This means that, as a conservative estimate, 1173 clinically recognized pregnancies will result in approximately 173 miscarriages, and 30 to 60 of the infants will have congenital anomalies in the remaining 1000 live births. The true incidence of pregnancy loss is much higher, but undocumented pregnancies are not included in this risk estimate. The 3% to 6% incidence of malformed offspring represents the background risk for human maldevelopment. Although we know little about the mechanisms which result in the in utero death of defective embryos, it is perhaps more important to understand the circumstances which permit abnormal embryos to survive to term.

Understanding the pathogenesis for the large group of malformations with unknown etiology will depend on identifying the genes involved in polygenic or pleurogenic processes, the interacting genetic and environmental determinants of multifactorial traits, and the statistical risks for error during embryonic development.

The known etiologies of teratogenesis include genetic and environmental factors that affect the embryo during development (e.g., drugs, chemicals, radiation,

* World Health Organization. Spontaneous and induced abortion. World Health Organization Technical Report Series, Number 461, Geneva World Health Organization, 1970.

hyperthermia, infections, abnormal maternal metabolic states, or mechanical factors). Environmental and genetic causes of malformations have different pathologic processes that result in abnormal development. Congenital malformations due to genetic etiology have a spectrum of pathologic processes that are the result of a gene deficiency, a gene abnormality, chromosome deletion, or chromosome excess. The pathologic nature of this process is determined before conception, or at least before differentiation, because of inherited or newly acquired genetic abnormalities present in all or most of the cells of the embryo. Although environmental factors may modify the development of the genetically abnormal embryo, the genetic abnormality is usually the predominant contributor to the pathologic process.

The remainder of this review will focus on prescription drugs and therapeutic agents which cause congenital malformations in the human. Although these agents account for less than 1% of all malformations, they are important because these exposures are preventable.

## OVERALL TERATOGENIC RISK

To clarify the difficulty in predicting the effect that an exposure to a drug or therapeutic agent will have on the developing embryo, we will briefly discuss factors which influence this prediction.

The baseline risk of human reproduction is based on epidemiological studies which have determined the incidence of fetal death and maldevelopment. Approximately 75% of all conceptions are lost before term, 50% within the first 3 weeks. Of the live-born infants, 3% to 6% will be recognized as congenitally malformed.

## ENVIRONMENTAL RISK PARAMETERS (OR MODIFIERS)

The susceptibility of an embryo or fetus to teratogenic influences is related to the stage of development at which the exposure occurs. The explanation for this phenomenon is that the fetus is constantly changing during development with respect to tissue receptors, metabolism, drug distribution, cell proliferation, etc. Thus, tissue response to an exposure and the ability of the fetus to recuperate from the insult vary during gestation. Although detrimental effects can be induced at any time during pregnancy, most major malformations result from exposures during days 18 to 40 of gestation in the human. However, the palate, central nervous system, and genital structures can be affected at later stages of development. Our knowledge of the time of resistance or susceptibility of the embryo to various environmental influences has expanded over the past 30 years. This information is of vital use in evaluating the significance of individual exposures or epidemiological studies.

Every teratogenic agent which has been validly tested has exhibited a dose-response relationship and a threshold dose response, that is, a dose below which there is no difference between the exposed and nonexposed in the incidence of malformations. The dose to which the fetus is exposed is determined by maternal pharmacokinetics, placental exchange, fetal and placental metabolism of the substance (and the teratogenic activity of the metabolites), fetal distribution of the

**TABLE 7-2.** Proposed Mechanisms of Teratogenesis

---

Cell death beyond recuperative capacity of the embryo/fetus
Mitotic delay: increase in the length of the cell cycle
Retarded differentiation: slowing or cessation in the process of differentiation
Physical constraint and vascular insufficiency
Interference with histogenesis by processes such as cell depletion, necrosis, calcification, or
  scarring
Inhibited cell migration and cell communication

---

From Beckman DA, Brent RL. Mechanism of known environmental teratogens: drugs and chemicals. Clin Perinatol 1986;13:649.

substance, and the presence of tissue-specific receptors. Factors which influence the response include maternal toxicity and drug-drug interactions. Additionally, more than 30 drug-related disorders are related to genotype, and although not proved in the human, genetic variations alter drug teratogenicity in experimental animals.

Finally, maternal disease states may produce deleterious effects on the fetus which are difficult to separate from a possible teratogenic effect of a therapeutic agent. This is an especially relevant consideration for long-standing conditions such as diabetes.

When counseling patients, especially in our litigious climate, three confounding influences are at work. One is the necessity to critically evaluate reported associations because of the anxiety created by unfounded reports and misinformation. The second is the fact that pregnancy is not without risk, and congenital malformations occur in the absence of drug or chemical exposures. The third is that there *are* teratogenic agents and new ones could be introduced.

## MECHANISMS OF TERATOGENESIS

Based on his review of the literature, Wilson (1979)† provided a format of theoretical teratogenic mechanisms: mutation; chromosomal aberrations; mitotic interference; altered nucleic acid synthesis and function; lack of precursors, substrates, or coenzymes for biosynthesis; altered energy sources; enzyme inhibition; osmolar imbalance, alterations in fluid pressures, viscosities, and osmotic pressures; and altered membrane characteristics. Even though an agent can produce one or more of these pathologic processes, exposure to such an agent does not guarantee that maldevelopment will occur. Furthermore, it is likely that a drug, chemical, or other agent can have more than one effect on the pregnant women and the developing conceptus, and therefore the nature of the drug or its biochemical or pharmacologic effects will not in themselves predict a human teratogenic effect. In fact, the discovery of human teratogens has come primarily from human epidemiological studies. Animal studies and in vitro studies can be very helpful in determining the mechanism of teratogenesis and the pharmacokinetics related to teratogenesis. We have proposed a list of mechanisms (Table 7-2) which we will

*Text continues on p. 59.*

---

† Wilson JG. Environment and birth defects. New York: Academic Press, 1973.

**TABLE 7-3.** Teratogenic Therapeutic Agents and Drugs.*

| Environmental Influence | Reported Effects or Associations | Comments |
| --- | --- | --- |
| Aminopterin, Methotrexate | Microcephalus, hydrocephalus, cleft palate, meningomyelocele, IUGR, abnormal cranial ossification, reduction in derivatives of first branchial arch, mental retardation, postnatal growth retardation. | Antimetabolic agents; folic acid antagonists that inhibit dihydrofolate reductase, resulting in cell death. |
| Androgens | Masculinization of female embryo: clitoromegaly with or without fusion of labia minora. Nongenital malformations are not a reported risk. | Effects are dose dependent; stimulates growth and differentiation of sex steroid receptor-containing tissue. |
| Angiotensin-converting Enzyme Inhibitors | Exposures may cause fetal and neonatal death, oligohydramnios, pulmonary hypoplasia, neonatal anuria, IUGR, and skull hypoplasia. | Antihypertensive agents; adverse fetal effects are related to severe fetal hypotension over a long period of time during the second or third trimester. Risk appears to be low. Can be used in a woman of reproductive age because therapy can be changed during the first trimester if the woman becomes pregnant without an increase in the risk of teratogenesis, since this group of drugs does not interfere with organogenesis. |
| Carbamazepine | Minor craniofacial defects (upslanting palpebral fissures, epicanthal folds, short nose with long philtrum), fingernail hypoplasia, and developmental delay. | Anticonvulsant; little is known concerning mechanism. Risk is not known but likely to be significant for minor defects |
| Coumarin | Nasal hypoplasia; stippling of secondary epiphysis; IUGR; anomalies of eyes, hands, neck; variable CNS anatomical defects, such as absent corpus callosum, hydrocephalus, or asymmetrical brain hypoplasia. | Anticoagulant; bleeding is an unlikely explanation for effects produced in the first trimester. Risk from exposure 10% to 25% during 8th to 14th week of gestation. CNS anatomical defects may occur anytime during second and third trimester and may be related to bleeding. |
| Cyclophosphamide | Growth retardation, ectrodactyly, syndactyly, cardiovascular anomalies, and other minor anomalies. | Alkylating agent; requires cytochrome P450 mono-oxydase activation; interacts with DNA, resulting in cell death. Magnitude of risk unknown. |

**TABLE 7-3.** (continued)

| Environmental Influence | Reported Effects or Associations | Comments |
|---|---|---|
| Diethylstilbestrol | Clear cell adenocarcinoma of the vagina occurs in between 1:1000 and 1:10,000 girls who were exposed in utero. Vaginal adinosis occurs much more frequently. Anomalies of the uterus and cervix may play a role in decreased fertility and an increased incidence of prematurity, although the majority of DES babies can conceive and deliver normal babies. Surprisingly, there are case reports of masculinization of the female fetus after high doses. The dose that increases risk of genitourinary abnormalities in the male is controversial. | Synthetic estrogen; stimulates estrogen receptor-containing tissue, may cause misplaced genital tissue, which has a greater propensity to develop cancer. Vaginal adenosis from exposures before 9th week of pregnancy, 75% risk; risk of adenocarcinoma is low (1 in 10,000). |
| Diphenylhydantoin | Hydantoin syndrome: microcephaly, mental retardation, cleft lip/palate, hypoplastic nails and distal phalanges; characteristic, but not diagnostic, facial features. | Anticonvulsant; direct effect on cell membranes, folate, and vitamin K metabolism. Metabolic intermediate (epoxide) has been suggested as the teratogenic agent. Wide variation in reported risk. Associations documented only with chronic exposure. |
| Lithium Carbonate | Although animal studies have demonstrated a clear teratogenic risk, the effect in humans is uncertain. Early reports indicated an increased incidence of Epstein's anomaly and other heart and great vessel defects, but as more studies are reported this association has diminished. | Antidepressant; mechanism has not been defined. Risk is low. |
| Oxazolidine-2,4-Diones (Trimethadione, Paramethadione) | Fetal trimethadione syndrome: V-shaped eyebrows, low-set ears with anteriorly folded helix, high-arched palate, irregular teeth, CNS anomalies, severe developmental delay. | Anticonvulsants; affects cell membrane permeability. Actual mechanism of action has not been determined. Wide variation in reported risk. Characteristic facial features are associations documented only with chronic exposure. |
| Penicillamine | Cutis laxa, hyperflexibility of joints. | Copper chelating agent; produces copper deficiency, inhibiting collagen synthesis and maturation. Condition appears to be reversible and the risk is low. |

| Progestins | Masculinization of female embryo exposed to *high* doses of some testosterone-derived progestins. The dose of progestins present in modern oral contraceptives presents no masculinization or feminization risks. All progestins present no risk for nongenital malformations. | Stimulates or interferes with sex steroid receptor-containing tissue. |
|---|---|---|
| Radioactive Isotopes | Tissue- and organ-specific damage dependent on radioisotope element and distribution; e.g., $^{131}$I administered to pregnant mother can cause fetal thyroid hypoplasia after the 8th week of development | Higher doses of radioisotopes can produce cell death and mitotic delay. Effect is dependent on dose, distribution, metabolism, and specificity of localization. |
| Radiation (External Irradiation) | Microcephaly, mental retardation, eye anomalies, IUGR, and visceral malformations depend on dose and stage of exposure | Diagnostic and therapeutic agents; produce cell death and mitotic delay. No measurable risk with exposures for 5 rad (0.05 Gy) or less of x-rays at any stage of pregnancy. |
| Retinoids (Etretinate, Isotretinoin) | Increased risk of central nervous system, cardioaortic, ear, and clefting defects. Microtia, anotia, thymic aplasia, and other branchial arch and aortic arch abnormalities. | Used in treatment of chronic dermatoses; retinoids can cause direct cytotoxicity and alter programmed cell death; after many cell types but neural cres; cells are particularly sensitive. |
| Sonography (Ultrasound) | No confirmed detrimental effects resulting from diagnostic medical sonography. | The levels and types of medical sonography that have been used in the past have no measurable risks. It would appear that if the embryonic temperature never exceeds 39°C, there is no measurable risk. |
| Tetracycline | Bone staining and tooth staining can occur with therapeutic doses. Persistent high doses can cause hypoplastic tooth enamel. No other congenital malformations are associated | Antibiotic; effects seen only if exposure is late in the first or during second or third trimester, since tetracylines have to interact with calcified tissue. |
| Thalidomide | Limb reduction defects (preaxial preferential effects, phocomelia), facial hemangioma, esophageal or duodenal atresia, anomalies of external ears, kidneys, and heart. The thalidomide syndrome, although characteristic and recognizable, can be mimicked by some genetic diseases. | Sedative-hypnotic agent; multiple theories have been proposed. Although it is likely that one or more of the theories have elements of the truth, the etiology of thalidomide teratogenesis has not been definitively determined. |

**TABLE 7-3.** (continued)

| Environmental Influence | Reported Effects or Associations | Comments |
|---|---|---|
| Thyroid: Iodine Deficiency, Iodides, Radioiodine, Antithyroid Drugs (Propylthiouracil) | Hypothyroidism or goiter; neurologic and aural damage is variable. | Fetopathic effect of endemic iodine occurs early in development. Fetopathic effect of iodides, antithyroid drugs, and radioiodine involves metabolic block, decreased thyroid hormone synthesis, and gland development. Maternal intake of 12 mg of iodide per day or more increases the risk of fetal goiter |
| Valproic Acid | Malformations are primarily facial dysmorphology and neural tube defects. Although there are some facial characteristics associated with this drug, they are not diagnostic. Small head size and developmental delay have been reported with high doses. | Anticonvulsant; little is known about the teratogenic action of valproic acid. The risk for spina bifida is about 1% but the risk for facial dysmorphology may be greater. |
| Vitamin A | The same malformations that have been reported with the retinoids have been reported with very high doses of vitamin A. Exposures below 10,000 IU present no risk to the fetus. | Retinoic acid is cytotoxic; it may interact with DNA to delay differentiation and/or inhibit protein synthesis. |
| Vitamin D | Large doses given in Vitamin D prophylaxis are possibly involved in the etiology of supravalvular aortic stenosis, elfin faces, and mental retardation. | Mechanism is likely to involve a disruption of cell calcium regulation. Genetic susceptibility and excessive doses are probably responsible. |
| Streptomycin | Hearing deficiency. | Although only rarely reported, streptomycin and a group of ototoxic drugs can interfere with hearing. It is a relatively low risk phenomenon and would be associated with long-duration maternal therapy during pregnancy |
| Bendectin (Doxylamine Succinate Pyridoxine) | Not teratogenic as used in doses to treat nausea and vomiting of pregnancy. | This drug is mentioned because it was involved in so much litigation as an alleged teratogen. It is a drug with no measurable risk. |

Modified from Beckman DA, Brent RL. Mechanism of known environmental teratogens: drugs and chemicals. Clin Perinatol 1986;13:649.

use in our discussion of the known teratogenic drugs and therapeutic agents in man. However, even if one understands the pathologic effects of an agent, one cannot predict the teratogenic risk of an exposure without taking into consideration the developmental stage, the magnitude of the exposure, and the reparability of the embryo.

## HUMAN TERATOGENIC DRUGS AND THERAPEUTIC AGENTS

What is known concerning the mechanism of action of drugs and therapeutic agents that have been shown to cause congenital malformations in man is summarized in Table 7-3. The table lists drugs and therapeutic agents that have been associated with an increased risk of reproductive toxicity. It gives the agent, the reported effects, and explanatory comments that clarify or highlight controversial issues. It is important to emphasize that the reproductive toxicity of these agents is dependent on the dose or magnitude of the exposure.

## OTHER HUMAN TERATOGENIC AGENTS: ALCOHOL

Table 7-4 lists other human reproductive toxins and teratogenic agents. Alcohol will be discussed briefly because of its relatively large social impact. Fetal alcohol syndrome (FAS) has been described in children with intrauterine growth retardation, microcephaly, mental retardation, maxillary hypoplasia, flat philtrum, thin upper lip, and reduction in the width of palpebral fissures (cardiac abnormalities also were seen). Many children of alcoholic mothers had FAS, and all of the affected children evidenced developmental delay.

**TABLE 7-4.** Other Environmental Reproductive Toxins and Teratogenic Agents Reported in the Human

---

Alcohol

Infectious agents
  Rubella
  Cytomegalovirus
  Herpes simplex
  Parvovirus B19
  Syphilis
  Toxoplasmosis
  Varicella zoster
  Venezuelan equine encephalitis

Maternal conditions
  Diabetes
  Phenylketonuria
  Endocrinopathies
  Nutritional deprivation

Mechanical problems

Methylmercury

Polychlorinated biphenyls

Smoking and nicotine

Cocaine

---

A period of greatest susceptibility and a dose-response relationship have not yet been established. Although we are reluctant to claim that malformations are due to single exposures to alcohol in the human, binge drinking early in pregnancy has been suggested to be associated with neural tube defects. Actually, the neural tube defects, if real, are a minor risk when compared to the risk of decreased brain growth and differentiation that results from high alcohol consumption during the second and third trimester. Chronic consumption of 6 oz of alcohol per day constitutes a high risk, but FAS is not likely when the mother drinks fewer than two drinks (equivalent to 2 oz of alcohol) per day. Reduction of alcohol consumption at any time in pregnancy reduces the severity of FAS but may not significantly reduce the risk of some degree of physical or behavioral impairment. The human syndrome is likely to involve the direct effects of ethanol and the indirect effects of genetic susceptibility and poor nutrition. Although alcoholic mothers frequently smoke and consume other drugs, there is little doubt that alcohol ingestion alone can have a disastrous effect on the developing embryo or fetus. It is estimated that there are at least several hundred children born each year with the full FAS and probably several thousand children with fetal alcohol effects.

## SUMMARY

Environmental causes of human malformations account for approximately 10% of malformations, and fewer than 1% of all human malformations are related to prescription drug exposure, chemicals, or radiation. However, malformations caused by prescription drugs and other therapeutic agents are important because these exposures are preventable. As we better understand the mechanisms of teratogenesis from all etiologies we may learn how to best predict and test for potential teratogenicity.

## ACKNOWLEDGEMENTS

We thank Mrs. Yvonne G. Edney and Mrs. Lisa A. Desmond for their assistance in the preparation of this manuscript. This work was supported in part by funds by NIH HD07075, NIH HD 18167, the Foerderer Foundation, and Harry Bock Charities.

---

# 8. NONPRESCRIPTION DRUGS AND ALCOHOL: ABUSE AND EFFECTS IN PREGNANCY

---

In modern American society the use of "recreational" drugs and alcohol has reached epidemic proportions, reaching pervasively into every socioeconomic class and becoming so important that presidential campaigns have seized on the drug problem as a major political issue. It is not the intent of the author of this chapter to describe the vast societal, legal, economic, and moral consequences of the use of illicit drugs. Rather, this chapter will be limited to a discussion of the effect of such chemicals on the mother and her fetus.

## ALCOHOL

### FETAL ALCOHOL SYNDROME

The term *fetal alcohol syndrome* (FAS) was coined by researchers in 1973 based on observations of 11 children of alcoholic mothers with characteristic features (Table 8-1). In 1980, specific criteria for FAS were proposed by the Fetal Alcohol Study Group of the Research Society on Alcoholism, requiring that at least one feature from each of three following categories be present for the diagnosis to be made:

1. Growth retardation before or after birth.
2. A pattern of abnormal features of the face and head (including small head circumference and small eyes) or evidence of retarded formation of the midfacial area (including a flattened bridge and short length of the nose, and flattening of the vertical groove between the nose and mouth—that is, the philtrum).
3. Evidence of central nervous system abnormality (e.g., abnormal neonatal behavior, mental retardation, or other evidence of abnormal neurobehavioral development).

### ALCOHOL-RELATED BIRTH DEFECTS

Other abnormalities associated with alcohol exposure in utero have subsequently been described, including ophthalmologic anomalies, otic anomalies, cardiac septal defects, hemangiomas, undescended testes, hernias, unusual fingerprint patterns, and palmar creases. The presence of any of these abnormalities in the offspring of an alcohol-using mother raises the question of a causal relationship. Because these abnormalities also occur in children who were not exposed to alcohol in utero, they can only be ascribed to maternal drinking when seen with the characteristic features of FAS. Another category of problems, "alcohol-related birth effects" (ARBE), consists of pregnancy complications and adverse outcomes that can be attributed to maternal alcohol use in the epidemiologic sense when potentially confounding variables have been controlled for. The birth of a small-for-dates baby to an alcoholic mother is an example of such an ARBE.

**TABLE 8-1.** Alcohol and the Fetus

---

Fetal alcohol syndrome: At least one from each of the following categories:
  Growth retardation
  Craniofacial abnormalities
  Central nervous system abnormalities
Alcohol-related birth effects: Any of the preceding problems in the offspring of an alcoholic individual

---

## PREVALENCE

The prevalence of FAS among the offspring of "heavy drinkers" (variously defined) ranges from 2.5% to 10% in prospective studies. Although it is difficult to obtain more specific data, it is clear that all cases of full-blown FAS have been reported in chronic alcoholic mothers who drank "heavily" throughout pregnancy.

## PATHOPHYSIOLOGY

The pathophysiologic mechanism for the adverse effects of alcohol on the developing fetus is poorly understood. It has been suggested that amniotic fluid may function as a reservoir, exposing the fetus to ethanol long after the mother has cleared it from her system. Either alcohol itself or acetaldehyde, or both, bear responsibility for the disruption of fetal growth and development. Alcohol is metabolized via a number of different systems, including alcohol dehydrogenase in the cytosol fraction of the liver, the hepatic microsomal ethanol-oxidizing system, and the peroxisomal-catalase system. There are genetic differences in some of these enzymes, and different individuals may induce such enzymes at different rates when exposed to the same concentrations of ethanol. Differential enzyme induction may lead to differential susceptibility to cell injury or disruption by other agents. Alternatively, ethanol or acetaldehyde may interfere with placental transport of vital nutrients such as amino acids, leading to a form of "fetal malnutrition."

## MANAGEMENT

There is no treatment or "cure" for fetal alcohol syndrome or alcohol-related birth effects. Therefore, the only possible strategy at the present time is prevention. The first component of prevention is education, so that women of childbearing age are aware of the risks of drinking during pregnancy.

To prevent fetal alcohol syndrome, it is first necessary to identify mothers at risk (those who are alcoholic). A number of approaches have been developed to taking an alcohol history, including the Ten Question Drinking History (TQDH) and the Michigan Alcohol Screening Test (MAST), which are standardized lists of questions to be asked. Perhaps the simplest and easiest to use is the CAGE approach, in which four basic questions are asked:

Have you ever:
Felt the need to Cut down drinking?
Felt Annoyed by criticism of your drinking?
Had Guilty feelings about drinking?
Taken a morning Eye-opener?

Depending on the study cited, either two or three positive answers (out of four) are highly suggestive of alcoholism. It is appropriate to administer the CAGE questions, or some other instrument for diagnosing alcoholism, to every patient at the time of obtaining a history.

Having identified the individual with a problem of alcohol intake, who is at increased risk for having a child with FAS, attention should next be turned to intervention.

The use of disulfiram to increase the motivation of alcoholics to avoid consumption of alcohol is generally considered contraindicated in pregnancy. A suspected but not proven teratogen, disulfiram, when taken in combination with alcohol, leads to very high circulating acetaldehyde concentrations.

Because alcohol has no known therapeutic value for either mother or fetus and because no threshold for adverse effects has been convincingly demonstrated, pregnant women should be advised to avoid alcohol altogether. However, this advice certainly should not be construed as suggesting interruption of pregnancy when a history of alcohol consumption has been elicited; the risks of low-level alcohol consumption, or even occasional binges of marked consumption, have not been demonstrated to date.

## COCAINE

### PHARMACOLOGY

Cocaine is an alkaloid originating in the leaves of the *Erythroxylon coca* plant that has a molecular weight of 339.81. It can be administered intranasally ("snorting"), orally, vaginally, sublingually, rectally, and by intravenous, subcutaneous, or intramuscular injection. Although at one time the most popular form of administration was intranasal, the emergence of a very inexpensive, pure, and portable form of cocaine ("crack cocaine") that when smoked gives a very immediate effect as it is absorbed by the pulmonary circulation has superseded the more traditional snorting. Cocaine is detoxified by cholinesterases, and cocaine and its metabolites are excreted in the urine, where they may be present for up to 3 days. Cocaine blocks the presynaptic reuptake of norepinephrine and dopamine, with the resultant accumulation of these neurotransmitters at receptor sites. Vasoconstriction, hypertension, myocardial irritability, and seizures may result. Euphoria may result from the accumulation of dopamine, a mechanism that may also be responsible for addiction.

### ADVERSE EFFECTS ON THE MOTHER

Medical complications reported with cocaine include acute myocardial infarction, cardiac arrhythmias, aortic rupture, subarachnoid hemorrhage, strokes, ischemic bowel damage, and various other problems. It would be expected that these same complications could occur in pregnant women, and a recent report of intracerebral hemorrhage during the postpartum period confirms that expectation (Table 8-2).

### ADVERSE EFFECTS ON THE PREGNANCY

Although not all studies have been confirmatory, it is highly likely that cocaine use can acutely trigger abruptio placentae by causing vasoconstriction in the uterine circulation, as evidenced by hypertension, with diminished placental perfusion. A number of other reports of increased perinatal morbidity in cocaine users have appeared. Types of morbidity include intrauterine growth retardation, preterm labor and delivery, premature rupture of membranes, meconium passage, and spontaneous abortion. Cerebral infarcts occurring in utero have been reported in offspring of cocaine-using mothers.

**TABLE 8-2.** Reported Effects of Cocaine on the Fetus and Pregnancy

---

Abruptio placentae
Intrauterine growth retardation
Preterm labor
Premature rupture of membranes
Meconium
Spontaneous abortion
Intrauterine cerebral infarctions
?Urinary tract abnormalities
Neurobehavioral disorders

---

## ADVERSE EFFECTS ON THE NEONATE

A further problem may be "behavioral teratogenesis," a condition in which cocaine-exposed newborns have been described as demonstrating poor organizational responses to their environment. Signs of possible withdrawal have been reported in cocaine-exposed neonates, as have long-lasting abnormalities of the electroencephalogram and abnormal visual-evoked potentials. Cocaine babies have been described as "difficult to comfort," perhaps because they do not respond normally to their environments.

## HEROIN

### PHARMACOLOGY

Heroin (diacetylmorphine) is not used medically in the United States. Its effects are similar to those of morphine, except that it appears to cross the blood-brain barrier more effectively than does morphine. Heroin is hydrolyzed to monoacetylmorphine and morphine and is excreted in the urine. Its effects are similar to those of other opioids, and physical dependence leading to abstinence-related withdrawal symptoms is induced with chronic use.

### FETAL EFFECTS

Heroin crosses the placenta, and addiction is common among fetuses of heroin-addicted mothers. Fetal withdrawal with intrauterine convulsions has been postulated. Heroin-addicted mothers are likely to deliver premature infants of low birth weight, although respiratory distress syndrome may actually occur with less frequency in such children. Teratogenicity has not been conclusively demonstrated. However, "behavioral teratogenicity" is highly likely, with neonates of heroin addicts demonstrating impairment of interactive abilities and motor changes (Table 8-3).

### NEONATAL ABSTINENCE SYNDROME

The most striking finding with perinatal heroin addiction is neonatal withdrawal, or abstinence syndrome. It occurs in infants both of mothers addicted to heroin

**TABLE 8-3.** Reported Effects of Heroin on Pregnancy

Fetal addiction
Intrauterine withdrawal
Neonatal abstinence syndrome
Low birth weight
Behavioral teratogenesis
Sudden infant death syndrome

and of mothers treated with methadone. This syndrome includes tremors, restlessness, hyperreflexia, high-pitched cry, sneezing, sleeplessness, tachypnea, yawning, sweating, fever, and, in severe cases, seizures. The onset of symptoms occurs from birth to as long as 2 weeks of age and may persist for up to 4 to 6 months. Treatment has ranged from supportive measures to the use of medications such as diazepam, barbiturates, and opioids such as paregoric and methadone. There is some evidence that withdrawal is less severe in infants whose mothers' methadone dose was down to 20 mg/day or less prior to delivery.

## TREATMENT IN PREGNANCY

The heroin-addicted mother is usually treated with methadone maintenance. There is no clear-cut advantage to methadone over heroin from the fetal point of view, and, in fact, methadone may be associated with worse withdrawal symptoms. However, heroin is not available for treatment in this country. Thus, the only way an addict can procure heroin is to do so illegally. Street heroin varies in its purity, and its availability depends on the ability of the addict to pay for it. Thus, the heroin addict is subject to periodic withdrawal symptoms that may put the fetus at risk.

## AIDS

The most significant problem facing intravenous drug users and their offspring now is the danger of acquired immunodeficiency syndrome (AIDS). Intravenous drug use accounts for the majority of HIV positivity among women, with some areas reporting a 50% seropositivity rate among IV drug users. Any patient acknowledging a history of IV drug use should be offered HIV testing early enough in gestation to allow an informed decision about whether to continue pregnancy.

## HALLUCINOGENS

Phencyclidine (PCP, or "angel dust") has apparently continued to be used as a hallucinogen to a greater extent than LSD. This drug was originally developed as an anesthetic agent but was not approved for human use because of its severe side effects. Patients recovering from phencyclidine anesthesia often manifested hallucinations, disorientation, agitation, and delirium. It is easy to produce PCP, and the drug is inexpensive on the street, so it has become a popular hallucinogen because of the very side effects that limited its use as an anesthetic agent. Animal studies demonstrated that phencyclidine readily crosses the placenta and appears in murine breast milk in concentrations 10 times those in maternal plasma. The drug has been shown to appear in umbilical cord plasma and amniotic fluid from human pregnancies, and the human placenta has been shown to be an active site for conversion of PCP to its metabolic products in vitro. In one case in which both maternal and umbilical cord levels were measured, the concentration of PCP in the fetus was double that in the mother. Animal studies have demonstrated reduced birth weight and embryotoxicity. Abnormal neonatal behavior in infants chronically exposed in utero to PCP has been described in case reports, but no epidemiologic studies have quantitated the risk. The possibility of structural or behavioral teratogenesis remains unproven.

## TOBACCO

There appears to be little disagreement that maternal smoking is associated with a significant reduction in birth weight of the offspring. There also appears to be an increased likelihood of preterm birth, antepartum hemorrhage, and perinatal mortality of low-birth-weight infants. Maternal smoking has been associated with reduced placental blood flow in humans. Nicotine administered to the mother has been associated with decreased uterine blood flow in the rhesus monkey, but in the human fetus it has been associated with increased umbilical blood flow. Its administration to the pregnant ewe is associated with a rapid fall in fetal $pO_2$ and a decline in the frequency of fetal breathing movements. Both standard cigarette smoke and smoke from nicotine-free cigarettes were associated with a drop in fetal $pO_2$ when inhaled by pregnant rhesus monkeys. This effect has been attributed to carbon monoxide, since carboxyhemoglobin is preferentially trapped on the fetal side of the placenta. The relative hypoxia induced by increased carboxyhemoglobin levels in the fetus could be responsible for a wide variety of adverse effects.

Maternal cigarette smoking has been implicated in the genesis of congenital malformations such as cleft lip and palate, but this association has not been universally present. A recent epidemiologic study suggests that only isolated oral clefts, unassociated with other birth defects, are increased in the offspring of cigarette smokers.

Some have suggested the term *fetal tobacco syndrome* to describe infants meeting the following four conditions:

1. A mother who smoked five or more cigarettes a day throughout the pregnancy.
2. No evidence of hypertension during the pregnancy.
3. Symmetrical growth retardation at term.
4. No other obvious cause of growth retardation.

Clearly, intervention is necessary to help women stop smoking. Encouraging developments have included a randomized intervention study, in which pregnant smoking women treated with a cessation program demonstrated a significant increase in birth weight and length of their offspring when compared to untreated smoking controls. It is clear that the major responsibility rests with caregivers for pregnant women. We must find out if our patients are smoking, educate them about the risks, and refer them to smoking cessation programs in our communities.

## CAFFEINE

Caffeine, a dioxypurine, is 1,3,7-trimethylxanthine. It is chemically related to the xanthines theophylline and theobromine. The xanthines exert most of their systemic effects by increasing intracellular cyclic AMP, altering ionized calcium levels, and potentiating the action of catecholamines. These systemic effects include central nervous system excitation, smooth muscle relaxation, increased heart rate, and increased cardiac output. There is also an increase in gastric acid secretion and diuresis. Caffeine is contained in coffee and tea (100 to 150 mg per average cup, but with wide variations), nondietetic cola drinks (35 to 55 mg per 12-oz serving), and cocoa (200 mg theobromine per average cup). Pregnant women near term have been shown to eliminate caffeine considerably more slowly than nonpregnant controls. Caffeine is fat soluble and has been demonstrated to cross the placenta in sheep and humans.

The administration of caffeine to pregnant sheep has been shown to result in a mild fall in uterine blood flow, but to have no effect on oxygenation or acid-base status. In human pregnancies near term, the maternal ingestion of two cups of coffee was associated with a small but significant fall in intervillous blood flow. A report of three pregnancies in which high maternal caffeine intake was associated with ectrodactyly in the offspring created a great deal of interest in the possibility; each mother was estimated to have consumed between 1100 and 1777 mg of caffeine on an average day during her pregnancy. However, at least three large epidemiologic studies in humans have failed to detect any increase in congenital anomalies related to caffeine intake among pregnant women.

In summary, there is no convincing evidence supporting a teratogenic or other adverse role on pregnancy for caffeine when taken in amounts equivalent to less than 10 cups of coffee per day. Pregnant women should be advised to use moderation in their caffeine intake, but it need not be avoided altogether.

---

# 9. RISK ASSESSMENT FOR DEVELOPMENTAL TOXICITY: EFFECTS OF DRUGS AND CHEMICALS ON THE FETUS

---

Structural or functional developmental defects complicate a significant number of pregnancies. Between 3% and 5% of all infants are born with a congenital malformation, and 1% to 2% have a severe malformation. There are three general causes:

1. The action of a mutated gene or chromosome anomaly (e.g., achondroplasia or maternal phenylketonuria).
2. The action of an environmental agent (e.g., congenital rubella, ionizing radiation, or aminopterin).
3. A combination of genetic and environmental factors (e.g., fetal phenytoin syndrome).

Among all congenital defects, 20% to 25% are associated with a chromosomal or genetic (spontaneous or Mendelian inheritance) anomaly, 7% to 10% are due to infection or maternal disease, and drugs and environmental chemicals account for approximately 2%. Approximately two-thirds of all developmental defects have no identifiable cause. It has been estimated that 7% to 10% of developmental defects are potentially preventable.

## PROBLEMS FACING OBSTETRICIANS

In defining the magnitude of the problems faced by obstetricians who want to provide accurate advice to patients concerning developmental toxicity, one should explore several issues: existing data on the developmental toxicity of drugs and chemicals in animals and humans, potential for occupational and environmental exposure, and potential for drug exposure.

## AVAILABLE DATA ON THE DEVELOPMENTAL TOXICITY OF CHEMICALS

It is estimated that there are approximately 90,000 chemicals in commerce in the United States. About 3000 of those chemicals have been tested for developmental toxicity in experimental animals and reported in the scientific literature. This means that many compounds of interest to the patient and her physician may have no published data from which any advice about the potential for developmental toxicity can be derived.

Of the approximately 3000 chemicals for which published data are available on developmental toxicity, between 500 and 1000 are teratogenic in animals. Of interest with respect to prediction of human risk for developmental toxicity, approximately 30 chemicals are thought to be developmental toxicants in humans.

## WOMEN IN THE WORK FORCE

It is estimated that approximately 44% of the work force (more than 45 million) are women. Of these, about 75% are between 16 and 44 years old and considered to be of reproductive age.

## DRUG USE DURING PREGNANCY

The common significant finding of these studies is that a large number of drugs are ingested during pregnancy. On average, 60% to 75% of pregnant women use from 3 to 10 medications during pregnancy. Excluded from these reviews were illicit and recreational drugs. Recent surveys have suggested that between 20% and 30% of pregnant women abuse some chemical substance during pregnancy.

Given the large number of women in the work force, the concern about environmental exposures in the home and neighboring environment, and the number of women who consume licit and illicit drugs during pregnancy, it would be an unusual obstetrical practice that did not generate one or two questions about the effect of these exposures on pregnancy each week.

## DEVELOPMENTAL TOXICANTS

A developmental toxicant is a drug, chemical, virus, bacteria, physical agent, or deficiency state that if present before conception, during the embryonic or fetal period, or during neonatal development alters the morphology or subsequent development or function of the newly formed individual. Developmental toxicology is the science that deals with the causes, mechanisms, manifestation, and prevention of developmental deviations of a structural or functional nature produced by developmental toxicants.

## PATTERNS OF DEVELOPMENTAL ABNORMALITY

When obstetricians are asked for advice on the relationship between environmental exposure and adverse developmental outcome, the questions typically represent one of two different concerns: "What is the effect of this exposure on my fetus?" or "My baby has a malformation. Was it caused by any exposures during my pregnancy?" To help understand approaches to both questions it is important to understand the types of malformations observed and the proposed etiologies of those malformations.

## MALFORMATION

"A malformation is a defect that results from an intrinsically abnormal developmental process." This implies that the developmental potential of the structure was abnormal from the beginning, at conception or very early in embryogenesis.

## DISRUPTION

"A disruption is a developmental defect that results from an extrinsic or intrinsic factor producing the breakdown of, or interference with, an originally normal developmental process." In the absence of the extrinsic or intrinsic factor (a deficiency state or chemical, biological, or physical exposure), development would have been normal.

## DEFORMATION

"A deformation is an abnormal form, shape, or position of a part of the body that is caused by mechanical forces acting on that part of the body during development."

## RISK ASSESSMENT FOR DEVELOPMENTAL TOXICITY

The process of risk assessment for human developmental toxicity encompasses four interrelated activities. The first is hazard identification: Can this agent produce adverse developmental effects in humans or experimental animals at any exposure short of a maternally toxic or lethal dose? If so, what type of effect is produced and what is the developmental window of susceptibility for the effect(s)? The second step is hazard characterization, which, at a minimum, requires dose-response data. Note that dose-response relationships in developmental toxicity can be complicated by multiple competing end points, such as reduced fetal weight, disruption of fetal development, and fetal death. Because of this, dose-response relationships may not have the familiar sigmoidal shape. In addition, because the use of the toxicity data in risk assessment implies extrapolation of animal data to humans, it is important to get as much information as possible on the site of toxicity and mechanism of action of the toxicant. The third step is exposure assessment: What is the likely amount of agent that the person was actually exposed to, and how much of the agent was absorbed and distributed to the fetus or placenta? The final step is risk characterization: How likely is the given exposure to result in an adverse developmental outcome, and what degree of uncertainty is inherent in that estimation?

## HAZARD IDENTIFICATION

### Timing of Exposure

One definition of developmental toxicity used by some regulatory agencies is "adverse effects on the developing organism that may result from exposure prior to conception to either parent, during prenatal development or if a result of prenatal exposure, postnatal to the time of sexual maturity." Most developmental toxicants, however, produce their effects during specific critical developmental periods, which vary across both compounds and species. A fundamental concept of developmental toxicology is that some stages of embryonic development are more vulnerable than others. The time of exposure to a developmental toxicant determines not only the severity of damage, but also the type of defect (Table 9-1).

## IMPACT OF DRUGS AND CHEMICALS ON THE FETUS

Using the approach outlined earlier, we have formulated a listing of drugs (Table 9-2) and chemicals (Table 9-3) and attempted to characterize their risk to the fetus,

*Text continues on page 75.*

**TABLE 9-1.** Critical Periods for Developmental Toxicity in the Human

| Days from LMP | Days from conception* | Biological Event |
|---|---|---|
| 14 | 0 | Ovulation |
| 15–16 | 1 | Conception |
| 19–21 | 5–7 | Implantation/Blastula |
| 38–39 | 24–25 | Anterior neuropore closes |
| 40–41 | 26–27 | Posterior neuropore closes |
| 41–42 | 27–28 | Upper limb bud develops |
| 43–44 | 29–30 | Lower limb bud develops |
| 51 | 37 | Crown-rump 10 mm |
| 60–61 | 46–47 | Heart septation |
| 70–72 | 56–58 | Palate closed |
| 98 | 84 | Second trimester begins |

*Based on 28-day menstrual cycle.

**TABLE 9-2.** Impact of Drugs on the Fetus

| Class and Compound | Risk | Comment |
|---|---|---|
| **Analgesics and Antipyretic** | | |
| Aspirin | S | Large doses may be toxic to mother and fetus |
| Acetaminophen | S | Fetal renal and maternal and fetal hepatic toxicity in large doses |
| **Narcotic Analgesics** | | |
| Codeine | C | Respiratory malformations, withdrawal |
| Pentazocine | S | Withdrawal with chronic use |
| Meperidine | S | Withdrawal with chronic use |
| **Antibiotics** | | |
| Penicillins | S | Routine use for infections during pregnancy |
| Cephalosporins | C | Probably safe, few epidemiologic studies |
| Tetracyclines | N | Incorporation in teeth and bones, maternal hepatic toxicity and acute fatty metamorphosis |
| Streptomycin | C | Ototoxicity at high doses, interaction with $MgSO_4$ |
| Gentamicin | C | Ototoxicity not reported, interaction with $MgSO_4$ |
| Tobramycin | C | Ototoxicity not reported, interaction with $MgSO_4$ |
| Amikacin | C | Ototoxicity not reported |
| Chloramphenicol | C | Cardiovascular collapse (gray syndrome) |
| Sulfonamides | S | Displace bilirubin from albumin hemolysis, anemia and hyperbilirubinemia in G6PD deficiency |
| Nitrofurantoin | S | |
| Metronidazole | C | Avoid during first trimester |
| Trimethoprim-Sulfamethoxazole | C | Folic acid antagonist |
| **Antituberculosis** | | |
| Isoniazid | S | Drug of choice for tuberculosis treatment during pregnancy |
| Rifampin | S | Drug of choice for tuberculosis treatment during pregnancy |
| Ethambutol | C | |
| para-Aminosalicylic acid | C | |
| **Immunizing Agents** | | |
| Live-virus vaccines | N | |
| Attenuated vaccines | N | |
| Killed-virus vaccines | S | |
| Tetanus toxoid | C | |
| Diphtheria toxoid | C | |
| **Antinauseant** | | |
| Cyclizine | S | |
| Buclizine | S | |
| Meclizine | S | |
| Prochlorperazine | S | |
| Trimethobenzamide | S | |

(continued)

**TABLE 9-2.** (continued)

| Class and Compound | Risk | Comment |
|---|---|---|
| **Antihistamines** | | |
| Diphenhydramine | C | Gentiourinary malformations |
| Chlorpheniramine | S | |
| Brompheniramine | S | |
| **Sedatives** | | |
| Barbiturates | C | Conflicting data on malformations, dependence with prolonged use |
| Ethanol | N | Fetal alcohol syndrome, craniofacial, and limb abnormalities, microcephaly |
| **Tranquilizers** | | |
| Chlordiazepoxide | C | Conflicting data on malformations, dependence with prolonged use |
| Meprobamate | C | Conflicting data on malformations, dependence with prolonged use |
| Diazepam | C | Oral clefts |
| **Antidepressants** | | |
| Lithium carbonate | N | Cardiovascular anomaly |
| Imipramine | C | Neonatal withdrawal |
| Amitriptyline | C | Neonatal withdrawal |
| Doxepin | C | |
| **Anesthetics** | | |
| Inhalational | C | Spontaneous abortion |
| **Anticonvulsants** | | |
| Phenytoin | C | Fetal hydantoin syndrome, define benefit : risk ratio |
| Carbamazepine | C | Conflicting data on malformations |
| Ethosuximide | C | Conflicting data on malformations, drug of choice for petit mal in pregnancy |
| Primidone | C | Conflicting data on malformations |
| Valproic acid | N | CNS, neural tube defects |
| Trimethadione | N | Congenital malformations, abortion |
| Paramethadione | N | Congenital malformations, abortion |
| **Aminophyllines** | | |
| Theophylline | S | Bronchodilator of choice in pregnancy |
| Diuretics | C | Initiation of use during pregnancy discouraged |
| **Reserpine and Rauwolfia Alkaloids** | | |
| Reserpine | C | |
| Methyldopa | C | |
| **Vasodilators** | | |
| Hydralizine | C | Drug of choice in preeclampsia, eclampsia |
| Sodium nitroprusside | C | Produces increased cyanide levels in fetus |
| Digitalis | S | |

(continued)

**TABLE 9-2.** (continued)

| Class and Compound | Risk | Comment |
|---|---|---|
| **Hypoglycemic** | | |
| Tolbutamide | N | Not indicated during pregnancy |
| **Antithyroid and Iodine** | | |
| Propylthiouracil | N | Mild fetal hypothyroidism and goiter, drug of choice for hyperthyroidism in pregnancy |
| Potassium iodide | N | Fetal hypothyroidism and goiter |
| Povidone-iodide | N | Fetal hypothyroidism and goiter |
| **Steroids** | | |
| Cortisone | C | |
| Betamethasone | C | Prevention of respiration distress |
| Diethylstilbestrol | N | Uterine and vaginal malformations (adenosis), epididymal cysts, hypotrophic testes, infertility |
| Estradiol | N | Congenital defects |
| Medroxyprogesterone | C | Possible congenital defects |
| Methyltestosterone | N | Masculinization |
| **Anticoagulants** | | |
| Heparin | S | Anticoagulant of choice, prolonged use associated with maternal osteopenia |
| Coumarins | N | Nasal hypoplasia, shortened extremities, abortion |
| **Antimalarials** | | |
| Chloroquine | C | Drug of choice for malaria, small increased risk for malformations |
| Quinine | C | Abortion, conflicting data on malformations |
| Pyrimethamine | C | Folic acid antagonist |
| **Cancer Chemotherapeutic** | | |
| Aminopterin | N/ | Malformations, spontaneous abortions |
| Busulfan | N | Multiple visceral malformations, abortion |
| Chlorambucil | N | Renal agenesis |
| Cyclophosphamide | N | Conflicting data on malformations, ovarian and testicular toxicity |
| Cytarabine | N | Malformations and chromosome abnormalities |
| 5-Fluorouracil | N | Multiple anomalies |
| Mechlorethamine | N | |
| Methotrexate | N | Malformations similar to aminopterin, folic acid antagonist |
| Procarbazine | N | Malformations, decreased spermatogenesis |
| **Antiacne** | | |
| Retinoids | N | Spontaneous abortion, hydrocephalus, microcephalus, ear and eye abnormalities, cardiovascular malformations |
| **Miscellaneous** | | |
| Penicillamine | N | Skin lesions (cutis laxa) |
| Disulfiram | N | Multiple anomalies |

S, Safe in normal exposure doses.
C, Caution, therapeutic indication should outweigh possible small risk.
N, Human developmental toxicant; use during pregnancy requires careful risk benefit analysis.

**TABLE 9-3.** Impact of Chemicals in Industry and the Environment on the Fetus

| Class and Compound | Risk | Comment |
|---|---|---|
| Methyl mercury | N | Microcephaly, mental retardation, cerebral palsy |
| Acetone | C | Sacral abnormalities, camptomelic syndrome |
| Benzene | C | Spontaneous abortions, premature births |
| Boric acid | C | Conflicting data on malformation rate |
| Carbon disulfide | C | Spontaneous abortions, sperm abnormalities, abnormal menses |
| Carbon monoxide | C | Stillbirth with maternal toxicity |
| Chloroprene | C | Possible mental defects, chromosomal abnormalities |
| 1,2-dibromo-3-chloropropane | C | Testicular toxicity, spontaneous abortion |
| Dichloromethane | C | Spontaneous abortion |
| Dinitrodipropylsulfanilamide | C | Miscarriage, heart defects |
| Ethylene dibromide | C | Decreased fertility |
| Formaldehyde | C | Spontaneous abortion |
| Hexachlorobenzene | C | Stillbirth |
| Lead | N | Increased abortion rate, stillbirth, central nervous system toxicity |
| Mercuric chloride | C | Spontaneous abortion |
| Methylethyl ketone | C | Spontaneous abortion |
| Methylparathion | C | Malformations |
| Polychlorinated biphenyls | N | Brown skin in newborns, growth retardation, exophthalmos |
| Sodium selenite | C | Spontaneous abortions, limb defects |
| Styrene | C | Spontaneous abortion |
| Toluene | C | Growth retardation, malformations |
| Trichloroethylene | C | Malformations, sacral agenesis |
| Vinyl chloride | C | Spontaneous abortions |
| Xylene | C | Sacral agenesis |

C = Caution; may pose risk of developmental toxicity during pregnancy.
N = Known human developmental toxicant.

if any. The data in these two tables reflect a qualitative attempt at hazard identification. It is important to reemphasize that existing data suggest that many more chemicals are developmental toxicants in experimental animals than have been identified as developmental toxicants in humans. This may reflect several factors, including differences in species sensitivity, level of exposure, or epidemiologic insensitivity.

# 10. VIRAL-INDUCED TERATOGENESIS

This chapter reviews five viruses known to be teratogenic to humans: cytomegalovirus, rubella, herpes simplex, Venezuelan equine encephalitis, and varicella viruses. Other viruses that can infect and produce disease or death of the fetus are influenza, rubeola, Western equine encephalitis, variola, vaccinia, hepatitis B, echoviruses, poliovirus, parvovirus B-19, and human immunodeficiency virus (HIV).

## CYTOMEGALOVIRUS

Maternal infections with cytomegalovirus are frequent. In most studies, 3% to 5% of women shed this virus at term. Severe damage due to congenital cytomegalovirus infection occurs at a rate of about 1 in 5000 to 1 in 20,000 births. Studies of asymptomatic infected newborns, however, suggest that as many as 10% to 15% of these children have some damage caused by this infection. The most frequent problems are low intelligence and some degree of deafness.

The most common cause of congenital infection is cytomegalovirus (CMV) (Table 10-1). Several serologic surveys in the United States have shown that approximately one-half of adult women have antibody to this virus. In addition, CMV can be isolated from the cervix or urine of 3% to 5% of pregnant women. The great majority of infected women are asymptomatic. Occasionally, cervicitis and illness resembling infectious mononucleosis are caused by infection with these viruses. Infection can be documented by isolation of the virus from the urine or cervical area, or by the production of antibody. The fluorescent and ELISA tests appear to be the most practical and reliable methods for detecting antibody and seroconversions. Congenital infection with CMV occurs in 0.5% to 1.5% of births. Present information indicates that as many as 10% to 15% of these children exhibit permanent damage in the form of mental or motor retardation or deafness. The severe form of cytomegalic inclusion disease occurs in 1 in 5000 to 1 in 20,000 live births. Congenital infection can be documented by isolation of the virus from the nasopharynx or urine. Specific IgM cytomegalovirus antibody is also present in many of the infected newborns.

A number of studies have shown that about 1% to 4% of pregnant women have a primary infection (seroconversion) with CMV. The reported annual rates are higher for low-income women (6.8%) and day care workers with young children in their care (11%).

## RUBELLA VIRUS

Rubella has almost disappeared in the United States, and no major epidemics have occurred since 1964. The great majority of children are immunized. At present, however, approximately 10% of women of childbearing age in the United States are at risk for this infection.

E. Albert Reece, John C. Hobbins, Maurice, J. Mahoney and Roy H. Petrie (Eds).
*Handbook of Medicine of the Fetus & Mother.* Copyright © 1995 by J.B. Lippincott Company

**TABLE 10-1.** Congenital Cytomegalovirus Infection

| | |
|---|---|
| Birth defects | Microcephaly, chorioretinitis, deafness, mental retardation, hepato-splenomegaly, epilepsy, hydrocephalus, cerebral palsy, death |
| Detection | |
| Mother | No clinical symptoms (rarely, infectious mononucleosis-like symptoms), virus isolation from urine and cervix, seroconversion (fluorescence, ELISA) |
| Child | Wide spectrum of clinical findings (listed above), only severely affected are usually recognized; lab tests—CMV-specific IgM, virus isolation from nasopharynx and urine |
| Prevention | Avoid contact, chemotherapy (?), vaccines (?) |

The defects due to congenital rubella are associated primarily with infection during the first 5 months of pregnancy (Table 10-2). The frequency of abnormal children following maternal infection is highest with rubella in the first month of gestation (50%), decreasing to 22% in the second month, 10% in the third month, and 6% in the fourth and fifth months. In the United States, approximately 10% of the women of childbearing age are at risk for rubella infection. With infections, clinical manifestations occur in approximately two-thirds of women of this age group. The most useful laboratory test is the ELISA method for antibody determination. With this method, susceptible individuals can be identified on the basis of absence of antibody, and seroconversions can be documented. IgM rubella-specific antibody is also detectable for a number of weeks following infection, so this determination can be used to document recent infection.

The usual manifestations of congenital rubella include malformations of the heart and great vessels, deafness, cataracts, microcephaly, and mental retardation. The newborns may also exhibit hepatosplenomegaly, hepatitis, pneumonitis, and encephalitis. Most infected newborns have rubella-specific IgM antibody, which persists for a number of months. Rubella vaccines are now used routinely in the United States. These vaccines produce a low incidence of side reactions, primarily arthritis and arthralgia, most marked in women of childbearing age. Immunity produced by the vaccines appears to be permanent.

## HERPES SIMPLEX VIRUS

In addition to the pain and discomfort associated with the infection, virus present in the vagina at term can be transmitted to the child during the birth process. In

**TABLE 10-2.** Congenital Rubella

| | |
|---|---|
| Defects | Malformations of heart and great vessels, microcephaly, deafness, cataracts, mental retardation, newborn bleeding, hepatosplenomegaly, pneumonitis, hepatitis, encephalitis, death |
| Detection | |
| Mother | Exposure, rash, nodes; lab tests—antibody response ELISA IgM specific antibody, virus isolation from nasopharynx |
| Child | Congenital rubella syndrome; lab tests—rubella-specific IgM, persisting rubella IgG antibody after 6 months of age, virus isolation from nasopharynx or cerebrospinal fluid |
| Prevention | Rubella vaccine, abortion |

over 50% of cases, this leads to severe, often fatal, disease in the newborn. The use of cesarean section for delivery significantly reduces the frequency of infections in the newborn.

Congenital herpes simplex virus (HSV) infections usually are acquired at birth (Table 10-3). Maternal infection is transmitted as a venereal disease, and 90% of such infections are due to HSV-2. HSV-1, conversely, usually affects the mouth, face, or upper part of the trunk. The congenital infections studied in detail in the Collaborative Perinatal Project Study were all related to primary HSV-2 infection occurring late in gestation. Other studies, however, have shown that HSV-1 can also result in severe fetal damage. Prior maternal infection with either strain does not completely protect the child; however, the severity of lesions is often reduced. Most women with vaginal HSV infection do not exhibit lesions; thus, infection is underreported. The diagnosis can be made by recognition of the typical inclusions in the cells of Papanicolaou smear, fluorescent staining, or by direct virus isolation.

The child with congenital infection usually appears normal at birth, but signs and symptoms of the disease develop during the first 1 to 3 weeks of life. The disease is manifested in three general forms:

1. Vesicular lesions of the skin or throat with or without conjunctivitis (15% of cases).
2. Central nervous system involvement, characterized by spinal fluid pleocytosis, elevated pressure, increased protein content, and convulsions (15% of cases).
3. Systemic disease, manifested by hepatitis, jaundice, pulmonary disease, hemolytic anemia, petechiae, hepatomegaly, and thrombocytopenia (70% of cases).

The prognosis in children with localized vesicular lesions (and conjunctivitis) is good, although about 50% of them progress to more extensive disseminated infection. Systemic infection is fatal in over 90% of cases. Laboratory tests useful in the diagnosis of HSV infection are the isolation of the virus from lesions, the pharynx, or the conjunctiva, or the presence of specific HSV IgM antibody.

**TABLE 10-3.** Perinatal Herpes Simplex Infection

| | |
|---|---|
| Defects | Three groups, <br> Limited—vesicular lesions on skin, throat, and sometimes conjunctivitis <br> Central nervous system—convulsions <br> Systematic—hepatitis, jaundice, hepatomegaly, thrombocytopenia, petechiae, hemolytic anemia, pulmonary disease |
| Detection | |
| Mother | Many asymptomatic and no herpetic lesions, virus isolation most sensitive, vaginal-cervical infection, some ulcerative lesions, husband may also have infection; lab tests—Papanicolaou smear often shows cells with inclusions, fluorescent tests often positive, antigen ELISA, virus isolation from cervix |
| Child | Often difficult to recognize initially, skin lesions present in about 50% of cases, most later develop severe brain or systemic disease (listed above); lab tests—isolation of virus from skin lesions, throat, eyes, or tissues; specific herpes IgM antibody |
| Prevention | Delivery by cesarean section, chemotherapy, particularly for limited infections; vaccines (?) |

Chemotherapy for congenital infection using acyclovir has been helpful. This drug reduces the frequency of morbidity and mortality. If there is only limited infection, the drug is particularly effective in reducing the number of permanent neurologic sequelae. Vaccines are not presently available, but are being investigated. Delivery by cesarean section is recommended in order to avoid contact between the child and the infected vaginal lesions, if these are found to be present near term.

## VENEZUELAN EQUINE ENCEPHALITIS VIRUS

Venezuelan equine encephalitis can be transmitted to humans during epidemics. This in turn can result in the spread of the virus to the baby, where severe infection of the brain and eyes can occur. Affected children may have hydrocephaly, porencephalic cysts, and cataracts. Most of the epidemics occur in the Caribbean or Central and South America.

The incubation period is approximately 2 to 5 days. The primary symptoms are headache, fever, malaise, and myalgia. Occasionally patients have seizures, mental confusion, coma, tremors, and encephalitis (Table 10-4).

Venezuelan equine encephalitis can be controlled by immunization of animals and quarantine. Vaccines for this virus have also been used in human beings. When administered directly to the rhesus fetuses, however, the vaccines produced severe damage to the brain and eyes. This should be considered, because the vaccine virus is being advocated for administration to women of childbearing age.

## VARICELLA VIRUS

Varicella (chickenpox) is recognized as a teratogen. Infection of the mother in the first half of pregnancy can lead to severe skeletal and brain damage of the child in

**TABLE 10-4.** Congenital Venezuelan Equine Encephalitis Infection

| | |
|---|---|
| Defects | Abortion, microphthalmia, absent cerebrum, massive CNS necrosis, hydrocephalus |
| Detection | |
| Mother | Exposure (epidemic in area), febrile illness, myalgia, encephalitis, specific antibody |
| Child | Microphthalmia, hydrocephalus, severe brain damage, specific antibody |
| Prevention | Vaccines to animals, possible danger of vaccines in pregnant women |

**TABLE 10-5.** Congenital Varicella

| | |
|---|---|
| Defects | Cataracts, microphthalmus, Horner's syndrome, anisocoria, optic atrophy, nystagmus, chorioretinitis, mental retardation, skin scarring, hypoplasia of limbs |
| Detection | |
| Mother | Rash, antibody response (fluorescence, ELISA) |
| Child | Defects (listed above); specific IgM antibody to varicella (some positive) |
| Prevention | Avoid exposure, vaccines (?), abortion (?) |

approximately 1% to 5% of cases. In addition, varicella at term can be transmitted intravenously to the child. This direct infection in the last few days of gestation may result in generalized varicella, which is fatal for approximately one-third of the infected children.

Varicella (chickenpox) and herpes zoster (shingles) are caused by the same virus. In the United States, approximately 15% of women of childbearing age are susceptible to varicella infection, and some of those infected during pregnancy have produced children with congenital defects (Table 10-5).

Varicella very late in pregnancy is often manifested at birth or in the newborn by the presence of the characteristic chickenpox skin lesion or severe pneumonia with other complications. Maternal infection 5 to 10 days before delivery may produce disease in the infant, and symptoms usually develop within 4 days of delivery. These infants usually escape severe effects of infection, presumably because maternal antibody confers some protection. However, maternal infection 0 to 5 days before delivery or 0 to 2 days after delivery may result in infection of the infant, and approximately 30% of infected children die of disseminated disease. The use of high-titered varicella zoster immune globulin (VZIG) shortly after birth prevents the disseminated disease.

# PART V. FETAL INFECTIONS OF MATERNAL ORIGIN AND TREATMENT

# 11.  TORCH VIRUS–INDUCED FETAL DISEASE

The acronym TORCH was coined to describe a group of perinatal infections with similar clinical features (Table 11-1). This group initially included *Toxoplasma gondii*, rubella virus, cytomegalovirus, and herpes simplex virus.

## TOXOPLASMOSIS

### EPIDEMIOLOGY

The incidence of toxoplasmosis varies throughout the world. Acute infection during pregnancy occurs in 10 in 1000 in France but in only 1.1 in 1000 in the United States.

**TABLE 11-1.** Torch-Virus Infections

|  | Toxoplasmosis | Rubella |
|---|---|---|
| **Laboratory Diagnosis** | | |
| Maternal | IgG seroconversion, T-IgM | IgG seroconversion, R-IgM virus isolation (throat) |
| Fetal/Neonatal | Cord IgM, placental histology, abnormal CSF | Cord IgM, IgG + >6 months |
| Fetal Signs | IUGR, NIH, microcephaly, anencephaly, hydranencephaly, cerebral calcifications | Microcephaly, IUGR, VSD |
| Neonatal Signs | Chorioretinitis, fever, hydrocephaly, hepatosplenomegaly, thrombocytopenia, seizures | Deafness, cataracts, mental retardation, hepatosplenomegaly, rash, thrombocytopenia |
| Treatment | Pyrimethamine 25 mg/d, sulfadiazine 1 g qid, spiramycin 3 g/d | No antiviral therapy |
| Prevention | Avoid raw meat, cat feces | Preconception testing and vaccine for susceptibles |

|  | Cytomegalovirus | Herpes |
|---|---|---|
| **Laboratory Diagnosis** | | |
| Maternal | Virus isolation, IgG seroconversion, C-IgM | Virus isolation (lesion, cervix) Tzanck smear, Pap smear |
| Fetal/Neonatal serology | Serology, virus Isolation (urine, possibly fetal blood) | Virus isolation (lesion, eye, CSF) Tzanck smear, H-IgM at <6 months |
| Fetal Signs | IUGR, NIH, microcephaly, hydrocephaly, cerebral calcifications, hepatosplenomegaly, SVT, heart block | Microcephaly, SAb, IUGR, cerebral calcifications |
| Neonatal signs | Hepatosplenomegaly, chorioretinitis, jaundice, purpura | Chorioretinitis, vesicles, jaundice, bleeding, CNS abnormalities |
| Treatment | Symptomatic for mother, no antiviral therapy | Acyclovir, vidarabine |
| Prevention | Hygienic measures vaccines being studied | Cesarean section if virus present at parturition |

C-IgM, CMV-specific IgM; CNS, central nervous system; CSF, cerebrospinal fluid; H-IgM, HSV IgM; IUGR, intrauterine growth retardation; NIH, nonimmune hydrops; R-IgM, rubella-specific IgM; SAb, spontaneous abortion; SVT, supraventricular tachycardia; T-IgM, toxoplasmosis-specific IgM; VSD, ventricular septal defect.

## TRANSMISSION

Fetal infection only occurs with acute maternal toxoplasmosis. Congenital toxoplasmosis is more frequent but usually less apparent when maternal infection occurs in later gestations. More than 90% of the infections acquired in the third trimester are asymptomatic.

## MICROBIOLOGY/IMMUNOLOGY

*Toxoplasma gondii* is a protozoan parasite with a complex life cycle: trophozoite (or tachyzoite), cyst, and oocyst. Trophozoites are the proliferative and invasive forms, whereas cysts are the latent forms, persisting in tissue for the lifetime of the host. Oocysts are found in cats that have ingested rodents infected with cysts. Humans become infected if they eat uncooked, or undercooked, fresh (never frozen) meat from infected animals. Human infection may also occur with hand-to-mouth contact with oocysts excreted in cat feces. Inhalation of aerosolized oocysts is another possible mechanism for infection. Parasitemia in a pregnant woman with acute toxoplasmosis may result in transplacental migration of the parasites, with subsequent fetal infection. An infected fetus can produce IgM antibodies to *Toxoplasma*, but this response may be suppressed by maternal IgG antibodies acquired transplacentally.

## CLINICAL MANIFESTATIONS: MATERNAL

An immunocompetent adult with acute toxoplasmosis is often only minimally symptomatic. When the disease is clinically apparent symptoms similar to infectious mononucleosis, including malaise, myalgias, sore throat, fever, and posterior cervical lymph node enlargement, may be present. Other findings include maculopapular rash, hepatosplenomegaly, and lymphocytosis. Ocular symptoms such as blurred vision, photophobia, and eye pain may be present with chronic disease. In the immunocompromised patient, severe disease with pulmonary and central nervous system involvement can be seen.

## CLINICAL MANIFESTATIONS: FETAL

Clinical manifestations that may prompt suspicion of infection include intrauterine growth retardation, nonimmune hydrops, hydrocephaly, microcephaly, anencephaly, and hydranencephaly.

## CLINICAL MANIFESTATIONS: NEONATAL

Most infants with congenital toxoplasmosis are asymptomatic in the newborn period. In a symptomatic infant, chorioretinitis is the most common finding. There are no pathognomonic findings; the classic triad of periventricular calcifications, chorioretinitis, and hydrocephaly is actually uncommon. Severe congenital toxoplasmosis, which complicates 1 in 4000 to 8000 pregnancies, may also be associated with fever, microcephaly, abnormal cerebrospinal fluid, jaundice, anemia, hepatosplenomegaly, thrombocytopenia, convulsions, lymphadenopathy, cataracts, microphthalmia, maculopapular rash, pneumonia, and diarrhea. Long-term complications include mental retardation, visual deficits, and seizures.

## DIAGNOSIS

Serologic techniques are the usual methods for diagnosis, but are some of the most error-prone assays. Traditionally, Sabin-Feldman dye test, indirect fluorescent assays (IFA), indirect hemagglutination assays (IHA), complement fixation (CF), and enzyme-linked immunosorbent assay (ELISA) tests have been used. Most labs no longer perform the Sabin-Feldman dye test. The assays that are used most commonly measure IgG, IgM, or both. IgM can appear as early as 1 week after an acute infection and can persist for several weeks or months. IgG usually does not appear until several weeks after the IgM rise, but low titers usually persist for years.

Optimally, IgG antibody to toxoplasmosis should be measured before conception; the presence of *Toxoplasma*-specific IgG would indicate protection from further infection. In pregnant women of unknown serologic status, the presence of a high *Toxoplasma* IgG titer should prompt testing for *Toxoplasma*-specific IgM. The presence of IgM is suggestive of a recent infection, especially if the titer is high, but it must be remembered that IgM may be present for up to 4 months when a fluorescent antibody test is used and for up to 8 months with an ELISA test. Prenatal diagnosis of congenital toxoplasmosis is possible using cordocentesis and amniocentesis with serologic tests for IgM and IgG on fetal blood and with isolation of the organism by inoculation into mice. However, IgM-specific antibodies may not be detected even in culture-proven cases because antibody synthesis may be delayed in the fetus and neonate.

## TREATMENT/PREVENTION

Usually, therapy is not necessary for toxoplasmosis in the mother and isolation is not required. Several medications are used to diminish the consequences of fetal infection, but the estimated efficacy of these is only approximately 50%. If acute toxoplasmosis is diagnosed early in pregnancy, the option of termination should be discussed. The combination of pyrimethamine (a folic acid antagonist) and sulfa drugs (sulfadiazine or triple sulfonamides) is the only effective medication generally available in the United States. Folic acid should be used with pyrimethamine to minimize its potential side effects of bone marrow depression and pancytopenia. Spiramycin, a macrolide antibiotic, used extensively in Europe but not approved for use in the United States, has been used frequently in the first trimester without adverse effects. Spiramycin crosses the placental barrier minimally; therefore, its effectiveness in the treatment of intrauterine infection is unclear.

The primary method of prevention of congenital toxoplasmosis is good hygiene. The pregnant woman should wash her hands thoroughly after contact with raw meat, cats, and materials potentially contaminated by cat feces. She should eat meat that has been cooked to ≥66†C, which is the temperature at which the cysts are rendered noninfectious.

## RUBELLA

### EPIDEMIOLOGY

Before the introduction of rubella vaccine in 1969, immunity to rubella through primary infection was acquired by 85% of the population by adolescence. Now 32% of all cases occur in the 15 to 29-year age group. The incidence of congenital rubella syndrome (CRS) has plateaued at approximately 0.05 per 100,000 live births. Despite immunization, 10% to 20% of the U.S. population is susceptible to rubella.

## TRANSMISSION

Rubella virus is spread by respiratory droplets in prolonged, close exposure. The virus is less communicable than varicella, with an 80% attack rate. Fetal infection requires maternal viremia and placental transmission. Serologic evidence of fetal exposure to rubella has been documented after inadvertent vaccination in pregnancy. To date, no cases of congenital defects of CRS have been reported due to vaccine. Nevertheless, vaccine administration is contraindicated in pregnancy because the theoretical risk of CRS following vaccination, although low, may not be zero. Virus is shed in breast milk as well; however, neonatal exposure to rubella during breast feeding has not been associated with morbidity.

The variable risk of CRS at different gestational ages has long been recognized. Rubella infection before implantation has been implicated in spontaneous abortion, stillbirth, neonatal death, and CRS. Rubella occurring from 12 days to 12 weeks after the last menstrual period (LMP) results in an 81% to 90% fetal infection rate. Gestational-age-specific rates of CRI ranged from 12% when infection occurs at 24 to 28 weeks to 58% at 36 to 40 weeks.

The type of malformation is gestational age specific. Cataracts and cardiac lesions are seen when infection occurs before 8 weeks. Deafness occurs with infection before 16 weeks; retinopathy, before 130 days.

Second and third trimester rubella infections are not without clinical consequence. Developmental delay, hearing loss, growth retardation, pulmonic stenosis, and thrombocytopenia can occur.

## MICROBIOLOGY/IMMUNOLOGY

Rubella is an RNA virus of the Togavirus family, measuring 40 to 50 nm. Infection causes cytolysis and decreased mitotic activity. Primary infection leads to production of rubella-specific IgM within 14 days. Viremia is characteristic in primary infection but may occur rarely with reinfection, as suggested by reports of CRS in those cases. Rubella-specific IgM persists for 3 months. IgG response is slower and usually persists indefinitely.

Seroconversion after vaccination occurs in 96% of patients. If antibody is measured by hemagglutination inhibition (HAI), 36% of patients may become seronegative with time. Detection of antibody by ELISA is more sensitive and therefore more predictive of immune status.

Congenital rubella leads to chronic, persistent infection and ongoing damage. Defective cell-mediated immunity may underlie the pathogenesis of some late effects of CRI.

## CLINICAL MANIFESTATIONS: MATERNAL

Postnatally acquired rubella is asymptomatic in 30% of adults. The incubation period is 14 to 21 days, with viral shedding beginning 1 week before onset of rash. The rash is macular and lasts 3 days. Malaise, fever, and postauricular and suboccipital adenopathy are also common. Arthralgias are common in adult women. Symptoms are nonspecific. Diagnosis should be made on serologic rather than clinical grounds.

## CLINICAL MANIFESTATIONS: FETAL/NEONATAL

First trimester rubella infection is believed to cause abortion. The Centers for Disease Control (CDC) classification of CRS is shown in Table 11-2.

Four major defects in CRS, in order of frequency, are deafness, mental retardation, heart lesions, and ophthalmologic abnormalities. The Collaborative Perinatal Research Study (CPRS) of 1964 reported that deafness was the most common single defect and is present in 100% of infants with multiple defects resulting from first trimester infection. Conversely, eye defects were present only with other abnormalities; cataracts and glaucoma were most frequent. Cardiac lesions include ventricular septal defect, patent ductus arteriosus, and peripheral pulmonic stenosis. Thrombocytopenic purpura (blueberry muffin rash), hepatosplenomegaly, osseous lesions, meningoencephalitis, and rubelliform rash may also be present in CRS.

Extended CRS includes cerebral palsy, mental retardation, developmental and language delay, seizures, cirrhosis, growth retardation, and immunologic disorders (e.g., hypogammaglobulinemia).

Delayed manifestations of CRI include endocrinopathies, late-onset deafness and ocular damage, renovascular hypertension, and encephalitis. There is a 20% incidence of diabetes mellitus by the age of 35. Other endocrinopathies include

---

**TABLE 11-2.** Classification of Congenital Rubella Syndrome
(National Congenital Rubella Syndrome Register)

---

1. CRS confirmed. Defects and one or more of the following present in the infant:
   Rubella virus isolated
   Rubella-specific IgM present
   Persistent rubella-specific IgG (ie, does not decrease at rate of one twofold dilution per month)
2. CRS compatible. Defects present but insufficient laboratory confirmation. Two defects from item a or one each from items a and b are necessary:
   a. Cataracts and/or congenital glaucoma, congenital heart disease, hearing loss, pigmentary retinopathy
   b. Purpura, splenomegaly, jaundice, microcephaly, mental retardation, meningoencephalitis, radiolucent bone disease
3. CRS possible. Clinical defects that do not fulfill criteria for CRS compatible
4. Congenital rubella infection only (CRI). Serologic evidence of infection without defects
5. Stillbirths: Stillbirths attributed to maternal rubella
6. Not CRS. The following laboratory findings are inconsistent with CRS in the absence of an immunodeficiency disease:
   Absent rubella antibody in child younger than 24 months of age
   Absent rubella antibody in the mother
   Rate of decline of rubella antibody consistent with decline of passively acquired antibody (one twofold dilution per month)

---

Adapted from CDC. Rubella and congenital rubella—United States, 1984–1986. MMWR 1987;36:664.

thyroid dysfunction and growth hormone deficiency. Delayed manifestations of CRS are thought to be due to circulating immune complexes.

Delayed manifestations occur in more than 20% of those with initially symptomatic CRS.

## DIAGNOSIS

Clinical diagnosis of postnatal infection is unreliable and must be confirmed by serology. Serologic evidence of maternal primary infection includes presence of rubella-specific IgM, or presence of a fourfold rise in HAI titer on acute and convalescent sera.

Prenatal diagnosis of congenital rubella infection is confirmed by the presence of rubella-specific IgM in fetal blood. Fetal immunocompetence is attained in the mid-second trimester; therefore, fetal blood sampling must be delayed until that time to avoid a false negative result. There are no abnormalities specific to rubella that are visible on prenatal ultrasound. The presence of nonspecific findings, such as VSD or microcephaly, in an at-risk pregnancy may aid in counseling the patient.

## PREVENTION/TREATMENT

Prevention of in utero rubella infection requires the acquisition of immunity by all persons before the childbearing years. Missed opportunities for vaccination of adults still occur and contribute to the continued existence of CRS.

There is no specific antiviral therapy for rubella infection. If in utero exposure to rubella virus is documented, the woman should be counseled as to the risks and consequences of CRI. Prenatal diagnosis is possible. With the potentially devastating effects of first trimester infection, a patient may choose to terminate the affected pregnancy if the diagnosis is made in a timely manner.

## CYTOMEGALOVIRUS

### EPIDEMIOLOGY

Cytomegalovirus (CMV) is the most common viral cause of congenital infection. An estimated 0.2% to 2.2% of all neonates are infected in utero, with 5% to 10% of these infants symptomatic at birth. Over 30,000 infants are born with congenital CMV infection in the United States every year. Primary CMV occurs in 1% to 2% of pregnant women. Approximately 50% of reproductive-age women are susceptible to CMV infection. CMV infection is spread through infected secretions or body fluids such as endocervical mucus, semen, blood, urine, saliva, breast milk, and tears. "High-risk" environments for exposure to CMV include child care centers, newborn nurseries, renal dialysis units, and areas of hospitals providing care for immunocompromised individuals.

### TRANSMISSION

Fetal infection can occur with both primary and recurrent maternal infection; however, the likelihood and severity of congenital disease appears to be greater with a primary infection. Transmission to the fetus occurs in approximately 40% of pregnancies with primary CMV. Transmission can occur at any time during pregnancy, but CMV infection acquired earlier in gestation may result in a more severely affected infant.

## MICROBIOLOGY/IMMUNOLOGY

Cytomegalovirus is an enveloped, double-stranded DNA virus of the herpesvirus family. IgG and IgM antibodies may be detectable several weeks after infection. Many different strains of cytomegalovirus have been identified by restriction endonuclease analysis. Studies indicate that recurrent infections and transmission to the fetus in immune women are more frequently due to reactivation than to reinfection.

## CLINICAL MANIFESTATIONS: MATERNAL

CMV infection in the immunocompetent mother is generally asymptomatic. In some patients a heterophile-negative mononucleosis-like syndrome may be present.

## CLINICAL MANIFESTATIONS: FETAL

Characteristics of fetal infection include intrauterine growth retardation, microcephaly, hydrocephaly, periventricular calcifications (Fig. 11-1), and hepatosplenomegaly. CMV has been reported to be the cause of nonimmune hydrops in 1.6% to 5% of cases. CMV has also been implicated in myocarditis; there have been reports of fetal heart block and of fetal supraventricular tachycardia.

**FIGURE 11-1.**
Ultrasound image of cytomegalovirus-induced intracranial calcifications. (Arrow indicates periventricular hyperechoic deposits.) (From Ghidini A, Sirtori M, Vergani P, et al. Fetal intracranial calcifications. Am J Obstet Gynecol 1989;160:86.)

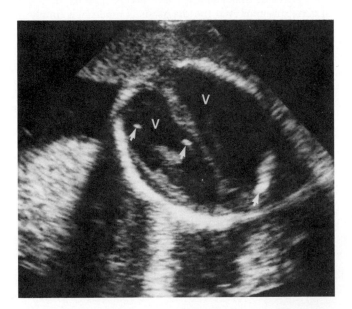

## CLINICAL MANIFESTATIONS: NEONATAL

Only approximately 10% of infants with congenital infection are symptomatic at birth. The clinical findings associated with cytomegalic inclusion disease (CID) include hepatosplenomegaly, growth retardation, microcephaly, hydrocephaly, cerebral calcifications, chorioretinitis, sensorineural hearing deficits, microphthalmia, jaundice, thrombocytopenia, purpura, mental retardation, and dental abnormalities. The mortality rate for the infants with clinical evidence of disease at birth is about 20%. Approximately 5% to 15% of the initially asymptomatic infants develop evidence of disease by 2 years of age, with sensorineural hearing deficits (5% to 10% of cases) and subsequent learning disabilities being the most important long-term sequelae.

## DIAGNOSIS

The most definitive method for diagnosis of CMV infection is by isolation of the virus, but the cytopathic effects of the virus may not be seen for 2 to 6 weeks. Serologic studies for the detection of antibody to CMV include indirect hemagglutination assay (IHA), enzyme-linked immunosorbent assay (ELISA), immunofluorescent assay (IFA), neutralization tests, and complement fixation (CF). CF assays are often inaccurate because of a high false-positive rate due to cross-reactivity with other herpesviruses. CMV-specific IgM antibody tests are helpful but of limited value because 30% of women with primary infections are initially seronegative and the test is positive in 10% of women with recurrent infection. The presence of cord blood CMV-specific IgM, which is detectable in 60% of infants with congenital infection, establishes the diagnosis. Cytomegalovirus has been isolated from amniotic fluid.

## TREATMENT/PREVENTION

No treatment other than symptomatic therapy is necessary for the immunocompetent adult with CMV infection. A variety of therapeutic agents have been administered for the treatment of congenital CMV infection, but none have been found to be satisfactory, because of toxicity or recurrence of infection after drug administration is terminated.

Routine antepartum serologic screening for CMV is not recommended at this time. The detection of maternal CMV antibody before conception indicates prior infection, but the degree of protection that this immunity provides against congenital infection in subsequent pregnancies is unclear.

## HERPES SIMPLEX VIRUS

### EPIDEMIOLOGY

Herpes simplex virus (HSV) infection is ubiquitous. Seropositivity to Type 1 HSV (HSV-1) is acquired by a majority of persons by age 7. The incidence of seropositivity to HSV-2 varies with age, sexual habits, and economic status. HSV-1 is the serotype found in most oral lesions; HSV-2 causes most lesions below the waist. Eighty-five percent of genital HSV in adults is due to HSV-2.

Excretion of HSV from the genital tract accompanies 0.1% to 0.4% of deliveries. The incidence of neonatal disease is 10 times lower, 0.01% to 0.04% of deliveries.

## TRANSMISSION

Transmission of genital HSV requires intimate contact of infectious secretions with susceptible mucous membranes or skin. There is a high rate of unsuspected genital transmission; 57% of partners of pregnant women had serologic evidence of HSV infection, yet only 6% had a history of HSV.

Neonatal transmission occurs intrapartum in the vast majority of cases—the virus is encountered in the infected maternal genital tract. Postnatal acquisition has been documented, especially in cases of HSV-1 neonatal infection.

Transplacental infection with HSV has been reported but is not well understood. Evidence for teratogenic potential of HSV is circumstantial. Reported cases of congenital HSV are rare, and serologic and virologic confirmation is incomplete. Cervical shedding of virus is more frequent in primary episodes: 87% versus 4% of recurrences. Duration of shedding and virus inoculum are also less in recurrent disease. These facts plus the transplacental passage of neutralizing antibody in recurrent infection may account for the lower risk of neonatal infection in recurrent episodes. Infection has been estimated to occur in over 50% of exposures during a primary infection versus less than 5% with recurrences.

## MICROBIOLOGY/IMMUNOLOGY

Herpes simplex virus is a double-stranded DNA virus of the same family as VZV, CMV, and EBV. HSV enters the host via skin or mucosa; after initial infection antibody is produced and the virus becomes latent in the ganglia of sensory neurons. Reactivation occurs in response to stimuli such as fever, ultraviolet light, menses, or emotional upset.

Most primary infections of external genitalia are symptomatic, but infection of the cervix may be subclinical.

Presence of antibody alters the course of disease in adults; transplacental antibody may also modify neonatal infection. Disseminated disease is rare in immunocompetent adults when compared to the neonate, especially the preterm infant.

Altered skin integrity may also be a factor in the higher infection rates and mortality of preterm neonates.

## CLINICAL MANIFESTATIONS: MATERNAL

Systemic symptoms such as fever, malaise, myalgia, and headache were present in 68% of women with primary infection and in 16% of recurrences. Local symptoms include pain, discharge, adenopathy, and dysuria. Lesions follow primary exposure in 2 to 10 days and are painful vesicles. These ulcerate and then heal without scarring. Lesions were present for a mean of 11 days in primary cases and for 7 days in recurrences. Viral shedding persists until the lesions heal. Cervical shedding is present with primary infection in over 80% of patients and in up to 30% of recurrences. Asymptomatic shedding occurs in less than 1% of pregnancies.

## CLINICAL MANIFESTATIONS: FETAL

Infection of the conceptus by transplacental spread of HSV has been linked with spontaneous abortion, preterm labor, and congenital malformations. The spectrum of anomalies is similar to congenital CMV infection. Microcephaly, periventricular calcifications, chorioretinitis, intrauterine growth retardation, and vesicular eruptions have been described. In most reports, virus isolation and serologic confirmation are incomplete. Complete prospective data are needed to define more clearly the congenital syndrome. Prenatal diagnosis of transplacental HSV is theoretically possible by demonstration of HSV IgM in fetal blood. Presently, the low risk of transmission may not justify invasive methods of prenatal diagnosis. Termination of pregnancy is not required in cases of first trimester primary HSV infection, because of the apparent low risk of fetal infection in those pregnancies that continue.

## CLINICAL MANIFESTATIONS: NEONATAL

Infection acquired intrapartum has an average incubation period of 6 to 12 days. Infection may be *localized* to the skin, eye, or oral mucosa; may be *disseminated*; or may involve the *central nervous system* (CNS). Neonatal HSV is rarely asymptomatic. Almost 50% of infections are in premature neonates.

Local infection occurs in 15% of cases. Signs include mucocutaneous vesicles, keratoconjunctivitis, and chorioretinitis. Mortality is lower than that for CNS or disseminated disease. Chorioretinitis or keratoconjunctivitis may result in blindness; 30% of infants with local disease develop major neurologic sequelae such as spastic quadriplegia or microcephaly. Seventy-five percent of localized infection will disseminate unless early therapy is instituted.

Neonatal HSV confined to the CNS occurs in 15% to 30% of cases. Onset is at 3 weeks of age; 65% have skin vesicles. Mortality is greater than 50% and devastating neurologic sequelae are the rule in survivors.

Disseminated infection occurs in 70% of neonates. Forty-five percent of affected neonates are premature. Onset is at 9 to 11 days of life; 90% have the characteristic vesicular rash. Involvement of liver and adrenal glands in 70% accounts for signs of jaundice, hemorrhage, and shock. CNS involvement occurs in 75%; pneumonitis is present in half of these infants. Mortality is over 50% and is usually due to disseminated intravascular coagulopathy or pneumonitis.

## DIAGNOSIS

A rapid assay for HSV with a high specificity and positive predictive value is needed to prevent neonatal transmission and infection. Virus identification by presence of cytopathic effect in tissue culture is the gold standard but necessarily takes time.

A potential benefit of rapid detection of HSV antigen in the maternal genital tract is the early identification of exposed neonates. Identification of virus in the maternal genital tract at the onset of labor or rupture of membranes should be the diagnostic goal. Antepartum HSV cultures do not predict either presence or absence of virus at the time of parturition. Virus is shed in 1.4% of parturients regardless of their antepartum culture status. Additionally, 50% of HSV-infected neonates are born to mothers with no history of genital herpes, thus discounting the value of screening only the high-risk patient.

The diagnosis of neonatal herpes is complicated by its nonspecific presentation and clinical resemblance to bacterial sepsis. Only half of infected neonates have skin lesions, and in the case of focal HSV encephalitis, virus may only be recoverable by brain biopsy.

## PREVENTION

A 1988 editorial by the Infectious Disease Society for Obstetrics and Gynecology proposed an alternate approach to the once standard practice of weekly HSV cultures after 32 weeks in patients with recurrent genital herpes. Their recommendations include the following: abandon weekly prenatal cultures; culture patients only when they are symptomatic. Obtain cultures of the mother or neonate at the time of delivery in all patients with a history of genital herpes or a partner with HSV, to identify potentially exposed neonates.

## TREATMENT

Acyclovir and vidarabine are specific antiviral therapies against HSV. Acyclovir has selective activity against herpes viruses, with little effect on uninfected cells. Its selectivity is due to activation by HSV-specific thymidine kinase. The activated form inhibits HSV DNA polymerase. Acyclovir is excreted primarily by the kidneys and has a wide margin of safety. Adverse reactions are rare with oral or topical forms.

Routine indications for antiviral therapy in pregnancy have not been established. Potential uses include treatment of cases of disseminated herpes and severe primary infection. Acyclovir is considered by many to be appropriate for treatment of disseminated HSV in pregnancy. Primary HSV infection in pregnancy increases the risk of adverse perinatal outcome (e.g., preterm delivery, intrauterine growth retardation, and congenital anomalies).

Both acyclovir and vidarabine have been used for neonatal HSV.

## EPSTEIN-BARR VIRUS

### EPIDEMIOLOGY

At least 95% of pregnant women demonstrate seroreactivity to EBV antigens. In general, prior infection and serologic conversion confer immunity and prevent reinfection.

### MICROBIOLOGY/IMMUNOLOGY

Epstein-Barr virus, a lymphotropic herpesvirus, is the etiologic agent of infectious mononucleosis. After a primary infection, viral excretion may continue for weeks or months. Antibodies to EBV viral capsid antigen (VCA) and early antigen (EA) develop early, whereas antibodies to EBV nuclear antigen (EBNA) may take weeks or months to develop. Reactivation of latent, persistent EBV infection has been found to occur more frequently in pregnancy, often occurring very early in gestation.

## TRANSMISSION

Transplacental transmission of EBV can occur but is very rare. Reactivation of latent, persistent EBV infection has not been associated with adverse perinatal outcome.

## CLINICAL MANIFESTATIONS: MATERNAL

More than half of all patients with primary EBV infections are asymptomatic. The most common clinical manifestations are the sore throat, fever, malaise, and lymph node enlargement characteristic of infectious mononucleosis.

## CLINICAL MANIFESTATIONS: FETAL/NEONATAL

There have thus far been no reported cases of antenatal diagnosis of EBV congenital infection. EBV has been implicated as the possible cause of congenital malformations (cardiovascular defects and cataracts) in several infants of mothers who developed infectious mononucleosis during the first trimester.

## DIAGNOSIS

Laboratory diagnosis of EBV infection depends primarily on serology. The detection of heterophil antibodies in a patient with clinical symptoms of infectious mononucleosis is usually diagnostic for an acute EBV infection. Antibodies to VCA are present in all individuals by the third week of infection. IgM-VCA declines over the next 3 months, whereas IgG-VCA persists for life. IgG-EA appears after the VCA antibodies and declines over the next 6 months. IgG-EBNA can sometimes be detected by the third to fourth week of infection and may persist indefinitely. IgM antibody to VCA is diagnostic for a primary EBV infection, but if there is no IgM-VCA, the presence of IgG antibody to VCA and EA, along with an absence of IgG to EBNA, is suggestive of primary or postacute infection.

## TREATMENT/PREVENTION

There are no specific treatment or preventative measures for EBV. Treatment of infectious mononucleosis is primarily supportive. Pregnant women should avoid contact with infectious mononucleosis patients to diminish their risks for infection, but even with intimate contact with EBV excreters, serosusceptible women may not necessarily acquire an infection. It is presently impossible to render an exact estimate of malformation risk to the fetus following documented EBV infection in pregnancy.

# 12. FETAL INFECTIONS FROM NON-TORCH VIRUSES

## HUMAN PAPILLOMA VIRUS

Human papilloma virus (HPV) is a common genital tract virus that causes anogenital warts. These viruses are of great interest not only because of a dramatic increase in frequency, but because of their potential roles in genital tract malignancy and juvenile respiratory papilloma virus. Although HPV has not yet been cultured, it is known to be a DNA virus. Presently, there are over 20 subtypes recognized, with the most common types being numbers 6, 11, and 16.

## EPIDEMIOLOGY

Within the last 15 years there has been a fully fourfold increase in genital warts (condylomata acuminata). If one considers the recently described cervical "flat warts," it is estimated that approximately 2% of reproductive-age females carry HPV. Contagion is thought to be relatively high, and condylomata acuminata have been reported on infants at birth. Respiratory papillomatosis results in warts of the larynx and trachea and is thought to result from contact with an infected maternal genital tract at delivery. Although the incubation period is variable, it is estimated to be relatively long—generally from about 3 to 8 months. Women who have genital warts may also be infected with other sexually transmitted diseases. Most women who have genital warts fall in the age range of 16 to 25.

## DIAGNOSIS

Classically, the genital wart appears as a soft verrucous lesion, several millimeters in diameter. With more common use of colposcopy, minute flat warts are now recognized commonly on the cervix. The diagnosis of condyloma acuminata is usually made on the basis of these classic clinical findings. However, condyloma of secondary syphilis should be ruled out by determining a serologic test for syphilis (i.e., VDRL). When the lesion appears atypical or if the diagnosis is suspect, a biopsy may be performed to confirm the diagnosis.

## JUVENILE RESPIRATORY PAPILLOMATOSIS

Respiratory papillomatosis has been recognized in both young children and adults, with approximately one-third of cases evident by age 5. The most frequent symptom is hoarseness due to involvement of the vocal cords. Over 90% of the HPV types are either 6 or 11.

Some researchers have concluded that in juvenile-onset respiratory papillomatosis, mother-to-infant transmission occurs most often during vaginal delivery but that in utero infection is also possible, since one child who developed respira-

E. Albert Reece, John C. Hobbins, Maurice, J. Mahoney and Roy H. Petrie (Eds). *Handbook of Medicine of the Fetus & Mother.* Copyright © 1995 by J.B. Lippincott Company

tory papillomatosis was born by cesarean section before membrane rupture. Further, in view of the frequency of genital warts and the rarity of juvenile respiratory papillomatosis, it was estimated that the risk of developing disease for a child born vaginally to an infected mother would be low, probably in the range of 1 in 80 to 1 in 1500. Based on this estimate, some might suggest that mothers with genital warts be delivered by cesarean section to prevent respiratory papillomatosis. There is little general support for this position, for three reasons:

1. The risk of transmission of the disease is very small.
2. Cesarean delivery does not offer a complete protection.
3. The risk of cesarean section for all women with any genital warts probably would outweigh the potential benefit.

## TREATMENT OF CONDYLOMATA ACUMINATA IN PREGNANCY

Specific treatment recommendations for the nonpregnant woman must be modified in pregnancy. Podophyllin should be avoided, since it may be absorbed if applied to large areas and may be toxic to the fetus. For an isolated large condyloma, surgical incision would be the most appropriate treatment. For smaller lesions, treatment may be performed with carbon dioxide laser, with electro-coagulation with curettage, or with cryotherapy.

## HEPATITIS

Of all hospitalized cases of hepatitis in pregnancy, approximately 80% are caused by hepatitis B. Hepatitis A is responsible for approximately 7%, and non-A, non-B hepatitis is responsible for the remainder.

## EPIDEMIOLOGY

Women in the United States most at risk for hepatitis B surface antigenemia (HBsAg) are as follows:

Asian Pacific Basin or Native Alaskan women, whether immigrants or U.S.-born, 15%

Haitian, Sub-Saharan African, Eastern European, Middle Eastern, Caribbean, Central or South American women, 15%

Women with occupational exposure (i.e., medical or dental), 0.5% to 1%

Women working or residing in custodial institutions, 3%

Women with acute or chronic liver disease, illicit drug users, or women with multiple blood transfusions, 7% to 10%

Women living in a household with an HBV-infected person, 6% to 13%.

The impact of HBV infection is immense. Its consequences include chronic hepatitis, cirrhosis, and primary hepatocellular carcinoma. Of an estimated 300,000 new cases yearly in the United States, 75,000 of these will become clinically ill, including 15,000 requiring hospitalization. A small number, estimated at 375, will die of fulminant disease. Six percent to 10% will become chronic carriers, and as many as 25% of these HBV carriers eventually will die of cirrhosis or hepatocellular carcinoma. Despite the availability of an effective vaccine, the incidence of HBV reported to the Centers for Disease Control (CDC) has continued to increase. In 1981, the incidence was 9.2 per 100,000, and in 1985 it was 11.5 per 100,000. The incidence of hepatitis B infection in pregnant women is the same as that in the general population, and the course of the disease in pregnancy is probably not altered.

HBV infection is spread by sexual transmission, blood transfusion, IV drug abuse, and intrauterine or perinatal transmission from the mother to the fetus or newborn (Table 12-1). The major concern in pregnancy is transmission to the infant. In the Far East, approximately 40% of HBV cases in mothers result in vertical transmission to the fetus or newborn. In the United States, the reported overall risk of perinatal HBV transmission from HBV surface antigen-positive mothers ranges from 20% to 50%, with the rate of transmission depending on population characteristics. These influencing characteristics include ethnic background, life-style, and persistence of the HBe antigen. Nonfulminant hepatitis probably does not increase fetal wastage but may be associated with an increased risk of prematurity. Finally, there is no apparent increase in congenital anomalies associated with maternal hepatitis B infection in pregnancy.

## VIROLOGY AND SEROLOGY OF HBV INFECTION

Hepatitis B virus is a DNA virus 42 nm in diameter. The outer protein coat is the so-called surface, the HBsAg. This antigen is produced in excess by the virus and appears in the serum of individuals with active infection. The central core contains DNA, a DNA polymerase, and the core antigen, HBcAg. The core antigen is found only in infected liver cells, not in the serum. The third antigen, HBeAg, is found in the serum and is a marker of high rates of perinatal transmission.

Each of these three HBV antigens has a corresponding antibody, called anti-HBs, anti-HBc, and anti-HBe. The serologic pattern that is followed in 90% of cases of HBV infection is that within 6 months of infection, all antigens are cleared from the serum. This individual becomes noninfectious. The antibodies to HBs and to HBc are lifelong markers of prior infection. In the remaining 10% of individuals with HBV infection, there is persistence of HBsAg beyond 6 months. Approximately 60% of these women with persistence of infection will develop chronic persistent hepatitis. About 10% will have asymptomatic HBsAg antigenemia, and approximately 30% will have chronic active hepatitis. All these groups are potentially infective of others, and pregnant women can transmit to the offspring. This is a group that is the target for prenatal screening. Transmission rates from the mother to the fetus or neonate are shown in Table 12-1.

**TABLE 12-1.** Hepatitis Transmission Rates from the Mother to the Fetus/Neonate

| Mother's Clinical and Serologic Status | Infection Rate in Infant (%) |
|---|---|
| Acute HBV in third trimester or within 1 month of delivery | 80–90 |
| Asymptomatic, HBeAG pos | 90 |
| Asymptomatic, HBeAG neg | 10–30 |
| Asymptomatic, anti-HBe pos | 0–10 |

## CLINICAL MANIFESTATIONS

After an incubation period of 45 to 160 days, hepatitis B may become clinically evident. Initial symptoms often include fever, headache, and abdominal pain, followed in several days by spontaneous resolution. At this point, the urine may become dark and jaundice may be evident. The liver is usually somewhat enlarged and tender. As the jaundice resolves, the patient spontaneously feels better and usually recovers rapidly. As noted, in approximately 10% of patients with hepatitis B, a form of chronic disease continues. Hepatitis B may present as an acute fulminated form that may become fatal, although this is quite rare in well-nourished Western populations. Fulminant hepatitis is heralded by a rapidly shrinking liver, rapidly rising bilirubin, and abnormalities in prothrombin time with development of encephalopathy and ascites. The mortality rate in such cases of fulminant hepatitis is greater than 80%.

In the neonate, the most frequent presentation of hepatitis infection is an asymptomatic child with chronic infection. Clinical illness is relatively infrequent with congenital hepatitis, but about 10% of neonates with asymptomatic disease become jaundiced within the first 3 to 4 months of life.

## TREATMENT

Most women with hepatitis B infection during pregnancy can be managed on an outpatient basis. There is no specific treatment, but supportive measures include increased bedrest and a high-protein, low-fat diet. Specific indications for hospitalization of women with viral hepatitis include severe anemia, diabetes, protracted nausea and vomiting, abnormalities in prothrombin time, a rapidly falling or low serum albumin level, and high serum bilirubin greater than approximately 15 mg/dL.

## PREVENTION

Women with a definite exposure to hepatitis B virus should be given hepatitis B immune globulin (HBIG) as soon as possible within a 7-day period of exposure, with a second dose 30 days after the first. Such passive immunization would be indicated for hospital exposures and inoculation with contaminated needles. Until June 1988, the Centers for Disease Control had recommended screening of pregnant women for asymptomatic hepatitis B infection on a selective basis.

However, in mid-1988, the Centers for Disease Control overhauled their recommendations based on several recent studies that demonstrated that selective screening identified only 50% of women who were HBsAg positive. The study populations were medically indigent women located in such cities as Cleveland, New Orleans, and Miami. In middle-class populations, the sensitivity of selective screening has not been well studied. Yet a cost analysis study carried out at the CDC concluded that even in extremely low prevalence populations (with a prevalence of less than 0.1%), the universal screening program would be cost effective.

The purpose of universal screening is to allow treatment of newborns of HBsAg-positive women with hepatitis B immune globulin (HBIG) and hepatitis B vaccine—a regimen that is 90% effective in preventing the development of HBV chronic carrier state in the newborn. The specifics of the recommendation are that women should be tested for HBsAg during an early prenatal visit. Testing for additional markers is considered unnecessary. Even though women who have HBeAg are at a much higher risk for perinatal transmission, there is still a risk of about 10% to 15% in perinatal transmission in women who do not have the antigen but who have HBsAg. If a woman is identified as being HBsAg positive, she should be evaluated for active liver disease. Infants born to HBsAg-positive women should receive HBIG (0.5 mL) IM once they are stable, preferably within 12 hours of birth. In addition, these infants should receive the recombinant HBV vaccine (5 μg per dose), or they may receive the plasma-derived vaccine (10 μg per dose). Either of these vaccines should be given intramuscularly in the following sequence of three doses: the first at birth, and the second and third at 1 and 6 months of age. It is estimated that the direct cost to prevent one newborn from becoming a chronic HBV carrier would be approximately $12,700 if the prevalence of HBsAg in a given population is approximately 5 in 1000.

Household members and sexual partners of women identified as being HBsAg positive should be tested to determine susceptibility to HBV infection. Susceptible individuals should receive the HBV vaccine.

Since few women in low-risk populations for HBV infection will have a change in the HBsAg antigen status during subsequent pregnancies, it may be argued that routine testing in each pregnancy is unnecessary. However, because of the expected benefits of routine testing and the possibility of omission if done selectively, the CDC currently recommends testing during each pregnancy. On the other hand, routine follow-up testing later in pregnancy is not necessary. Women who deliver without prenatal care should be tested as early as possible on delivery admission so that infants at risk can begin to receive their prophylaxis within 48 hours after birth. It is further recommended that hospitals that cannot rapidly test for HBsAg either develop this capability or test at another laboratory.

As a further preventive measure it is recommended that during delivery of HBsAg-positive women, gloves, masks, and glasses or goggles be worn by delivery room personnel to keep infectious fluids away from mouth, nose, eyes, and breaks in the skin. All these precautions are equally important in guarding against HBV infection and in preventing transmission of the AIDS virus. Thus, to prevent both of these serious infections, universal blood and body fluid precautions are the best measures of preventing nosocomial transmission.

## VARICELLA

A member of the herpesvirus group, varicella zoster (VZ) virus is a DNA virus that exhibits a viral latency. Primary infection usually occurs in childhood, clinically presenting as chickenpox. As a highly contagious disorder, varicella zoster infection is acquired by most children in the United States prior to reproductive age and is generally a self-limited disease characterized by typical skin lesions. It is recognized that when adults contract the disease both constitutional and pulmonary symptoms may be more severe. Reactivation of latent zoster infection clinically presents as shingles, generally occurring in the older population or in immunocompromised individuals. Zoster presents as painful crops of vesicular lesions occurring along the distribution of a segmental dermatome.

The remainder of this discussion will be limited to the effects of VZ infection in pregnancy. There are two major concerns for the perinatologist. The first is the risk the infection imposes for the mother; the second is the risk of either teratogenesis or perinatal acquisition to the fetus or neonate.

## EPIDEMIOLOGY

Over 150,000 cases of chickenpox occur annually in the United States. Yet, because of widespread underreporting, it is estimated that the actual number of cases is 2 to 3 million. Over 90% of the population has been infected during childhood. The incidence of varicella zoster infection in pregnancy is estimated at approximately 5 in 10,000 pregnancies.

## CLINICAL PRESENTATION

After an incubation period of from 10 to 20 days (usually 13 to 17 days), fever and rash commonly occur simultaneously in children. In adults, fever and generalized malaise usually precede the rash by several days. The rash usually begins on the face and scalp and then spreads to the trunk. There is usually minimal involvement of the extremities. The skin lesion begins as a macule and proceeds to a vesicular and then pustular stage. Healing is heralded by the presentation of crusts and scabs. The prominent feature of the disease is itching. Over a period of 2 to 5 days, new crops of lesions occur, and lesions in various stages of progression usually are present at the same time.

Bacterial infection of the skin is the common secondary complication of chickenpox. Encephalitis, meningitis, myocarditis, glomerulonephritis, and arthritis are all rare complications in childhood. The most serious complication of varicella infection is pneumonia. It occurs more commonly in adults, but the pneumonia does not appear to have an increased prevalence in pregnant women as opposed to other adults. Currently, it is estimated that approximately 5% to 10% of adults with chickenpox develop pneumonia. In a review of the literature on varicella pneumonia in pregnancy, Young and Gershon noted in 1983 that of 77 cases of chickenpox in pregnancy, 29% developed pneumonia.* Because of selectivity, we estimate that this incidence of varicella pneumonia in pregnancy is high. Ten deaths occurred—all in women who had pneumonia. The mortality of varicella pneumonia in this series was 45%. There were no severe complications in women who did not develop pneumonia. Accordingly, it appears that uncomplicated chickenpox poses no major threat to the pregnant woman, especially in view of current critical care abilities to manage severe respiratory distress and failure. We believe that mortality now would be improved.

For the clinician, the main objective is to maintain a high index of suspicion for pneumonia in women who have varicella infection in pregnancy. Pulmonary symptoms usually begin on the second to sixth day after appearance of the rash and usually present with a mild nonproductive cough. If the disease is more severe, there may be additional symptoms, including hemoptysis, dyspnea, pleuritic chest pain, or progression to frank cyanosis. Physical examination in women who develop pneumonia would find fever, rales, and wheezes. The chest

---

*Young NA, Gershon AA. Chicken pox, measles, and mumps. In: Remington JS, Klein JO, eds. Infectious disease of the fetus and newborn. Philadelphia: WB Saunders, 1983:375.

x-ray characteristically shows a miliary pattern or a diffuse nodular pattern. On the chest x-ray, the perihilar regions are more likely to be involved. Women who have varicella infection without complications in pregnancy do not need to be hospitalized. However, women with this infection must be warned to contact their physician immediately in the event of any pulmonary symptoms, including a mild cough. At this point, hospitalization with full respiratory support, if necessary, should be indicated.

In a recent series of 43 pregnancies complicated by maternal varicella, Paryani and Arvin noted that 9 women had developed associated morbidity.[†] Varicella pneumonia developed in 4 of these women (9%), 1 of whom died. Premature labor developed in 4 out of 42 (10%), with premature delivery occurring in 2 (5%). Another woman developed herpes zoster infection. If a pregnant woman is exposed to varicella infection, it is very likely that she is immune, but if she is not immune, it is most probable that she will become infected. McGregor and colleagues recently pointed out that most pregnant women have detectable antibody even if they have a negative history of chickenpox.[‡] In their series, 12 out of 17 (71%) of such women were already antibody immune. Of those women with indeterminate histories, approximately 90% were immune. On the basis of these data, it appears appropriate and cost effective to test for maternal antibody by any of the following antibody tests: fluorescent antibody to membrane antigen (FAMA), enzyme-linked immunosorbent assay (ELISA), enhanced neutralization test, and immune adherence hemagglutination.

If it is found that a woman has been exposed and is susceptible, varicella zoster immune globulin (VZIG) may be given. When administered intramuscularly within 3 days of exposure, it is likely that VZIG ameliorates the course of the maternal disease as it does in children. However, it is not at all certain that passive immunization with VZIG prevents fetal infection. Currently, there is no reason to believe that VZIG in pregnancy is harmful. Thus, the only disadvantage of providing VZIG to nonimmune pregnant women with exposure to varicella is the cost, currently a few hundred dollars.

## VARICELLA IN THE NEWBORN

Acquisition by the fetus of maternal antibody usually is protective. However, in an infant born after maternal viremia but before maternal development of antibodies, the infant is at high risk for potentially life-threatening neonatal varicella infection. Infants at risk are those whose mothers develop clinical varicella within 5 days of birth or within the first 5 days after delivery. Congenital varicella infection has been reported in approximately 20% of term infants born to mothers with varicella within this time frame, and the case fatality has been reported at approximately 30%. Infants born 5 or more days after maternal development of clinical illness develop either a mild varicella infection or none whatsoever. Both zoster immunoglobulin (ZIG) and varicella zoster immunoglobulin (VZIG) have been shown to modify or prevent varicella in normal children, leading one researcher to recommend their use in preventing severe neonatal infections.

† Paryani SG, Arvin AM. Intrauterine infection with varicella zoster virus after maternal varicella. N Engl J Med 1986;314:1542.

‡ McGregor JA, Mark S, Crawford GP, et al. Varicella zoster antibody testing in the care of pregnant women exposed to varicella. Am J Obstet Gynecol 1987;157:281.

Accordingly, infants at risk, as outlined earlier, should receive ZIG or VZIG as passive immunization at a dose of 1.25 mL. Weibel and colleagues have recently reported excellent results using a live attenuated varicella vaccine.[§] The seroconversion rate was 94% and the vaccine was 100% effective in preventing varicella. In a placebo-controlled group, approximately 10% of children developed varicella.

## EFFECT OF ZOSTER VARICELLA INFECTION IN EARLY PREGNANCY

Congenital birth defects due to varicella in early pregnancy were not recognized until about 40 years ago. The syndrome of congenital varicella infection consists of limb hypoplasia, cicatricial skin lesions, atrophic digits, psychomotor retardation, growth retardation, and even bilateral cortical atrophy. We now recognize that maternal varicella infection in the first trimester of pregnancy may be responsible for such a syndrome, but the risk of the fetus developing these anomalies with first trimester chickenpox has only recently been recognized. Of 11 infants of women with first trimester varicella, 1 (9%) developed findings consistent with congenital varicella syndrome.

## EFFECT OF ZOSTER IN PREGNANCY

Herpes zoster infection, as noted, is caused by the same virus that causes clinical chickenpox. Zoster occurs very rarely in pregnancy, and because it is a reactivation, maternal antibodies are already present. In healthy women, zoster poses no special threat to the fetus or newborn.

## MEASLES (RUBEOLA)

Measles is a common acute illness, most likely occurring in childhood. Among the most communicable of childhood exanthems, rubeola is characterized by fever, coryza, cough, maculopapular rash, and conjunctivitis. Rubeola virus is an RNA virus belonging to the paramyxovirus group.

## EPIDEMIOLOGY

With an incubation time between 10 and 14 days, measles is spread chiefly by droplets expectorated by infected persons. The virus gains access to susceptible individuals via the nose, oropharynx, and conjunctiva. It is most communicable during the prodromal as well as catarrhal stages of infection. Three-fourths of exposed susceptible individuals develop the infection. Prior to the availability of live measles vaccines, epidemics occurred in the United States at 2- to 3-year intervals. Since 1963, the introduction of the attenuated measles vaccine has had a major impact in decreasing measles in the United States.

Occurring less frequency than either chickenpox or mumps in pregnancy, measles has a rate of approximately of 0.4 to 0.6 per 10,000 pregnancies.

§ Weibel RE, Neff BJ, Kuter BJ, et al. Live attenuated varicella virus vaccine. Efficacy trial in healthy children. N Engl J Med 1984;310:1409.

## CLINICAL MANIFESTATIONS

The clinical prodrome that consists of fever and malaise usually begins 10 to 11 days after exposure. The coryza, sneezing, conjunctivitis, and cough usually begin approximately 24 hours later. This catarrhal phase worsens over the next few days, often leading to marked conjunctivitis and photophobia. The so-called Koplik's spots, pathognomonic of measles, appear at the end of the prodrome. These characteristic lesions are tiny granular, slightly raised, white lesions surrounded by erythema and located on the lateral buccal mucosa. The characteristic rash begins 12 to 14 days after exposure and begins on the head and neck, especially in the posterior auricular region. The rash, maculopapular in character, spreads to the trunk, upper extremities, and finally the lower extremities.

Pulmonary complications are the most frequent complications of measles, with otitis media and croup also occurring frequently. Bacterial pneumonia is the complication with most frequent association with mortality. Encephalitis is a less common serious complication, occurring in an estimated 1 case of measles out of 1000. Rare complications of measles include thrombocytopenic purpura, myocarditis, and subacute sclerosing panencephalitis.

## EFFECTS OF MEASLES ON THE MOTHER

It is unclear whether pregnant women with measles are at greater risk for serious complications or death than nonpregnant adults. Recent studies have noted that measles in pregnant women is very rarely associated with major complications such as pneumonia.

## EFFECT OF MEASLES ON THE FETUS

Recent reviews of the literature note that there is an increased rate of prematurity in pregnancies complicated by measles, especially when the disease occurs in the third trimester. However, measles does not appear associated with an increased risk for spontaneous abortion. No fetal syndrome of abnormalities has been found among the sporadic instances of congenital defects occurring in women who reported maternal measles. Thus, if there is any increased risk of congenital malformations from measles occurring in pregnancy, the risk appears to be very small. When measles becomes clinically apparent in the first 10 days of life, it is considered to be congenital, that is, transplacental in origin. Cases becoming clinically evident at 14 days or after are considered to be acquired postnatally. Postnatally acquired measles is usually a very mild disorder, whereas the spectrum of congenital measles varies from a mild illness to a rapidly fatal disease. We note that the presence of maternal measles immediately prior to delivery usually does not involve the fetus and neonate. In cases of congenital measles, a mortality rate of 32% has been reported (7 out of 22). Premature infants with congenital measles have a significantly higher death rate (56%) than do term infected infants (20%). We do not know whether transplacentally acquired antibodies to measles virus diminish the case fatality rate in congenital measles if the mother's rash occurs more than 48 hours before delivery. It is important to note that the reported cases of mortality due to congenital measles all occurred in the preantibiotic era. Accordingly, with antimicrobial therapy effective against secondary bacterial pneumonia and modern support, we anticipate that fatal outcomes of rubeola infection are much less likely.

## DIAGNOSIS

Diagnosis of measles relies on the clinical history and typical clinical presentation. Elements in the differential diagnosis include rubella, scarlet fever, meningococcemia, roseola, Rocky Mountain spotted fever, infectious mononucleosis, other enterovirus infections, toxoplasmosis, and drug eruptions.

## TREATMENT

Uncomplicated measles is treated symptomatically. If secondary otitis media or pneumonia occurs, then an appropriate antibiotic should be instituted.

## PREVENTION

Susceptible exposed pregnant women, neonates, and their contacts should receive passive immunization. Immune serum globulin (ISG) in a dose of 0.25 mg/kg as soon as possible after an exposure may prevent or at least modify the infection. Children born to women who have measles in the last week of pregnancy or first week postpartum should also be given the immune serum globulin as soon as possible in the same dose.

## MUMPS

Mumps is an acute generalized infection in childhood that has a predilection for the parotid and salivary glands. There is no characteristic rash. The mumps virus is also an RNA virus and a member of the paramyxovirus family.

## EPIDEMIOLOGY

The virus is spread by saliva and droplet contamination. It has been recovered from salivary and respiratory secretions from approximately 7 days before the onset of clinical parotitis until 9 days afterward. The usual incubation period runs approximately 2 to 2.5 weeks. Only approximately 10% of cases occur after the age of 15, because most adults are immune as a consequence of childhood illness. Approximately one-third of cases are subclinical. Mumps is less contagious than measles or chickenpox, and the attack rate, even among exposed, susceptible household members, is low. Mumps occurs more frequently in pregnant women than measles or chickenpox, with an estimated incidence of approximately 0.8 to 10 cases per 10,000 pregnancies.

## CLINICAL MANIFESTATIONS

Mumps begins with a prodrome of fever, malaise, myalgia, and anorexia and then develops into parotitis within approximately 24 hours. This stage is characterized by tender, painful, swollen parotid glands. On physical examination, the orifice of Stenson's duct is red and swollen. Most commonly, parotitis is bilateral. The submaxillary glands are less involved and never become involved without parotid gland involvement. It is unusual for sublingual glands to be affected. Mumps is usually self-limited, and complications are rare.

In approximately 20% of postpubertal males, orchitis occurs. This is the most common manifestation other than parotitis in this group. Oophoritis is much less common and presents with adnexal pain. Aseptic meningitis is a rare but recognized neurologic complication of mumps. Mumps meningitis is almost always benign and self-limited. Rare complications of mumps include pancreatitis, mastitis, thyroiditis, myocarditis, arthritis, and nephritis.

## EFFECT ON MOTHER AND FETUS

In pregnancy, mumps is generally benign and not more involved than in nonpregnant patients. Similarly, asymptomatic meningitis in pregnant patients is neither more frequent nor severe. Mortality is extremely rare in both pregnant and nonpregnant adults.

In retrospective studies, mumps occurring in the first trimester of pregnancy has been associated with a twofold increase in the rate of spontaneous abortion. Mumps, however, has not been associated with prematurity, growth retardation, or excess perinatal mortality. It is uncertain whether mumps leads to any congenital disease. Definite evidence of teratogenic potential for mumps virus in humans has not been presented. In a controlled prospective study, Siegal noted that congenital malformations were no more common in neonates whose mothers had mumps during pregnancy than in controls.[||] In both groups of studies, the rates of congenital anomalies were approximately 2%.

Of concern in the past decade and a half has been the purported association between maternal mumps infection and development of the congenital cardiac defect endocardial fibroelastosis. Data are currently conflicting, and the low incidence of mumps in pregnancy makes it unlikely that prospective and controlled data will be gathered in the near future.

## DIAGNOSIS

As with measles, the diagnosis of mumps is usually made on clinical grounds. The diagnosis is straightforward with the typical presentation of acute bilateral parotitis and the history of recent exposure. In more difficult cases, the diagnosis may depend on virus isolation or on demonstration of a rising antibody of the complement fixation, hemagglutination inhibition, or neutralizing antibody type.

## TREATMENT

Again, the treatment of mumps is symptomatic in both pregnant and nonpregnant individuals. Supportive treatment includes bedrest, application of cold or heat to the parotids, and analgesics. Maternal mumps is not an indication for termination of pregnancy.

Live attenuated mumps vaccine has been effective in preventing primary mumps,

[||] Siegal M. Congenital malformations following chicken pox, measles, mumps, and hepatitis. Results of a cohort study. JAMA 1973;226:1521.

because 95% of susceptible individuals develop antibodies. Clinical adverse reactions have been infrequent and mild. Immunization of mumps with live-virus vaccine in pregnancy is contraindicated on the theoretical grounds that the developing fetus might be harmed. Although the risk to the fetus seems negligible, the innocuous nature of mumps in pregnancy suggests that any risk from vaccination should be avoided.

## INFLUENZA

Influenza viruses belong to the myxovirus group and cause the clinical entity of influenza that occurs in epidemics. Type A influenza is responsible for most epidemics and is associated with more severe disease, whereas types B and C occur less frequently.

### EPIDEMIOLOGY

The frequency and severity of influenza outbreaks have been related to changes in the viral antigens. The major antigenic changes occur at 10- to 30-year intervals and are associated with severe infection because of the absence of protective antibodies.

Two major pandemics occurred in 1918 and in 1957–1958. More than 20 million deaths occurred worldwide during the pandemic of 1918.

### CLINICAL PRESENTATION

With a short incubation period of 1 to 4 days, influenza presents with abrupt onset of an upper respiratory infection, fever, malaise, myalgia, and headache. With wide clinical variability, the major portion of the disease lasts approximately 3 days in most cases.

Definitive diagnosis can be made by isolation of virus from throat washings during acute illness or by serologic confirmation of a fourfold rise in antibody. Although these antibodies are of either the complement fixation or hemagglutination inhibition types, they are rarely indicated clinically.

### MATERNAL EFFECTS OF INFLUENZA

For the obstetrician, the major concern of influenza infection in pregnancy is the increased likelihood for potentially life-threatening pneumonia. From reports of epidemics in both 1918 and 1957, it appears that pregnant women were disproportionately represented in individuals dying of influenza. In addition, reported estimates of maternal mortality rate are approximately 27%, with a mortality rate of almost 50% in cases complicated by pneumonia. It is not certain, however, whether pregnant women are more likely to develop influenza or whether they are more likely to develop influenza pneumonia. Yet if influenza pneumonia develops in pregnancy, then it is more severe. Deaths among pregnant women with influenza may result from secondary bacterial infection and from primary influenza pneumonia without secondary superinfection.

## EFFECTS OF INFLUENZA ON THE FETUS

Contradictory data address the issues of the effect of influenza on abortion, prematurity, and congenital anomalies. These studies may be summarized as noting that the vast majority of women who have influenza in pregnancy have normal outcomes and that there seems to be little influence on congenital abnormalities, intrauterine growth, prematurity, or stillbirth.

## TREATMENT

As in other adults, management of uncomplicated pregnant women with influenza is symptomatic, consisting of bedrest, analgesics, liberal fluid intake, and antipyretics (acetaminophen). If signs of pneumonia occur in pregnant women with influenza, prompt evaluation and hospitalization are indicated. Broad-spectrum antibiotic coverage for presumed bacterial superinfection is required.

In nonpregnant individuals, use of amantadine, a blocker of the replication of influenza A virus, has been efficacious in preventing symptoms, shortening the clinical disease, and improving pulmonary function. Since this drug has been associated with teratogenic effects in animals, it is not recommended for use in pregnant women.

## PREVENTION

In years of epidemics, it is generally considered advisable to vaccinate pregnant women. However, during the 1977 swine flu vaccination program, pregnancy (in and of itself) was not considered among the high-risk conditions. Influenza vaccines are as immunogenic in pregnant women as in other adults, and no specific complications have been encountered in pregnant women. Because the vaccines are killed virus preparations, they are safe for use during pregnancy.

## HUMAN PARVOVIRUS INFECTION IN PREGNANCY

Human parvovirus (B19) infection, recently recognized as a cause of fetal death, has caused great concern in physicians, public health officials, and pregnant women. Information has been developing rapidly, and this chapter will attempt to summarize the current state of knowledge.

B19, first discovered in England in 1975, is now recognized as the causative agent of erythema infectiosum, a worldwide illness most common in children. B19 is also the primary etiologic agent of transient aplastic crisis in patients with chronic hemolytic anemias. As noted, B19 has been associated with both spontaneous abortions and stillbirths and may be involved in acute arthralgia and arthritis as well as chronic anemia in immunodeficient patients. The virus is a member of the Parvoviridae family.

## CLINICAL FEATURES OF B19 INFECTION

Erythema infectiosum is characterized by a facial rash commonly referred to as "slapped cheek" appearance. There is also a lace-like rash on the trunk and extremities. The rash may also reappear several weeks later, following exposure to temperature, sunlight, and emotional stress. Otherwise, the patient is well at the onset of the rash but may give a history of mild systemic symptoms a few days before the rash's onset. Pruritus may be a common feature in some outbreaks. Erythema infectiosum is more common in the winter and spring and usually lasts approximately 5 to 9 days in children. Headache, fever, anorexia, sore throat, and gastrointestinal symptoms occur in a minority of children. Complications such as lymphadenopathy, arthralgia, or arthropathy rarely occur in children. As with other viral infections (e.g., rubella), erythema infectiosum (also known as "fifth disease") tends to be more severe in adults. Here fatigue, fever, adenopathy, and arthritis are common. There have also been reports of more serious complications, such as encephalitis, pneumonia, and hemolytic anemia.

In investigations of outbreaks, asymptomatic infection has been reported in up to 20% of adults and children. B19 infection is also associated with a condition known as transient aplastic crisis with asymmetrical peripheral polyarthropathy and with severe chronic anemia in patients who are immunodeficient.

The major concern for the obstetrician, however, is infection with B19 in pregnant women. In most of the reported B19 infections during pregnancy, there has been no adverse outcome. However, in some cases fetal death, usually involving hydrops fetalis, has occurred. Preliminary results are now being gathered to estimate the risk of fetal death after maternal B19 exposure.

Studies in both the United States and the United Kingdom have suggested that the risk of fetal death in a woman with documented B19 infection is less than 10%. In data cited by the CDC, a British study reported on 174 pregnant women with IgM antibody to B19, followed prospectively toward delivery.[*] Fetal loss occurred in 17%, but not all fetal deaths resulted directly from B19 infection. An estimate of the number of fetal deaths linked to B19 infection was made by determining whether fetal tissues contained B19 DNA. Tests for B19 DNA were available on a subset of infants who died. By extrapolating these results to all fetal deaths, researchers estimated that fewer than 10% of the 174 B19-infected women might have had a B19-associated fetal loss. In the United States, studies are also ongoing to determine the rate of fetal death. At this time, with 95 pregnant women with IgM antibody to B19 being followed, fetal deaths have so far occurred in 4% of 49 women followed to term, but it is not known whether these fetal deaths were caused by B19 infection. In one instance, the fetus was hydropic. Since antibody status of women may not be commonly available, it is important to estimate the risk of fetal death after exposure. These estimates must take into account the rate of susceptibility in the general population and the risk of infection after exposure. The CDC estimates that if these factors were taken into account, the risk of fetal death would be less than 2.5% after exposure of a pregnant woman to a household member with a documented infection. The upper limit of the risk of fetal death would be less than 1.5% in a pregnant woman who has prolonged exposure to B19 infection in the workplace. Further, it is estimated that the upper limit of risk of fetal death occurring in pregnant women with other types of exposure (e.g., limited exposure to students with erythema infectiosum) would be substantially less.

[*] Centers for Disease Control. Risks associated with human parvovirus B19 infection. MWMR 1989;38(6):81.

Current data suggest that B19 is not responsible for a substantial proportion of fetal deaths in the general population. As noted by Kinney and colleagues, the rate of serologically confirmed B19 infection was the same in a group of 96 stillbirths and in controls (1% each group).** Further, in a survey of 50 fetuses with nonimmune hydrops fetalis, 4 (8%) had positive tests for B19 DNA. There is currently no evidence that the rate of congenital anomalies exceeds background rates following B19 infection. Tissues that are positive for B19 DNA have been identified in 20 fetal deaths and in 17 cases with associated pathologic findings; nonimmune hydrops fetalis was present in all. The mechanism of fetal death is undetermined, but it is likely that severe anemia may precipitate congestive heart failure and hydrops. The fetus appears to be especially vulnerable to B19 infection because fetuses have short red blood cell survival time and the fetal red cell volume expands rapidly.

DNA specific for B19 has been identified in respiratory secretions of viremic patients, suggesting this as a major mode of spread. At the time that erythema infectiosum develops, however, patients are probably past the point of greatest infectiousness. After close contact exposure, the virus appears to be transmitted effectively; during school outbreaks, 10% to 60% of students develop erythema infectiosum. In the settings of outbreaks it is not clear whether the major mode of transmission involves direct contact from person to person, large-particle droplets; small-particle droplets; or fomites. It is also known that the virus can be transmitted parenterally through transfusion and vertically from mother to fetus.

## DIAGNOSIS

Diagnostic testing is available in only a few sites—primarily research laboratories—and through the Centers for Disease Control. At the time of writing, however, the CDC is accepting specimens from only selected patients, including pregnant women exposed to B19 or with symptoms suggestive of B19 and from cases of nonimmune hydrops fetalis probably related to B19 infection. The CDC is not accepting specimens for routine antibody testing. B19 antibody assays are available, with the most sensitive test to detect recent infection being the IgM antibody assay. This can be performed by a captured antibody radioimmunoassay or by enzyme immunoassay. There is also an IgG, B19 antibody assay that is usually positive by the seventh day of illness. IgG persists for years. The IgM antibody, on the other hand, begins to decline after 30 to 60 days. The most sensitive test for detecting the virus is the B19 DNA nucleic acid hybridization.

## TREATMENT AND PREVENTION

Currently, no treatment is available in individuals with presumed B19 infection. They are treated with supportive measures. In otherwise healthy individuals, B19 infection usually produces a mild self-limited infection.

Further, there is no vaccine to prevent B19 infection and no studies have been conducted to assess the value of commercially available immunoglobulin. At this

---

** Kinney JS, Anderson LJ, Farrar J, et al. Risk of adverse outcomes of pregnancy human parvovirus B19 infection. J Infect Dis 1968;157:663.

point, the CDC does not recommend routine prophylaxis with immunoglobulin. In health care settings where exposures to B19 may be possible through contact with patients with B19 infection (such as transient aplastic crisis), the CDC has recommended infection control measures such as admission of patients with transient aplastic crisis due to chronic B19 infection to private rooms. It is noteworthy that most patients with erythema infectiosum are past their period of infectiousness by the time clinical symptoms develop, and these individuals do not present a risk for further transmission. Thus, isolation precautions are not necessary.

Hospital personnel who may be pregnant or who might wish to become pregnant should know about the potential risks to their fetus from exposure to B19 infection. In homes, school, and the workplace, the greatest risk of transmitting B19 occurs before the symptoms of erythema infectiosum develop. Therefore, transmission cannot truly be prevented by excluding contact with persons who have erythema infectiosum. The only measure that is currently recommended is hand washing.

## MANAGEMENT OF THE PREGNANT WOMAN WITH DOCUMENTED INFECTION

For women with documented infection, diagnostic ultrasound examinations and maternal serum α-fetoprotein levels have been employed in an attempt to identify the adversely affected fetus. It is uncertain whether these tests have high sensitivity and specificity. Intrauterine blood transfusion to the fetus has been attempted for the fetus with B19-induced severe anemia, but the benefits of this approach are not yet evaluated. In view of the recentness of the association between B19 infection and adverse pregnancy outcome, there is great concern in the community. Because of great and intensive interest, it is likely that new information will develop shortly.

---

# 13. BACTERIAL, PARASITIC, AND MICROBIAL INFECTIONS IN THE FETUS

---

For practical purposes, there are only two important routes of fetal infection: the ascending, or transcervical route; and the transplacental route. The ascending route, by far the more common, results in intra-amniotic infection and transorificial fetal infections. It is characterized histologically by a polymorphonuclear leukocytic infiltration of the chorion and amnion—"chorioamnionitis," often associated with acute umbilical angiitis. The etiologic agents are usually bacteria.

Transplacentally acquired fetal infections are nearly always secondary to maternal bloodstream infections but may rarely result from spread from the decidua to the fetus, either from a focus of dormant endometritis or by the ascending decidual pathway. Parenchymal placental lesions, chiefly villous inflammation, are the hallmark of transplacental fetal infections. The great majority of transplacental infections are caused by viruses, but bacteria, fungi, protozoa, and helminths have been implicated as well (Table 13-1). (For a more thorough discussion of this topic, please see Chapter 27 in Reece EA, Hobbins JC, Mahoney MJ, and Petrie RH, eds. Medicine of the fetus & mother. J.B. Lippincott, 1992.)

## TRANSPLACENTALLY ACQUIRED BACTERIAL INFECTIONS

## LISTERIOSIS

*Listeria monocytogenes* is a small, aerobic, non-spore-forming, gram-positive rod that is beta-hemolytic on blood agar. Major serotypes causing infection are Ia, Ib, IVa, and IVb. *L. monocytogenes* is widely distributed in the environment and in animals, but the source of human infections is poorly understood. Food-borne outbreaks have been traced to soft cheeses, milk, raw vegetables, and shellfish. Although most maternal infections are mild, *Listeria* infection in pregnancy may result in abortion, preterm labor, and fetal infection, with reported rates of neonatal mortality ranging from 7% to more than 50%.

**TABLE 13-1.** Nonviral Transplacental Fetal Infections

**Bacteria**
*Listeria monocytogenes*
*Mycobacterium tuberculosis*
*Mycobacterium leprae*
*Campylobacter fetus and C. jejuni*
*Salmonella typhi*
*Francisella tularensis*
*Treponema pallidum*
*Borrelia burgdorferi*
*Borrelia hermsii*
*Leptospira*
*Brucella abortus and B. melitensis*
*Yersinia pestis*
*Bacillus anthracis*
*Staphylococcus aureus*
*Coxiella burnetii*

**Protozoa**
*Toxoplasma gondii*
*Plasmodia*
Trypanosomes
*Leishmania donovani*
*Babesia microti*

**Helminths**
*Ascaris lumbricoides*
*Ancylostoma duodenale and Necator americanus*
*Trichinella spiralis*
Schistosomes

**Fungi**
*Cryptococcus neoformans*
*Coccidioides immitis*

Maternal infection with *Listeria* is often asymptomatic, but patients may present with a flu-like syndrome characterized by chills, fever, and back pain, occasionally mimicking a pyelonephritis. Although diarrhea is commonly believed to be a symptom of listeriosis, it was not reported by any pregnant patients in a recent outbreak. Most infected gravidas present with fever, active preterm labor, and brown-stained amniotic fluid that is frequently mistaken for meconium. Intrapartum fetal monitoring commonly shows nonspecific abnormalities.

Both early- and late-onset forms of neonatal listeriosis occur, similar to group B streptococcal infection. The early type presents within 2 days of birth with signs of septicemia and is felt to be due to transplacental infection. The late form of the disease appears after the fifth day of life and usually presents as meningitis.

Maternal listeriosis should be suspected in a pregnant woman with a flu-like syndrome, especially if she has back pain and premature labor. Blood cultures, which are often positive, and vaginal cultures and gram stains should be performed as part of the evaluation of such a patient. Antimicrobial therapy (ampicillin plus gentamicin) of infection diagnosed during pregnancy is essential, since it may prevent fetal infection and its consequences.

Congenital listeriosis should be considered in the differential diagnosis of a depressed preterm infant after a labor complicated by fetal distress and meconium or brown-stained amniotic fluid. A gram stain should be performed of amniotic fluid, the newborn's throat and skin, or eye lesions. Gram stain of a fecal smear from an infected newborn may show the organism in profusion.

Presumptive diagnosis of *Listeria* by gram stain demands immediate institution of therapy. Initial therapy with ampicillin plus gentamicin is recommended, because this combination is highly effective in animal models of *Listeria* infection.

## TUBERCULOSIS

Three prerequisites must be met to establish the diagnosis of congenital tuberculosis:

1. The primary tuberculous complex must be present in the liver.
2. Extrauterine acquisition of infection must be definitely excluded.
3. The tuberculous lesions must be present at birth.

One researcher advises that the diagnosis of congenital tuberculosis be actively sought in neonates born to women with active cavitary, pelvic, or military tuberculosis who are not receiving therapy. Findings in the newborn include loss of appetite, failure to gain weight, progressive bilateral interstitial pneumonia (without abnormal chest auscultation), and ascites.

If the infant is suspected of having congenital tuberculosis, 5 tuberculin units of purified protein derivative (TU PPD) skin testing and chest x-rays should be obtained promptly. Cutaneous tuberculin reactivity is unlikely before 4 to 6 weeks of life and can be delayed for many months. Regardless of the skin test results, treatment of the infant should be initiated promptly with isoniazid and rifampin.

## CAMPYLOBACTER INFECTIONS

The major pathogen of humans, *Campylobacter jejuni*, causes acute enteritis.

*Campylobacter fetus* more commonly causes a prolonged relapsing illness characterized by fevers, chills, myalgias, bacteremia, meningitis, and vascular infections. Infections during pregnancy typically present with upper respiratory symptoms, pneumonitis, fever, and bacteremia. In a review of reported cases of *Campylobacter* infection in pregnancy, some have concluded that abortion, stillbirth, and early neonatal meningitis are due to transplacental spread.

*Campylobacter* enteric infections are treated with fluid and electrolyte replacement and erythromycin. The need for treating septic or bacteremic episodes with agents other than erythromycin has not been established. For patients who appear very toxic, and those with endovascular infections, gentamicin is probably the agent of choice.

## SALMONELLOSIS

Nearly all cases of neonatal salmonellosis are acquired during the perinatal period via the ascending route. Transplacental infection is extremely rare, but it has been reported and is almost exclusively due to *Salmonella typhi*. In uncomplicated gastroenteritis caused by nontyphi *Salmonella* species, antimicrobials do not shorten the duration of disease. In invasive *Salmonella* disease, such as typhoid fever, non–*S. typhi* bacteremia, or *S. choleraesuis* infections, chloramphenicol, ampicillin, or amoxicillin is indicated, depending on susceptibility studies. Chloramphenicol should be avoided near delivery because of "gray syndrome."

Typhoid vaccine is a killed bacterial vaccine that offers some protection for those working or traveling in endemic areas. However, its use is commonly associated with systemic febrile reactions. Since febrile illness has been linked with spontaneous pregnancy loss, typhoid vaccine is not routinely recommended during pregnancy. Emphasis should be placed on water purification techniques and a safe supply of drinking water rather than on typhoid immunization.

## TULAREMIA

*Francisella tularensis*, the causative agent of tularemia, is a small gram-negative coccobacillus. In the United States rabbits are the most important reservoir. Transmission is by indirect contact via insect bites; direct contact with infected animals; ingestion of contaminated, inadequately cooked meat or water; or inhalation of contaminated particles by laboratory technicians working with this highly infectious organism.

Several cases of tularemia during pregnancy, with maternal recovery and subsequent delivery of a normal infant, have been reported. A review of the literature, however, identified only a single case of transplacentally acquired congenital tularemia.

## RELAPSING FEVER

Relapsing fever is a vector-borne bacterial infection characterized by recurring febrile attacks separated by periods of relative well-being. Spirochetes of the genus *Borrelia* cause the disease. Most cases in the United States are caused by *B. hermsii*, transmitted by infective ticks in forested western mountain areas.

Acute infection with relapsing fever during pregnancy often results in spontaneous abortion; in one study 92% of women aborted. The diagnosis of congenital infection requires both the onset of disease prior to the third day of life (the incubation prior of relapsing fever is 3 to 10 days), and the demonstration of spirochetes in peripheral blood smears or placental tissue. Some recommend examining stained placental sections in suspected cases of congenital relapsing fever as a rapid and sensitive method for accurate diagnosis of this disease. Warthin-Starry silver stains and a standard acridine orange stain are both effective.

## LYME DISEASE

Lyme disease is a tick-borne illness caused by a newly identified spirochete, *Borrelia burgdorferi*. In the United States there are three distinct foci of Lyme disease: the northeastern states from Massachusetts to Maryland, the upper midwestern states of Minnesota and Wisconsin, and four western states, including parts of California, Oregon, Nevada, and Utah. Lyme disease usually begins with a characteristic skin lesion, erythema chronicum migrans, accompanied by a flu-like syndrome and neurologic abnormalities, including headache, photophobia, dysesthesias, and stiff neck. Some patients later develop cardiac abnormalities, such as atrioventricular heart block or myopericarditis, neurologic complications, or intermittent attacks of arthritis.

Because Lyme disease is caused by a spirochete, there has been understandable concern about the effect of maternal Lyme disease on the fetus and the risk of transplacental transmission of infection. Preliminary epidemiologic data have begun to emerge.

Twenty-two cases of Lyme disease in pregnancy have been reported to date. Although these 22 cases undoubtedly represent an incomplete picture of the impact of Lyme disease on pregnancy, several observations seem appropriate:

1. The frequency of adverse outcomes in reported cases, 7 of 22, or 32%, warrants close surveillance and epidemiologic and laboratory studies of pregnant women with Lyme disease.
2. Although no specific congenital anomaly has been associated with Lyme disease, cardiac abnormality would appear the most likely candidate.
3. Although antibiotic treatment of gravidas with Lyme disease is strongly endorsed, such treatment apparently will not always ensure a normal outcome.
4. Even classical symptoms or signs of Lyme disease may be overlooked by the patient and her physician unless they are informed about disease manifestations and the potential implications in pregnancy.
5. Because results of serologic tests for Lyme disease are often negative during the first several weeks of infection, the diagnosis of Lyme disease should be made on the basis of clinical criteria, and treatment should be begun immediately. Many obstetricians now regularly prescribe prophylactic treatment for deer tick bites during pregnancy. Antibiotic therapy for clinical disease is often chosen according to the stage of disease. Oral antibiotics are administered for the rash and flu-like symptoms of early Lyme disease; intravenous antibiotics are used if the disease is recognized later, when the patient is suffering from arthritic or neurologic complications. However, other physi-

cians feel it is best to administer intravenous treatment immediately to a pregnant woman with Lyme disease at any stage. The most common oral regimen is amoxicillin 500 mg tid or penicillin V 500 mg qid, given for 3 or more weeks. Intravenous therapy can be either 20 million units of penicillin G given in divided doses every 4 hours for 2 to 3 weeks, or ceftriaxone 2 g once daily for 14 to 21 days.

It would seem prudent for pregnant women to avoid tick exposure assiduously in endemic areas.

At the time of delivery of women who have acquired Lyme disease during pregnancy, the placenta should be examined microscopically for spirochetes.

## LEPTOSPIROSIS

*Leptospira* produce a group of syndromes with protean manifestations, including fever, headache, chills, severe malaise, vomiting, myalgia, and conjunctivitis. Intrauterine infection of the human fetus has been demonstrated. Although case reports clearly document the occasional occurrence of transplacental infection, it is likely that the majority of fetal wastage observed is secondary to maternal disease rather than to direct fetal involvement.

## BRUCELLOSIS

The rarity of human fetal wastage resulting from maternal *Brucella* infection, as compared with the common problem in domestic animals, may be explained by the lack of the carbohydrate erythritol in the human placenta. This substance is the preferred nutrient for growth of the brucellae species and is present in the placentas of animal hosts who commonly abort as a major manifestation of the illness.

## PLAGUE

The fetal wastage resulting from maternal infection with plague probably results from the systemic effects of illness rather than from direct placental or fetal infection. However, true intrauterine infection with *Yersinia pestis*, the plague bacillus, has been described.

## ANTHRAX

In 1923, a case of probable transplacental *Bacillus anthracis* infection was reported with the following documentation: positive maternal cultures at necropsy, positive cultures from fetal heart blood and liver, and typical long gram-positive bacilli in the microscopic sections of fetal liver.

## COMMON AEROBIC BACTERIA

Although aerobic bacteria such as group B streptococci and *Escherichia coli* are by far the commonest causes of ascending fetal infection, they are virtually unmentioned in the etiology of transplacental infection. A single report, published in

1951, describes a case of intrauterine meningitis and hydrocephalus caused by *Staphylococcus aureus*.

Whether the common aerobic bacteria are truly rare causes of transplacental fetal infection or transplacental infection caused by them is mistakenly interpreted as resulting from ascending infection is not addressed in the literature.

## Q FEVER

Q fever is a zoonosis caused by the rickettsia *Coxiella burnetii*. In humans the illness is characterized by fever to 40°C (104°F), chills, malaise, myalgia, chest pain, and occasionally pneumonia and hepatitis. Humans are usually infected by inhaling infectious aerosols.

*C. burnetii* has been isolated from placentas and breast milk of mothers who acquired Q fever from 3 years to 2 months before delivery. The most compelling evidence for transplacental infection in humans was given by a report in which the cord serum of four infants had high levels of IgM antibodies specific for *C. burnetii*. The children were normal at birth. A recent report describes a 19-year-old woman with a history of spontaneous abortions and delivery of abnormal children. At 29 weeks gestation she gave birth to an infant who died at 6 days of age. An elevated titer of antibody to phase II antigen was demonstrated in the serum obtained from the infant's blood. Serum from the mother had positive titers of both phase I and phase II antigens.

## TRANSPLACENTALLY ACQUIRED PROTOZOAL AND HELMINTHIC INFECTIONS

### MALARIA

Malaria causes an increased rate of abortions and is the most important cause of low birth weight in the tropics. Premature labor may begin during a malarial attack or shortly thereafter, probably as a response to maternal fever and systemic illness.

Evidence that malaria causes stillbirths is sparse. Fetal distress is said to be common in mothers with acute malaria and may be caused by high fever or hypoglycemia.

Congenital malaria has been reported for all four species of *Plasmodia* and is more common among infants of women who have clinical attacks of malaria during pregnancy than in those with chronic subclinical infections. Additionally, placental infection is much more common than congenital infection, indicating that the placenta serves as a relatively effective barrier to fetal infection.

For most North American women, travel represents the only real threat of acquiring malaria. In areas where chloroquine-sensitive *P. falciparum* is present, prophylactic regimens that are safe in pregnancy have been developed. Pregnant women must realize, however, that no prophylactic regimen can ensure complete protection against malaria, that the most severe complications of malaria are more common in pregnant women, and that these drug regimens occasionally produce unwanted side effects.

In areas where chloroquine-resistant *P. falciparum* is present there is no safe regimen for pregnant women and travel should be avoided unless the need is imperative. Barry has recently reviewed malarial prophylaxis in pregnancy. Detailed recommendations for the prevention of malaria may be obtained 24 hours a day by calling the CDC Malaria Hotline at (404) 332-4555.

## AFRICAN SLEEPING SICKNESS

African trypanosomiasis (African sleeping sickness) is caused by *Trypanosoma brucei gambiense* or *Trypanosoma brucei rhodesiense*. Congenital transmission of African trypanosomiasis has infrequently been reported, with most cases caused by *T. gambiense* infection. Vertical transmission of the parasite is proved if the infant of an infected mother has never been in an endemic area or if the parasite is found in the newborn within 5 days of birth.

The diagnosis of congenital infection can be made if parasites are found in the infant's peripheral blood or cerebrospinal fluid (CSF). High IgM levels in serum and CSF are also noted, although newborns may have normal CSF IgM levels in spite of the presence of parasites in the CSF.

## CHAGAS' DISEASE

Chagas' disease (American trypanosomiasis) is caused by the flagellate *Trypanosoma cruzi*. It occurs from the southern portion of the United States to Argentina. *T. cruzi* is transmitted to humans by insect vectors, by blood transfusion, and transplacentally.

Congenital transmission may occur during any stage of maternal disease. Maternal parasitemia is greatest in the acute phase of the infection, but this period of intense parasitemia is brief. Thus, most congenital infections occur in infants born to women who may be asymptomatic but have the chronic form of the disease.

Congenital Chagas' disease may cause abortion, prematurity, intrauterine growth retardation, and intrauterine and neonatal death. Congenital infections occur in 1% to 4% of women with serologic evidence of having had Chagas' disease and are very rare among infants with a birth weight of greater than 2500 g. Congenitally infected low-birth-weight infants can be either premature or small for gestational age. Symptoms may be present from birth or develop days, weeks, or even months later. Early-onset jaundice, anemia, and petechiae are common. Hepatosplenomegaly, cardiomegaly with congestive heart failure, esophageal involvement with regurgitation, myxedematous edema, and encephalitis with convulsions have been described in congenitally infected infants.

The diagnosis of congenital Chagas' disease in the newborn is based on the demonstration of trypomastigotes in the circulating blood. When available, cord blood should be centrifuged and examined directly. Otherwise the leukocyte layer obtained from a microhematocrit tube should be examined. In stillbirths and neonatal deaths, the diagnosis is based upon histologic examination of the placenta and fetal tissues.

No satisfactory chemotherapy for Chagas' disease is currently available; nifurtimox is being evaluated. Information regarding treatment can be obtained from the Parasitic Disease Division, Centers for Disease Control, Atlanta, Georgia.

## VISCERAL LEISHMANIASIS (KALA-AZAR)

Leishmaniasis is the general name given to infection caused by any member of the protozoan genus *Leishmania* and includes visceral, cutaneous, and mucocutaneous syndromes. *L. donovani* is the etiologic agent responsible for visceral leishmaniasis (kala-azar, Dumdum fever, Assam fever, or infantile splenomegaly), which is characterized by a subacute or chronic course with fever, hepatosplenomegaly, anemia, leukopenia, hyperglobulinemia, and progressive emaciation.

Two probable cases of transplacentally acquired visceral leishmaniasis have been reported.

## AMEBIASIS

Amebiasis is caused by a protozoan, *Entamoeba histolytica*, that is found in all areas of the world. There are no reported cases of congenital amebiasis and no well-documented data on direct fetal morbidity due to maternal amebiasis. Amebiasis affects the fetus indirectly, causing premature labor and possibly stillbirth, when severe electrolyte imbalances or shock occur in the mother.

## BABESIOSIS

Babesiosis is a protozoan tick-borne disease of domestic and wild animals that is occasionally transmitted to humans. Most case reports in the United States have come from Long Island, Nantucket, and Martha's Vineyard. A single case of transplacentally acquired babesiosis has recently been reported. The infant was delivered by cesarean section 1 week after the mother was bitten by a tick. Although the mother remained asymptomatic, the infant became ill 1 month after birth, developing fever, hepatosplenomegaly, anemia, and thrombocytopenia. *Babesia microti* organisms were found in the infant's erythrocytes, although the mother's peripheral blood smears at the time of delivery and 1 month later revealed no parasites.

## ASCARIASIS

A single case of congenital ascariasis was reported in 1972. Thus, the most plausible explanation seems to be transplacental transmission—migration of the larvae from the mother's intestine to the maternal lymphatics and bloodstream, to the placenta and into the fetal circulation, then to the fetus's small intestine, where they developed into adult worms.

## OTHER INTESTINAL NEMATODES

Neither whipworm infection (*Trichuris trichiura*) nor pinworm infestation (*Enterobius vermicularis*) is associated with transplacental transmission, since systemic migration of larvae does not occur. Congenital hookworm infection (*Ancylostoma duodenale, Necator americanus*) was first reported in 1917.

## TRICHINOSIS

Trichinosis is a well-known zoonotic parasitic infection caused by the tissue nematode *Trichinella spiralis*. Infection results from the consumption of undercooked meat of animals infected with *T. spiralis* cysts. *T. spiralis* has been identified in the placenta, and sporadic reports of intrauterine infection by *Trichinella* have been published.

## SCHISTOSOMIASIS

Several trematodes (blood flukes) of the genus *Schistosoma* can infect human beings. The most frequently encountered species are *S. haematobium, S. japonicum*, and *S. mansoni*. *Schistosoma* infection of the placenta has been sporadically reported. Although the frequency of placental infection is as high as 25% in endemic areas, the infestations are light and cause little histologic reaction. A cause-and-effect relationship between schistosomiasis and abortion, prematurity, and intra-uterine growth retardation has yet to be clearly demonstrated.

## OTHER TREMATODE INFECTIONS

Trematode infections other than schistosomiasis (i.e., fasciolopsiasis, heterophyiasis, metagonimiasis, clonorchiasis, opisthorchiasis, fascioliasis, and paragonimiasis) produce no known adverse effects on the fetus.

## CANDIDIASIS

Despite the frequency with which *Candida* species colonize the pregnant vagina, reports of fetal *Candida* infections are rare. Only 50 cases have been reported since the first definite case was described in 1958. The method of transmission is not entirely clear, but ascending infection through either ruptured or even intact membranes seems most likely. Although candidemia has been reported during pregnancy, hematogenous transmission from mother to fetus has never been described. Thus, fetal *Candida* infections are *not* transplacentally acquired.

The hallmark of fetal *Candida* infection is the presence of discrete rounded yellow plaques, varying in size from 0.5 to 2 mm, on the surface of the umbilical cord and membranes.

One additional feature of congenital fetal *Candida* infection is worthy of note. The majority of such gestations are complicated by the presence of an intrauterine foreign body, either a retained intrauterine contraceptive device or, less commonly, a cervical suture.

## TRANSPLACENTALLY ACQUIRED FUNGAL INFECTIONS

### CRYPTOCOCCOSIS

Infection with *Cryptococcus neoformans* follows inhalation of the fungus; the respiratory tract is the primary focus of infection. Hematogenous dissemination may then occur to any organ in the body, the central nervous system being the most common site of infection following dissemination. The fact that bloodstream dissemination occurs suggests the potential for transplacental spread in pregnancy. Data regarding congenital cryptococcosis are extremely scanty, but six infants who developed this infection in the first month of life have been reported. All these neonates died, and in each, organisms with the morphologic appearance of *Cryptococcus* were identified by microscopic examination of tissue obtained at autopsy or by culture. Miller has reviewed these cases.

## COCCIDIOIDOMYCOSIS

Coccidioidomycosis is caused by *Coccidioides immitis,* a dimorphic fungus.

Primary infection may be entirely asymptomatic or may resemble an acute influenzal illness with fever, chills, cough, and pleural pain. Disseminated coccidioidomycosis is a progressive, frequently fatal granulomatous disease characterized by lesions and abscesses throughout the body, especially in subcutaneous tissues, skin, bone, peritoneum, thyroid, and the CNS. An estimated 1 in every 1000 cases of symptomatic coccidioidomycosis becomes disseminated. Dissemination is more common in blacks, in Filipinos, and during pregnancy. In pregnancy both the incidence of dissemination (10%) and its resultant mortality (90%) rise markedly.

Although coccidioidal dissemination occurs frequently during pregnancy, with occasional invasion of the placenta, infants are nearly always born free of infection. A few cases of transplacental fetal coccidioidomycosis have been reported. It has been speculated that the infrequency of congenital infection reflects the limitation of infection to the placenta because of either the size of the coccidioidal spherules, resulting in their physical exclusion from the fetal circulation, or the severity of the host reaction, resulting in thrombosis of the adjacent vascular spaces and generation of an acute inflammatory response.

# 14. ANTIBIOTICS AND OTHER ANTIMICROBIAL AGENTS IN PREGNANCY AND DURING LACTATION

## PENICILLINS

The penicillins have a wide margin of safety and lack toxicity for both the pregnant woman and the fetus. Adverse effects, however, may include nausea, epigastric distress, diarrhea, and candidal vaginitis. (For a more thorough discussion of antibiotics and antimicrobial agents in pregnancy and during lactation, please see Chapter 28 in Reece EA, Hobbins JC, Mahoney MJ, and Petrie RH, eds. Medicine of the fetus & mother. J.B. Lippincott, 1992.)

There is no evidence that penicillin or its derivatives are teratogenic. There is little experience in pregnancy with the new penicillins such as piperacillin, mezlocillin, and azlocillin. These drugs, therefore, should be used in pregnancy only when another, better-studied antibiotic is not effective.

## PHARMACOLOGY

The pharmacokinetics of the penicillin group of antibiotics have been relatively well studied. Several studies have revealed that the serum levels of these drugs are lower and their renal clearance is higher throughout pregnancy when compared to the nonpregnant state.

The transplacental passage of penicillin is by simple diffusion. The free circulating portion of the antibiotic crosses the placenta, resulting in a lower maternal serum level of the unbound portion of the drug.

At term maternal serum and amniotic fluid concentrations of penicillin G are equal at 60 to 90 minutes after intravenous administration, representing rapid passage into the fetal circulation and amniotic fluid. Continuous intravenous infusions have caused equal concentrations of penicillin G at 20 hours in maternal serum, cord serum, and amniotic fluid. Ampicillin rapidly crosses the placenta, and fetal serum levels can be detected within 30 minutes, and equilibrate in an hour.

Amoxicillin is similar to ampicillin in its spectrum of activity but is stable in the presence of gastric acid and may be given without regard to meals. It has been used effectively as a 3-g single dose to treat bacteriuria in pregnancy.

Methicillin crosses rapidly into the fetal circulation and amniotic fluid. Following a 500-mg intravenous dose over 10 to 15 minutes, equilibration has occurred within 1 hour in fetal tissues.

Carbenicillin crosses the placenta and distributes to fetal tissues. Following a 4-g intramuscular dose, mean peak concentrations in cord and maternal serum have occurred at 2 hours and have been similar. Ticarcillin rapidly crosses the placenta into the fetal circulation and amniotic fluid.

Oxacillin and dicloxacillin cross the placenta only in low concentrations because of the high degree of maternal protein binding. Cord serum and amniotic fluid levels of oxacillin were less than 0.3 µg/mL in 15 of 18 patients given 500 mg orally 0.5 to 4 hours prior to cesarean section. Following a 500-mg intravenous dose of dicloxacillin, the peak fetal serum level was only 8% of the maternal peak level.

Most penicillins are primarily excreted unchanged in the urine with only small amounts being inactivated in the liver. This is of significance in patients with impaired renal function, which requires reduction in dosage.

## BREAST-FEEDING

Penicillin G and ampicillin are excreted into breast milk in low concentrations. There are three problems that theoretically might be seen in the nursing infant:

1. Modification of bowel flora (possible diarrhea, candidiasis)
2. Allergic response
3. Interference with the interpretation of culture results

The benefits of continued breast-feeding usually outweigh these potential risks.

# CEPHALOSPORINS

The use of cephalosporins in obstetrics has been extensive. They are used as prophylactic agents in cesarean section and in the treatment of septic abortion, pyelonephritis, and amnionitis.

There is no evidence of teratogenicity of these agents. The third-generation agents have had limited use during pregnancy.

## PHARMACOLOGY

Maternal serum levels attained with these drugs during pregnancy are lower than those in nonpregnant patients receiving equivalent dosages, due to a shorter half-life in pregnancy and an increased volume of distribution. This is true not only for well-established cephalosporin drugs (e.g., cephalothin, cephalexin, and cephazolin), but also for the newer cephalosporins (e.g., cephoxitin, cephradine, and cefuroxime).

These drugs readily cross the placenta to the fetal bloodstream and ultimately the amniotic fluid.

Transplacental transfer of these drugs is fairly rapid, and adequate bactericidal concentrations are attained in both fetal soft tissues and the amniotic fluid. Repeated high-bolus doses of cephalosporins have been shown to result in higher levels in fetal serum and amniotic fluid than continuous intravenous infusions of the same amount of drug.

## BREAST-FEEDING

The cephalosporins are excreted into breast milk in sufficiently low concentrations that the infant receives an insignificant dose. Although the same theoretical concerns exist as with penicillins, the advantages of continued breast-feeding during treatment usually outweigh these risks.

## SULFONAMIDES

The sulfonamides are often used for treatment of urinary tract infections in pregnancy. Among 1455 human infants exposed to sulfonamides during the first trimester, no teratogenic effects were noted (Heinonen, Slone, and Shapiro, 1977).*

The administration of sulfonamides should be avoided in glucose-6-phosphate dehydrogenase-deficient women. A dose-related toxic reaction may occur in these individuals, resulting in red cell hemolysis.

The sulfonamides compete with bilirubin for binding sites on albumin, thus raising the levels of free bilirubin in the serum and increasing the risk of hyper-bilirubinemia or kernicterus in the neonate. For that reason it is recommended that an alternate antibiotic be used in the third trimester, if possible.

---

* Heinonen PO, Slone D, Shapiro S. Birth defects and drugs in pregnancy. Littletone, MA: Publishing Sciences Group, 1977.

## PHARMACOLOGY

The sulfonamides are easily absorbed orally, and they readily cross the placenta, achieving fetal plasma levels 50% to 90% of those attained in the maternal plasma.

## USE WITH TRIMETHOPRIM

Sulfa is often given with trimethoprim in treatment of urinary tract infections. Controlled trials have failed to show any increased risk of birth defects after first trimester exposure.

## SULFASALAZINE

Sulfasalazine is used for treatment of ulcerative colitis and Crohn's disease because of its relatively poor oral absorption. However, it does cross the placenta to the fetal circulation, with fetal concentrations approximately the same as maternal concentrations, although both are low. Neither kernicterus nor severe neonatal jaundice has been reported following maternal use of sulfasalazine, even when the drug was given up to the time of delivery.

## BREAST-FEEDING

Sulfonamides are excreted into breast milk in low concentrations (less than 1% of the maternal dose) and so breast-feeding is usually continued during administration of these drugs.

## NITROFURANTOIN

Nitrofurantoin is an antimicrobial agent used in the treatment of acute uncomplicated lower urinary tract infections as well as for long-term suppression in patients with chronic bacteriuria. Nitrofurantoin is capable of inducing hemolytic anemia in patients deficient in G6PD. No reports linking the use of nitrofurantoin with congenital defects have been located.

## PHARMACOLOGY

Nitrofurantoin absorption from the gastrointestinal tract varies with the form administered. The macrocrystalline form is absorbed more slowly than the crystalline and is associated with less gastrointestinal intolerance. Therapeutic serum levels are not achieved; therefore, this drug is not indicated when there is a possibility of bacteremia.

## BREAST-FEEDING

Nitrofurantoin is excreted into breast milk in very low concentrations.

## TETRACYCLINES

The tetracyclines readily cross the placenta and are firmly bound by chelating to calcium in developing bone and tooth structures. This produces brown discoloration of the teeth, hypoplasia of the enamel, inhibition of bone growth, and other skeletal abnormalities. The yellowish brown staining of the teeth usually occurs in the second or third trimesters of pregnancy after 24 weeks. Alternate antibiotics are currently recommended during pregnancy. Hepatotoxicity has been presumed to be an overdose effect and has not been reported with brief courses of therapy at lower doses. First trimester exposure to tetracycline has not been found to have any teratogenic risk in the Collaborative Perinatal Project.

## BREAST-FEEDING

Tetracycline is excreted into breast milk in low plasma concentrations. There is high binding of the drug to calcium and protein, limiting absorption from the milk.

## AMINOGLYCOSIDES

Aminoglycosides are commonly used with penicillin or clindamycin in the treatment of postpartum endometritis, septic abortion, or endometritis. They should be given during pregnancy only when serious gram-negative infections are suspected. Gentamicin is preferred over tobramycin and amikacin, since it has been more extensively studied.

Streptomycin and kanamycin have been associated with congenital deafness in the offspring of mothers who took these drugs during pregnancy. Ototoxicity may be increased with simultaneous use of ethacrynic acid.

Nephrotoxicity may be increased when the drug is given in combination with cephalosporins, and this should be avoided. Neuromuscular blockade may be potentiated by the combined use of these drugs and curariform drugs. Potentiation of magnesium sulfate-induced neuromuscular weakness has also been reported in a neonate exposed to magnesium sulfate and gentamicin. No known teratogenic effect is associated with the use of these drugs in the first trimester other than ototoxicity.

## PHARMACOLOGY

The aminoglycosides are poorly absorbed after oral administration and are rapidly excreted by the normal kidney. Because the rate of clearance is related to the glomerular filtration rate, dosage must be reduced in the face of abnormal renal function.

The serum aminoglycoside levels are usually lower in pregnant than in non-pregnant patients receiving equivalent doses due to more rapid elimination. Thus, it is important to monitor levels to prevent subtherapeutic dosing.

## BREAST-FEEDING

Aminoglycosides are known to be excreted in low levels into breast milk. Since oral absorption of these drugs by the infant is poor, ototoxicity or other side effects would not be expected.

## ERYTHROMYCIN

Erythromycin is the alternate drug of choice to penicillin for many diseases in pregnancy, including gonorrhea or syphilis, and is used for primary treatment for other diseases, such as mycoplasma and chlamydia. It is also an adequate substitute in the treatment of urinary tract infection, provided the urine can be adequately alkalized.

Erythromycin estolate has been associated with subclinical reversible hepatotoxicity during pregnancy. Thus, other forms that are felt to be relatively nontoxic are usually recommended. No teratogenic risk of erythromycin has been reported.

## PHARMACOLOGY

Erythromycin and its salts are not consistently absorbed from the gastrointestinal tract of pregnant women, and their transplacental passage is unpredictable. Both maternal and fetal serum levels achieved after the administration of the drug in pregnancy are low and vary considerably. Thus, some authors have recommended that penicillin be administered to every newborn whose mother has received erythromycin for the treatment of syphilis.

## BREAST-FEEDING

Erythromycin is excreted into breast milk in small amounts.

## CLINDAMYCIN

Clindamycin should be used in pregnancy only when anaerobic infections are suspected that are not sensitive to other antibiotics. If diarrhea develops during the administration of this drug, the patient should be evaluated for the possibility of pseudomembranous colitis, which has been reported in up to 10% of patients. No reports linking the use of clindamycin with congenital defects have been noted.

## PHARMACOLOGY

Clindamycin crosses the placenta, achieving maximum cord serum levels of about 50% of the maternal serum. It is 90% bound to serum protein, and fetal tissue levels increase following multiple dosing. Maternal serum levels after dosing at various stages of pregnancy are similar to those of nonpregnant patients.

## BREAST-FEEDING

Clindamycin is excreted into breast milk in low levels, and nursing is usually continued during administration of this drug.

## METRONIDAZOLE

Several studies have failed to show any increase in the incidence of congenital defects or other adverse pregnancy outcomes among newborn infants of mothers treated with metronidazole during pregnancy. Because of the controversy surrounding this drug, deferring therapy until after the first trimester is probably wise.

## PHARMACOLOGY

Metronidazole crosses the placenta to the fetus throughout gestation with a cord: maternal plasma ratio at term of approximately 1.0.

## BREAST-FEEDING

Metronidazole is excreted into breast milk in small amounts. The American Academy of Pediatrics recommends interrupting breast-feeding after a single 2 g oral dose for 12 to 24 hours to allow clearance of the drug.

## LINDANE (QUELL)

Toxicity in humans after topical use of 1% lindane has been observed almost exclusively after overexposure to the agent. However, about 10% of the dose is recovered in the urine after application to the skin. Since this drug is a potent neurotoxin, its use during pregnancy should be limited. The manufacturer recommends no more than two treatments during pregnancy. Pregnant women should be advised to wear gloves when shampooing their children's hair. Alternate drugs are usually recommended, specifically pyrethrins with piperonyl butoxide (RID).

## PHARMACOLOGY

## BREAST-FEEDING

No reports describing the use of lindane in lactating women have been noted. However, the amount of lindane ingested in breast milk would be less than the amount absorbed from direct topical application to the infant.

## PYRETHRINS WITH PIPERONYL BUTOXIDE (RID)

Topical absorption is poor, so potential toxicity should be less than that with lindane.

## ANTIFUNGAL AGENTS

No risk has been confirmed with use in pregnancy. Clotrimazole has not been implicated as a teratogen. Miconazole is also absorbed in small amounts from the vagina. Use in pregnancy is not known to be associated with congenital malformations. Use of these drugs should be postponed until after the first trimester, if possible, for theoretical reasons.

# PART VI. FETAL DIESEASES: GENETIC DISORDERS

## 15. DISORDERS OF FETAL HEMOGLOBIN AND BLOOD CELLS

### BLOOD AND BLOOD-FORMING TISSUES

#### PRODUCTION SITES

Embryonic red blood cell production starts by 2 weeks after conception. The original site of production is the yolk sac, but at 7 to 9 fetal weeks (9 to 11 menstrual weeks) production switches to the fetal liver, and production of white blood cells and platelets begins. At midgestation, hematopoiesis begins in the bone marrow and rapidly increases to fill the marrow; concurrently, hematopoiesis in the liver decreases. The site changes are thought to occur by progressive seeding of totipotential stem cells, first from the yolk sac to the liver and then from the liver to the bone marrow.

#### HEMOGLOBIN

The peripheral red blood cell is one of the most specialized cells in the body: 95% of its protein is hemoglobin. Hemoglobin has four subunits, each containing one iron atom attached to a porphyrin ring to form heme, which is attached to a globin chain. Each hemoglobin molecule's four globins consists of two pairs of identical chains.

The globins are divided into the alpha-like globins, with genes located on chromosome 16, and the beta-like globins, with genes located on chromosome 11. The alpha-like family includes an embryonic form (zeta) and an adult form (alpha). The beta-like family includes an embryonic form (epsilon), a fetal form (gamma), a major adult form (beta), and a minor adult form (delta). Through development there is a progression from embryonic hemoglobins, Gower I ($\zeta_2\epsilon_2$), Portland ($\zeta_2\gamma_2$), and Gower II ($\alpha_2\epsilon_2$), to fetal hemoglobin ($\alpha_2\gamma_2$), to adult hemoglobins ($\alpha_2\beta_2$ and $\alpha_2\delta_2$).

#### COAGULATION

##### Hemophilia A (Factor VIII Deficiency)

Hemophilia A is the most common example of a coagulation-factor deficiency that produces severe clinical manifestations. Its estimated incidence is 1 in 10,000 Caucasian male births. It is transmitted as an X-linked deficiency of factor VIII.

 E. Albert Reece, John C. Hobbins, Maurice, J. Mahoney and Roy H. Petrie (Eds). *Handbook of Medicine of the Fetus & Mother.* Copyright © 1995 by J.B. Lippincott Company

Despite greatly improved replacement therapy, hemophilia A continues to exact a heavy medical and socioeconomic cost. This has produced an increased demand for prenatal diagnosis.

Originally, prenatal diagnosis of hemophilia A was done by fetal blood sampling and determining factor VIII activity by coagulant and antigen determinants. More than 200 male fetuses at risk were tested using this method. However, since the isolation of the factor VIII gene, almost all prenatal diagnoses of hemophilia A have been made using recombinant DNA techniques.

### Hemophilia B (Factor IX Deficiency)
About 15% of patients with hemophilia have hemophilia B. Its clinical manifestations are similar to those of hemophilia A, and the disease is also inherited as an X-linked trait. Dozens of at-risk fetuses have been tested using immunologic and coagulant tests. The gene for factor IX has been cloned and intragenic probes used for recombinant DNA prenatal diagnoses. More recently, gene amplification by the polymerase chain reaction, followed by DNA sequencing to identify the mutation in specific families, has been applied to carrier testing and prenatal diagnosis.

### Von Willebrand's Disease
Von Willebrand's disease, a relatively common and usually mild autosomal dominant trait, is characterized by a prolonged bleeding time and abnormalities of the factor VIII complex. Rarely, homozygosity for the von Willebrand's gene or a severe form of the disease leads to a request for prenatal diagnosis. Fetal blood samples have been used successfully to identify both unaffected and affected fetuses, using coagulant activity and immunologic measurements.

## RED BLOOD CELLS

## HEMOGLOBINOPATHIES

### Alpha Thalassemia
The thalassemias are hereditary microcytic anemias caused by defects in the rate of hemoglobin synthesis. Each thalassemia is named for the globin chain that is insufficiently produced. The diseases are inherited as autosomal recessive traits; thalassemia minor is the carrier state, thalassemia major the affected homozygote.

Alpha thalassemia major is a lethal fetal disorder; only a few liveborns have been reported. The hydrops fetalis and markedly enlarged edematous placenta associated with the fetal disorder produces a 50% incidence of preeclampsia in the mother. This has been a significant factor in the drive to provide prenatal diagnosis for women with at-risk pregnancies. Originally, prenatal diagnosis was done by analyzing fetal blood samples for globin chain synthesis and composition by carboxymethyl cellulose columns, electrophoresis, or high-performance liquid chromatography. However, the advent of recombinant DNA techniques has caused a drop in the number of diagnoses made by fetal blood sampling and an increase in prenatal diagnoses for alpha thalassemia.

### Beta Thalassemia
The fetus with beta thalassemia major does well in utero because gamma globin is the predominant beta-like globin produced, but the switch to beta globin produc-

tion after birth causes a corresponding decrease in hemoglobin level. The infant rapidly becomes dependent on transfusions.

The severity of this disorder has led to prenatal diagnosis of more than 10,000 at-risk fetuses. Prenatal diagnosis methods are essentially the same as for alpha thalassemia and have progressed from globin chain synthesis in fetal blood samples to recombinant DNA techniques.

### Structurally Abnormal Hemoglobins

The most significant clinically is sickle-cell disease. This includes homozygotes for hemoglobin S and also the mixed heterozygotes for hemoglobin S and either another beta globin structural variant or one of the beta thalassemias.

The methodology for prenatal diagnosis has undergone the same changes as described for the thalassemias.

### Methemoglobinemia

Congenital methemoglobinemia is due to homozygous deficiency of red blood cell NADH-diaphorase (methemoglobin reductase), which normally reduces methemoglobin. The disease has two presentations. Type I, which is due to an enzyme deficiency only in red blood cells, is a benign treatable condition. Type II, which is due to an enzyme deficiency in all cells, is associated with a progressive neurologic disorder that is lethal. Because the status of the fetus at risk for type II methemoglobinemia is reflected in amniocytes, prenatal diagnosis is possible.

## MEMBRANE ABNORMALITIES

### Spherocytosis

In the United States the incidence is about 1 in 4500. Spherocytosis is most likely due to a structural or functional abnormality in spectrin. The hemolytic anemia is successfully treated by splenectomy. The trait is inherited in an autosomal dominant fashion.

### Elliptocytosis

These include disorders inherited in an autosomal dominant mode and are generally clinically mild.

## METABOLIC ABNORMALITIES

### Hexose Monophosphate Shunt

The most common enzyme deficiency of this group is X-linked glucose-6-phosphate dehydrogenase deficiency.

### Glycolysis Disorders

There are eight enzymes in the Embden-Meyerhof glycolysis pathway whose deficiencies produce variable hemolysis. All are inherited as autosomal recessive traits (except phosphoglycerate kinase, which is X-linked).

## OTHER DISORDERS

### Fanconi Anemia

Fanconi anemia is an autosomal recessive disorder characterized clinically by progressive pancytopenia, variable physical abnormalities, and a predisposition to the development of malignancies. Prenatal diagnoses have been done on dozens of at-risk fetuses by examining amniocytes or chorionic villus cells for spontaneous and diepoxybutane-induced chromosome breakage.

### Blackfan-Diamond Syndrome

Blackfan-Diamond syndrome is an autosomal recessive disorder characterized by pure red blood cell anemia due to a congenital deficiency of erythroid precursors.

## LYMPHOCYTES

### Bare Lymphocyte Syndrome

The bare lymphocyte syndrome, characterized by an absence of lymphocyte surface antigens, has been diagnosed by membrane immunofluorescence using monoclonal antibodies for HLA class I and II molecules.

### Agammaglobulinemia

X-linked agammaglobulinemia has been excluded by examining B lymphocytes with a monoclonal antibody in fetal blood.

### Severe Combined Immunodeficiency

The diagnosis of severe combined immunodeficiency (SCID) has been reported by fetal blood analysis. This diagnosis is performed by enumeration of T and B lymphocytes using specific monoclonal antibodies and functional evaluation of phytohemagglutinin-induced T-cell proliferation in fetal blood obtained at 18 to 20 menstrual weeks. Because of the heterogenous nature of this disorder, the specific defect must be well characterized in a specific family.

## GRANULOCYTES

### Chronic Granulomatous Disease

Chronic granulomatous disease causes recurrent pyogenic infections with catalase-positive organisms due to impaired activation of neutrophil oxygen metabolism. This disorder has been diagnosed using fetal granulocytes' presence or absence of nitroblue tetrazolium reduction, which measures superoxide production.

### Chédiak-Higashi Disease

Chédiak-Higashi syndrome, a generalized disorder of cellular dysfunction, is characterized by large neutrophil cytoplasmic granules and an increased susceptibility to pyogenic infections. This autosomal recessive disorder has been excluded in three at-risk fetuses.

## PLATELETS

### Thrombocytopenia Absent Radius Syndrome

Thrombocytopenia absent radius syndrome is an autosomal recessive disorder that may also include bilateral aplasia of the radii, renal and cardiac malformations, and an allergy to cow's milk. This disorder has been prenatally diagnosed by demonstration of absent radii at 16 to 20 menstrual weeks.

### Wiskott-Aldrich Syndrome

Wiskott-Aldrich syndrome is an X-linked disorder that presents in the first year of life with thrombocytopenia, eczema, and recurrent infections. Fatal hemorrhage, infection, or a malignant reticuloendothelioma is common. Recently, the gene for Wiskott-Aldrich has been mapped to a 20-centimorgan region on the X chromosome. Schwartz and coworkers have reported first trimester prenatal diagnoses of the syndrome by using flanking markers (DXS7 and DXS14) with more than 98% accuracy.*

### Glanzmann Thrombasthenia

Glanzmann thrombasthenia, a rare autosomal recessive disorder, is characterized by a normal platelet count but a lack of ADP-induced platelet aggregation, causing severe bleeding. This abnormality has been analyzed by fetal blood sampling for prenatal diagnosis.

### Bernard-Soulier Syndrome

Bernard-Soulier syndrome, an autosomal recessive disorder of platelet adhesion, is characterized by a prolonged bleeding time and very large platelets.

### Grey Platelet Syndrome

The Grey platelet syndrome, a rare defect of platelet alpha granules, has been prenatally excluded by measuring platelet beta thromboglobulin, which is reduced in this disorder.

---

*Schwartz M, Mibashan RS, Nicolaides KH, et al. First-trimester diagnosis of Wiskott-Aldrich syndrome by DNA markers. Lancet 2:1405.

# PART VII. FETAL DISEASES: PRENATAL DIAGNOSIS OF CONGENITAL ANOMALIES

## 16. PRENATAL DIAGNOSIS OF ANOMALIES OF THE HEAD AND NECK AND CENTRAL NERVOUS SYSTEM

### HYDROCEPHALUS

#### INCIDENCE AND CLASSIFICATION

The incidence of congenital hydrocephalus ranges between 0.3 and 1.5 in 1000 births in different series. Hydrocephalus can result from pathologic entities that differ both in etiology and clinical course. In our experience, fetal ventriculomegaly usually enters one of three main entities: triventricular hydrocephalus (which may result from both aqueductal stenosis or communicating hydrocephalus), Dandy-Walker malformation, and hydrocephalus associated with other cerebral anomalies (most frequently, disorders of dorsal induction, disorders of ventral induction, and disruptive lesions).

#### ETIOLOGY AND RECURRENCE RISK

Congenital infections and genetic factors are both involved in the pathogenesis of aqueductal stenosis. Infectious agents include toxoplasmosis, syphilis, cytomegalovirus, mumps, and influenza virus. Many familial cases indicate an X-linked pattern of transmission that is thought to account for 25% of lesions occurring in males. Multifactorial etiology has also been suggested. Congenital tumors such as gliomas, pinealomas, and meningiomas cause aqueductal stenosis by external compression.

Communicating hydrocephalus usually results from failure of reabsorption of cerebrospinal fluid. A multifactorial etiology with a recurrence risk of 1% to 2% has been suggested. Communicating hydrocephalus in its most typical manifestation is characterized by a variable degree of enlargement of the entire ventricular system associated with dilatation of the subarachnoid spaces.

The etiology of Dandy-Walker malformation is still unclear. Genetic factors probably play a major role. An autosomal recessive transmission is implicated in at least some instances. More recently, this view has been challenged, and a multi-

E. Albert Reece, John C. Hobbins, Maurice, J. Mahoney and Roy H. Petrie (Eds). *Handbook of Medicine of the Fetus & Mother*. Copyright © 1995 by J.B. Lippincott Company

factorial etiology with an empiric recurrence risk of 1% to 5% has been advocated. Dandy-Walker malformation is frequently associated with other nervous system abnormalities, such as agenesis of corpus callosum, systemic anomalies such as congenital heart disease (mainly ventricular septal defects), polydactyly-syndactyly, cleft palate, and polycystic kidneys. It may also be related to a number of genetic and nongenetic syndromes that have been extensively reviewed.

## PATHOLOGY

In aqueductal stenosis, outlet obstruction of the third ventricle results in severe enlargement of the lateral and third ventricles (triventricular hydrocephalus). In communicating hydrocephalus, at least in early stages, distention of the lateral, third, and fourth ventricles (tetraventricular hydrocephalus) is seen in association with enlarged subarachnoid cisterns. In advanced stages, however, the fourth ventricle and subarachnoid cisterns may appear normal or even small, probably as a consequence of the compression operated by the large lateral ventricles.

Dandy-Walker malformation is featured by the association of three distinct anomalies: hydrocephalus, a retrocerebellar cyst, and a defect in the cerebellar vermis through which the posterior fossa cyst communicates with the fourth ventricle.

Despite the classical definition, it has been demonstrated that in 80% of cases hydrocephalus is absent at birth and develops only after several months or years.

## PRENATAL DIAGNOSIS

Since macrocrania usually does not develop until late in gestation, head measurements are unreliable, and the identification of hydrocephalus should depend on the direct demonstration of enlargement of the ventricular system. Nomograms of the normal size of frontal horns, atria, and occipital horns of the lateral ventricles throughout gestation are now available. Several authors have demonstrated that a qualitative evaluation of the intracranial structures is most useful in cases of early hydrocephalus. In early hydrocephalus, the choroid plexus cyst is shrunken and anteriorly displaced, thus being clearly detached from the medial wall (Fig. 16-1). This simple approach is very effective in screening for fetal hydrocephalus.

Once hydrocephalus has been recognized, the site of the obstruction may be inferred by identifying the enlarged portion of the ventricular system. Marked dilatation of the lateral and third ventricles suggests aqueductal stenosis (Fig. 16-2). Tetraventricular enlargement in the presence of a normal cerebellar vermis associated with distention of the subarachnoid cisterns suggests communicating hydrocephalus (Fig. 16-3). A defect in the cerebellar vermis through which the fourth ventricle communicates with a posterior fossa cyst indicates Dandy-Walker malformation (Fig. 16-4). An attempt to differentiate the anatomical type of hydrocephalus should always be made, since each form carries a different prognosis. In most cases, however, distinction between aqueductal stenosis and communicating hydrocephalus is not possible, as has been demonstrated by noncontrast computed tomographic studies in infants.

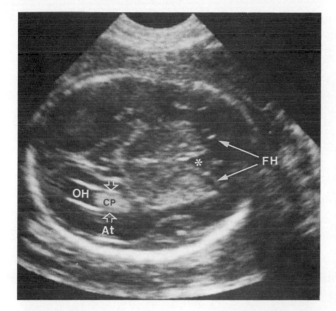

**FIGURE 16-1.** Axial scan of the fetal head at the level of frontal horns (FH), atria (At), and occipital horns (OH) of lateral ventricles. The choroid plexus (CP) fills the atrium entirely, being closely apposed to both the medial and lateral wall (*open arrows*). (*, cavum septi pellucidum.)

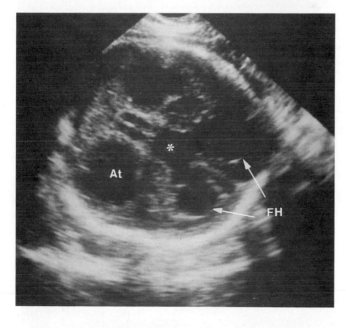

**FIGURE 16-2.** Fetal triventricular hydrocephalus. Gross enlargement of the lateral ventricles and particularly of the third ventricle (*). The fourth ventricle appeared small. The infant was found at birth to have aqueductal stenosis. (FH, frontal horns; At, atria of lateral ventricles).

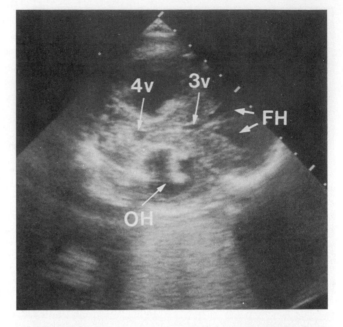

**FIGURE 16-3.** Fetal tetraventricular hydrocephalus. Enlargement of the frontal and occipital horns of lateral ventricles (FH, OH) and of the third ventricle (3v) is attested to by this scan. There is also questionable enlargement of the fourth ventricle (4v). This infant was found at birth to have communicating hydrocephalus.

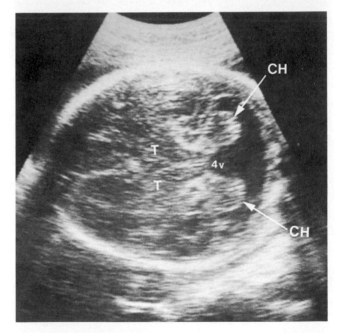

**FIGURE 16-4.** Fetal Dandy-Walker malformation. A wide defect is seen at the level of the cerebellar vermis. Through this defect the cystic cisterna magna amply communicates with the area of the fourth ventricle (4v). The cerebellar hemispheres (CH) are widely separated. (T, thalami.)

## PROGNOSIS AND MANAGEMENT

Neurosurgical studies of infants with aqueductal stenosis indicate a mortality rate ranging between 10% and 30%. According to recent experience, isolated communicating hydrocephalus carries a good prognosis. Infants with Dandy-Walker malformation have an overall mortality rate ranging between 12% and 26% and an IQ above 80 in 30% to 40% of cases. Much work has been done trying to correlate the outcome of ventriculomegalic infants with the extent of ventricular enlargement. At present, the outcome of affected infants seems to depend more on the nature of the underlying lesion than on the degree of ventriculomegaly.

Difficulties in establishing a reliable prognosis in utero are reflected in uncertainties in electing the proper obstetrical management. When the diagnosis of hydrocephalus is made prior to viability, many parents would probably request termination of pregnancy. When this option is not accepted, and in those cases recognized later on in pregnancy, a thorough discussion with the couple of the possible choices is recommended. Many authors feel that delivery as soon as fetal maturity is achieved and prompt neurologic treatment will maximize the chances of survival and normal development for the affected infants. A cesarean section is recommended in those cases with associated macrocrania. As a chance of normal intellectual development appears possible, cephalocentesis to allow vaginal delivery in cases of fetopelvic disproportion is strongly contraindicated, in view of the significant risk associated with such procedure.

## DISORDERS OF DORSAL INDUCTION

### INCIDENCE

The incidence of neural tube defects varies considerably according to geographic and ethnic factors. A figure of 1 in 1000 to 2000 births is commonly quoted for the general population. In South Wales, the frequency rises to about 7 in 1000 births.

### ETIOLOGY AND PATHOGENESIS

Failure of closure of the anterior (anencephaly) or posterior (spina bifida) neuropore has been advocated by the vast majority of authors.

### PATHOLOGY

Spina bifida is subdivided into occulta and aperta. Spina bifida occulta is characterized by vertebral schisis covered by normal soft tissues. Spina bifida aperta is characterized by a defect of the skin, underlying soft tissues, and vertebral arches exposing the neural canal. The defect may be covered by a thin meningeal membrane (meningocele). In the presence of neural tissue inside the sac the lesion is defined as a *myelomeningocele*, a term often used to indicate all cases of spina bifida aperta. The defect may vary considerably in size. The lumbar, thoracolumbar, or sacrolumbar areas are most frequently affected. Spina bifida aperta is almost always associated with a typical intracranial malformation (Arnold-Chiari type II) consisting of displacement of the cerebellar vermis, fourth ventricle, and medulla oblongata through the foramen magnum inside the upper cervical canal.

The term *cephalocele* indicates a protrusion of intracranial contents through a bony defect of the skull. Encephaloceles are characterized by the presence of brain tissue inside the lesion. When only meninges protrude, the term *cranial meningocele* should be used. Cephaloceles often cause impaired cerebrospinal fluid circulation and hydrocephalus. Massive encephaloceles may be associated with microcephaly.

## PRENATAL DIAGNOSIS

Anencephaly was the first congenital anomaly recognized in utero by ultrasound. The diagnosis is easy and relies on the demonstration of the absence of the cranial vault. Because the fetal head can be positively identified by modern ultrasound equipment as early as the first trimester, anencephaly is recognizable at that time.

We are not aware of cases of spina bifida occulta diagnosed in utero by ultrasound. Open defects can be recognized by demonstrating the defect of the neural arches and overlying soft tissues. The accuracy of ultrasound in predicting fetal spinal lesions is a critical issue. The predictive value of the technique largely depends on the quality of the equipment, the experience of the operator, and the amount of time dedicated to any single patient. No data are available with regard to level 1 or basic untargeted examinations. However, there is little doubt that the sensitivity of these examinations is quite low. Level 2 examinations on patients at risk because of either familial history or elevated α-fetoprotein are much more accurate.

Sonologists have focused recently on the evaluation of intracranial anatomy in fetuses with spina bifida. Several reports indicate that typical cranial signs are consistently found. These findings include frontal bossing (the "lemon sign"), hypoplasia of the posterior fossa structures, attested by an abnormal configuration of the cerebellum (the "banana sign"), an abnormally reduced transverse cerebellar diameter, failure to recognize the cerebellum, and obliteration of the cisterna magna. These signs can be demonstrated easily even by less experienced sonographers and are therefore potentially useful for sonographic mass screening of spina bifida.

Fetal cephaloceles should be suspected when a paracranial mass is seen on sonography. The diagnosis of encephaloceles is easy, since the presence of brain tissue inside the sac is striking on ultrasound. Differentiation of a cranial meningocele from soft-tissue edema or a cystic hygroma of the neck may be difficult. Demonstration of the bony defect in the skull would allow a proper diagnosis, but cranial meningoceles are often associated with extremely small (a few millimeters) defects that are not amenable to antenatal sonographic recognition. Certain clues can assist a correct diagnosis. Cranial cephaloceles are very often associated with ventriculomegaly. Cystic hygromas arise from the region of the neck, have multiple internal septations and a thick wall, and are often associated with generalized soft-tissue edema and hydrops. Some cephaloceles protrude through the base of skull inside the pharynx. These lesions are obviously inaccessible to prenatal ultrasound identification unless derangement of intracranial morphology is present. Becaue cephaloceles are often associated with other anomalies, a careful investigation of the entire fetal anatomy is recommended.

## PROGNOSIS AND MANAGEMENT

Anencephaly is invariably fatal. The outcome for infants with spina bifida is dictated by the site and extension of the lesion. The mortality is high, with the 7-year survival rate being only 40% despite early treatment. Many of the survivors will suffer from significant disabilities, such as lower limb paralysis or dysfunction and incontinence. The association of spina bifida and severe hydrocephalus was traditionally considered a poor prognostic factor for intellectual development More recent studies indicate that in many cases control of intracranial hypertension by shunting results in a normal and even superior intelligence.

The outcome of infants with cephalocele is primarily related to the presence or absence of brain tissue inside the lesion. Encephaloceles carry a neonatal mortality rate of about 40% and an incidence of intellectual impairment and neurologic sequelae of 80%. Infants with cranial meningoceles develop a normal intelligence in 60% of cases.

Since anencephaly is an invariably fatal lesion, termination of pregnancy can be offered at any time in pregnancy. When the diagnosis of spina bifida is made prior to viability, termination of pregnancy can be offered to the parents. When this is refused, and in those cases recognized later or in gestation, an attempt to identify the site and the extent of the lesion should be made to give a tentative prognosis. Options should be discussed with the couple. Several reports indicate that birth injury is frequent in fetuses with spina bifida and represents a major prognostic shortcoming. Therefore, cesarean delivery is recommended.

When a prenatal diagnosis of cephalocele is made, termination of pregnancy can be offered prior to viability. In continuing pregnancies, a cesarean section should be considered to avoid birth trauma. However, since infants with massive encephaloceles and microcephaly have a dismal prognosis, conservative management can be offered in these cases.

## DISORDERS OF VENTRAL INDUCTION

The term *ventral induction* refers to the interrelated developmental events that occur in the embryonic forebrain starting from the fifth week of gestation and that lead to the separation of the cerebral hemispheres and to the formation of the midline structures. The differentiation of these nervous structures is closely related to the development of the midface. Disorders of ventral induction include a group of midline cerebral defects that encompass a wide spectrum of severity and are typically associated with craniofacial malformations.

## HOLOPROSENCEPHALY

### INCIDENCE

The incidence of holoprosencephaly is unknown because milder forms are probably unrecognized. An incidence of 4 in 1000 abortions has also been reported, suggesting a high intrauterine fatality rate from this defect.

### PRENATAL DIAGNOSIS

Several cases of sonographic antenatal diagnosis of holoprosencephaly have been reported in the literature. A variety of findings has been described. In our experience, the most valuable finding was the demonstration of the single primitive ventricle, which was possible in all cases. We were also able to recognize the dorsal sac, when present, and to predict facial anomalies such as cyclopia, hypotelorism, anophthalmia, arhinia, and proboscis and median cleft lip. Demonstration of facial anomalies strengthens the diagnosis of holoprosencephaly based on central nervous system findings. Conversely, should any of the aforementioned facial features be serendipitously encountered, a careful examination of the intracranial contents is recommended.

### PROGNOSIS AND MANAGEMENT

The invariably poor prognosis for infants affected by alobar and semilobar holoprosencephaly is well established. Although precise prognostic figures are not available, infants with the lobar variety may have both a normal lifespan and a normal intelligence.

When either alobar or semilobar holoprosencephaly is identified in utero, termination of pregnancy can be offered prior to viability. A conservative management is strongly recommended in continuing pregnancies. The prognosis of lobar holoprosencephaly is unclear, and this is reflected in uncertainties about obstetric management.

## AGENESIS OF THE CORPUS CALLOSUM

### INCIDENCE

The incidence of agenesis of the corpus callosum is highly controversial and depends mainly on the techniques used to ascertain it. Figures ranging from 1 in 100 to 1 in 19,000 have been reported.

### ETIOLOGY

The etiology is unknown.

### PRENATAL DIAGNOSIS

The criteria for the postnatal diagnosis of agenesis of the corpus callosum by diagnostic imaging techniques, such as ventriculography, computed tomography, and ultrasound, are well established. The bodies of the lateral ventricles are invariably widely separated, and the atria and occipital horns are enlarged (colpocephaly). The third ventricle is frequently enlarged and dorsally extended, being found at the same level as or higher than the bodies of lateral ventricles (Fig. 16-5).

## PROGNOSIS AND MANAGEMENT

Establishing a reliable prognosis for agenesis of the corpus callosum is extremely difficult. Many patients suffer from mental retardation and neurologic abnormalities—including increased muscle tone and seizures—and are psychologically abnormal. However, in some cases the condition is totally asymptomatic. Difficulties in assessing the prognosis are reflected in uncertainties as to parental counselling and obstetrical management.

A careful search for associated anomalies, including echocardiography and karyotyping, is mandatory. Termination of pregnancy can be offered prior to viability, but the parents should be informed that there is a chance of entirely normal intellectual and neurologic development. In continuing pregnancies, no specific obstetric management is required. Agenesis of the corpus callosum may be associated with macrocephaly. In these cases, a cesarean delivery is definitely indicated.

## DESTRUCTIVE CEREBRAL LESIONS
### PORENCEPHALY

#### Incidence and Etiology
The incidence of porencephaly is rare. The etiology is unknown. The acquired form may be the consequence of thrombosis of cerebral vessels resulting from embolization or infection.

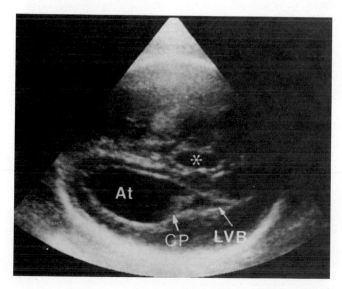

**FIGURE 16-5.** Colpocephaly demonstrated by an axial scan of the head in a fetus with agenesis of the corpus callosum. The atria of lateral ventricles (At) are considerably enlarged; the bodies of lateral ventricles (LVB) are normal in size but widely separated. The third ventricle is enlarged and displaced upward, thus resulting in a median cystic structure (*) that can be seen at the same level as the bodies of the lateral ventricles. (CP, choroid plexus.)

## Pathology

The term *porencephaly* refers to a condition in which cystic cavities are found within the brain matter. It may be either the consequence of a morphogenetic disorder (true porencephaly or schizencephaly) or the result of an intrauterine or postnatal destructive process (pseudoporencephaly or encephaloclastic porencephaly).

## Prenatal Diagnosis

Prenatal sonographic identification of intracerebral cystic cavities is easy (Fig. 16-6), but the differential diagnosis with intracranial cysts of different nature, such as arachnoid cysts and congenital tumors, may be impossible.

## Prognosis and Management

Both true porencephaly and congenital pseudoporencephaly are severe anomalies with a dismal prognosis. The vast majority of patients are affected by severe mental retardation and important neurologic sequelae such as blindness and tetraplegia.

When a confident diagnosis of porencephaly is made prior to viability, termination of pregnancy should be offered to the parents. In continuing pregnancies, conservative obstetric management is recommended.

## HYDRANENCEPHALY

### Incidence

Hydranencephaly is very rare.

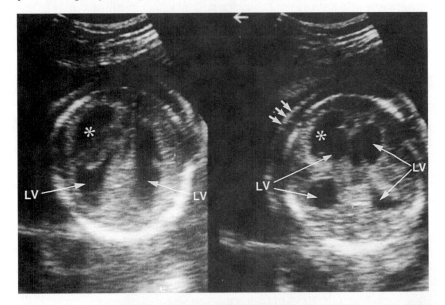

**FIGURE 16-6.** Porencephaly in a second trimester fetus with multiple anomalies and nonimmune hydrops. The lateral ventricles are enlarged (LV) and loss of cerebral tissue in the parietal region can be appreciated (*). Significant scalp edema is present (*arrowhead*).

## Etiology and Pathogenesis
Hydranencephaly is thought to result from an intrauterine destructive process and may be considered an extreme form of pseudoporencephaly.

## Prenatal Diagnosis
Even if replacement of intracranial structures with fluid is easily detected by antenatal sonography, certain identification of hydranencephaly may be difficult. The differential diagnosis includes severe hydrocephalus and holoprosencephaly. However, even in the most devastating forms of ventriculomegaly, it is possible to demonstrate the falx cerebri and some spared cortex. In alobar holoprosencephaly, the falx is absent, but a crescent-shaped frontal cortex can usually be seen. In hydranencephaly, the falx is absent or incomplete in the vast majority of cases. In our experience, the most valuable finding for a specific diagnosis is the demonstration of the bulb-like brain stem, which, in the absence of the surrounding cortex, bulges inside the fluid-filled intracranial cavity (Fig. 16-7). The sonographic appearance is somewhat similar to that of the hypoplastic thalami that can be seen in cases of alobar or semilobar holoprosencephaly. Obviously, confusion between holoprosencephaly and hydranencephaly is without serious consequences, since both conditions share a dismal prognosis and the obstetrical management does not differ.

## Prognosis and Management
Prognosis is poor. Long survival has been reported. However, these infants are obviously incapable of any intellectual achievement. When a confident diagnosis of hydranencephaly is made in a fetus, conservative management is suggested.

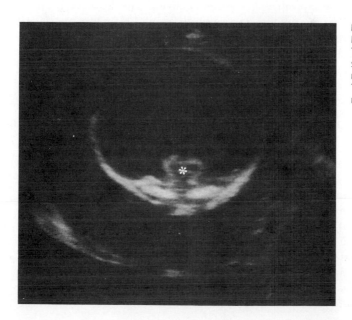

**FIGURE 16-7.**
Hydranencephaly. The cerebral hemispheres are entirely replaced by fluid. The brain stem (*) is relatively spared.

## MICROCEPHALY

### DEFINITION AND INCIDENCE

Some authors suggest that we use as a diagnostic criterion a head circumference two standard deviations below the mean. Others believe that a threshold of three standard deviations below the mean should be used. Differences in diagnostic modalities probably account for the wide variability of the incidence of this condition reported in different studies. Figures ranging from 1.6 in 1000 births to 1 in 25,000 to 50,000 can be found in the literature.

### ETIOLOGY

The etiology is extremely heterogeneous. Microcephaly should be considered not as a separate entity but as a symptom of many etiologic disturbances. Genetic and environmental causative factors are both well accepted, and the reader is referred to the extensive reviews on the subject.

### PRENATAL DIAGNOSIS

Many difficulties arise in attempting to identify fetal microcephaly. The utility of head measurements alone is limited, since these can be markedly biased by factors such as incorrect dating or intrauterine growth retardation. Furthermore, the natural history of fetal microcephaly is largely unknown. A comparison of biometric parameters, such as the ratio of head circumference to abdominal circumference and the ratio of femur length to biparietal diameter, has been suggested. Nevertheless, both false-positive and false-negative diagnoses have been reported. It is clear that the predictive value of ultrasound biometry has several limitations at present. A qualitative evaluation of the intracranial structures is a very useful adjunct to biometry, since cerebral malformations are found in a significant proportion of infants with microcephaly. Measurement of the fetal frontal lobe may assist the diagnosis (Fig. 16-8).

### PROGNOSIS AND MANAGEMENT

Establishing a reliable prognosis for infants affected by microcephaly is difficult. Associated anomalies obviously have a major influence on the outcome. Controversial clinical data exist with regard to isolated microcephaly. Even if it is hard to derive precise prognostic figures, there is evidence that a small head size does not necessarily imply mental retardation.

When a confident prenatal diagnosis of microcephaly is made in a pregnancy at risk, the couple will most likely request termination of pregnancy. A conservative management is certainly indicated also in cases of fetal microcephaly with associated cerebral or extracerebral anomalies. A confident diagnosis of isolated microcephaly in a pregnant patient who has no risk factors occurs quite rarely in our experience. The infrequency of these observations is responsible for an uncer-

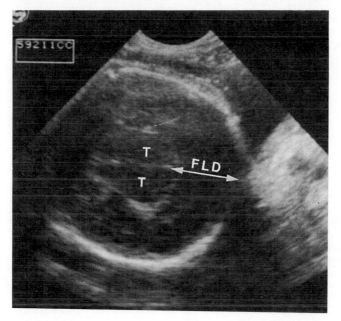

**FIGURE 16-8.** Reduction of the frontal lobe distance (FLD) in a fetus with severe microcephaly. (T, thalami.)

tainty in obstetrical management. In any case, it is necessary to remember that infants with a small head may have a normal intelligence and that at present there is no established correlation between head measurement and intellectual development.

## CHOROID PLEXUS CYSTS

### INCIDENCE

Prenatal sonographic identification of choroid plexus cysts has been reported with increasing frequency (Fig. 16-9). Although other authors have reported a very low incidence of fetal choroid plexus cysts, we have documented this finding in almost 3% of routine second trimester sonograms.

### ETIOLOGY

The etiology is unknown.

### PATHOLOGY

Although choroid plexus cysts are a frequent finding in antenatal sonography, there are no pathologic studies in the literature. It is commonly assumed that fetal choroid plexus cysts demonstrated with sonography are probably the same entity as the "neuroepithelial" cysts that have been described in autopsy studies of adults (i.e., simple fluid-filled cysts lined by normal choroid plexus tissue).

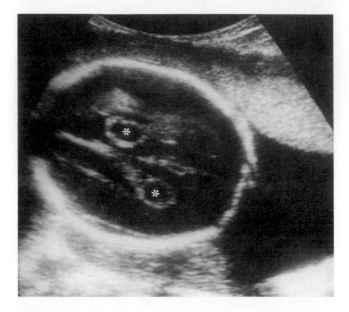

**FIGURE 16-9.** Bilateral choroid plexus cysts in a second trimester fetus.

## PRENATAL DIAGNOSIS

Choroid plexus cysts can be easily demonstrated with sonography (see Fig. 16-4). In most cases, the cyst is single and unilateral. However, bilateral cysts are very frequently seen. Rarely, bizarre clusters of multiple cysts can be found.

## PROGNOSIS AND MANAGEMENT

Although the pediatric literature indicates that small choroid plexus cysts have no clinical significance, their detection in utero may increase the risk of chromosomal aberrations, and specifically of trisomy 18.

In our early experience, all cases with choroid plexus cysts and trisomy 18 had associated malformations that were easily detected with ultrasound (congenital heart disease and skeletal abnormalities were the most frequent findings). Identification of a choroid plexus cyst is an indication for a careful survey of fetal anatomy. Current experience indicates that in the presence of a normal karyotype the prognosis is excellent. However, serial sonographic examinations are suggested, since a disproportionate increase of the cyst with symptoms of intracranial pressure has been described in rare cases.

# 17. FETAL THORACIC MALFORMATIONS

Fetal thoracic malformations represent a relatively rare group of potentially lethal congenital anomalies. Traditionally, these conditions have received relatively little attention, possibly because they are rare or because sonographic visualization of these structures is complicated by acoustic shadowing of the fetal limbs, making prenatal diagnosis difficult. However, in recent years improvement in real-time ultrasonography has permitted the prenatal diagnosis of a variety of congenital malformations, including thoracic anomalies, and this has led to the increasing interest in this group of developmental abnormalities.

Aberrant development in the normal sequence of events will result in a variety of malformations, as outlined in Table 17-1.

## BRONCHOGENIC CYSTS

### ETIOPATHOLOGY

Bronchogenic cysts arise from abnormal budding of the laryngotracheal tube. They often remain attached to the tracheobronchial tree and are found in the area of the trachea, mediastinum, or pulmonary lung tissue. When aberrant budding occurs in early bronchial development, these cysts assume a periesophageal or mediastinal location in about 30% of cases. If development occurs later, intra-parenchymal lesions are observed in about 70% of the cases. These cysts may be single or multiple, contain a mucoid fluid, and are lined by pseudostratified columnar epithelium. The lower lobes are more often involved than the upper lobes; however, right and left lung fields and male and female fetuses are equally affected.

### PRENATAL DIAGNOSIS

Sonographic diagnosis of intraparenchymal lesions requires identification of thin-walled sonolucent cysts without associated diaphragmatic defect or echodense septae (Fig. 17-1). When these lesions are suspected, other potential defects should be excluded, such as diaphragmatic hernia or macrocystic adenomatoid malformations. If the lesion is mediastinal, a greater challenge may be experienced, because midline lesions such as goiters, teratomas, and vascular malformations must be excluded.

### MEDICAL MANAGEMENT AND OUTCOME

Prenatal diagnosis of intrathoracic cysts should not evoke a need for any special medical management. Ultrasound examinations throughout pregnancy are advised in order to look for evidence of hydrops or polyhydramnios. It is most important that these infants be immediately evaluated postnatally so that, if

E. Albert Reece, John C. Hobbins, Maurice, J. Mahoney and Roy H. Petrie (Eds).
*Handbook of Medicine of the Fetus & Mother*. Copyright © 1995 by J.B. Lippincott Company

**TABLE 17-1.** Intrinsic Intrathoracic Malformations

Bronchogenic cysts
  Isolated
  Coexisting cardiac and thoracic anomalies
Congenital cystic adenomatoid malformations
  Macrocystic
  Microcystic
Bronchopulmonary sequestration
  Intralobar
  Extralobar
Primary pulmonary hypoplasia (scimitar syndrome)
Congenital pleural effusion (chylothorax/hydrothorax)
  Idiopathic
  Inheritable (possibly X-linked)

Modified from Reece EA, Lockwood CJ, Rizzo N, Pilu G, Boviccelli L, Hobbins JC. Intrinsic intrathoracic malformations of the fetus: sonographic detection and clinical presentation. Obstet Gynecol 1987;70:627, with permission.

necessary, respiratory assistance can be initiated immediately and medical or surgical management promptly instituted.

Bronchogenic cysts may be well tolerated, especially if they appear as isolated lesions. They can, however, cause postnatal obstruction of bronchioles, leading to recurrent respiratory tract infection or airway compression. Following surgical excision of these lesions, infants often do very well.

## CYSTIC ADENOMATOID MALFORMATION

### ETIOPATHOLOGY

This is a unilateral hamartoma that usually presents during the first day of life, often as a serious respiratory emergency. These patients present clinically in three

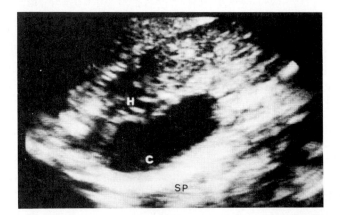

**FIGURE 17-1.** Bronchogenic cyst. Longitudinal section of the fetal chest demonstrating a large unilocular cyst (C) posterior to the heart (H). Spine (SP) is located posterior to the cyst. (From Reece EA, Lockwood CJ, Rizzo N, Pilu G, Bovicelli L, Hobbins JC. Intrinsic intrathoracic malformations of the fetus: sonographic detection and clinical presentation. Obstet Gynecol 1987;70:628.)

ways: stillborn, or neonatal or perinatal death; progressive respiratory distress in the newborn; and acute or chronic pulmonary infection in the older infant and child. Fetal anasarca and maternal polyhydramnios are characteristically associated antepartum features of this lesion.

Morphologically and pathologically this lesion has been categorized into three subtypes. Type I typically has one large cystic cavity with trabeculations of the wall, with smaller cavities adjacent to normal lung parenchyma. In type II, there are multiple small cysts of up to 1 cm in diameter. Type III is predominantly solid. All three types share common histologic features: an adenomatoid increase in terminal bronchiolar structures; a polypoid configuration of the cuboidal/columnar epithelium lining the cystic structures; an increase in elastic tissue in areas lined by cuboidal/columnar epithelium, often associated with polypoid projections; and absence of inflammation.

There is aberrant lymphatic drainage with this lesion, resulting in pleural effusion and hydrops. Progressive worsening of this disorder with increased fluid accumulation would enhance the likelihood of pulmonary hypoplasia.

Polyhydramnios is a commonly associated feature of cystic adenomatoid malformations resulting from either esophageal obstruction or excessive lung fluid production. There has also been an association between maternal hydramnios and fetal anasarca. The reported incidence of maternal hydramnios occurring in association with cystic adenomatoid malformation varies from 30% to as much as 80%.

## PRENATAL DIAGNOSIS

Prenatal diagnosis of macrocystic tumors requires identifying small peripheral cysts (Fig. 17-2). The microcystic variety poses more of a challenge and appears as an echodense mass replacing the lung (Fig. 17-3). Both types may result in a significant shift of the mediastinum with cardiac displacement.

Type III cystic adenomatoid malformations have been described previously. The finding of a solid, space-occupying lung lesion with gross mediastinal shift and often associated with maternal polyhydramnios and fetal hydrops but without other detectable associated anomalies should raise the possibility of congenital cystic adenomatoid malformation.

## MEDICAL MANAGEMENT AND OUTCOME

Respiratory distress and cyanosis are the common initial signs in the vast majority of children born with cystic adenomatoid malformation. The respiratory distress is believed to be due to compression and displacement of the normal pulmonary tissue. Management will depend on the time of diagnosis and the presence or absence of hydrops or polyhydramnios. In the absence of hydrops or polyhydramnios, the outcome is quite good, and repeated thoracentesis has been shown to improve the chance of survival. The fetus, however, that is anomalous and has hydrops or associated polyhydramnios has an extremely poor prognosis.

The prognosis is better for patients with the macrocystic variety, who have an overall survival rate as high as 70% compared to 20% with the microcystic lesion. Fetuses without associated anomalies, hydrops, or pulmonary hypoplasia tend to

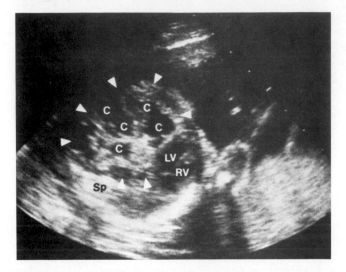

**FIGURE 17-2.** Macrocystic adenomatoid malformation. Transverse section through the fetal thorax demonstrating dextrorotation of the fetal heart (LV, left ventricle; RV, right ventricle) caused by a large, multilocular cystic mass (C) (*outlined by arrowheads*). Spine (SP) is located posteriorly. (Romero R, Chervenak FA, Kotzen J, et al. Antenatal sonographic findings of extralobar pulmonary sequestrations. J Ultrasound Med 1982;1:131.)

have a better outcome. The survival rate for the type I lesion is 69%, whereas the mortality rate for type III has been almost 100%. The mortality rate for the latter appears to be related to the extreme mediastinal shift associated with circulatory and respiratory embarrassment.

Almost all infants with congenital adenomatoid malformation have respiratory distress. Respiratory functions compromised by pulmonary hypoplasia or by compression of the thoracic viscera can result in heart failure.

There is a tendency for this cystic mass to expand progressively after birth, leading to air trapping. Immediate surgical decompression, the treatment of choice, has been shown to be well tolerated by infants. Survival depends on both the extent of the hypoplasia and the state of lung maturation.

## BRONCHOPULMONARY SEQUESTRATION

### ETIOPATHOLOGY

Bronchopulmonary sequestration is a rare thoracic defect in which a systemic artery supplies an accessory or dysplastic segment of lung.

The sequestration of pulmonary tissue has been defined as masses of pulmonary tissue that have no communication with the bronchial tree. Within the subgroups there are three types:

1. Intralobar, that is, part of the lobe of a lung
2. Extralobar, that is, a separate lobe still attached to the main pulmonary mass
3. Complete sequestration, that is, entirely independent of the lungs

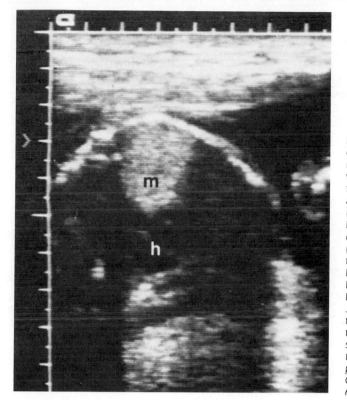

**FIGURE 17-3.** Microcystic adenomatoid malformation. Transverse section of the fetus demonstrating an echodense mass (m) filling the right hemithorax. The mediastinum and heart (h) are deviated to the left. (From Reece EA, Lockwood CJ, Rizzo N, Pilu G, Bovicelli L, Hobbins JC. Intrinsic intrathoracic malformations of the fetus: sonographic detection and clinical presentation. Obstet Gynecol 1987;70: 631.)

## PRENATAL DIAGNOSIS

Sonographic prenatal diagnosis of either form (intralobar or extralobar), although possible, may be difficult and requires a certain degree of sophistication. The extralobar lesion may present as a discrete, echodense lesion in the left costaphrenic sulcus (Fig. 17-4). Prenatal diagnosis of the intralobar variety does not seem feasible at this time.

## MEDICAL MANAGEMENT AND OUTCOME

Lung masses of significant size associated with or without pleural effusion and diagnosed prior to 24 weeks tend to have a poor outcome. Therefore, pregnancy termination may be offered in such circumstances. Of course, adequate diagnosis and workup will be necessary in order to provide appropriate counseling. If this diagnosis is made after 24 weeks, the prognosis would be related to whether or not there is polyhydramnios, pleural effusion, fetal hydrops, or mediastinal shift.

Fetal outcome in the presence of the above complications is uniformly poor, with mortality rates as high as 100%.

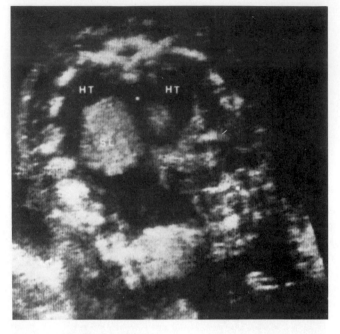

**FIGURE 17-4.** Bronchopulmonary sequestration. Transverse section through the fetal thorax demonstrating sequestered extralobar lung segment (SL) and hydrothorax (HT). (From Romero R, Chervenak FA, Kotzen J, et al. Antenatal sonographic findings of extralobar pulmonary sequestrations. J Ultrasound Med 1982;1:131.)

## PRIMARY PULMONARY HYPOPLASIA (THE SCIMITAR SYNDROME)

### ETIOPATHOLOGY

Primary pulmonary hypoplasia is a very rare thoracic anomaly characterized by total anomalous pulmonary venous drainage with connection to the left innominate vein by a vertical or scimitar vein.

This pulmonary malformation is frequently associated with hypoplasia of the right lung with bronchial anomalies, dextropositon or dextrorotation of the heart, hypoplasia of the right pulmonary artery, and anomalous systemic arterial supply to the lower lobe of the right lung directly from the aorta or its main branches. The term *scimitar syndrome* has been coined to describe this complex of defects.

### PRENATAL DIAGNOSIS

Sonographic diagnosis may be suspected with the identification of severe dextrocardia, mediastinal shift, or intrinsic cardiac defects.

### MEDICAL MANAGEMENT AND OUTCOME

If such a diagnosis is suspected and there are other congenital anomalies, the option of pregnancy termination may be advised. For example, cardiac defects, most commonly ventricular septal defects, frequently coexist and may significantly influence the prognosis. In general, the prognosis is poor.

# CONGENITAL CHYLOTHORAX

## ETIOPATHOLOGY

Although pleural effusions are unusual during fetal or even early neonatal life, chylothorax is the most common form of thoracic effusion encountered in the prenatal period. This disorder occurs at an incidence of 1 in 10,000, with males affected twice as commonly as females. About 60% of effusions appear on the right, but occasionally bilateral collection of fluid occurs. Chylothorax represents accumulation within the pleural cavity of a fluid called chyle, which is clear, with abundant lymphocytes of about 60% (Table 17-2).

The cause of chylothorax is unknown. Some investigators have indicated that this disorder may result from rupture or failed fusion of the thoracic lymphatic channels. Chylothorax has also been reported in the presence of monosomy X or trisomy 21, or occurring in each male offspring within families, indicating a possible X-linked inheritance.

## PRENATAL DIAGNOSIS

Sonographic findings include unilateral or rarely bilateral effusion, with or without collapsed lungs (Fig. 17-5). It should be pointed out, however, that these sonographic findings are indistinguishable from nonchylothorax effusion. Thoracentesis has been used to demonstrate a marked lymphocytosis, with the fluid remaining clear before birth but becoming cloudy neonatally following feeding. The precise prenatal diagnosis using these hematologic indices remains unsettled.

Tachypnea, retractions, and cyanosis occur with many pulmonary disorders in the newborn. When these symptoms occur in association with maternal polyhydramnios, the diagnosis of spontaneous chylothorax should be considered.

## MEDICAL MANAGEMENT AND OUTCOME

Management depends on the severity of the disorder and the gestational age at which it is identified. As indicated previously, chylothorax may be associated with

**TABLE 17-2.** Congenital Chylothorax

| |
|---|
| Characteristics of chyle |
|   Milky appearance |
|   Separated into two distinct layers on standing |
|   Clear when fat is extracted by alkali and ether |
|   Most of the fat present is neutral fat |
|   Odorless |
|   Sterile |
|   Bacteria static |
|   Alkaline reaction |
|   Fat content 0.4 to 4 grams per 100 mL |
|   Specific gravity greater than 1.012 |
|   Protein content generally between 1.0 and 6 grams per 100 mL |

From Diwan RV, Brennan JN, Philipson EH, Jain S, Bellon EM. Ultrasonic prenatal diagnosis of type III congenital cystic adenomatoid malformation of lung. J Clin Ultrasound 1983;11:218, with permission.

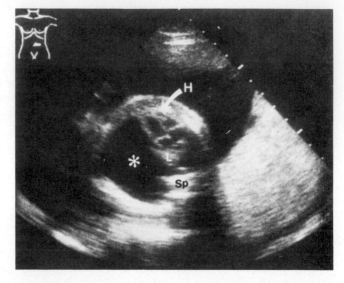

**FIGURE 17-5.**
Chylothorax/hydrothorax. Transverse section of the fetal thorax demonstrating the fetal heart (H), lung (L), and spine (Sp). Fluid surrounding the heart (*) represents idiopathic hydrothorax or chylothorax. (From Romero R, Pilu G, Ghidini A, et al. Prenatal diagnosis of congenital anomalies. Norwalk, CT: Appleton & Lange, 1987:196.)

chromosomal abnormalities. Therefore, if this lesion is identified prior to 24 weeks, karyotypic analysis ought to be conducted and appropriate counseling given based on the laboratory results. The accumulation of fluid before 24 weeks might adversely affect lung development and, therefore, might lead to pulmonary hypoplasia and neonatal death, even in the otherwise normal fetus. If the diagnosis is made at or beyond 24 weeks, such fetuses should be managed expectantly. Thoracentesis should be performed as fluid accumulation increases. In our experience, such procedures might prevent the development of pulmonic hypoplasia.

Spontaneous resolution of these effusions is rare, so the prognosis for these fetuses, especially when this condition occurs early in pregnancy, is poor. Mortality statistics range from 15% to 50%. Fetuses, however, that survive the initial neonatal period might expect to have resolution of chylothorax with surgical ligation of the thoracic duct.

# 18. PRENATAL DIAGNOSIS OF CARDIOVASCULAR ANOMALIES

## INCIDENCE AND ETIOLOGY OF CONGENITAL HEART DISEASE

Congenital heart defects (CHD) are among the most frequent malformations encountered at birth. They are currently estimated to occur in 8% to 9% of live births, and an even higher frequency has been documented in spontaneous abortions. Spontaneous selection of fetuses with severe CHD, chromosomal aberrations, or multiple anomalies most likely accounts for the discrepancy between prenatal and postnatal series.

Congenital heart disease probably results from a wide variety of causes. Chromosomal aberrations are found in 4% to 5%. Mendelian transmission and environmental factors have been documented, but they probably account for only a minority of cases. An unusually high frequency of cardiac anomalies has been reported recently in children of mothers with CHD. These observations have prompted the hypothesis that cytoplasmic inheritance or teratogens may play a major role in the etiology of CHD. Table 18-1 reports the recurrence risks of CHD.

## THE TECHNIQUE OF FETAL ECHOCARDIOGRAPHY

Fetal echocardiography is necessarily used only in a selected number of pregnancies carrying a higher than normal risk of fetal cardiac anomalies. A tentative list of indications is reported in Table 18-2.

By using a high-frequency transducer (5 to 7 MHz), the main cardiac connections can be consistently imaged starting from 14 weeks of gestation. From a technical point of the view, however, the optimal time for fetal echocardiography is between 20 and 26 weeks. In later gestation, increasing calcification of the fetal ribs and relative decrease in amniotic fluid volume hinder the examination, and it is rare that this can be satisfyingly accomplished at term.

The sequential approach to the evaluation of cardiac anatomy, originally suggested for pathologic and angiographic studies, is very suitable for fetal echocardiography. The left and right sides of the fetus are assessed by determining the position of the head and spine. The visceral situs is then assessed by demonstrating the relative position of the stomach, hepatic vessels, abdominal aorta, and inferior vena cava (Fig. 18-1). A transverse cross section of the fetal chest provides a four-chamber view (Fig. 18-2). This view is easily obtained even by sonographers who do not have specific training in fetal echocardiography, and it permits the identification of many cardiac anomalies. The elements that are relevant in the analysis of the four-chamber view are as follows: position of the heart inside the thorax (the heart is normally positioned in the left side of the chest, with the apex pointing to the left); integrity of the ventricular and atrial septum; and equal size of the left and right ventricles and atria. The patency of the atrioventricular

E. Albert Reece, John C. Hobbins, Maurice, J. Mahoney and Roy H. Petrie (Eds). *Handbook of Medicine of the Fetus & Mother.* Copyright © 1995 by J.B. Lippincott Company

**TABLE 18-1.** Recurrence Risks of Congenital Heart Disease

| Defect | Recurrence Risks (Percentage) | | |
|---|---|---|---|
| | One Sibling Affected* | Father Affected† | Mother Affected† |
| Aortic stenosis | 2 | 3 | 13–18 |
| Atrial septal defect | 2.5 | 1.5 | 5–4.5 |
| Atrioventricular canal | 2 | 1 | 14 |
| Coarctation | 2 | 2 | 4 |
| Patent ductus arteriosus | 3 | 2.5 | 3.5–4 |
| Pulmonary stenosis | 2 | 2 | 4–6.5 |
| Tetralogy of Fallot | 2.5 | 1.5 | 2.5 |
| Ventricular septal defect | 3 | 2 | 6–10 |

* Data derived from Nora JJ, Nora AH. Genetics and counseling in cardiovascular disease. Springfield, IL: Charles C Thomas, 1978.
† Data derived from Nora JJ, Nora AH: Maternal transmission of congenital heart disease: new recurrence risk figures and the questions of cytoplasmic inheritance and vulnerability to teratogens. Am J Cardiol 1987; 59:459.

**TABLE 18-2.** Indications for Fetal Echocardiography

**Maternal and Familial Indications**
Familial history of congenital heart disease
Maternal diabetes
Maternal drug exposure during pregnancy*
Maternal infections during pregnancy*
Maternal alcoholism*
Maternal connective tissue disease
Maternal phenylketonuria

**Fetal Indications**
Polyhydramnios
Nonimmune hydrops
Dysrhythmias
Extracardiac anomalies*
Chromosomal aberrations*
Symmetrical intrauterine growth retardation

* The interested reader is referred to Copel JA, Pilu G, Kleinman CS. Congenital heart disease and extracardiac malformations. Associations and indications for fetal echocardiography. Am J Obstet Gynecol 1986;154:1121.

valves can be demonstrated by real-time imaging of the movements of the leaflets. Additional elements that can be visualized in the four-chamber view include the more apical insertion of the tricuspid valve with regard to the mitral valve and the presence of the moderator band of the trabeculae septomarginalis at the apex of the right ventricle. These elements are both of value in distinguishing the morphologic left ventricle from the morphologic right ventricle.

Tilting the transducer cephalad, the left and right ventriculoarterial connection can be identified, and further angulation allows the visualization of the right outflow tract and main pulmonary artery, ductus arteriosus, and aortic arch. M-mode ultrasound evaluation of the fetal heart is easily performed by using the

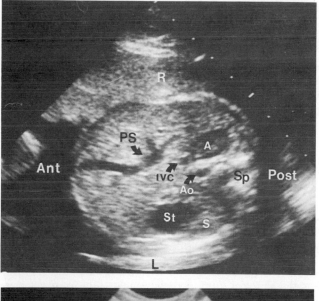

**FIGURE 18-1.**
Transverse cross section of the upper abdomen in a second trimester fetus, demonstrating visceral situs. The portal situs (PS), the anatomical landmark of the hilus of the liver, can be clearly recognized. The stomach (St), spleen (S), inferior vena cava (IVC), and abdominal aorta (Ao) are demonstrated. (Ant, anterior; Post, posterior; R, right; L, left; A, right adrenal gland.)

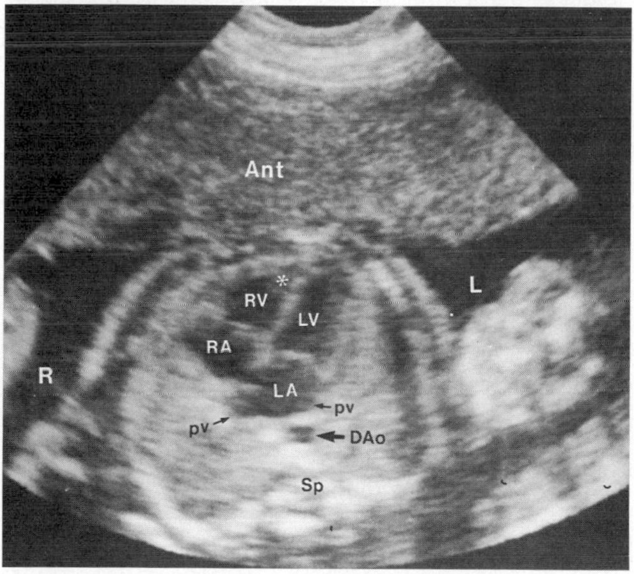

**FIGURE 18-2.** Four-chamber view of the heart in a second trimester fetus. (RV, right ventricle; LV, left ventricle; RA, right atrium; La, left atrium; PV, pulmonary veins; DAo, descending aorta; Sp, spine; *, the moderator band of the trabecula septomarginalis. Other abbreviations are as in previous figure.)

currently available real-time directed M-mode apparatuses. Movements of the cardiac valves and walls can be studied with this technique.

Pulsed Doppler ultrasound evaluation has recently been applied to the study of the heart function in the live human fetus. Adequate recordings of velocity waveforms of the blood flow through the atrioventricular valves, great vessels, and inferior vena cava can be obtained in almost all cases after 18 to 20 weeks gestation. Several authors have pointed out remarkable differences between in utero and postnatal Doppler studies. The higher velocity in the flow at the ventricular inlet that is dependent on atrial contraction when compared to passive venous filling has been interpreted as a sign of the physiologic "stiffness" of the fetal myocardium. Pulsed Doppler ultrasound, in combination with two-dimensional and M-mode sonography, has proved useful in the evaluation of both fetal dysrhythmias and structural anomalies. In this regard, Doppler is of value for documenting atrioventricular valve insufficiency. It has been demonstrated recently that the association of structural heart disease, hydrops, and atrioventricular valve insufficiency carries a very poor prognosis. It has also been found that in normal fetuses, the peak velocity in both the ascending aorta and pulmonary artery is less than 1 m/s. This observation is relevant for the prenatal diagnosis of pulmonic and aortic stenosis, which are associated with poststenotic turbulence. However, the use of Doppler in the fetus is still an area of ongoing research. Sophisticated analyses of cardiac function are appearing with increasing frequency.

## ATRIAL AND VENTRICULAR SEPTAL DEFECTS

Atrial septal defects (ASD) are commonly divided into *primum* and *secundum* types. Primum ASD is the simplest form of the atrioventricular septal defects, which cover a wide spectrum of severity, the most severe of which is the complete atrioventricular defect. Atrioventricular septal defects (according to a different terminology, *atrioventricular canals*) are found in more than 50% of infants with trisomy 21. Secundum ASD may be a part of the Holt-Oram syndrome, with autosomal dominant transmission.

Complete atrioventricular septal defects have an ASD with a ventricular septal defect and a common atrioventricular valve (Fig. 18-3).

**FIGURE 18-3.** Complete atrioventricular septal defect. A common atrium (CA) is demonstrated in association with a common atrioventricular valve with central opening (*arrows*) and a large ventricular septal defect. (Other abbreviations as in the previous figures.)

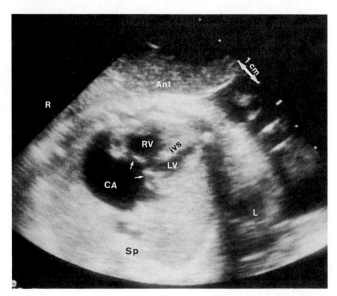

Atrioventricular septal defects are among the most frequent types of CHD found in cardiosplenic syndromes (asplenia and polysplenia, also defined as right and left isomerism, respectively). Diagnosis of these conditions is possible by evaluation of the visceral situs.

Ventricular septal defects (VSD) are probably the most common form of CHD. The echocardiographic diagnosis depends on the demonstration of a dropout of echoes in the ventricular septum (Figure 18-4).

## PULMONARY AND AORTIC STENOSIS

Pulmonic stenosis increases both the work of the right ventricle and the pressure, leading to myocardial hypertrophy. In the most severe cases, right ventricular overload may cause insufficiency of the tricuspid valve and congestive heart failure. Aortic stenosis includes three different lesions: subaortic stenosis, valvar stenosis, and supravalvular stenosis. Subaortic stenosis includes a fixed type, which is the consequence of a fibrous or fibromuscular obstruction, and a dynamic type, which is due to a thickened ventricular septum obstructing the outflow tract of the left ventricle.

Postnatal ultrasound diagnosis of pulmonary or aortic stenosis depends on demonstration of doming of the cusps with real-time and poststenotic turbulence detected by Doppler ultrasound. Prenatal diagnosis is probably difficult, since only a few, very severe cases have been described thus far, mainly in association with enlargement of the ventricles or poststenotic enlargement or hypoplasia of the great vessels.

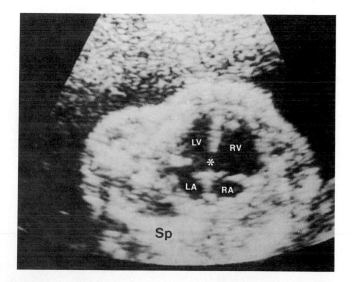

**FIGURE 18-4.** Four-chamber view in a second-trimester fetus with a large perimembranous ventricular septal defect (*). There is evidence indicating that ventricular septal defects are well tolerated during intrauterine life. However, in our experience large defects are often associated with some degree of enlargement of the right ventricle. Color Doppler has revealed that in these cases a left-to-right shunt is a frequent finding even prior to birth. (Abbreviations as in previous figures.)

## TETRALOGY OF FALLOT

Tetralogy of Fallot is defined by the association of a ventricular septal defect (usually in the perimembranous area), infundibular pulmonic stenosis, aortic valve overriding the ventricular septum, and hypertrophy of the right ventricle.

Associated defects, including atrial septal defects and bicuspid or absent pulmonary valve, are frequently seen. The main factor affecting hemodynamics is the degree of hypoplasia of the right ventricular outflow tract, since this causes both a decrease in pulmonary blood flow and a right-to-left shunt at the level of the ascending aorta, with decreased oxygen saturation. However, tetralogy of Fallot does not seem to cause hemodynamic compromise in utero. Even in the case of very tight infundibular stenosis or pulmonary atresia, the combined output of both ventricles will be directed toward the aorta, and the pulmonary vascular bed will be supplied by reverse flow through the ductus arteriosus. This concept is supported by the observation of normal intrauterine fetal growth in affected fetuses. Congestive heart failure is very rarely seen in neonates, and it usually occurs only in those with an absent pulmonary valve.

Echocardiographic diagnosis can be made by demonstrating the aorta overriding the ventricular septum (Fig. 18-5).

## TRANSPOSITION OF THE GREAT ARTERIES

Transposition of the great arteries (TGA) includes two anatomical forms: complete TGA and corrected TGA. In complete TGA, the aorta arises from the morphologic right ventricle and the pulmonary artery arises from the left ventricle in the presence of a normal atrioventricular connection.

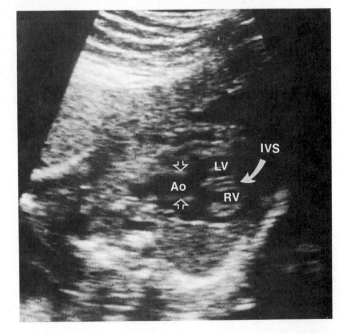

**FIGURE 18-5.** Tetralogy of Fallot. A large aortic root (Ao) is clearly seen overriding by almost 50% the ventricular septum (IVS). (Other abbreviations as in previous figures.)

Fetal echocardiography allows us to identify abnormalities of the ventriculoarterial connection, but meticulous scanning is required. In both complete and corrected transposition, the two great vessels arise parallel from the base of the heart. By careful scanning, the aorta and pulmonic artery can be identified and their relationship with each ventricle can be assessed.

Fetuses with uncomplicated complete transposition should not undergo hemodynamic compromise in utero. Survival after birth depends on the persistence of fetal circulation. In corrected transposition, discordance between atrioventricular and ventriculoarterial connection cancel each other, and ideally there should not be any hemodynamic imbalance. Corrected transposition may indeed be an occasional finding at autopsy. However, important associated cardiac anomalies are found in the vast majority of cases (ventricular septal defects, pulmonic stenosis, abnormalities of the atrioventricular valves, atrioventricular block).

## DOUBLE-OUTLET RIGHT VENTRICLE

Double-outlet right ventricle (DORV) is commonly defined as a cardiac lesion in which most of the aorta and the pulmonary artery arise from the right ventricle. The relative position of the two great vessels is variable. A defect of the ventricular septum is almost always associated, as are other anomalies, such as atrial septal defects, pulmonary stenosis, and abnormalities of the atrioventricular valves. By definition, the term *DORV* includes those cases of tetralogy of Fallot in which the aorta arises predominantly from the right ventricle. Prenatal diagnosis of DORV has been reported.

## HYPOPLASTIC LEFT HEART SYNDROME

Hypoplastic left heart syndrome (HLHS) is characterized by a very small left ventricle, with mitral and/or aortic atresia. HLHS is frequently associated with intrauterine heart failure. The prognosis has classically been regarded as extremely poor. Untreated infants usually die in the very first days of life.

Ultrasound recognition of HLHS in the fetus depends on the demonstration of a small left ventricle. The ascending aorta is severely hypoplastic. The right ventricle, right atrium, and pulmonary artery are usually enlarged. By the use of pulsed Doppler ultrasound it may be possible to demonstrate retrograde blood flow in the ascending aorta and a systolic regurgitant jet within the right atrium in those cases with tricuspid insufficiency.

## PULMONARY ATRESIA WITH INTACT VENTRICULAR SEPTUM

Pulmonary atresia with intact ventricular septum (PA:IVS) in infants is usually associated with a hypoplastic right ventricle. In fetuses, cases with enlarged right ventricle and atrium have been described with unusual frequency. Prenatal diagnosis of PA:IVS relies on the demonstration of a small pulmonary artery with an atretic pulmonary valve.

## UNIVENTRICULAR HEART

The term *univentricular heart* defines a group of anomalies unified by the presence of an atrioventricular junction that is entirely connected to only one chamber in the ventricular mass. The main ventricular chamber may be either of left or right type, and in some cases may be of indeterminate type. A rudimentary ventricular chamber lacking atrioventricular connection is a frequent but not constant finding. Antenatal echocardiographic diagnosis is usually easy.

## CARDIOMYOPATHIES

Congenital cardiomyopathies include a heterogeneous group of myocardial disorders, commonly subdivided into nonobstructive and obstructive forms. The etiology of the former type includes inborn errors of metabolism, muscular dystrophies, and infections.

Cardiomyopathies of both obstructive and nonobstructive types share in common, either since a consequence of pump failure or valvular regurgitation or as a consequence of obstruction of ventricular outflow, a more or less marked tendency to congestive heart failure.

Echocardiographic diagnosis of nonobstructive forms relies on demonstration of cardiomegaly and poor contractility of ventricular chambers. In obstructive forms, thickening of the interventricular septum and free walls of the ventricles has been reported (Fig. 18-6).

## COARCTATION OF THE AORTA

A discrete shelf between the isthmus and the descending aorta is the most common finding at anatomical dissection. Tubular hypoplasia of a segment of the aortic arch is seen less frequently. Coarctation may be a postnatal event, and this limits prenatal diagnosis in many cases. However, this anomaly has been described in the fetus, although only in late pregnancy.

## FETAL DYSRHYTHMIAS

The fetal electrocardiogram is of little value in the prenatal diagnosis of dysrhythmias, as a satisfactory transabdominal recording can be obtained in a minority of cases. At present, M-mode and pulsed Doppler ultrasound are the most suitable techniques for the assessment of irregular fetal heart rhythm.

## PREMATURE ATRIAL AND VENTRICULAR CONTRACTIONS

Premature atrial and ventricular contractions are the most frequent fetal dysrhythmias. Repeated premature contractions can give rise to complex rhythm patterns. Premature atrial contractions may be either conducted to the ventricles or blocked, depending on the time of the cardiac cycle in which they occur, thus resulting in either an increased or a decreased ventricular rate. Blocked premature atrial contractions must be differentiated from atrioventricular block. Premature atrial and ventricular contractions are considered a benign condition. However, because there is at least a theoretical possibility that in a few cases an ectopic beat could trigger a reentrant tachyarrhythmia, serial monitoring of the fetal heart during pregnancy is suggested. Prenatal diagnosis of fetal extrasystoles is easy by using TM-mode. Pulsed Doppler ultrasound evaluation of blood flow in fetuses with

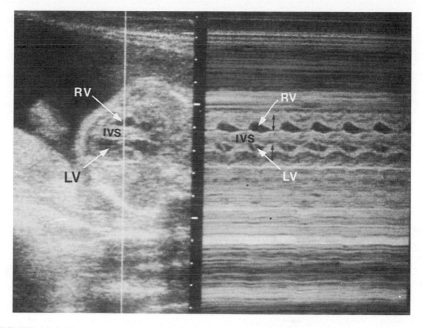

**FIGURE 18-6.** Hypertrophic cardiomyopathy in a second trimester fetus. Thickened free walls of the ventricles and ventricular septum (IVS) are clearly demonstrated in both real-time and TM-mode sonograms. The ventricular cavities (RV, LV) are significantly reduced in size.

premature beats suggests that the fetal heart is capable of postextrasystolic potentiation and that the Frank-Starling mechanism is operative beginning in the early stages of fetal development.

## SUPRAVENTRICULAR TACHYARRHYTHMIAS

Supraventricular tachyarrhythmias include supraventricular paroxysmal tachycardia (SVT), atrial flutter, and atrial fibrillation. SVT is characterized by an atrial frequency between 200 and 300 beats per minute (bpm) and a 1:1 atrioventricular conduction rate (Fig. 18-7).

Diagnosis of fetal tachyarrhythmia can be accomplished easily by direct auscultation or continuous Doppler examination. M-mode and/or pulsed Doppler ultrasound allow us to identify the precise heart rate and to recognize the atrioventricular sequence of contraction.

The association between fetal tachyarrhythmia and nonimmune hydrops is well established. It has been postulated that a fast ventricular rate results in suboptimal filling of the ventricle. This would lead to decreased cardiac output, right atrial overload, and congestive heart failure.

## ATRIOVENTRICULAR BLOCK

Third-degree, or complete, AV block involves complete dissociation of atria and ventricles, usually with independent and slow activation of the ventricles (Fig.

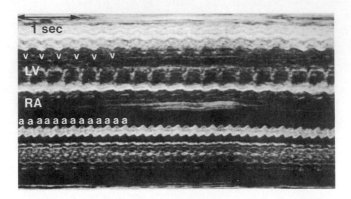

**FIGURE 18-7.** Supraventricular tachycardia in a third trimester fetus. The TM-mode sonogram indicates an atrial rhythm of about 220 bpm and a one-to-one ventricular response (v). Return to a normal sinus rhythm was noted following maternal administration of a daily dose of 240 mg of verapamil. Digoxin and procainamide had been previously administered without any beneficial effect.

18-8). Third-degree AV block is widely reported to be associated in over half of the cases with cardiac structural anomalies, including corrected transposition, univentricular heart, cardiac tumors, and cardiomyopathies. Although in the cases without structural cardiac disease the etiology is unknown, growing evidence suggests an association with the presence of maternal antibodies against SSA and SSB antigens. Transplacental passage of these antibodies would lead to inflammation and damage of the conduction system. Anti-SSA antibodies have been reported in over 80% of mothers that delivered infants with AV block, although

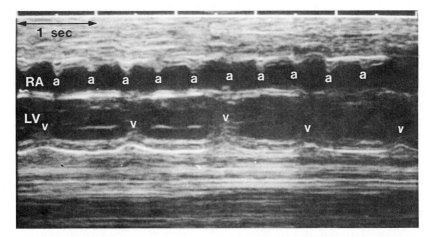

**FIGURE 18-8.** Complete atrioventricular block. The TM-mode sonogram reveals a regular atrial activity (a) with a frequency of about 120 bpm and a slow, independent ventricular activity (v) with a frequency of about 60 bpm. This infant was delivered at term by cesarean section. A pacemaker had to be installed on the third day of life.

only 30% had clinical evidence of connective tissue disease (mostly lupus erythematosus).

## OBSTETRIC MANAGEMENT OF PREGNANCIES WITH FETAL STRUCTURAL CHD

Currently, most series of prenatally diagnosed CHD include mainly cases that were referred because of either associated extracardiac anomalies or very severe cardiac alterations resulting in gross cardiomegaly or intrauterine heart failure. It is not surprising that the outcome of these cases has generally proved to be dismal. Nevertheless, the experience thus far seems to indicate that fetal echocardiography has great potential in accurately identifying correctable cardiac defects whose prognosis could be ameliorated by prompt neonatal assistance. Although these cases are a minority at present, there is reason to believe that their number will grow in the near future.

# 19. GASTROINTESTINAL AND GENITOURINARY ANOMALIES

## GASTROINTESTINAL ANOMALIES

Structural anomalies of the gastrointestinal (GI) tract are relatively common. Fetuses with GI anomalies, which often allow a good quality of life after postnatal surgical correction, largely benefit from prenatal diagnosis. Anomalies can be subdivided into two groups: intestinal obstructions and ventral wall defects.

## OBSTRUCTIONS

The echo-free areas resulting from fluid collection and progressive dilation of the bowel cranial to the obstruction site are easily detected by ultrasound. Furthermore, a GI obstruction is often associated with hydramnios, allowing a better visualization. A proximal obstruction can be expected in approximately 1 in 15 pregnancies with polyhydramnios. GI obstructions can involve the esophagus, duodenum, and small bowel; they can be intrinsic or extrinsic (e.g., intrathoracic cyst or annular pancreas). Conversely, distal obstructions are not usually associated with hydramnios, and their detection is rather more difficult.

### Esophageal Atresia

**Pathogenesis.** Esophageal atresia is a relatively frequent anomaly, occurring in 1 in 3000 to 3500 live births. It is caused by an impairment in the process of recanalization of the primitive esophagus. An abnormal connection between trachea and esophagus is usually derived from an imperfect development of the respiratory diverticulum (Fig. 19-1). In the most common type of fistula (90% to

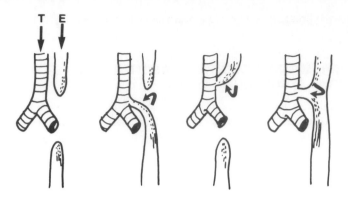

**FIGURE 19-1.** Different types of esophageal atresia with and without tracheoesophageal fistula. Esophageal atresia without fistula, atresia of the upper esophagus with a fistula connecting the lower portion of the esophagus and the trachea (more common), atresia of the lower esophagus with a fistula connecting the upper portion of the esophagus and the trachea, and double fistula (upper and lower portions of the esophagus) ending in the trachea.

95%), the upper portion of the esophagus ends blindly (esophageal atresia), and the lower portion develops from the trachea near the bifurcation. The two portions of the esophagus may be connected by a solid cord.

**Associated Anomalies.** Severe structural anomalies are associated in nearly 50% of the cases, including heart, GI, and genitourinary (GU) tract anomalies; skeletal deformities; cleft defects of the face; and central nervous system (CNS) lesions such as meningoceles or hydrocephalus. Chromosomal anomalies, particularly trisomy 21, are also commonly present.

**Prenatal Diagnosis.** Prenatal diagnosis is based on indirect findings. Rarely, an elongated upper mediastinal and retrocardiac anechoic structure, interpreted as the dilated proximal esophageal pouch, can be observed (Fig. 19-2). Ultrasound criteria for diagnosis are polyhydramnios and failed visualization of the stomach. The bowel appears uniformly echogenic, even in late pregnancy, due to the absence of amniotic fluid. In the majority of the cases, a fistula between the respiratory and the GI tract distal to the obstruction allows ingestion of amniotic fluid. Conversely, absence of amniotic fluid in the GI tract does not mean absence of tracheo-esophageal fistula, because a small quantity of fluid cannot be seen with ultrasound or a fistula may be obstructed in utero.

**Prognosis and Management.** We are not aware of any case of esophageal atresia that was diagnosed or even suspected earlier than during the early third trimester of pregnancy. Because the prognosis of the affected newborn is worse if severe congenital anomalies are associated with it, an accurate ultrasound examination of the entire fetal anatomy should be performed. Time and mode of delivery are not influenced by prenatal diagnosis. Delay in postnatal recognition, however, results in increased neonatal morbidity and mortality. Prenatal diagnosis alerts the pediatrician, facilitates prompt neonatal diagnostic confirmation, and allows for prevention of possible complications, such as aspiration pneumonia, which can be lethal.

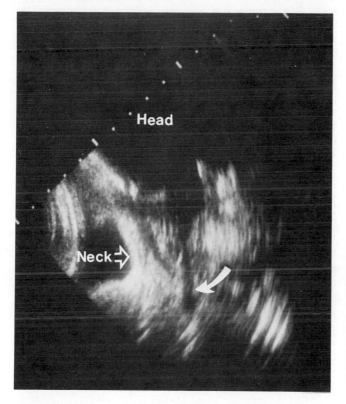

**FIGURE 19-2.** Coronal section of the neck in a fetus with esophageal atresia, showing the blind end of the esophagus (*arrow*). (From Romero et al. Prenatal diagnosis of congenital anomalies. Norwalk, CT: Appleton and Lange, 1988:235.)

## Duodenal Obstruction

**Pathogenesis.** Duodenal obstruction occurs in approximately 1 in 7500 to 10,000 live births. The anomaly can be either intrinsic or extrinsic. Extrinsic lesions are mainly the consequence of a compression of the duodenum by the surrounding annular pancreas or by peritoneal fibrous bands. With intrinsic obstructions in duodenal atresia or stenosis, either defect derives from an incomplete developmental process during the second and third month of fetal life.

**Associated Anomalies.** Duodenal atresia is very often associated with other malformations. Nearly 30% of the fetuses have trisomy 21. Other common anomalies include structural cardiac anomalies (20%), malrotation of the colon (22%) and, less frequently, tracheo-esophageal fistula and renal malformations.

**Prenatal Diagnosis.** Detection of two echo-free areas inside the abdomen ("double-bubble" sign), representing the dilated stomach and first portion of the duodenum, is crucial for prenatal diagnosis (Figure 19-3). Polyhydramnios is a constant associated finding. Bovicelli and associates (1983) reported a prenatal ultrasound diagnosis at 26 weeks gestation;[*] previous ultrasound examinations had revealed normal fetal anatomy until 23 weeks. It would be interesting to

---

[*]Bovicelli L, Rizzo N, Orsini LF, Pilu G. Prenatal diagnosis and management of fetal gastrointestinal anomalies. Semin Perinatol 1983;7:109.

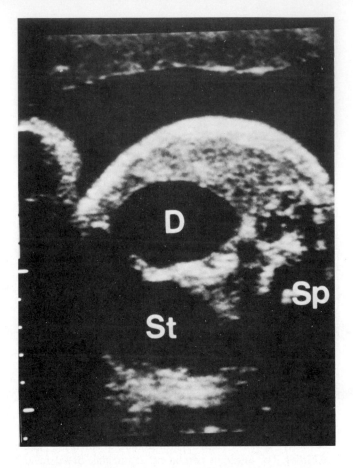

**FIGURE 19-3.**
Transverse scan of the upper fetal abdomen in case of duodenal atresia. The double-bubble sign is evident. (St, stomach; D, dilated duodenal bulb; Sp, spine.)

determine whether that gestational age represents a threshold for ultrasound in utero detection of duodenal atresia. In summary, prenatal diagnosis of duodenal atresia on the basis of the double-bubble sign mostly depends on the sonographer's expertise.

**Prognosis and Management.** Postnatal prognosis of duodenal atresia depends mainly on the following: associated anomalies, birth weight, and prompt confirmation of prenatal diagnosis.

Prenatal detection of the anomaly allows for prevention of neonatal vomiting or aspiration pneumonia through early aspiration of gastric contents.

## Intestinal Obstructions (Below the Level of the Duodenum)

**Pathogenesis.** Intestinal obstructions are a quite common congenital anomaly, occurring in 1 in 300 to 1500 live births. Obstructions can be intrinsic or extrinsic. Intrinsic lesions result from absent (atresia) or partial (stenosis) recanalization of the intestine. Extrinsic obstructions are caused by malrotation of colon with volvulus, peritoneal bands, meconium ileus, and agangliosis (Hirschsprung's disease).

**Associated Anomalies.** Intestinal atresias or stenosis are infrequently associated with other anomalies.

**Prenatal Diagnosis.** With GI obstructions below the level of the duodenum, multiple echo-free areas within the distended fetal abdomen are usually seen (Fig. 19-4). The more distal the site of the obstruction, the greater is the number of anechoic structures. The severity of the polyhydramnios depends on the level of the obstruction: "high" obstructions are often associated with a certain degree of polyhydramnios, whereas obstructions of the colon are generally not accompanied with increased volume of amniotic fluid.

Perforation as a consequence of impaired blood supply to the distended bowel can be suspected by ultrasound demonstrating ascites that was previously absent. Because meconium begins to accumulate in fetal bowel at 4 months, any perforation occurring after that time could bring the outflow of meconium into the peritoneal cavity. As a result, an intense reaction occurs, leading to extensive adhesions. If it is localized at the site of perforation, a calcified mass develops. At ultrasound, this appears as a highly echogenic mass, often visible near the liver.

**Prognosis and Management.** When prenatal diagnosis is made, delivery should be planned in a center where prompt postnatal correction can be performed, thus improving the infant's prognosis.

The survival rate of surgically treated infants depends on prematurity and associated anomalies. Associated anomalies are far less common than in cases of duodenal atresia. Chromosomal anomalies are also rare. In case of meconium ileus, cystic fibrosis is a possibility.

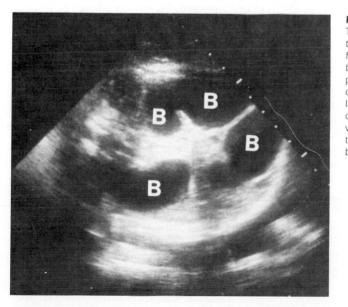

**FIGURE 19-4.**
Transverse scan of the abdomen in a fetus with small bowel atresia. Multiple distended loops of bowel are visible. In real time, increased peristalsis was noted. (B, distended loops of bowel.)

Fetuses with uncomplicated intestinal obstruction can be delivered vaginally at term. Induction of preterm delivery should be considered when perforation occurs and ascites are seen.

## ABDOMINAL WALL DEFECTS

Congenital abdominal wall defects are always associated with external herniation of viscera. Depending on the site and extent of the lesion, two separate pathologic entities are described—omphalocele, or exomphalos, and gastroschisis. Omphalocele is a herniation of the bowel through the umbilical ring. Gastroschisis is a lateral abdominal wall defect with eviscerated bowel and intact umbilicus. Congenital abdominal wall defects can be successfully corrected after birth. Intrauterine diagnosis allows appropriate management of the affected fetus.

### Omphalocele

**Pathogenesis.** Omphalocele is a sporadic anomaly with a risk of occurrence of 1 in 6000 live births. It results from an alteration of the vital mechanism of closing of the body of the embryo. Impaired embryonic folding at the level of the lateral folds causes a herniation of intra-abdominal contents through the open umbilical ring into the base of the umbilical cord. Protrusion is covered by a translucent, avascular membrane consisting of peritoneum inside and amniotic membrane outside, separated by Wharton's jelly.

**Associated Anomalies.** Omphalocele is often associated with other abnormalities, as a result of general interference with embryonic development during early gestation. Malrotation of the gut and duodenal obstruction are frequent. GU anomalies, including exstrophy of the bladder, penile anomalies, and undescended testes, are also very common. Congenital heart diseases are frequent and represent the most important cause of death for the affected child. Chromosomal anomalies occasionally occur, particularly trisomies 13, 18, and 21. If macrosomia is present, one should suspect Beckwith-Wiedemann syndrome.

**Prenatal Diagnosis.** Omphalocele is relatively easy to detect with ultrasound from early midtrimester. Since normal migration of the midgut back into the abdomen occurs between the ninth and 12th gestational weeks, the diagnosis of ventral wall defects should not be made before 14 weeks. Protrusion generally consists of bowel alone, but in severe cases, liver and stomach can also be herniated (Fig. 19-5). Polyhydramnios is often present.

**Prognosis and Management.** Omphalocele, unlike gastroschisis, is often associated with additional congenital anomalies (45% versus 5%); the mortality rate is therefore higher (34% versus 12.7%). Cardiovascular malformations are present in 40% of the cases. They are more common in cases of trisomy 18, whereas the association of holoprosencephaly with omphalocele suggests the diagnosis of trisomy 13. Thus, in cases of omphalocele, a thorough sonographic evaluation of the fetus and fetal karyotype should be performed.

When prenatal diagnosis of a giant omphalocele is made, or when multiple malformations are found, termination of pregnancy may be considered. If pregnancy is continued, the obstetrician should be able to select the most appropriate time and mode of delivery and plan adequate therapy for the newborn and

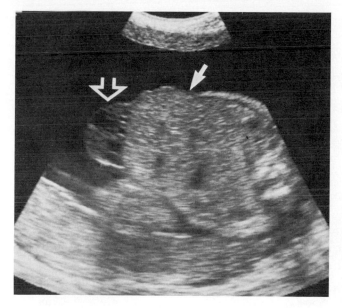

**FIGURE 19-5.**
Transverse section of a 30-week fetus with large omphalocele. The solid arrow is pointing at the defect in the abdominal wall; the open arrow indicates the amnioperitoneal membrane surrounding the herniated viscera.

subsequent surgical correction. In cases of small defects or isolated anomaly, if the omphalocele is intact, there appears to be no need to anticipate early delivery. In cases of ruptured omphalocele, a preterm cesarean section is suggested to avoid the pathologic alterations of the bowel being exposed to the amniotic fluid, which can compromise the outcome of postnatal surgical correction. Because the mortality rate of newborns affected by abdominal wall defects largely depends on the clinical condition of the malformed baby at the time of admission, maternal transport to a specialized center and an accurately planned cesarean delivery would probably avoid the risks of a sudden, unexpected delivery leading to a delay in surgical care.

## Gastroschisis

**Pathogenesis.** Gastroschisis represents the herniation of some of the intraabdominal content through a paraumbilical defect of the abdominal wall. The umbilical cord is normally inserted and no sac is visible. Occasionally, only a short tract of the intestine is herniated; in most cases, however, all of the small and large intestines protrude. Chemical peritonitis is an ominous complication due to amniotic fluid exposure of eviscerated abdominal contents.

**Associated Anomalies.** Associated anomalies are uncommon in gastroschisis compared to omphalocele.

**Prenatal Diagnosis.** Multiple rounded, thick-walled, echo-free structures within the amniotic cavity along the anterior surface of the fetal abdomen, representing freely floating herniated loops of bowel, suggest a diagnosis of gastroschisis (Fig. 19-6). Polyhydramnios is a common feature. An impairment of fetal growth is often associated with gastroschisis. On this occasion, the volume of amniotic fluid can be reduced and visualization is suboptimal.

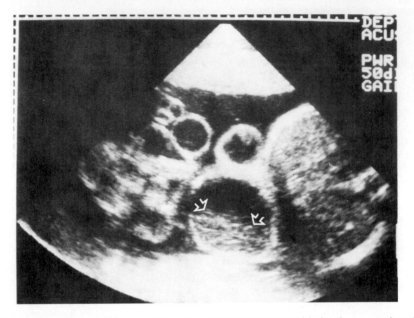

**FIGURE 19-6.** Free-floating loops of bowel in a fetus with gastroschisis. Levels are seen into the lumen of the loops (*arrow*).

## PROGNOSIS AND MANAGEMENT.

Prognosis for a fetus affected by gastroschisis has improved dramatically during the last three decades. Perinatal mortality decreased from 82% in 1960 to less than 10% in 1984. This is likely to be attributable to improved surgical technique and the use of parenteral nutrition. Gastroschisis is less frequently associated with other congenital anomalies than omphalocele. As with omphalocele, it can be a part of amniotic band syndrome. Unlike omphalocele, gastroschisis is often associated with IUGR and oligohydramnios.

In light of the association with IUGR, risks connected to prematurity should be balanced with benefits of decreasing the time of exposure to the action of amniotic fluid. As with omphalocele, a fetus affected by gastroschisis should preferably be delivered by cesarean section in a center where the neonate can receive intensive care and where neonatal surgical correction is promptly available. Delay in pediatric care, in fact, increases the risk of sepsis and may be the cause of severe dehydration and rapid heat loss, which may compromise the outcome of surgical correction. Long-term follow-up of survivors is excellent: children show normal growth and development in follow-up to 5 years of age.

## URINARY TRACT ANOMALIES

Antenatal ultrasonography permits accurate identification of the fetal urinary tract. The antenatal sonographic detection of urinary tract anomalies is dramatically important for choosing the appropriate prenatal and postnatal management, and has improved the prognosis of children affected by these anomalies.

## BILATERAL RENAL AGENESIS

Bilateral renal agenesis is a condition occurring in 1% to 3% of live-born infants.

### Pathogenesis
The anomaly can be isolated, or it can feature a genetic syndrome. When isolated the empiric risk for incidence in sibs has been estimated at 3.5%. However, hereditary renal adysplasia (HRA) is an autosomal dominant trait with incomplete penetrance (50% to 90%). It has been suggested that HRA may account for most cases of bilateral renal agenesis when parents are apparently normal. Thus, in offspring of affected or obligate heterozygotes for HRA, the empiric risk of severe bilateral renal aplasia is 15% to 20%.

### Associated Anomalies
Renal agenesis can be part of Potter's syndrome, which includes pulmonary hypoplasia, skeletal deformities, and typical facies, characterized by low-set ears. Oligohydramnios is considered responsible for pulmonary hypoplasia and skeletal deformities.

### Prenatal Diagnosis
Failed visualization of kidneys and bladder, associated with oligohydramnios and IUGR, prompts the diagnosis of bilateral renal agenesis (Fig. 19-7). Prenatal diagnosis can be rather difficult due to the lack of amniotic fluid and to the posture of the fetus, which impairs detection of the kidneys. Additionally, adrenals are usually hypertrophic in cases of bilateral renal agenesis and can be confused with normal kidneys. Identification of the renal capsule and renal pelvis allows the two structures to be distinguished.

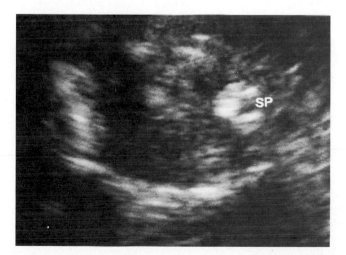

**FIGURE 19-7.**
Transverse section of the abdomen of a fetus with bilateral renal agenesis. Note the empty renal fossa. (SP, spine.)

### Prognosis and Management

Prognosis is poor, because bilateral renal agenesis is not compatible with life; affected fetuses die either in utero or soon after birth due to pulmonary hypoplasia.

Termination of pregnancy can be offered to the couple when diagnosis is made during the second trimester, whereas conservative management is the treatment of choice in the infrequent cases of third trimester diagnosis, particularly when the diagnosis is uncertain.

## INFANTILE POLYCYSTIC KIDNEY DISEASE

Infantile polycystic kidney (IPKD), or Potter's Type I dysplasia, invariably involves both kidneys, which appear symmetrically enlarged and contain multiple minute cysts.

### Pathogenesis

IPKD is an autosomal recessive disease, with a recurrence risk of 25% in a subsequent pregnancy after an affected child. A defect of the collecting system seems to be responsible for the anomaly.

### Associated Anomalies

In severe cases, compromised renal function leads to a marked oligohydramnios, which in turn is responsible for the pulmonary hypoplasia and skeletal deformities typical of Potter's syndrome.

### Prenatal Diagnosis

On ultrasound, both kidneys usually appear extremely enlarged and hyperechogenic (Fig. 19-8). The hyperechogenicity seems to be due to multiple minute cysts, which fall below the resolution power of the ultrasound equipment, thus increasing the acoustic transmission. In severe cases, the bladder is absent and oligohydramnios is extreme.

### Prognosis and Management

Prognosis of IPKD (Potter's Type I cystic dysplasia) is poor, depending on the severity of the disease. If diagnosis is made within the second trimester, termination of pregnancy is an option that can be offered to the parents. If diagnosis is made in the third trimester, conservative management is advisable. Occasionally, when the fetal abdomen is excessively distended, a cesarean section should be performed to avoid the risk of soft-tissue dystocia.

## MULTICYSTIC DYSPLASTIC KIDNEY DISEASE

Multicystic dysplastic kidney disease (MDKD) or Potter's Type IIA renal dysplasia is one of the most common congenital renal anomalies. Renal parenchyma is replaced by a number of cysts of variable size. One kidney is affected in the vast majority of cases, although bilateral renal involvement has been reported. The prevalence of unilateral MDKD is unknown; bilateral involvement is estimated to occur in 1 out of 1000 live births.

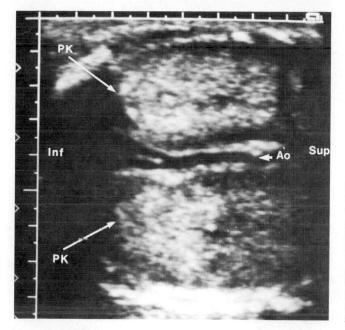

**FIGURE 19-8.** Coronal section of a fetus with infantile polycystic kidney disease (IPKD). Kidneys appear enlarged and hyperechogenic at both sides of the fetal aorta (Ao). (PK, polycystic kidney; Inf, inferior; Sup, superior.)

## Pathogenesis

MDKD is a sporadic disease. However, few examples of familial cases have been described. MDKD also can be a feature of genetic syndromes, usually as a secondary event. The anomaly is secondary to atresia of either the ureter or the pelvis or both during the metanephric stage of development.

## Associated Anomalies

MDKD is often associated with other congenital anomalies. Zerres and Fodisch reported an incidence of 50%; we recently reported an incidence of 37%.[†] Associated anomalies include CNS, GI, and congenital heart diseases, and chromosomal aberrations.

## Prenatal Diagnosis

The criteria for prenatal ultrasound diagnosis are multiple cysts of various sizes, separated by thin layers of hyperechoic tissue (Fig. 19-9). Affected kidneys are usually extremely enlarged. The hypoplastic or atretic collecting system is undetectable by ultrasound. In the unilateral variant, contralateral kidney and bladder are normal, as is the amount of amniotic fluid. Occasionally, the contralateral renal pelvis appears slightly enlarged due to compensatory urine flow. When both kidneys are affected, the bladder is not detected and amniotic fluid is decreased.

Distinction between MDKD and obstructions at the UPJ in prenatal sonograms can be extremely difficult. Coronal scans seem to be most specific, because in UPJ obstructions they clearly demonstrate the connection between the renal pelvis and

---

[†] Rizzo N, Gabrielli S, Pilu G, et al. Prenatal diagnosis and obstetrical management of multicystic dysplastic kidney disease. Prenat Diagn 1987;7:109.

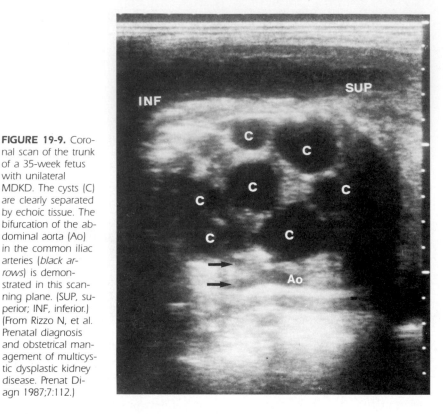

**FIGURE 19-9.** Coronal scan of the trunk of a 35-week fetus with unilateral MDKD. The cysts (C) are clearly separated by echoic tissue. The bifurcation of the abdominal aorta (Ao) in the common iliac arteries (*black arrows*) is demonstrated in this scanning plane. (SUP, superior; INF, inferior.) (From Rizzo N, et al. Prenatal diagnosis and obstetrical management of multicystic dysplastic kidney disease. Prenat Diagn 1987;7:112.)

the dilated calyceal system (Fig. 19-10). Conversely, in MDKD the cysts are separated. Similarly, differential diagnosis between UVJ and MDKD is rather difficult, frequently leading to misinterpretations of the ultrasound picture.

## Prognosis and Management

In cases of unilateral MDKD, with no sign of failure of renal function and no associated anomalies, prognosis is good and the fetus can be safely delivered vaginally at term.

Bilateral MDKD has an invariably poor prognosis, and termination of pregnancy can be offered to the couple when diagnosis is made prior to viability.

When other anomalies are associated, prognosis and management vary according to the type and severity of the diseases. In these cases, we recommend a detailed survey to exclude associated anomalies, and performing fetal karyotype.

## ADULT POLYCYSTIC KIDNEY DISEASE

Adult polycystic kidney disease (APKD), or Potter's Type III renal dysplasia, almost invariably affects both kidneys, although often asymmetrically. Although the malformation process begins in utero, in most cases the disease is clinically manifested in adulthood, or more rarely in early infancy.

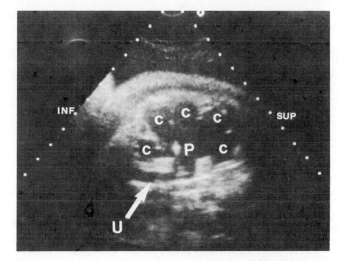

**FIGURE 19-10.** A coronal scan of the fetal trunk demonstrating renal cysts (C) radially distributed and communicating with an enlarged renal pelvis (P). The proximal portion of the dilated ureter (U) is also visualized in this scanning plane. The contralateral kidney appeared normal on ultrasound. A diagnosis of unilateral ureterovesical junction obstruction was made at this point and confirmed after birth. (INF, inferior; SUP, superior.) (From Rizzo N, et al. Prenatal diagnosis and management of multicystic dysplastic kidney disease. Prenat Diagn 1987;7:115.

## Pathogenesis

APKD may be inherited as an autosomal dominant trait, and it may be a feature of genetic and nongenetic syndromes. Sporadic diseases have also been reported in the literature.

## Prenatal Diagnosis

APKD has been detected in the third trimester. We were able to make a diagnosis during the second trimester. Ultrasound revealed a grossly enlarged left kidney, which contained multiple cysts of variable size intermixed with well-represented, hyperechogenic solid tissue. The contralateral kidney and the bladder were normal. The amniotic fluid was within normal range. Careful survey of fetal anatomy did not reveal other abnormalities.

In other cases, bilateral involvement can occur. Differential diagnosis between MDKD and APKD is possible, because in APKD renal parenchyma interposed between the cysts is well preserved in most cases. When APKD has been found in a newborn or in a fetus, both parents should be carefully examined. Using a highly polymorphic DNA probe genetically linked to the mutant gene, prenatal diagnosis is possible.

## Associated Anomalies

APKD is often part of malformation complexes, which have been extensively reviewed. Detection of Potter's Type III cystic dysplasia associated with occipital encephalocele allows for the diagnosis of Meckel-Gruber syndrome, which is a lethal anomaly occurring in an autosomal recessive manner (25% recurrence risk for subsequent pregnancies). Therefore, careful survey of the entire fetal anatomy is mandatory.

## Prognosis and Management

Because experience with prenatal diagnosis is limited, no data regarding the natural history of the disease are available. Based on postnatal course, APKD is a chronic disease that can be asymptomatic and detected at autopsy only. It can manifest itself at any age, from the newborn period to adulthood.

Parents at risk should be informed of the possibility of first trimester prenatal diagnosis. When diagnosis is made before viability, the option to terminate the pregnancy can be offered to the couple. Conservative management should be the rule when diagnosis is made after viability.

## OBSTRUCTIVE UROPATHIES

GU tract obstructions are among the most common congenital anomalies. The prevalence of obstructive uropathies is unknown, although it has been estimated in 1 out of 6000 live births. These anomalies are usually sporadic, but a few familial cases also have been described. Prenatal ultrasound diagnosis is based on the recognition of a dilated GU tract. Prognosis and management vary considerably according to the type and severity of the obstruction, and also in relation to associated anomalies. According to the level of the obstruction, it is possible to distinguish high (at the level of the ureteropelvic junction), median (at the level of the ureterovesical junction), and low (at the level of the urethra) obstructions. High and median obstructions can be either bilateral or unilateral.

### Ureteropelvic Junction Obstruction

The prevalence of the disease is unknown. Male neonates seem to be more frequently affected (male to female ratio, 5:1).

**Pathogenesis.** In most cases sporadic, familial occurrence or autosomal dominant cases have been reported.

**Associated Anomalies.** Urinary anomalies, such as vesicoureteral reflux, kidney duplication, contralateral renal agenesis, and meatal stenosis, are commonly associated. GI and cardiac anomalies and neural tube defects are variably present in association.

**Prenatal Diagnosis.** Prenatal ultrasound diagnosis is based on the finding of a dilated renal pelvis. Particularly at advanced gestational age, a slightly enlarged pelvis is fairly common. Quantitative criteria for diagnosis have been suggested: anteroposterior diameter >1 cm, and the ratio between maximal transverse diameter of the pelvis and renal diameter measured at the same level (>0.5). The severity of the anomaly varies from mild dilation to enormous cystic masses, without any chance of recognizing the calyces. If unilateral, the contralateral kidney is normal, the bladder is visible, and the amniotic fluid is preserved. Bilateral diseases, when severe, may determine compromised renal function. Occasionally, mild hydronephrosis detected by ultrasound in utero has not been confirmed on postnatal examination; therefore, spontaneous resolution can occur. Differential diagnosis has to be established with multicystic kidney (see the earlier section on MDKD). In late gestation, it is sometimes impossible to distinguish the two conditions; however, neither of them requires alteration of standard obstetric management. Duplication of the kidney is commonly associated with dilation of one or both renal pelves.

**Prognosis and Management.** Prognosis is good, unless associated anomalies are present. In most cases, obstruction is not particularly tight and probably develops late in gestation. Rarely, and particularly in cases of bilateral involvement, the process progresses to compromised renal function. There is generally no need to alter standard obstetric management; affected fetuses should be vaginally delivered at term.

## Ureterovesical Junction Obstruction

**Pathogenesis.** Ureterovesical junction (UVJ) obstruction is a sporadic disease in most cases. It can be unilateral or bilateral. The anomaly is caused by a deficiency of muscular fibers at the distal end of the ureter, limiting peristalsis, or by the presence of fibrous tissue instead of muscular fibers in the ureter wall. Urine, therefore, cannot enter the bladder, accumulating in the proximal portion of the ureter, and eventually causing dilation of the renal pelvis.

**Associated Anomalies.** Various urinary anomalies can be associated with UVJ obstruction, such as contralateral renal agenesis, ectopic kidney, renal cystic dysplasia, and horseshoe kidney. Cardiac and GI anomalies can occasionally occur.

**Prenatal Diagnosis.** In cases of UVJ obstruction, the ureter is dilated and tortuous, and on ultrasound appears as a collection of cysts of variable size localized between the renal pelvis, which is variably dilated, and the bladder, which is of normal morphology and dimensions. Amniotic fluid is present in normal amounts.

**Prognosis and Management.** Prognosis is good, unless in cases of bilateral involvement renal function deteriorates. In most cases, obstetrical management remains unchanged. When the pathological process worsens along with gestation, preterm induction of labor can be attempted so that postnatal surgical correction can be performed soon after birth.

## Urethral-Level Obstruction

**Pathogenesis.** The anomaly is generally sporadic; however, in some cases it has a genetic basis. Obstruction is usually caused by two semicircular membranous plicae at the level of the verumontanum. Those plicae, as urine flows from the bladder, adhere and close the upper portion of the urethra. The upper urinary tract anatomy (bladder, ureters, and renal pelvis) is dilated. Increased upstream pressure with time is responsible for kidney dysplasia. An early obstruction is more likely to determine compromised renal function, compared with cases that are diagnosed only in late pregnancy.

**Prenatal Diagnosis.** Urethral valves cannot be detected by ultrasound. Diagnosis has been suggested by dilation of the entire GU tract in a male fetus. The urinary bladder is overdistended, often reaching the transverse umbilical line. The initial portion of the urethra is often visible, giving a peculiar "keyhole" image (Fig. 19-11). Ureters are usually moderately dilated and tortuous. The renal pelvis can be only minimally dilated, particularly in cases of compromised renal function. The increased pressure in the urinary system may lead to a severe kidney

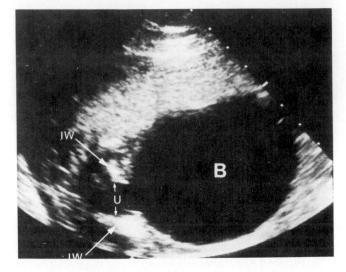

**FIGURE 19-11.** Longitudinal scan of the lower abdomen in a fetus with lower obstructive uropathy (Potter IV). The dilatation of the proximal tract of the urethra (U) is evident. (B, enlarged bladder; IW, iliac wings.)

dysplasia, which is characterized by hyperechogenicity of the kidneys and the presence of cortical cysts. More or less severe oligohydramnios is present. The association of low obstructive uropathy and ascites is typical of the so-called prune-belly syndrome, which is also characterized by a distended abdomen and abdominal wall hypoplasia.

**Associated Anomalies.** Associated anomalies are present in a minority of cases of low obstructive uropathies.

**Prognosis and Management.** Among fetal kidneys with obstructive uropathies, sonographic demonstration of renal dysplasia indicates irreversible renal damage that is probably consequent to elevated pressures within the developing nephron system. The presence of cortical cysts is suggestive of dysplasia. However, absence of the cysts does not exclude renal dysplasia, because not all dysplastic kidneys have cysts, or the cysts may be smaller than the ultrasound resolution power. An increased renal echogenicity is occasionally found in cases of renal dysplasia, due to the presence of abundant fibrous tissue. Not all the dysplastic kidneys are hyperechogenic and, conversely, 20% of hyperechogenic kidneys are not dysplastic. Therefore, increased renal echogenicity cannot predict renal dysplasia with certainty. Because ultrasound has a limited accuracy, evaluation of renal function is enhanced by analysis of the urine sampled by intrauterine cystocentesis. A poor prognostic factor is a decreased output (<2 mL/hr) of isotonic urine (osmolarity, >210 mOsm; sodium, >100 mEq/mL; chloride, >90 mEq/mL). Conversely, normal glomerular and tubular function is implied by hypotonic fetal urine. When in utero diagnosis of low obstructive uropathies is made, prognosis is relatively poor. Affected neonates carry a high risk for death (32% to 50%) as a consequence of pulmonary hypoplasia, associated congenital anomalies, renal failure, and surgical complications after decompressive surgery. Most patients show an improvement in renal function after surgery, although progressive renal failure may occur despite correction.

Obstetrical management depends on associated congenital anomalies, gestational age at diagnosis, and status of renal function. Careful survey of the anatomy is mandatory, although it is hampered by oligohydramnios. Infusion of saline may be useful. Fetal karyotype by amniocentesis or, when this is not feasible, by cordocentesis, should be undertaken, because various prevalences of associated chromosomal anomalies (up to 23% of the cases) are reported in the literature. When an anatomical or chromosomal defect that is incompatible with life is diagnosed, the option of terminating the pregnancy can be offered to the couple. Next, renal function needs to be studied. Poor prognostic factors are oligohydramnios, the presence of cortical cysts, and the urine parameters reported above. With poor prognostic criteria, termination of pregnancy or conservative management are the available options. If prognosis is good, further management depends on gestational age at diagnosis. If diagnosis is made during the third trimester and fetal lung maturity is proved by an L/S ratio, the fetus should be delivered vaginally, if not clinically contraindicated, where pediatric surgery is available. If the diagnosis is made after viability but before lung maturity, preventive in utero decompression may be attempted, or, in cases of decreasing amniotic fluid, conservative management and intervention only may be chosen. The outcome of infants who have undergone vesicoamniotic shunt is reported in the Registry of the International Fetal Medicine and Surgery Society.[‡] Forty percent (35/87) of the fetuses with obstructive uropathies who underwent in utero surgery survived. Because the vesicoamniotic shunt cannot be the ideal long-term treatment for obstructive uropathies, Harrison and coworkers, with a small group of five patients, have used a technique for open fetal urinary tract decompression.[§] All fetuses were delivered by cesarean section at 32 to 35 weeks. Three fetuses showed normal pulmonary function at birth. Two fetuses died soon after birth of pulmonary hypoplasia. Of the three surviving infants, two had normal renal function, but one required renal transplantation for worsening of renal function. Open fetal surgery is therefore feasible, and may prevent pulmonary hypoplasia at birth; however, the effect of decompression on the development of renal dysplasia and ultimate renal function is still unknown.

## FETAL OVARIAN CYSTS

Ovarian cysts are one of the most common causes of abdominal mass in the female neonate. They are the most significant genital anomaly presenting in the prenatal period.

### Pathogenesis
Although classically related to hormonal stimulation, the cause of the anomaly is still uncertain. Interestingly, congenital ovarian cysts have occurred in association with hypothyroidism.

---

[‡] Evans M. Newsletter, International Fetal Medicine and Surgery Society, 1989.
[§] Crombleholme TM, Harrison MR, Langer JC, et al. Early experience with open fetal surgery for congenital hydronephrosis. J Pediatr Surg 1988;23:1114.

## Prenatal Diagnosis

Prenatal ultrasound diagnosis is possible from the second trimester of pregnancy. Cystic mass in the fetal lower abdomen, integrity of GI and GU tracts, and female sex are the main ultrasound criteria for diagnosis of fetal ovarian cyst. In the majority of cases, the cyst is completely fluid; sometimes it is septated. Polyhydramnios is often present. However, diagnosis is always presumptive, because rare conditions, including mesenteric and urachal cysts, enteric duplication anomalies, cystic teratoma, and low intestinal obstructions, cannot be ruled out with certainty in utero. Serial examinations of the anomaly allow the detection of structural changes of the cyst, which prompt the diagnosis of a complication of the cyst.

## Associated Anomalies

Associated anomalies are uncommon, although an increased amniotic fluid is often present, probably secondary to partial GI obstruction.

## Prognosis and Management

Prognosis and management of fetal ovarian cysts depends largely on the natural history of the mass. The cyst may increase in size, decrease, or even disappear, or lead to complications such as torsion, infarction, and rupture. In this light, once prenatal ultrasound diagnosis has been made, serial examinations should be performed throughout gestation to detect any structural change in the mass. Enlargement of the mass, causing distension of the fetal abdomen, is an indication for cesarean section to avoid the risk of soft tissue dystocia. Ultrasound-guided fine-needle aspiration of large fetal ovarian cysts may eliminate the need for a cesarean section and theoretically may diminish the risk of intrauterine torsion. However, the benefit of such an invasive procedure is unclear, and it may possibly cause intraperitoneal bleeding. Sudden development of intense hyperechogenicity within the mass, followed by a complex, heterogeneous appearance, should be considered to result from an intrauterine torsion of the cyst with infarction. When this occurs, immediate delivery should be considered. Conversely, small cysts detected in utero can subsequently disappear and may not be present on a postnatal ultrasound evaluation.

In summary, prenatal diagnosis of fetal ovarian cysts per se should not modify standard obstetrical management, whereas complications occurring during gestation, such as torsion and rupture, may require active obstetric intervention. Fetuses with confirmed diagnosis often require postnatal ovariectomy soon after birth.

# 20. FETAL SKELETAL ANOMALIES

Skeletal dysplasias are a heterogeneous group of disorders that affect the development of chondro-osseous tissues and result in abnormalities in the size and shape of different segments of the skeleton. Little is known about their etiology, but genetic factors are clearly important, because a Mendelian pattern of inheritance has been described in many of these conditions. Sporadic cases suggest the appearance of new spontaneous mutations or environmental factors. Exposure to drugs (e.g., thalidomide, warfarin), ionic radiation, hyperthermia, hyperglycemia (diabetes mellitus), mechanical factors, and vascular disruption with hypoperfusion of specific areas in the embryo have been implicated in the etiology of some skeletal dysplasias. Prevalence of skeletal dysplasias is given in Table 20-1.

## BIRTH PREVALENCE AND CONTRIBUTION TO PERINATAL MORTALITY

The birth prevalence of skeletal dysplasias, excluding limb amputations, recognizable in the neonatal period has been estimated to be 2.4 of 10,000 births. In a large series, 23% of affected infants were stillborn, and 32% died during the first week of life. Thanatophoric dysplasia and achondrogenesis accounted for 62% of all lethal skeletal dysplasias. The most common nonlethal skeletal dysplasia was achondroplasia.

## CLASSIFICATION OF SKELETAL DYSPLASIAS

1. Osteochondrodysplasias—abnormalities of cartilage and/or bone growth and development
2. Dysostoses—malformations of individual bones singly or in combination
3. Idiopathic osteolysis—disorders associated with multifocal resorption of bone
4. Skeletal disorders associated with chromosomal aberrations
5. Primary metabolic disorders

## TERMINOLOGY FREQUENTLY USED IN THE DESCRIPTION OF BONE DYSPLASIAS

Shortening of the extremities can involve the entire limb (micromelia), the proximal segment (rhizomelia), the intermediate segment (mesomelia), or the distal segment (acromelia). The diagnosis of rhizomelia or mesomelia requires the comparison of the dimensions of the bones of the legs and forearm with those of the thigh and arm. The relationship between the humerus and ulna, and the femur and tibia, can be used in the assessment of rhizomelia and acromesomelia. Table 20-2 presents skeletal dysplasias characterized by rhizomelia, mesomelia, acromelia, and micromelia.

E. Albert Reece, John C. Hobbins, Maurice, J. Mahoney and Roy H. Petrie (Eds). *Handbook of Medicine of the Fetus & Mother.* Copyright © 1995 by J.B. Lippincott Company

**TABLE 20-1.** Birth Prevalence (per 10,000 Total Births) of Skeletal Dysplasias

|  | Birth Prevalence (per 10,000) | Frequency Among Perinatal Deaths |
|---|---|---|
| Thanatophoric dysplasia | 0.69 | 1:246 |
| Achondroplasia | 0.37 | — |
| Achondrogenesis | 0.23 | 1:639 |
| Osteogenesis imperfecta type II | 0.18 | 1:799 |
| Osteogenesis imperfecta (other types) | 0.18 | — |
| Asphyxiating thoracic dysplasia | 0.14 | 1:3196 |
| Chondrodysplasia punctata | 0.09 | — |
| Camptomelic dysplasia | 0.05 | 1:3196 |
| Chondroectodermal dysplasia | 0.05 | 1:3196 |
| Larsen syndrome | 0.05 | — |
| Mesomelic dysplasia (Langer's type) | 0.05 | — |
| Others | 0.46 | 1:800 |
| Total skeletal dysplasias | 2.44 | 1:110 |

Camera G, Mastroiacova P. Birth prevalence of skeletal dysplasias in the Italian multicentric monitoring system for birth defects. In: Papadatos CJ, Bartsocas CS, eds. Skeletal dysplasias. New York: Alan R. Liss, 1982:441.

**TABLE 20-2.** Classification of Skeletal Dysplasias by Rhizomelia, Mesomelia, Acromelia, and Micromelia

**Rhizomelia**
Thanatophoric dysplasia
Atelosteogenesis
Chondrodysplasia punctata (rhizomelic type)
Diastrophic dysplasia
Congenital short femur
Achondroplasia

**Mesomelia**
Mesomelic dysplasia (Langer, Reinhardt, and Robinow types)
COVESDEM association

**Acromelia**
Ellis-van Creveld syndrome (Chondroectodermal dysplasia)

**Micromelia**
Achondrogenesis
Atelosteogenesis
Short-rib–polydactyly syndrome (type I and type II)
Diastrophic dysplasia
Fibrochondrogenesis
Osteogenesis imperfecta (type III)
Kniest dysplasia
Dyssegmental dysplasia
Roberts syndrome

Reproduced with permission from Romero R, Athanassiadis AP, Sirtori M, Inati M. Fetal skeletal anomalies. In: Fleischer AC, Romero R, Manning FA, Jeanty P, James AE Jr, eds. The principles and practice of ultrasonography in obstetrics and gynecology, 4th ed. Norwalk, CT: Appleton & Lange, 1991:286.

Several skeletal dysplasias feature alterations of the hands and feet. The term *polydactyly* refers to the presence of more than five digits. It is classified as postaxial if the extra digits are on the ulnar or fibular side, and preaxial if they are located on the radial or tibial side. Syndactyly refers to soft-tissue or bony fusion of adjacent digits. Clinodactyly consists of deviation of a finger (or fingers). The most common spinal abnormality seen in skeletal dysplasias is platyspondylia, which consists of flattening of the vertebrae. Kyphosis and scoliosis can also be identified in utero. Prenatal diagnosis of hemivertebra and coronal clefting of vertebral bodies has been made.

## BIOMETRY OF THE FETAL SKELETON IN THE DIAGNOSIS OF BONE DYSPLASIAS

The type of nomogram required to assess the normality of bone dimensions uses gestational age as the independent variable and the long bone as the dependent variable. For the proper use of these nomograms, the clinician must accurately know the gestational age of the fetus. Tables 20-3 and 20-4 present nomograms for the assessment of limb biometry for the upper and lower extremities, respectively. For those patients presenting with uncertain gestational age, comparisons between limb dimensions and the head perimeter can be used (Figs. 20-1 and 20-2).

## CLINICAL PRESENTATION

Clinical presentation usually involves (1) a patient who has delivered an infant with a skeletal dysplasia and desires antenatal assessment of a subsequent pregnancy; or (2) the incidental finding of a shortened, bowed, or anomalous extremity during a routine sonographic examination.

Despite these difficulties and limitations, there are good medical reasons for attempting an accurate prenatal diagnosis of skeletal dysplasias. A number of these disorders are uniformly lethal, and a confident antenatal diagnosis would present the patient with options for the termination of the pregnancy. Table 20-5 lists such disorders. Other skeletal dysplasias are associated with mental retardation, and this information is important in prenatal counseling. There is a group of disorders associated with thrombocytopenia. Vaginal delivery may expose these infants to the risk of intracranial hemorrhage.

## APPROACH TO THE DIAGNOSIS OF SKELETAL DYSPLASIAS

1. *Evaluation of long bones.* All long bones should be measured in all extremities. Comparisons with other segments should be performed to establish whether the limb shortening is predominantly rhizomelic, mesomelic, or acromelic, or whether it involves all segments (Fig. 20-3). A detailed examination of each bone is necessary to exclude the absence or hypoplasia of individual bones (fibula, tibia, scapula, radius), which are frequently absent in certain conditions.

   An attempt should be made to characterize the degree of mineralization. This can be assessed by examining the acoustic shadow behind the bone and the echogenicity of the bone itself. Signs of demineralization are the visual-

**TABLE 20-3.** Normal Values for the ARM (mm)

| Week | Humerus | | | Ulna | | |
|---|---|---|---|---|---|---|
| | Percentile | | | Percentile | | |
| | 5th | 50th | 95th | 5th | 50th | 95th |
| 12 | — | 9 | — | — | 7 | — |
| 13 | 6 | 11 | 16 | 5 | 10 | 15 |
| 14 | 9 | 14 | 19 | 8 | 13 | 18 |
| 15 | 12 | 17 | 22 | 11 | 16 | 21 |
| 16 | 15 | 20 | 25 | 13 | 18 | 23 |
| 17 | 18 | 22 | 27 | 16 | 21 | 26 |
| 18 | 20 | 25 | 30 | 19 | 24 | 29 |
| 19 | 23 | 28 | 33 | 21 | 26 | 31 |
| 20 | 25 | 30 | 35 | 24 | 29 | 34 |
| 21 | 28 | 33 | 38 | 26 | 31 | 36 |
| 22 | 30 | 35 | 40 | 28 | 33 | 38 |
| 23 | 33 | 38 | 42 | 31 | 36 | 41 |
| 24 | 35 | 40 | 45 | 33 | 38 | 43 |
| 25 | 37 | 42 | 47 | 35 | 40 | 45 |
| 26 | 39 | 44 | 49 | 37 | 42 | 47 |
| 27 | 41 | 46 | 51 | 39 | 44 | 49 |
| 28 | 43 | 48 | 53 | 41 | 46 | 51 |
| 29 | 45 | 50 | 55 | 43 | 48 | 53 |
| 30 | 47 | 51 | 56 | 44 | 49 | 54 |
| 31 | 48 | 53 | 58 | 46 | 51 | 56 |
| 32 | 50 | 55 | 60 | 48 | 53 | 58 |
| 33 | 51 | 56 | 61 | 49 | 54 | 59 |
| 34 | 53 | 58 | 63 | 51 | 56 | 61 |
| 35 | 54 | 59 | 64 | 52 | 57 | 62 |
| 36 | 56 | 61 | 65 | 53 | 58 | 63 |
| 37 | 57 | 62 | 67 | 55 | 60 | 65 |
| 38 | 59 | 63 | 68 | 56 | 61 | 66 |
| 39 | 60 | 65 | 70 | 57 | 62 | 67 |
| 40 | 61 | 66 | 71 | 58 | 63 | 68 |
| | mm | mm | mm | mm | mm | mm |

Modified from Romero R, Athanassiadis AP, Sirtori M, Inati M. Fetal skeletal anomalies. In: Fleischer AC, Romero R, Manning FA, Jeanty P, James AE Jr, eds. The principles and practice of ultrasonography in obstetrics and gynecology, 4th ed. Norwalk, Ct: Appleton & Lange, 1991:283.

ization of an unusually prominent falx and the absent or decreased echogenicity of the spine. It should be stressed that there are limitations in the sonographic evaluation of mineralization of long bones and that other structures, such as the skull, may be better suited for this assessment (Fig. 20-4). The degree of long-bone curvature should be examined. At present, there is no objective means of assessing this sign, and experience is the only means

**TABLE 20-4.** Normal Values for the Leg (mm)

| Week | Tibia | | | Femur | | |
|------|-------|-------|-------|-------|-------|-------|
| | Percentile | | | Percentile | | |
| | 5th | 50th | 95th | 5th | 50th | 95th |
| 12 | — | 7 | — | 4 | 8 | 13 |
| 13 | — | 10 | — | 6 | 11 | 16 |
| 14 | 7 | 12 | 17 | 9 | 14 | 18 |
| 15 | 9 | 15 | 20 | 12 | 17 | 21 |
| 16 | 12 | 17 | 22 | 15 | 20 | 24 |
| 17 | 15 | 20 | 25 | 18 | 23 | 27 |
| 18 | 17 | 22 | 27 | 21 | 25 | 30 |
| 19 | 20 | 25 | 30 | 24 | 28 | 33 |
| 20 | 22 | 27 | 33 | 26 | 31 | 36 |
| 21 | 25 | 30 | 35 | 29 | 34 | 38 |
| 22 | 27 | 32 | 38 | 32 | 36 | 41 |
| 23 | 30 | 35 | 40 | 35 | 39 | 44 |
| 24 | 32 | 37 | 42 | 37 | 42 | 46 |
| 25 | 34 | 40 | 45 | 40 | 44 | 49 |
| 26 | 37 | 42 | 47 | 42 | 47 | 51 |
| 27 | 39 | 44 | 49 | 45 | 49 | 54 |
| 28 | 41 | 46 | 51 | 47 | 52 | 56 |
| 29 | 43 | 48 | 53 | 50 | 54 | 59 |
| 30 | 45 | 50 | 55 | 52 | 56 | 61 |
| 31 | 47 | 52 | 57 | 54 | 59 | 63 |
| 32 | 48 | 54 | 59 | 56 | 61 | 65 |
| 33 | 50 | 55 | 60 | 58 | 63 | 67 |
| 34 | 52 | 57 | 62 | 60 | 65 | 69 |
| 35 | 53 | 58 | 64 | 62 | 67 | 71 |
| 36 | 55 | 60 | 65 | 64 | 68 | 73 |
| 37 | 56 | 61 | 67 | 65 | 70 | 74 |
| 38 | 58 | 63 | 68 | 67 | 71 | 76 |
| 39 | 59 | 64 | 69 | 68 | 73 | 77 |
| 40 | 61 | 66 | 71 | 70 | 74 | 79 |
| | mm | mm | mm | mm | mm | mm |

Modified from Romero R, Athanassiadis AP, Sirtori M, Inati M. Fetal skeletal anomalies. In: Fleischer AC, Romero R, Manning FA, Jeanty P, James AE Jr, eds. The principles and practice of ultrasonography in obstetrics and gynecology, 4th ed. Norwalk, Ct: Appleton & Lange, 1991:284.

by which the operator can discern the boundary between normality and abnormality (Fig. 20-5). Finally, the possibility of fractures should also be considered (e.g., osteogenesis imperfecta) (Fig. 20-6). The fractures may be extremely subtle or may lead to angulation and separation of the segments of the affected bone (Fig. 20-7).

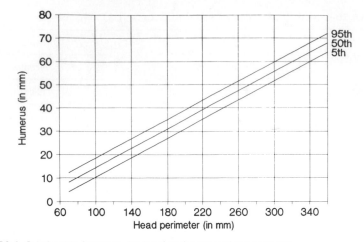

**FIGURE 20-1.** Relationship between the head perimeter and the humerus.

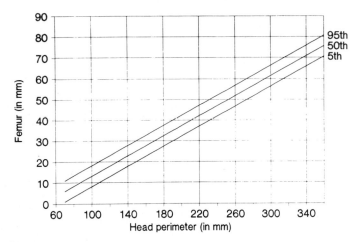

**FIGURE 20-2.** Relationship between the head perimeter and the femur.

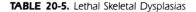

**TABLE 20-5.** Lethal Skeletal Dysplasias

Achondrogenesis
Thanatophoric dysplasia
Short-rib–polydactyly syndromes (types I, II, and III)
Fibrochondrogenesis
Atelosteogenesis
Homozygous achondroplasia
Osteogenesis imperfecta, perinatal type
Hypophosphatasia

Romero R, Athanassiadis AP, Sirtori M, Inati M. Fetal skeletal anomalies. In: Fleischer AC, Romero R, Manning FA, Jeanty P, James AE Jr, eds. The principles and practice of ultrasonography in obstetrics and gynecology. 4th ed. Norwalk, CT: Appleton & Lange, 1991:287.

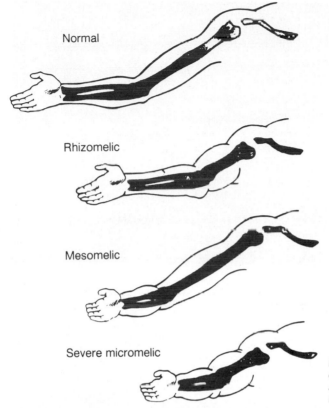

Normal

Rhizomelic

Mesomelic

Severe micromelic

**FIGURE 20-3.** Varieties of short-limb dysplasia according to the segment involved.

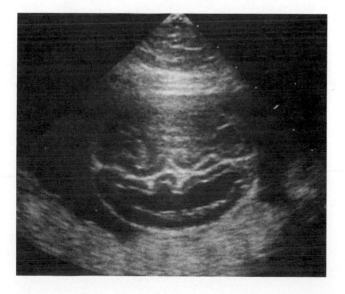

**FIGURE 20-4.** Demineralization of the skull in a case of congenital hypophosphatasia.

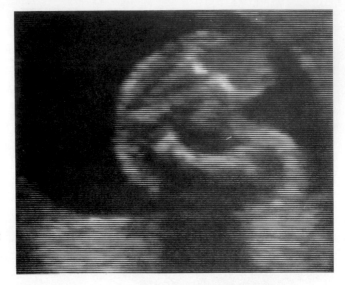

**FIGURE 20-5.** Shortening and bowing of the humerus with short but straight ulna and radius in a fetus with micromelia.

**FIGURE 20-6.** Osteogenesis imperfecta type II. Multiple fractures in long bones and ribs are present. Note the severe bowing and shortening of both femurs.

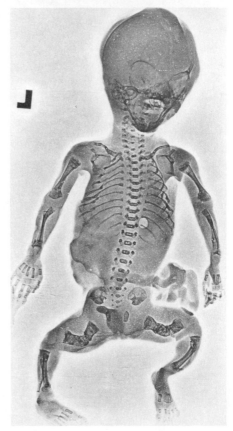

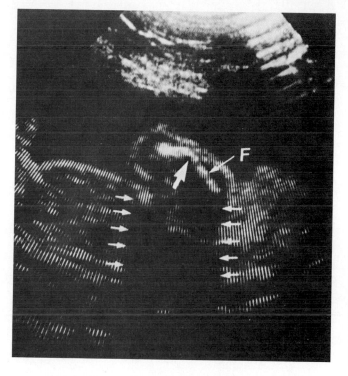

**FIGURE 20-7.** In utero fracture in a case of osteogenesis imperfecta. The large arrow corresponds to the fracture site. The small arrows outline the decreased shadowing cast by the bone. (F, femur.)

2. *Evaluation of thoracic dimensions.* Several skeletal dysplasias are associated with a hypoplastic thorax. The appropriateness of thoracic dimensions can be assessed by measuring the thoracic circumference at the level of the four-chamber view of the heart. The thoracic circumference can be measured or calculated using the following formula: thoracic circumference = (antero-posterior diameter + transverse diameter) × 1.57. The thoracic length is measured from the boundary between the neck and the chest to the diaphragm. Tables 20-6 and 20-7 illustrate nomograms used to evaluate the thoracic dimensions in fetuses with known gestational age. The thoracic-to-abdominal circumference ratio (normal value: 0.77–1.01) and the thoracic-to-head circumference ratio (normal value: 0.56–1.04) permit evaluation of the transverse thoracic dimensions.

   Evaluation of thoracic dimensions is a critical part of the workup because the cause of death in most lethal skeletal dysplasias is pulmonary hypoplasia secondary to an underdeveloped rib cage (Fig. 20-8). Table 20-8 displays skeletal dysplasias associated with alteration of thoracic dimensions.

3. *Evaluation of hands and feet.* Hands and feet should be examined to exclude polydactyly, brachydactyly, and extreme postural deformities. Table 20-9 shows a nomogram of the fetal foot size throughout gestation. Table 20-10 displays disorders associated with hand and foot deformities. Disproportion between hands and feet and the other parts of the extremity may also be a sign of a skeletal dysplasia. Figure 20-9 illustrates the relationship between

**TABLE 20-6.** Fetal Thoracic Circumference Measurements (in cm)

| Gestational Age (wk) | No. | Predictive Percentiles | | | |
|---|---|---|---|---|---|
| | | 5 | 25 | 75 | 95 |
| 16 | 6 | 6.4 | 8.0 | 10.3 | 11.9 |
| 17 | 22 | 7.3 | 8.9 | 11.2 | 12.8 |
| 18 | 31 | 8.2 | 9.8 | 12.1 | 13.7 |
| 19 | 21 | 9.1 | 10.7 | 13.0 | 14.6 |
| 20 | 20 | 10.0 | 11.7 | 13.9 | 15.5 |
| 21 | 30 | 11.0 | 12.6 | 14.8 | 16.4 |
| 22 | 18 | 11.9 | 13.5 | 15.7 | 17.3 |
| 23 | 21 | 12.8 | 14.4 | 16.6 | 18.2 |
| 24 | 27 | 13.7 | 15.3 | 17.5 | 19.1 |
| 25 | 20 | 14.6 | 16.2 | 18.4 | 20.0 |
| 26 | 25 | 15.5 | 17.1 | 19.3 | 21.0 |
| 27 | 24 | 16.4 | 18.0 | 20.2 | 21.9 |
| 28 | 24 | 17.3 | 18.9 | 21.2 | 22.8 |
| 29 | 24 | 18.2 | 19.8 | 22.1 | 23.7 |
| 30 | 27 | 19.1 | 20.7 | 23.0 | 24.6 |
| 31 | 24 | 20.0 | 21.6 | 23.9 | 25.5 |
| 32 | 28 | 20.9 | 22.6 | 24.8 | 26.4 |
| 33 | 27 | 21.8 | 23.5 | 25.7 | 27.3 |
| 34 | 25 | 22.8 | 24.4 | 26.6 | 28.2 |
| 35 | 20 | 23.7 | 25.3 | 27.5 | 29.1 |
| 36 | 23 | 24.6 | 26.2 | 28.4 | 30.0 |
| 37 | 22 | 25.5 | 27.1 | 29.3 | 30.9 |
| 38 | 21 | 26.4 | 28.0 | 30.2 | 31.9 |
| 39 | 7 | 27.3 | 28.9 | 31.1 | 32.8 |
| 40 | 6 | 28.2 | 29.8 | 32.1 | 33.7 |

Modified from Chitkara U, Rosenberg J, Chervenak FA, et al. Prenatal sonographic assessment of the fetal thorax: normal values. Am J Obstet Gynecol 1987;156:1069.

femur length and foot length. The femur length/foot length ratio is nearly constant from the 14th to the 40th week.

4. *Evaluation of the fetal cranium.* Orbits should be measured to exclude hypertelorism. Other findings that should be searched for are micrognathia, short upper lip, abnormally shaped ear, frontal bossing, and cloverleaf skull deformity.

5. *Evaluation of the internal organs.* Some syndromes present with specific abnormalities of the internal organs, thus helping in the differential diagnoses of these entities.

Despite all efforts to establish an accurate prenatal diagnosis, a careful study of the newborn will be required in all instances. Examination of the skeletal radiographs will permit precise diagnoses in the overwhelming majority of cases, since the classification of skeletal dysplasias is largely based on radiographic findings. In lethal skeletal dysplasias, histologic examination of the chondro-osseous tissue

**TABLE 20-7.** Fetal Thoracic Circumference Measurements (in cm)

| Gestational Age (wk) | No. | Predictive Percentiles | | | |
|---|---|---|---|---|---|
| | | 5 | 25 | 75 | 95 |
| 16 | 6 | 1.1 | 1.6 | 2.4 | 3.0 |
| 17 | 22 | 1.3 | 1.8 | 2.6 | 3.2 |
| 18 | 31 | 1.4 | 2.0 | 2.8 | 3.4 |
| 19 | 21 | 1.6 | 2.2 | 3.0 | 3.6 |
| 20 | 20 | 1.8 | 2.4 | 3.2 | 3.8 |
| 21 | 30 | 2.0 | 2.6 | 3.4 | 4.0 |
| 22 | 18 | 2.2 | 2.8 | 3.6 | 4.1 |
| 23 | 21 | 2.4 | 3.0 | 3.8 | 4.3 |
| 24 | 27 | 2.6 | 3.1 | 3.9 | 4.5 |
| 25 | 20 | 2.8 | 3.3 | 4.1 | 4.7 |
| 26 | 25 | 2.9 | 3.5 | 4.3 | 4.9 |
| 27 | 24 | 3.1 | 3.7 | 4.5 | 5.1 |
| 28 | 24 | 3.3 | 3.9 | 4.7 | 5.4 |
| 29 | 24 | 3.5 | 4.1 | 4.9 | 5.5 |
| 30 | 27 | 3.7 | 4.3 | 5.1 | 5.6 |
| 31 | 24 | 3.9 | 4.5 | 5.3 | 5.8 |
| 32 | 28 | 4.1 | 4.6 | 5.4 | 6.0 |
| 33 | 27 | 4.3 | 4.8 | 5.6 | 6.2 |
| 34 | 25 | 4.4 | 5.0 | 5.8 | 6.4 |
| 35 | 20 | 4.6 | 5.2 | 6.0 | 6.6 |
| 36 | 23 | 4.8 | 5.4 | 6.2 | 6.8 |
| 37 | 22 | 5.0 | 5.6 | 6.4 | 7.0 |
| 38 | 21 | 5.2 | 5.8 | 6.6 | 7.1 |
| 39 | 7 | 5.4 | 6.0 | 6.8 | 7.3 |
| 40 | 6 | 5.6 | 6.1 | 6.9 | 7.5 |

Modified from Chitkara U, Rosenberg J, Chervenak FA, et al. Prenatal sonographic assessment of the fetal thorax: normal values. Am J. Obstet Gynecol 1987;156:1069.

should be performed, since this information may help reach a specific diagnosis. Chromosomal studies should be included, because there is a specific group of constitutional bone disorders associated with cytogenetic abnormalities. Biochemical studies are helpful in rare instances.

## OSTEOCHONDRODYSPLASIAS

### THANATOPHORIC DYSPLASIA, FIBROCHONDROGENESIS, ATELOSTEOGENESIS

Thanatophoric dysplasia is the most common lethal skeletal dysplasia in fetuses and neonates. It is characterized by extreme rhizomelia, a normal trunk length with a narrow thorax, and a large head with a prominent forehead.

It occurs in 0.24 to 0.69 of 10,000 births. Two subtypes have been identified: type 1, with typical bowed "telephone receiver" femurs and without cloverleaf skull;

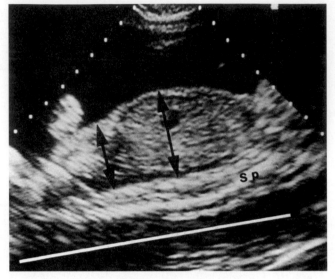

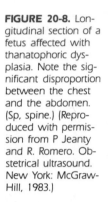

**FIGURE 20-8.** Longitudinal section of a fetus affected with thanatophoric dysplasia. Note the significant disproportion between the chest and the abdomen. (Sp, spine.) (Reproduced with permission from P Jeanty and R. Romero. Obstetrical ultrasound. New York: McGraw-Hill, 1983.)

**TABLE 20-8.** Skeletal Dysplasias Associated with Altered Thoracic Dimensions

---

**Long, Narrow Thorax**
Asphyxiating thoracic dysplasia (Jeune)
Chondroectodermal dysplasia (Ellis–van Creveld)
Metatropic dysplasia
Fibrochondrogenesis
Atelosteogenesis
Campomelic dysplasia
Jarcho-Levin syndrome
Achondrogenesis
Osteogenesis imperfecta congenita
Hypophosphatasia
Dyssegmental dysplasia
Cleidocranial dysplasia

**Short Thorax**
Osteogenesis imperfecta (type II)
Kniest dysplasia (metatropic dysplasia type II)
Pena-Shokeir syndrome

**Hypoplastic Thorax**
Short-rib–polydactyly syndrome (type I, type II)
Thanatophoric dysplasia
Cerebro-costo-mandibular syndrome
Cleidocranial dysostosis syndrome
Homozygous achondroplasia
Melnick-Needles syndrome (osteodysplasty)
Fibrochondrogenesis
Otopalatodigital syndrome type II

---

Modified from Romero R, Athanassiadis AP, Sirtori M, Inati M. Fetal skeletal anomalies. In: Fleischer AC, Romero R, Manning FA, Jeanty P, James AE Jr, eds. The principles and practice of ultrasonography in obstetrics and gynecology. 4th ed. Norwalk, CT: Appleton & Lange, 1991:292.

**TABLE 20-9.** Nomogram of Fetal Foot Size Throughout Gestation (mm)

| Gestational Age Week | Percentile | | |
|---|---|---|---|
| | 10th | 50th | 90th |
| 14 | 16 | 18 | 21 |
| 15 | 16 | 19 | 22 |
| 16 | 18 | 22 | 28 |
| 17 | 19 | 22 | 22 |
| 18 | 19 | 27 | 30 |
| 19 | 25 | 30 | 39 |
| 20 | 33 | 33 | 33 |
| 21 | 24 | 24 | 24 |
| 22 | 25 | 36 | 40 |
| 23 | 41 | 41 | 40 |
| 24 | 46 | 46 | 46 |
| 25 | 40 | 47 | 53 |
| 26 | 40 | 47 | 54 |
| 27 | 45 | 50 | 56 |
| 28 | 51 | 53 | 55 |
| 29 | 49 | 54 | 58 |
| 30 | 61 | 61 | 61 |
| 31 | 51 | 56 | 52 |
| 32 | 54 | 57 | 62 |
| 33 | 59 | 59 | 59 |
| 34 | 60 | 65 | 71 |
| 35 | 71 | 71 | 71 |

Romero R, Athanassiadis AP, Sirtori M, Inati M. Fetal skeletal anomalies. In: Fleischer AC, Romero R, Manning FA, Jeanty P, James AE Jr, eds. The principles and practice of ultrasonography in obstetrics and gynecology. 4th ed. Norwalk, CT: Appleton & Lange, 1991:294.

and type 2, with cloverleaf skull and short, straight long bones. The majority of cases of thanatophoric dysplasia (all type 1 and most cases of type 2) are sporadic. Some familial cases of type 2 have been reported.

The association of cloverleaf skull and micromelia is specific for thanatophoric dysplasia. There is a relatively large calvarium with a prominent forehead, a saddle nose, and hypertelorism. Additional findings are short ribs, platyspondylia, and short and broad tubular bones in hands and feet.

Fibrochondrogenesis is a lethal chondrodysplasia inherited with an autosomal recessive pattern and characterized by micromelia with significant metaphyseal flaring, normal head size, undermineralized skull, platyspondylia, clefting of the vertebral bodies, and narrow and bell-shaped thorax.

Atelosteogenesis is also a lethal chondrodysplasia characterized by severe micromelia (with hypoplasia of the distal segments of the humerus and femur), bowing of long bones, narrow chest with short ribs, coronal and sagittal vertebral clefts, and dislocation at the level of the elbow and knee.

**TABLE 20-10.** Skeletal Dysplasias Associated with Polydactyly and Syndactyly

---

**Postaxial Polydactyly**
Chondroectodermal dysplasia
Short-rib–polydactyly syndrome (type I, type II)
Asphyxiating thoracic dysplasia
Otopalatodigital syndrome
Mesomelic dysplasia, Werner type (associated with absence of thumbs)

**Preaxial Polydactyly**
Chondroectodermal dysplasia
Short-rib–polydactyly syndrome, type II
Carpenter syndrome

**Syndactyly**
Poland syndrome
Acrocephalosyndactylies (Carpenter syndrome, Apert syndrome)
Otopalatodigital syndrome, type II
Mesomelic dysplasia, Werner type
TAR syndrome
Jarcho-Levin syndrome
Roberts syndrome

**Brachydactyly**
Mesomelic dysplasia, Robinow type
Otopalatodigital syndrome

**Hitchhiker Thumbs**
Diastrophic dysplasia

**Clubfoot Deformity**
Diastrophic dysplasia
Osteogenesis imperfecta
Kniest dysplasia
Spondyloepiphyseal congenita
Metatropic dysplasia
Mesomelic dysplasia Nievergelt type
Chondrodysplasia punctata
Larsen syndrome
Roberts syndrome
TAR syndrome
Pena-Shokeir syndrome

---

Romero R, Athanassiadis AP, Sirtori M, Inati M. Fetal skeletal anomalies. In: Fleischer AC, Romero R, Manning FA, Jeanty P, James AE Jr, eds. The principles and practice of ultrasonography in obstetrics and gynecology. 4th ed. Norwalk, CT: Appleton & Lange, 1991:294.

## ACHONDROGENESIS

Achondrogenesis, or anosteogenesis, is a lethal chondrodystrophy characterized by extreme micromelia, short trunk, and macrocrania. Traditionally, this disorder has been classified into two types: the more severe form, which is type I achondrogenesis (Parenti-Fraccaro), and type II achondrogenesis (Langer-Saldino). Recently, type I has been subdivided into two subtypes: type IA (Houston-Harris) and type IB (Fraccaro). Evidence now suggests that hypochondrogenesis and achondrogenesis type II are phenotypic variants of the same disorder. Indeed, clinically and radiologically, achondrogenesis type II, hypochondrogenesis, and

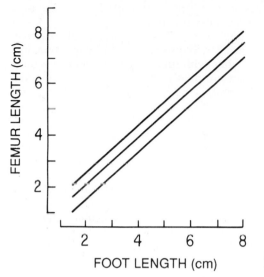

FOOT LENGTH (cm)

**FIGURE 20-9.** Relationship between the femur length and the foot length.

neonatal spondyloepiphyseal dysplasia congenita form a continuum spectrum of disease.

Prenatal diagnosis should be suspected on the basis of micromelia, lack of vertebral ossification, and a large head with various degrees of ossification of the calvarium. Achondrogenesis type IA and type IB are inherited with an autosomal recessive pattern, whereas most cases of achondrogenesis type II and hypochondrogenesis have been sporadic (new autosomal dominant mutations).

## ACHONDROPLASIA

The most common nonlethal skeletal dysplasia is achondroplasia. It is characterized by rhizomelic shortening, limb bowing, lordotic spine, and enlarged head. It is inherited with an autosomal dominant pattern, and its prevalence is 1 out of 66,000. Advanced paternal age is a risk factor for achondroplasia. The major difficulty in the antenatal diagnosis is that the long-bone growth in this disease is not clearly appreciated in most cases until the third trimester of pregnancy. Heterozygous achondroplasia is compatible with a normal life and intellectual development. The disease is lethal in the homozygous state.

Hypochondroplasia is a disorder that resembles achondroplasia. The differential diagnosis between these two conditions is based on the sparing of the head and the lack of tibial bowing in hypochondroplasia.

## OSTEOGENESIS IMPERFECTA AND HYPOPHOSPHATASIA

In type I (autosomal dominant) of osteogenesis imperfecta, patients have bone fragility, blue sclera (all ages), and hearing loss. There is osteoporosis and a normal calvarium; fractures range from none to multiple. Type II (new dominant mutations; less than 5% autosomal recessive) is also known as the perinatal variety and is uniformly lethal. There is almost no ossification of the skull; beaded ribs; shortened, crumpled long bones; and multiple fractures in utero. The thorax is short but not narrow. Type II is subclassified into three subtypes—IIA, IIB, and IIC—according to radiologic criteria (Fig. 20-10). Type III (autosomal recessive, rare) is a nonlethal variety characterized by blue sclera and multiple fractures present at birth. The sclera becomes white with time. The membranous skull is severely deossified and the long bones are mildly shortened but with marked angulations. Type IV (autosomal dominant) is the mildest form. Long bones and sclera are normal. There is mild to moderate osseous fragility, and 25% of the newborns have fractures. There is significant heterogeneity in the expression of the disease even within the same family. Linkage analysis has been used effectively for prenatal diagnosis. Hypophosphatasia is a group of disorders characterized by demineralization of bones and low alkaline phosphatase in serum and other tissues.

Fetuses with congenital hypophosphatasia have generalized demineralization of the skeleton, with shortening and bowing of tubular bones. Multiple fractures are present. The marked demineralization of the cranial vault results in deformation of the skull after external compression. Prenatal diagnosis of this condition has been reported with ultrasound and by assaying alkaline phosphatase in tissue obtained by chorionic villus sampling and alkaline phosphatase in amniotic fluid cell culture.

## SKELETAL DYSPLASIAS CHARACTERIZED BY A HYPOPLASTIC THORAX

There is a specific group of dysplasias in which thoracic hypoplasia is a cardinal feature. These include asphyxiating thoracic dysplasia, Ellis-van Creveld syndrome, short-rib–polydactyly syndrome, and campomelic syndrome. Other disorders presenting with altered thoracic dimensions are thanatophoric dysplasia, atelosteogenesis, fibrochondrogenesis, achondrogenesis, and Jarcho-Levin syndrome.

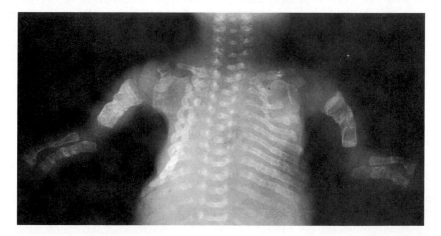

**FIGURE 20-10.** Osteogenesis imperfecta type IIA. Multiple skeletal fractures are present. Note the contiguous beading of the ribs and other long bones. The spine shows platyspondyly.

## Asphyxiating Thoracic Dysplasia

Asphyxiating thoracic dysplasia, known as Jeune syndrome, is rare. Its prevalence is 0.14 in 10,000 births, and it is inherited in an autosomal recessive pattern. It is characterized by a narrow and "bell-shaped" thorax, with short, horizontal ribs. Long bones are normal or mildly shortened. Asphyxiating thoracic dysplasia has a wide spectrum of clinical manifestations varying from lethal to mild forms.

## Short-Rib–Polydactyly Syndromes

Short-rib—polydactyly syndromes are a group of disorders characterized by micromelia, constricted thorax, and postaxial polydactyly.

## Chondroectodermal Dysplasia

Chondroectodermal dysplasia, also known as Ellis-van Creveld syndrome, is inherited with an autosomal recessive pattern. There is a high incidence in Amish communities. It is characterized by acromesomelia with normal spine and skull, postaxial polydactyly long and narrow thorax with short ribs, and congenital heart disease (60% of the cases).

## Campomelic Dysplasia

Campomelic dysplasia is characterized by bowing of the long bones of the lower extremities, an enlarged and elongated skull with a peculiar small facies, hypoplastic scapulae, and several associated anomalies, such as cleft palate, micrognathia, hydrocephalus, hydronephrosis, and congenital heart defects. Sporadic cases as well as some with an autosomal recessive pattern of inheritance have been described.

## Diastrophic Dysplasia

Diastrophic dysplasia is characterized by micromelia, clubfoot, hand deformities, multiple joint flexion contractures, and scoliosis. This disorder is inherited as an autosomal recessive trait. The clinical features include rhizomelic-type micromelia, contractures, hand deformities with abducted position of the thumbs ("hitchhiker thumb"), and severe talipes equinovarus.

This disease is not lethal, and intellectual development is unaffected. Pseudodiastrophic dysplasia has a similar presentation as diastrophic dysplasia and is inherited with an autosomal recessive pattern.

## Kniest Syndrome

Kniest syndrome is an autosomal dominant disorder characterized by involvement of the spine (platyspondylia and coronal clefts) and the tubular bones (shortened and metaphyseal flaring), with a broad and short thorax.

Two distinct types of dyssegmental dysplasia have been recognized: the mild, Rolland-Desbuquois form and the lethal Silverman-Handmaker. The latter is characterized by anarchic ossification of the vertebral bodies, metaphyseal flaring, and severe bowing of the long bones. The Rolland-Desbuquois type has essentially the same features, but the defects are much milder. The disease is autosomal recessive.

## LIMB DEFICIENCY OR CONGENITAL AMPUTATIONS

On occasion, the only identifiable anomaly is the absence of an extremity (limb deficiency) or a segment of an extremity (congenital amputation) (Table 20-11). Limb deficiencies can present alone or as part of a specific syndrome.

## SYNDROMES WITH ABSENT LIMBS AND FACIAL ANOMALIES

The aglossia-adactylia syndrome consists of transverse amputations of the limbs and malformations of the mouth, including micrognathia, vestigial tongue (hypoglossia), dental abnormalities, and ankylosis of the tongue to the hard palate, the floor of the mouth, or the lips (glossopalatine ankylosis). The condition is sporadic and has been attributed to a vascular accident.

The Möbius sequence consists of a number of facial anomalies attributed to paralysis of the sixth and seventh cranial nerves. The Möbius sequence is generally sporadic. The associated limb reduction anomalies (25% of cases) are

**TABLE 20-11.** Congenital Amputations

Absent limb(s) only
  Single absent limb
  Multiple absent limbs
Absent limbs with rings
  Congenital ring constriction syndrome
Absent limbs and face anomaly
  Aglossia–adactylia syndrome
  Möbius syndrome
Absent limbs with other anomalies
  Ichthyosiform skin (CHILD syndrome)
  Fibula agenesis–complex brachydactyly (Dupan syndrome)
  Splenogonadal fusion
  Skull and scalp defects (Adams-Oliver syndrome)
Phocomelia
  Thalidomide
  Thrombocytopenia with absent radii (TAR) syndrome
  Roberts pseudothalidomide-SC syndrome
  Grebe syndrome
Proximal femoral focal deficiency
  Femoral hypoplasia–unusual facies syndrome
  Femur–fibula–ulna complex
  Femur–tibia–radius complex
Split-hand/split-foot (SH/SF) syndromes
  Only split hand/split foot
  SH/SF and absent long bones
  Ectrodactyly, ectodermal dysplasia, cleft lip/palate (EEC syndrome)
  Some others
    Split foot and triphalangeal thumb, autosomal dominant
    Split foot, or split hand and central polydactyly (see central polydactyly)
    SH/SF and congenital nystagmus (Karsch-Neugebauer syndrome)
    SH/SF and renal malformations (acrorenal syndrome)
    Split foot and mandibulofacial dysostosis (Fontaine syndrome), autosomal dominant

Goldberg MD. The dysmorphic child: an orthopedic perspective. New York: Raven Press, 1987.

generally present in the upper extremities and range from transverse deficiencies to absent digits.

### Limb Reduction Defects Associated With Other Anomalies

Congenital hemidysplasia with ichthyosiform erythroderma and limb defects (CHILD syndrome) is a defect characterized by strict demarcation of the skin lesions to one side of the midline. The presence of unilateral defects of long bones is an important feature of the syndrome. The CHILD syndrome affects females predominantly (by a ratio of 19:1).

Fibula aplasia–complex brachydactyly (Du Pan syndrome) is an extremely rare condition characterized by bilateral agenesis of the fibula with abnormalities of the metacarpals and proximal phalanges.

The splenogonadal fusion syndrome is characterized by limb reduction defects and splenogonadal fusion. Most reported cases have occurred in males. Typically, there is a mass in the scrotum, and an ectopic spleen is identified during surgery.

The Adams Oliver syndrome is a group of disorders characterized by the association of limb reduction defects and scalp anomalies (aplasia cutis and deficiency of bony calvarium). Sporadic and familial cases have been reported.

### Phocomelia

Typically in phocomelia, the hands and feet are present, but the intervening arms and legs are absent.

Robert's syndrome is an autosomal recessive disorder characterized by the association of tetraphocomelia and facial dysmorphisms (hypertelorism, facial clefting defects, hypoplastic nasal alae). The upper extremities are generally more severely affected than the lower extremities.

Grebe syndrome is an autosomal recessive disorder characterized by marked hypomelia of upper and lower limbs increasing in severity from proximal to distal segments.

### Proximal Femoral Focal Deficiency, or Congenital Short Femur

Proximal femoral focal deficiency, or congenital short femur has been classified into five groups: type I, simple hypoplasia of the femur; type II, short femur with angulated shaft; type III, short femur with coxa vara (the most common); type IV, absent or defective proximal femur; and type V, absent or rudimentary femur. Femoral hypoplasia can be associated with unusual face syndrome B, which consists of bilateral femoral hypoplasia and facial defects, including short nose with broad tip, long philtrum, micrognathia, and cleft palate. The syndrome is sporadic and has been associated with maternal diabetes mellitus. A familiar form has been described.

If the defect is unilateral, it may correspond to the femur-fibula-ulna or femur-tibia-radius complex.

### Split-Hand-and-Foot Deformities

The term *split-hand-and-foot syndrome* is used to refer to a group of disorders characterized by splitting of the hand and foot into two parts. Split-hand-and-foot deformities can occur as isolated anomalies or as part of a more complex syndrome.

The split-hand-and-foot and absent-long-bones syndromes include two conditions in which there is split hand and aplasia of the tibia or split foot with aplasia of the ulna. The ectrodactyly-ectodermal dysplasia–cleft lip/palate syndrome (EEC syndrome) generally involves the four extremities, with more severe deformities of the hands. The pattern of inheritance is autosomal dominant. Intelligence is generally normal.

## CLUBHANDS

Radial clubhand includes a wide spectrum of disorders that encompass absent thumb, thumb hypoplasia, thin first metacarpal, and absent radius. Ulnar clubhand is much less frequent than radial clubhand and ranges from mild deviations of the hand of the ulnar side of the forearm to complete absence of the ulna. A fetal karyotype is indicated because several chromosomal abnormalities (e.g., trisomy 18, trisomy 21, and other structural aberrations) have been reported in association with clubhand deformities.

### Radial Clubhand

Fanconi's anemia (pancytopenia) is an autosomal recessive disease characterized by the association of bone marrow failure (anemia, leukopenia, and thrombocytopenia) and skeletal anomalies, including a radial clubhand with absent thumbs, radial hypoplasia, and a high frequency of chromosomal instability. Approximately 25% of affected individuals do not have limb reduction anomalies. Up to 25% of the patients will show some degree of mental deficiency.

TAR syndrome is an autosomal recessive disorder characterized by thrombocytopenia (platelet count of less than 100,000/mm$^3$) and bilateral absence of the radius. Congenital heart disease is present in 33% of the cases.

Aase syndrome is an autosomal recessive condition characterized by congenital hypoplastic anemia and a radial clubhand with bilateral triphalangeal thumb and a hypoplastic distal radius.

Holt-Oram syndrome is an autosomal dominant disorder characterized by congenital heart disease (mainly atrial septal defects, secundum type, and ventricular septal defects), aplasia or hypoplasia of the radius, and triphalangeal or absent thumbs.

The VATER association is the result of a defective mesodermal development during embryogenesis before the 35th day of gestation. The typical findings are vertebral segmentation (70%), anal atresia (80%), tracheo-esophageal fistula (70%), esophageal atresia, and radial and renal defects (65% and 53%, respectively). Other anomalies include a single umbilical artery (35%) and congenital heart disease, occurring in nearly 50% of the patients. The VATER association occurs sporadically, although recurrence within a sibship has been reported.

The Goldenhar syndrome is characterized by hemifacial microsomia, vertebral anomalies, and radial defects.

## POLYDACTYLY

Polydactyly can be classified as postaxial (the most common form), preaxial, and central (see Table 20-10). Postaxial polydactyly occurs on the ulnar side of the hand

**TABLE 20-12.** Disorders of the Developing Motor
System on All Levels, Leading to Immobilization

**Disorders of the Developing Neuromuscular System**
Loss of anterior horn cells
Radicular disease with collagen proliferation
Peripheral neuropathy with neurofibromatosis
Congenital myasthenia
Neonatal myasthenia (maternal myasthenia gravis)
Amyoplasia congenita
Congenital muscular dystrophy
Central core disease
Congenital myotonic dystrophy
Glycogen accumulation myopathy

**Disorders of Developing Connective Tissue or Connective Tissue Disease**
Muscular and articular connective tissue dystrophy
Articular defects by mesenchymal dysplasia
Increased collagen synthesis

**Disorders of Developing Medulla or Medullar Disease**
Congenital spinal epidural hemorrhage
Congenital duplication of the spinal canal

**Disorders of Brain Development (e.g., Porencephaly or Brain Disease)**
Congenital encephalopathy

Romero R, Athanassiadis AP, Sirtori M, Inati M. Fetal skeletal anomalies. In: Fleischer AC, Romero R, Manning FA, Jeanty P, James AE Jr, eds. The principles and practice of ultrasonography in obstetrics and gynecology. 4th ed. Norwalk, CT: Appleton & Lange, 1991:303.

and fibular side of the foot. Preaxial polydactyly is present on the radial side of the hand and the tibial side of the foot.

The majority are isolated conditions with an autosomal dominant mode of inheritance. Some of them are part of a syndrome, usually an autosomal recessive one.

## ARTHROGRYPOSIS

The term *arthrogryposis multiplex congenita* (AMC) refers to multiple joint contractures present at birth. Neurologic, muscular, connective tissue, skeletal abnormalities, or intrauterine crowding can lead to impaired fetal motion and AMC. Table 20-12 lists motor systems that can lead to AMC. The pattern of inheritance depends on the specific cause of AMC. In a series of 350 cases, 46% of cases corresponded to a syndrome with no recurrence risk, 23% corresponded to disorders inherited with a mendelian pattern (autosomal dominant, recessive, or X-linked), 20% were unknown conditions, 6% were associated with environmental disorders, 3% were chromosomal, and 2% were multifactorial in origin.

Ten percent of patients with AMC have associated anomalies of the central nervous system.

The cardinal findings are absent fetal movement on real-time examination and severe flexion deformities.

# 21. FETAL NEOPLASM

Neoplasms may be divided into five main categories: tumors of the head and neck, brain, heart, chest, and abdominal/pelvic areas (Table 21-1). Since tumors of the chest are described in detail in Chapter 17, they will not be discussed here.

## TUMORS OF THE HEAD AND NECK

### CYSTIC HYGROMA

#### Etiopathology

Cystic hygroma, the most frequent fetal tumor of the head and neck, is found in 1 in 200 spontaneous abortuses. These lesions result from lymphatic system abnormalities, in which the jugular lymphatic sacs fail to drain into the internal jugular vein, resulting in dilated lymphatic channels and giving a cystic appearance sonographically. These cysts present as sacs with or without multiple septations (Fig. 21-1).

The lymphatic system is a complex network of thin-walled vessels that return tissue fluid to the jugular lymphatic sac, which in turn empties into the jugular vein. This system is established as early as the sixth week of pregnancy, and obstruction of these channels alters the development of the vessel systems, causing dilation of the lymphatic channels with back-up of tissue fluid. When this obstructive process occurs at the level of the jugular lymphatics, it leads to dilation of these vessels and results in the characteristic cystic hygroma. It is also believed that a more severe obstructive process with failure in communication can lead to progressive, severe lymphedema or nonimmune hydrops. The persistence of redundant skin folds is seen at birth as webbing of the neck (pterygium coli), which is also observed in Turner's syndrome, Noonan syndrome, or familial pterygium coli.

#### Prenatal Diagnosis

Prenatal diagnosis of cystic hygromas is not very difficult and can be made as early as the first trimester of pregnancy (see Fig. 21-1).

Because cystic hygroma is associated with a number of other abnormalities, both structural and chromosomal, it is important to carry out a careful anatomical survey of the entire fetal anatomy. Renal abnormalities, cardiac anomalies, single umbilical artery, and adrenal masses should all be ruled out. Fetal karyotyping should also be performed, since this lesion is associated with Turner's syndrome in about half of the cases. The differential diagnosis includes other cervical abnormalities, such as cephalocele, cystic teratoma of the neck, or cephalomeningocele.

#### Medical Management and Outcome

Medical management depends largely on the karyotypic and sonographic findings. If the diagnosis of cystic hygroma is made in the first trimester and karyo-

E. Albert Reece, John C. Hobbins, Maurice, J. Mahoney and Roy H. Petrie (Eds). *Handbook of Medicine of the Fetus & Mother.* Copyright © 1995 by J.B. Lippincott Company

**TABLE 21-1.** Prenatal Ultrasound Diagnosis of Fetal Tumors

**Head and Neck Tumors**
Cystic hygroma
Epignathus
Goiter
Hemangioma
Neuroblastoma
Proboscis
Thyroid teratoma

**Intracranial Tumors**
Choroid plexus papilloma
Choroid plexus cyst
Craniopharyngioma
Glioblastoma
Teratoma

**Cardiac Tumors**
Fibroma
Rhabdomyoma

**Chest Tumors**
Bronchogenic cyst
Cystic adenomatoid malformation
Extralobar sequestration

**Abdominal and Pelvic Tumors**
Appendiceal abscess
Cavernous hemangioma
Choledochal cyst
Extrathoracic pulmonary sequestration
Meconium ileus
Mesoblastic nephroma
Neuroblastoma
Ovarian cyst and teratoma
Multicystic kidney disease
Polycystic kidney disease
Sacrococcygeal teratoma
Urachal cyst

Modified from Kurjak A, Zalud I, Jurkovic D, et al. Ultrasound diagnosis and evaluation of fetal tumors. J Perinat Med 1989; 17:173.

typic analysis reveals trisomy 18, then pregnancy termination may be offered to the patient. Similarly, if the diagnosis is made later, but before 24 weeks, and there are multiple congenital malformations or nonimmune hydrops, pregnancy termination may also be considered. When this diagnosis is made after 24 weeks and neither major congenital malformations nor nonimmune hydrops are present and the karyotype is normal (which occurs in 25% of cases), then such patients should be followed expectantly with serial ultrasound examinations.

## EPIGNATHUS

### Etiopathology
An epignathus is a large, disfiguring teratoma that arises out of the fetal mouth and may involve the sphenoid bone, pharynx, tongue, and/or jaw.

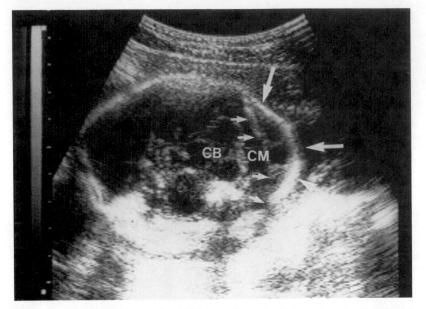

**FIGURE 21-1.** Fetal head scan at a level slightly inferior to the thalami, depicting the cerebellum (CB) and the cisterna magna (CM). Posterior to these structures is a septated echolucent sac representing a cystic hygroma.

## Prenatal Diagnosis

Epignathuses are rare lesions, and prenatal diagnosis has only been reported twice. Both cases were described as huge masses emanating from the mouth, containing solid and cystic components.

## Medical Management and Outcome

Since these lesions can be of variable size and involve multiple structures, management depends on both size and location. For example, some lesions may alter the facial anatomy significantly or grow into the face or head. If such cases are diagnosed before 24 weeks gestation, termination may be offered; otherwise management should be expectant.

## FETAL GOITER

### Etiopathology

Fetal goiter is an enlargement of the thyroid gland, presenting as a solid neck mass with some echolucent areas when observed with ultrasound. The usual cause is maternal ingestion of iodine preparations. Fetal goiter may also be caused by maternal diseases such as Graves' disease or the treatment of hyperthyroidism with iodine or, rarely, with propylthiouracil.

Goiters resulting from maternal hypothyroidism may be caused by treatment given to the mother, deficiency of iodine, or a congenital metabolic disorder of thyroid synthesis. Congenital hypothyroidism, however, is rare. Another cause of hypothyroidism includes thyroid hormone-enzyme deficiency, which can also result in goiter with varying effects, ranging from hypothyroidism to a euthyroid state.

## Prenatal Diagnosis

The antenatal diagnosis of fetal goiter may be difficult but is based solely on the identification of a mass in the neck region of the fetus that causes hyperextension of the fetal head.

## Medical Management and Outcome

Medical management depends largely on the cause of the fetal goiter. For example, fetal goiter resulting from aggressive maternal propylthiouracil therapy would be best managed by a significant reduction in medication, and in patients taking iodide would require discontinuation of the drug. Similarly, the prognosis is relative to the cause of the fetal goiter. If hypothyroidism is diagnosed at birth, then aggressive supplemental treatment is necessary, since prolonged hypothyroidism may be associated with severe mental retardation.

## INTRACRANIAL TUMORS

## CHOROID PLEXUS PAPILLOMA

### Etiopathology

Papillomas are usually benign tumors of variable size attached to the normal choroid plexus, occurring in one or both of the cerebral ventricles. However, in the majority of cases, the lesion is unilateral and found in the atrial portion of the lateral ventricle.

### Prenatal Diagnosis

Papillomas are often recognized following the diagnosis of hydrocephalus. A unilateral dilation of the lateral ventricle, associated with an echogenic mass in the ipsilateral atrium of the lateral ventricle, would be highly indicative of a choroid plexus papilloma (Fig. 21-2).

### Medical Management and Outcome

If the diagnosis is made antenatally, obstetric management should be unaltered. Patients should be allowed to go full term, or if severe hydrocephalus and polyhydramnios exist, pregnancy should be continued until there is pulmonic maturity.

## CHOROID PLEXUS CYST

### Etiopathology

Choroid plexus cysts are thought to result from the folding of the neuroepithelium, which becomes filled with fluid and cellular debris. The pediatric literature reports that many choroid plexus cysts occur as asymptomatic findings in children; however, some are reportedly associated with chromosomal anomalies, particularly trisomy 18.

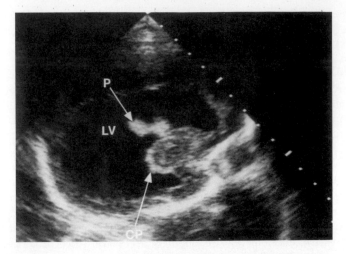

**FIGURE 21-2.** Parasagittal scan in a 30-week fetus with hydrocephalus secondary to a choroid plexus papilloma. The papilloma (P) is seen as an echogenic mass attached to the normal choroid plexus (CP) and protruding inside the dilated lateral ventricle (LV). (Pilu G, Rizzo N, Orsini LF, et al. Antenatal recognition of the cerebral anomalies. Ultrasound Med Biol 1986;12:319.

### Prenatal Diagnosis
Choroid plexus cysts are usually located in the atrium of the lateral ventricle, in a location similar to where the choroid plexus papilloma are found (Fig. 21-3).

### Medical Management and Outcome
Choroid plexus cysts are believed to be benign, and serial ultrasound examinations are recommended to exclude the development of hydrocephalus. Otherwise, obstetric care should remain unaltered. It has been reported that these cysts are associated with aneuploidy.

## TERATOMAS

### Etiopathology
Teratomas are the most frequent intracranial tumors, accounting for 0.5% of all intracranial neoplasms. Other teratomas diagnosed prenatally include the sacrococcygeal teratoma which is discussed in the section on Abdominal and Pelvic Tumors.

### Prenatal Diagnosis
Fetuses with teratomas usually present with a sudden onset of large-for-dates size in otherwise normal pregnancies. The rapid growth in maternal abdominal girth usually results from the development of associated polyhydramnios. An enlarged mass with distortion of the anatomy is usually present in prenatally diagnosed cases. Multiple cystic spaces within a solid tumor were described in some of the reported cases. Calcification was noted by ultrasound in others; however, varying echodensities within the tumors were common features.

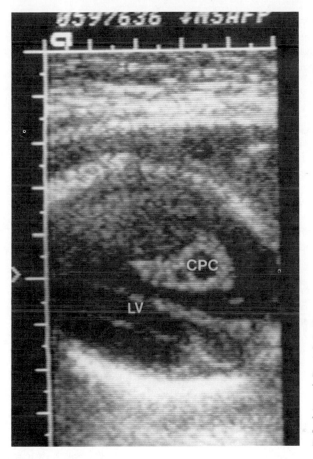

**FIGURE 21-3.** Scan of fetal head at the level of the lateral ventricles. In the near field is shown the choroid plexus containing a cystic area, choroid plexus cyst (CPC). In the far field, the lateral wall of the lateral ventricle can be seen delineating the borders of the lateral ventricle.

## Medical Management and Outcome

In light of the poor prognosis associated with this lesion, termination of pregnancy should be offered to those patients who have not yet reached 24 weeks gestation. Beyond the latter gestational age, obstetric care should be otherwise unaltered. A pediatric surgeon should be consulted, because attempts should be made to resect the tumor postnatally. Although long-term survival may be possible, the risk of neurologic impairment is high.

## CARDIAC TUMORS

### Etiopathology

The most frequent cardiac tumor in the fetus or neonate is rhabdomyoma, which typically arises from the interventricular septum and interrupts electrical conduction within the heart.

The overwhelming majority of primary cardiac tumors are benign and are usually incidental findings at autopsy. They include lipoma, fibroma, leiomyoma, hamartoma, myxoma, rhabdomyoma, and hemangioma. In the fetus, a cardiac mass may produce congestive heart failure and hydrops, which may lead to fetal demise. Cardiac masses may be associated with arrhythmia, pericardial infusion, obliteration of the cardiac chamber, and embolic phenomena. Higher complication rates are expected with rapidly growing malignancies, such as rhabdomyosarcoma.

### Prenatal Diagnosis

Prenatal sonographic diagnosis of cardiac tumors has been reported. The usual findings include a solid echogenic mass in the right ventricle that abuts on the intraventricular septum. The likelihood of poor outcome is increased when there is coexistent structural heart disease.

### Medical Management and Outcome

Cardiac neoplasm in the fetus may result in stillbirth or early neonatal death. These rare tumors are almost exclusively rhabdomyomas, although atrial hemangioma has been described.

## ABDOMINAL AND PELVIC TUMORS

Abdominal masses can represent neoplasms, as well as displaced or enlarged organs, such as the spleen, kidneys, or lungs. Many of these lesions are part of systemic abnormalities (e.g., multicystic kidney disease, the most common of all neonatal abdominal masses).

### OVARIAN CYST

### Etiopathology

Ovarian cysts are one of the most common causes of abdominal-pelvic masses in female neonates. These cysts are unilateral and unilocular with a high variation in size. The cause of this disease is still uncertain; however, excessive ovarian stimulation by gonadotropins is considered to be a likely cause.

### Prenatal Diagnosis

Ovarian cysts should be considered when a fetus presents with a unilateral, unilocular, echolucent structure in the abdominal-pelvic region, especially if the bladder and stomach can be seen separately. Prenatal diagnosis of large fetal ovarian cysts with ultrasonography has been reported on several occasions based on the following criteria: presence of a cystic structure that is symmetrical in shape, usually unilateral, and separate from the gastrointestinal and urinary tracts in a female fetus.

### Medical Management and Outcome

Following the prenatal diagnosis of a probable ovarian cyst, serial ultrasound examinations can be used to detect any structural changes in the mass. An increase in size can cause distention of the fetal abdomen and, if persistent, may result in prune belly syndrome. If the mass is enlarged and the fetal abdomen is distended, it may be necessary to remove excess fluid by needle aspiration, thereby relieving the pressure on the abdominal wall and preventing the development of pulmonic hypoplasia. Cesarean section was performed routinely for these conditions in the past; however, sonographically guided needle aspiration may be conducted so as to permit normal vaginal delivery.

## SACROCOCCYGEAL TERATOMA

### Etiopathology

Sacrococcygeal teratoma is one of the most common tumors seen in the newborn; of affected infants, 80% are female. It is observed in the perinatal period, with approximately 60% arising from the sacrococcygeal region. These tumors are true neoplasms, arising from the presacral area and composed of cells representative of more than one germ layer. They are thought to be derived embryologically from multipotential cells segregated from primitive Hensen's node. A classification system developed by the surgical section of the American Academy of Pediatrics is as follows: type I lesion is external and has no identifiable pelvic extension; type II shows an intrapelvic component, but the majority of the mass is external; type III, the presacral component, predominates over the external portion; and type IV, teratomas, is entirely intrapelvic and not externally identifiable. The combination of cystic and solid areas within the mass is the most common presentation. Scattered calcifications are frequently present in these tumors, which probably represent fragments of bone. Type I and type II account for more than 80% of the cases. Although in 5% to 25% of cases there are associated anomalies, no specific types have been identified. These anomalies include spina bifida, obstructive uropathy, and cleft palate.

The reported incidence of sacrococcygeal teratoma is 1 in 35,000 live births. Most of these cases are asymptomatic during pregnancy and are frequently not diagnosed until birth. Although chromosomal abnormalities or associated life-threatening congenital anomalies are rare, the mortality rate is very high, appearing to result from a secondary effect of the tumor. Preterm labor with premature delivery is also common and associated with polyhydramnios. Other complications connected with this lesion include massive hemorrhage into the tumor with secondary high-output cardiac failure or fetal exsanguination, occurring both in utero and intrapartum.

### Prenatal Diagnosis

Prenatal diagnosis of types I, II, and III involves the identification of the external mass arising from the sacral area. This mass, as mentioned earlier, may be multicystic with solid components and areas of calcification. The presence of fetal hydrops is a very poor prognostic sign. Amniotic fluid alpha-fetoprotein and acetylcholinesterase enzyme values have been reported to be either high-normal or elevated, making it difficult to distinguish between neural tube defects and sacrococcygeal teratoma.

### Medical Management and Outcome

Appropriate treatment for fetal sacrococcygeal teratoma remains undefined. For cases diagnosed after 30 weeks, cesarean section is indicated following pulmonic maturity to avoid dystocia, uterine rupture, fetal hemorrhage of the tumor, or traumatic injury to the mother and fetus. When these lesions are diagnosed prior to 30 weeks, a high fetal death rate is observed and is often associated with the development of hydrops and placentomegaly. In both cases, serial ultrasound examinations should be done, provided neither hydrops nor placentomegaly has occurred, and attempts should be made to carry all pregnancies to pulmonic maturity. There may be an evolving role for in utero surgical intervention.

# 22.  FIRST-TRIMESTER PRENATAL DIAGNOSIS

The virtual explosion of technology in the last 10 years has given physicians special insight into fetal growth and development. This chapter is devoted to only one portion of the unfolding fetal story: early development. (For a more thorough discussion of this topic, please see Chapter 41 in Reece EA, Hobbins JC, Mahoney MJ, and Petrie RH, eds. Medicine of the fetus & mother. J.B. Lippincott, 1992.)

The major factor responsible for our enhanced ability to diagnose abnormal fetal development has been the exponential improvement in ultrasound imagery. These changes have enabled physicians to perform invasive procedures safely and obtain samples of amniotic fluid, chorionic villi, and fetal blood.

## ULTRASOUND

This chapter will focus on the comprehensive first trimester evaluation.

Over the past 7 years significant improvements in gray-scale imagery have enabled us to scrutinize the embryo in detail. The newest technology uses a transvaginal approach to the ultrasound evaluation of the first trimester conceptus. The transvaginal probe can be directed to within a few centimeters of the embryo, and since there is less dissipation of sound over a shorter pathway, very high frequency probes can be used. Coupled with the ability to use highly focused transducers, this technology dramatically improves both axial and lateral resolution. Remarkable detail can be obtained with transvaginal ultrasound examination of embryos magnified several times.

## CROWN-RUMP LENGTH

Using transvaginal probes, the gestational sac and embryo can be visualized at about 4 to 5 menstrual weeks (Fig. 22-1). By 7 menstrual weeks, the investigator should be able to distinguish two fetal poles and to measure the CRL by both transabdominal and transvaginal techniques. CRL correlates closely with gestational age until about 12 weeks; after that, the measurement is less reliable.

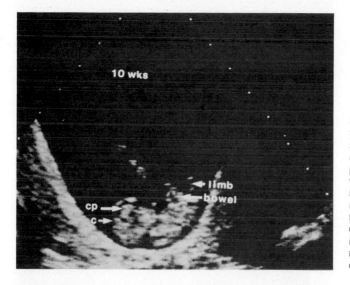

**FIGURE 22-1.** First trimester fetus. Some structures are recognizable: choroid plexus (cp), calvarium (c), herniated bowel, cord (extending anteriorly), and the lower limbs. Crown–rump length is measured from the calvarium to the end of the rump.

## YOLK SAC

The early secondary yolk sac produces the gonadocytes, blood vessels and red blood cells, and the epithelia for the digestive and respiratory tracts, and invaginates to generate portions of the midgut. The yolk sac is also the site of early protein synthesis; alpha fetoprotein is the principal protein synthesized.

Unfortunately, the vestigial remnant of the secondary yolk sac seems to convey little information about early embryonic or fetal development. There are, however, data to suggest that failing to visualize a yolk sac or finding one either less than 2 mm in diameter or solid in appearance may be associated with a missed abortion or a fetal anomaly. An association between a yolk sac greater than 5 mm in diameter and fetal abnormalities has also been noted.

## ULTRASOUND DIAGNOSIS OF CONGENITAL ANOMALIES

### Cranial Anomalies

In the first trimester the fetal cranium undergoes some developmental changes that can easily be chronicled with ultrasound. Between 6 and 8 menstrual weeks, a large echospared area can normally be seen in the posterior cranium, reflecting the confluence of the third and fourth ventricles. This completely normal finding can be mistaken for a posterior fossa cyst. Throughout the first and early second trimesters, the lateral ventricles appear large, leading the inexperienced observer to suspect ventriculomegaly. In addition, the earliest we have noted the calvarium to be well demonstrated is at 10 menstrual weeks, so anencephaly is a diagnosis best made beyond this gestational age. Despite the potential difficulties encountered in diagnosing cranial abnormalities in the first trimester, many cephalic anomalies can be identified, such as acrania, encephalocele, and anencephaly (Fig. 22-2).

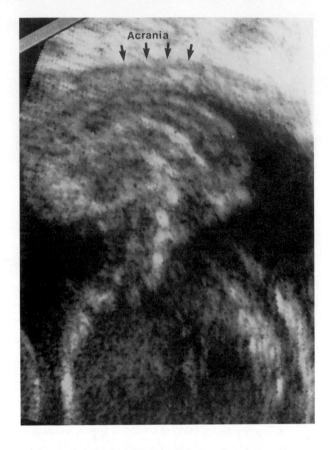

**FIGURE 22-2.** Ultrasound picture of a fetus with acrania. The calvarium calcifies at about 10 weeks; therefore, the absence of a calcified skull (*black arrows*) suggests a diagnosis of acrania.

It has become apparent that there are many variations on the cystic hygroma theme. When first using the vaginal probe, we occasionally began seeing a posterior nuchal membrane that extended from the fetal occiput to the upper dorsal surface of the fetus. Since then, we have observed lateral nuchal cysts, large septated echolucent cysts (classic cystic hygroma), and general body-wall edema.

Because the fate of embryos displaying these "abnormalities" had not been clarified in the literature, we collected cases from Yale University and combined them with those identified by our colleagues at the University of Bologna, Italy. Thus far, we have outcome data on 30 such embryos. Karyotypic information was available on 29: 15 had aneuploidy, and 14 had normal chromosomes. Six patients chose to terminate pregnancy, and 8 continued the pregnancy, delivering morphologically normal infants at term.

## Cardiac Anomalies

Using the transvaginal transducer, the beating heart can be observed inside the embryo's chest cavity as early as 7 menstrual weeks. Using the same technique, a four-chamber view of the heart has been obtained as early as 12 menstrual weeks, allowing the diagnosis of major cardiac defects by the end of the first trimester in some cases.

With transvaginal scanning, gross cardiac anomalies such as large interventricular septal defects and hypoplastic chambers could well be identified before 14 weeks of gestation. Obviously, however, this theoretical possibility must be borne out by further investigation. Ventricular hypoplasia, which may represent a late change, cannot be excluded by a first trimester examination. Conversely, there is a suspicion that some interventricular septal defects may close in late gestation.

### Abdominal Anomalies

Fetal kidneys can be visualized as early as 10 weeks (Fig. 22-3), and the fetal bladder can be seen by 12 weeks in most cases. Renal agenesis may be easier to diagnose in the first trimester because at that time there is enough amniotic fluid to aid in imaging intra-abdominal structures. On two recent occasions megacystis has been identified at or before 13 menstrual weeks.

### Spinal/Skeletal Anomalies

Neural tube defects can be definitively diagnosed as early as the late first trimester. Both lateral pedicles and the spinal body ossify by the 10th menstrual week, allowing the visualization of the spinal column and potential defects (Fig. 22-4). Our group has identified a low sacral defect at 11 weeks using transvaginal sonography. Long bone lengths can consistently be measured by the 12th week of gestation. Although severe skeletal dysplasias (e.g., phocomelia, amniotic band syndrome) could well be diagnosed at this time, little is known about the early development of many of the other short-limb dysplasias (e.g., osteogenesis imperfecta, thanatophoric dysplasia, camptomelic dysplasia). With transvaginal sonography, fetal hands, feet, and even digits can be visualized by the 12th menstrual week.

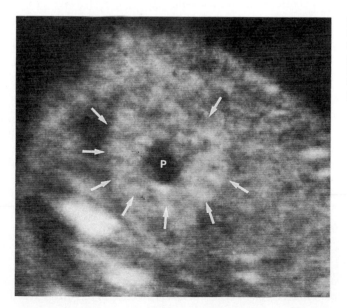

**FIGURE 22-3.** Kidney in an 11-week-old fetus with a dense echogenic rim (*arrows*) and a slightly dilated renal pelvis (P).

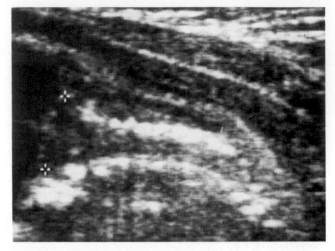

**FIGURE 22-4.** A 12-week-old fetus with spine depicted as parallel lines extending from the neck to the sacrum. At the posterior aspect of the head can be seen the cerebellum (*asterisks*).

A variety of conditions such as amniotic band syndrome, tibular radial aplasia syndrome, and body stalk anomalies have been diagnosed with ultrasound in the first trimester.

## BIOCHEMICAL SCREENING

Maternal serum alpha fetoprotein (MSAFP) screening has become almost uniformly accepted as an efficacious way to identify patients at greater risk of having a fetus with a neural tube defect. High MSAFP levels have also been associated with fetal conditions such as ventral wall defects, renal agenesis, obstructive uropathies, and gastrointestinal obstructions, all of which can be potentially diagnosed with ultrasound.

Since MSAFP can be quantified with very sensitive assays before 14 weeks, it was originally hoped that MSAFP screening could be pushed back into the first trimester, but initial results have been inconsistent.

## CHORIONIC VILLUS SAMPLING

Because the placental villi and the fetus are derived from the same tissue, villi sampling has become an attractive source of data for genetic studies on the fetus. Further, these cells are actively growing; they come from a single cell line, and tissue culture of these cells can be obtained more rapidly than that of amniotic fluid cells. The indications for CVS are similar to those for amniocentesis. The specimens obtained can be directly examined for karyotyping, or cultured for biochemical studies, gene mapping, or karyotypic analysis.

### TRANSCERVICAL CVS

This procedure involves advancing a catheter under ultrasound direction to the thickest part of the placenta (Fig. 22-5). Trophoblast is then aspirated through the

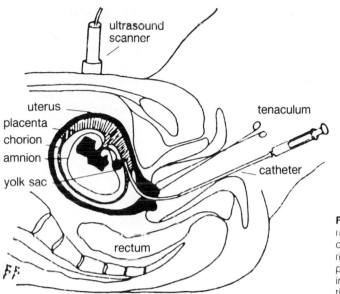

**FIGURE 22-5.** Schematic representation of transvaginal chorionic villus sampling, showing instruments and pertinent landmarks.

catheter into a syringe attached to the hub of the catheter. Generally, 5 mg or more is needed for direct chromosome analysis, but results can be obtained after cell culture with a sample of less than 5 mg.

## TRANSABDOMINAL CVS

The major advantage of this technique is that the cervix, which may be responsible for infectious morbidity, is circumvented. The transabdominal CVS procedure is a modification of an amniocentesis technique. Either a needle-aspiration transducer or a freehand technique can be used. The operator simply places a needle tangentially through the placental substance under ultrasound guidance. While aspirating through a syringe attached to the hub of the needle, the needle tip is moved up and down through the placenta until adequate tissue is obtained for analysis. Some investigators prefer to use a double-needle technique in which a smaller needle is advanced through an "introducer" needle.

## ADVANTAGES AND DISADVANTAGES

There have been two prospective clinical trials, one in the United States and one in Canada. The results from the six-center American trial indicate a 0.7% greater risk for transcervical CVS when compared with second trimester amniocentesis. A Canadian randomized clinical trial yielded similar results. However, since some patients in the chromosomally normal CVS group chose to terminate their pregnancies, if the study subject denominator were adjusted accordingly, the increased risk of CVS could reach 1.7%. From these data it appears that CVS carries a slightly higher risk of pregnancy loss than does second trimester amniocentesis.

Recent reports also suggest a higher rate of transverse limb defects and jaw level deformities after CVS. The rate, however, of these defects still is below 1 per 1000.

## AMNIOCENTESIS

In 1966, it became clear that fetal cells obtained from amniotic fluid could be cultured and later karyotyped. This stimulated some institutions to offer second trimester amniocentesis to women at significant risk for fetal chromosomal abnormalities.

Today, few women over age 35 are not offered amniocentesis. Stimulated by the demand to provide earlier information to couples at risk for fetal conditions that were generally diagnosed by second trimester amniocentesis and frustrated by the governmental regulatory aspects of CVS investigation, some investigators began exploring the possibility of performing early amniocentesis before the 14th week of gestation.

### RISKS OF SECOND TRIMESTER AMNIOCENTESIS

Since few studies deal with the risks of early amniocentesis, it is useful to review the results of second trimester studies. Those who counsel patients weighing their diagnostic options may have the impression that the risks of second trimester amniocentesis are small. But it has been difficult to quantify these risks precisely, primarily because there is little information on spontaneous fetal loss rates. Many studies deal with the risks of amniocentesis, but many of these suffer from insufficient numbers or inadequate control data; sometimes older techniques of amniocentesis were used.

Since 1979, 17 studies have emerged on the risk of second trimester amniocentesis. Most offer no control data. The average total fetal loss rate was 3.3% (2.4% to 5.2%), and the spontaneous abortion rate was 1.3% (0.1% to 1.5%).

Amniocentesis is not an innocuous procedure and results in spontaneous abortion in up to 1 percent of cases. In addition, infants born to mothers undergoing amniocentesis had a higher rate of respiratory difficulties (respiratory distress syndrome and pneumonia) than other pregnancies not receiving amniocentesis. The most likely mechanism for respiratory difficulties would be the effect on the developing lung of a sudden decrease in amniotic fluid volume.

### RISKS OF EARLY AMNIOCENTESIS

Although the gestational age of study populations varies, "early" amniocenteses have generally been performed between 10 and 14 weeks of gestation. Initial results have suggested fetal loss rates comparable to those of second trimester amniocentesis. However, the studies have problems that make the results difficult to evaluate. Only after more studies can we confidently counsel patients who wish to have an early amniocentesis about the potential risk of the procedure.

### EMBRYOSCOPY

Endoscopic techniques for direct visualization of the fetus allow detailed, direct observations of fetal anatomical structures and integument. Current approaches

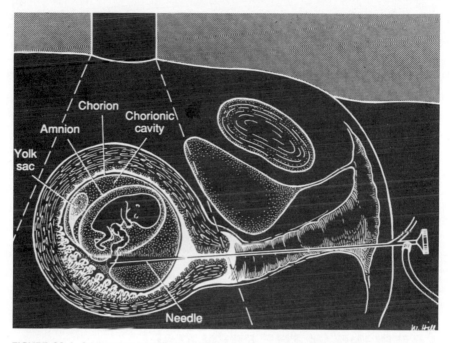

**FIGURE 22-6.** Schematic representation of embryoscopy, with the endoscope inserted transvaginally under ultrasound guidance. Pertinent anatomical landmarks are labelled.

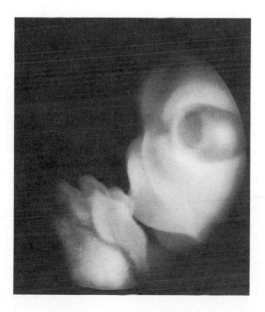

**FIGURE 22-7.** The face of a 10-week-old fetus visualized via embryoscopy.

include fetoscopy in the second trimester and the recently developed embryo-scopy in the first trimester.

Embryoscopy, however, is a relatively new and evolving procedure in which a rigid endoscope is inserted transcervically. We use ultrasound to guide the rigid endoscope through the cervix and chorion into the extracoelomic cavity. The chorion is ruptured with the tip of the endoscope, but the amnion remains intact. The yolk sac and placenta are directly visualized, and the embryo is seen through the amnion. The embryo can be seen directly through the endoscopic eyepiece or via a video camera and monitor (Figs. 22-6, 22-7).

We find the most important current application of embryoscopy to be in the confirmation of anomalies diagnosed by ultrasound before elective pregnancy termination. Additionally, with embryoscopy we can gain access into the embry-onic circulation through the vitelline vessels that course through the extraembry-onic coelom. This would allow for injection of hemopoietic stem cells or cloned genes into embryos with hemoglobinopathies or single-gene defects.

# 23. AMNIOCENTESIS, SKIN BIOPSY, AND UMBILICAL CORD BLOOD SAMPLING IN THE PRENATAL DIAGNOSIS OF GENETIC DISEASES

## AMNIOCENTESIS

This chapter discusses the technique, risks, and complications of genetic amnio-centesis. (For a more thorough discussion of this topic, please see Chapter 42 in Reece EA, Hobbins JC, Mahoney MJ, and Petrie RH, eds. Medicine of the Fetus & Mother. J.B. Lippincott, 1992.)

## TECHNIQUE

Genetic amniocentesis is most commonly performed at approximately 16 weeks of gestation. At this time the uterus has enlarged sufficiently so that amniotic fluid can easily be aspirated transabdominally. In addition, the ratio of viable to non-viable cells is greatest at this gestational age. However, this procedure has been successfully performed as early as 9 weeks of menstrual age.

Before performing an amniocentesis a thorough ultrasound examination should be performed for the following reasons:

1. To document fetal viability
2. To determine the number of fetuses
3. To detect major fetal structural abnormalities
4. To locate the placenta

5. To confirm gestational age
6. To confirm adequate amniotic fluid volume
7. To select an optimal pocket of fluid for sampling
8. To rule out significant uterine or adnexal pathology

After a thorough ultrasound examination is performed, the optimal site for needle placement is selected. Ideally, this site should be one where there is adequate amniotic fluid volume, no fetal parts are present, and the placenta does not have to be traversed to reach the fluid. The area where the umbilical cord inserts into the placenta should always be avoided because of the possibility of perforating one of the large chorionic plate vessels that abound in this location.

Once the sampling site has been selected, the abdominal wall is thoroughly cleansed with iodine solution. The ultrasound transducer is then placed in a sterile plastic bag or glove. Sterile gel is placed on the abdomen, and again the appropriateness of the selected site is reassessed. Using the freehand technique while observing the ultrasound screen, a 20- to 22-gauge needle is introduced under direct visualization. Once satisfactory placement of the needle is obtained, the stylet is removed and in most instances free flow of amniotic fluid will follow. A 10- to 30-mL syringe is attached to the needle and 20 to 30 mL of fluid are removed. Occasionally, the fluid will be blood-tinged initially, in which case syringes should be changed and the bloody fluid discarded. If fluid cannot be aspirated, the needle can be rotated in place or the stylet replaced to reposition the tip. One cause of failure to obtain fluid is tenting of the membranes, which usually can be seen by ultrasound. Often this can be overcome by withdrawing the needle a few centimeters and then thrusting it forward in a quick, controlled motion to the desired depth. Care must be taken not to "overshoot" the targeted area when performing this maneuver. Inability to pierce the membranes despite attempting this approach should prompt the operator to remove the needle and select another insertion site. If the flow of fluid stops during the procedure, it is often because the negative pressure created by aspiration of the fluid causes obstruction of the tip with membranes, cord, or fetal skin. In this situation rotating the needle 90° to 180° often solves the problem. In some cases cessation of flow may be due to a uterine contraction at the insertion site. In these cases the stylet should be replaced and the needle repositioned. Once the fluid has been obtained, fetal cardiac activity within the normal range should be visualized and shown to the patient for her reassurance.

If an initial attempt is unsuccessful, a second needle can be inserted in another location. However, no more than two needle insertions should be performed on any given occasion, and the procedure should not be reattempted until several days or a week later. If the patient is Rh negative, she should be given Rh-immune globulin (300 $\mu$g) unless the father has also been documented to be Rh negative. After the procedure the patient can resume normal activities.

## RISKS AND COMPLICATIONS

The older collaborative studies, with the exception of that performed in Britain, reported loss rates due to amniocentesis of approximately 0.3% to 0.5% (Table 23-1). These studies, however, were conducted when amniocentesis was a relatively new procedure, ultrasound was not uniformly used, and none of them were

**TABLE 23-1.** Risks and Complications of Late Amniocentesis

| Studies | Number of Subjects | Total Pregnancy Loss | Comments |
|---|---|---|---|
| United States Collaborative Study 1971–1973 | Cases N = 1040 Controls N = 992 | 3.5% | Pregnancy loss included spontaneous abortions, stillbirths, and neonatal deaths. |
| Canadian Collaborative Study 1973–1976 | N = 1020 | 5.2% | Not statistically different from control group. |
| British Collaborative Study 1973–1976 | Cases N = 2428 Matched controls N = 2428 | Fetal loss rate was 1–1.5% higher in the study group. | Infants from the study group had a higher incidence of respiratory difficulties and orthopedic postural abnormalities. |
| University of California Center for the Health Sciences Study 1975–1978 | Cases N = 2000 Controls N = 2000 | 2.7% 2.2% | No difference in neonatal respiratory difficulties or orthopedic abnormalities. |
| Danish Collaborative Study 1980–1984 | N = 4606 | Study group 1.7% Controls .7% | This difference was statistically significant. |

randomized. Technical factors that may be associated with higher risk of spontaneous abortion are needle gauges larger than 20, placental perforation, and more than two needle insertions at any given time. Other factors include raised alpha-fetoprotein before the procedure and the presence of discolored amniotic fluid.

## SPECIFIC RISK FACTORS

### Placental Localization
The available data suggest that the placenta should be avoided whenever possible and that, when this is not possible, its thinnest portion should be traversed. To achieve this, ultrasound localization is necessary to select the optimal sampling site.

### Rhesus Isoimmunization
Disruption of the fetal-maternal circulation during amniocentesis can cause isoimmunization in Rh-negative women carrying Rh-positive fetuses. It appears that approximately 1% of Rh-negative women at risk will become sensitized as a result of amniocentesis if Rh-immune globulin is not given. The American College of Obstetricians and Gynecologists recommends administration of 300 μg of Rh-immune globulin following second trimester procedures. If further amniocenteses are performed 6 or more weeks after the initial procedure, Bowman and Pollock (1985), recommend a second dose of 300 μg of Rh-immune globulin.*

*Bowman JM, Pollock JM. Transplacental fetal hemorrhage after amniocentesis. Obstet Gynecol 1985;66:749.

## Discolored Amniotic Fluid

Discolored amniotic fluid has been reported in 1% to 7% of midtrimester amnio-centeses. Brown or green discoloration has been found to be due to the presence of soluble blood breakdown products in the vast majority of cases, although meconi-um also has been detected in a small number. A history of vaginal bleeding prior to the amniocentesis has been reported in 38% to 75% of these cases. In recent controlled studies where amniocentesis was preceded by ultrasound examina-tion, fetal loss rates between 7% and 16% have been reported for women with discolored fluids. These rates were significantly higher than those of the controls. Other authors have reported no difference in fetal losses among patients with this finding. Thus, it appears that discolored amniotic fluid may imply a greater risk of fetal loss, and these pregnancies should be monitored accordingly.

## MATERNAL RISKS

The risks of life-threatening maternal complications after amniocentesis are al-most nonexistent. The incidence of amnionitis secondary to the procedure is approximately 1 per 1000 women.

## OTHER PREGNANCY COMPLICATIONS

Complications occurring shortly after amniocentesis are not uncommon, but they are usually self-limited. Postprocedure amniotic fluid leakage occurs in 1% to 2% of patients. Since leakage of fluid is transient in most cases, these patients should be managed expectantly. Ultrasound examinations should be performed peri-odically to evaluate amniotic fluid volume and appropriate fetal growth. Persistent leakage and severe oligohydramnios are probably associated with a much worse prognosis than when amniotic fluid volume is normal. Vaginal spotting and uterine contractions are also not uncommon, but they are almost always transient and of little consequence.

## AMNIOCENTESIS IN MULTIPLE GESTATIONS

Genetic amniocenteses in twin pregnancies are relatively common. The counsel-ing issues in twins are more complicated than those in singletons. The first point is that the risk of an abnormal result is doubled. Furthermore, the risk of losing the pregnancy may be increased because of the necessity of having a minimum of two needle insertions. A more complicated issue is the possibility of discordant results (i.e., finding that one fetus is normal while the other is not). The couple should at least consider what they would do under these circumstances. At the present time three options are available: continuation of the pregnancy, termination of both fetuses, or selective termination of the affected twin.

As is true for singletons, the technique of amniocentesis in twins requires a careful ultrasound exam before the procedure. In addition to the usual parame-ters, one must identify the membrane separating the sacs and the lie of each fetus within its sac. The needle should be introduced into the first sac under ultrasound guidance; after aspiration of the amniotic fluid sample, a small amount of dye is injected before the needle is removed. Indigo carmine is the dye most commonly used. Methylene blue should be avoided because it can cause methemoglobinemia. The other sac is then entered with a different needle; aspiration of clear fluid indicates that the initial reservoir has not been resampled. Blue amniotic fluid, on the other hand, indicates that the same sac has been sampled twice, although a slight blue tinge may result from transmembranous diffusion of the dye in monochorionic pregnancies. If the same sac has been sampled twice, the needle should be removed, a different area identified, and another amniocentesis performed in an attempt to aspirate clear fluid. No more than four needle insertions should be attempted at any given time. It is difficult to quantify the risks of amniocentesis in twin pregnancies because all of the studies report a small number of patients and none of them have a group of matched controls.

## EARLY AMNIOCENTESIS

Although genetic amniocentesis is usually performed at approximately 16 weeks gestation, it has been done as early as 9 weeks. The safety and success rate in obtaining a diagnosis in these early procedures are still unknown, as is the volume of fluid that can be removed safely from the uterus. With the advent of chorionic villus sampling (CVS), which is performed at 8 to 12 weeks, physicians are being asked to perform genetic testing earlier in pregnancy. Of particular concern in this regard are those patients who present at a gestational age too advanced for first trimester CVS but too early for the more traditional amniocentesis.

## FETAL BLOOD SAMPLING

### FETAL KARYOTYPING

Karyotyping cultured amniocytes can take anywhere from 1 to 3 weeks. However, quicker results are sometimes necessary. Results from karyotypes performed on fetal white blood cells are usually available within 48 to 72 hours. Common indications for rapid fetal karyotyping are the detection of structural malformations or intrauterine growth retardation because management decisions may need to be made within days. If the need for karyotyping arises at a critical gestational age (i.e., close to the time when a legal termination of pregnancy is no longer possible, or if delivery is imminent), analysis of fetal blood is also indicated. Another indication for karyotyping fetal white blood cells is mosaicism in amniotic fluid or chorionic villus sampling.

## FETAL BLOOD DISORDERS

Although the majority of hemoglobinopathies and coagulopathies can be diagnosed by analyzing DNA obtained by amniocentesis or chorionic villus sampling, there are still situations in which fetal blood sampling is necessary. Examples are those families that are not informative for the DNA probes available, or cases in which the affected individuals are deceased. Congenital thrombocytopenias can also be diagnosed by fetal platelet count determination.

## FETAL INFECTION

Direct isolation of an organism in fetal blood or amniotic fluid is the most reliable evidence of fetal infection. This, however, is not always possible because culturing techniques may be either very difficult to perform or extremely lengthy. In these cases other evidence of infection may be helpful. As in the adult, fetal responses to infection may be either specific or nonspecific. The former response includes production of IgM antibodies that are directed specifically at the offending organism. The production of such antibodies, however, depends on the maturity of the fetal immune system, and consequently, gestational age. In most cases detection of this marker of infection has proved to be very reliable when present, but its absence does not rule out fetal exposure to the organism. Nonspecific evidence of infection has proved to be very useful in these cases. Some of these signs include thrombocytopenia, erythroblastosis, leukocytosis, eosinophilia, elevated γ-glutamyltransferase, and lactic dehydrogenase and elevated total IgM. These findings are not pathognomonic of fetal infection, and some of them can be seen in other fetal conditions, such as intrauterine growth retardation. Nevertheless, when fetal infection is a possibility, positive nonspecific findings may be very helpful in either expediting a positive isolation of the organism or informing the patient that the chances of infection are high.

## TECHNIQUE

Fetal blood can be aspirated from the cord root, free-floating loops of cord, or the hepatic vein within the fetal liver. The placental insertion of the cord root is usually the preferred site. After identification of the cord insertion site the maternal abdomen is cleaned with an antiseptic solution and the transducer is placed in a sterile plastic bag. A 20- to 22-gauge needle is introduced under direct ultrasound guidance through the maternal abdominal wall into the targeted vessel. Once the needle is in place a 1-mL disposable syringe that has been flushed with heparin is attached to the needle. Gentle aspiration will yield pure fetal blood if the needle is placed correctly. Once blood has been aspirated its fetal origin should be confirmed. The volume of blood withdrawn depends on the indication for sampling and the gestational age. In general, we do not exceed 4 mL during the second trimester and 6 mL during the third. Once an adequate sample is obtained, the needle is withdrawn and the duration of bleeding from the puncture site is determined. Fetal cardiac activity should be assessed during and after the procedure.

When the placenta is posterior and the needle has to traverse the amniotic cavity, fetal movements may dislodge the needle, possibly tearing the cord vessel and causing significant fetal bleeding. Some authors have advocated paralyzing the fetus with a neuromuscular blocking agent immediately after entry into the vessel to avoid this complication. Fetal paralysis can also be achieved by administering the drug intramuscularly into the fetal thigh or buttock before the cord is punctured. Several neuromuscular blocking agents have been used, including d-tubocurarine (1.5 to 3 mg/kg), pancuronium (0.3 mg/kg), and atracurium besylate (0.4 mg/kg). Although paralyzing the fetus appears to be safe, it is usually unnecessary for fetal blood sampling because the sampling time is usually short. However, during longer procedures, such as intravascular transfusions, fetal paralysis is often very helpful.

## ASSESSMENT OF FETAL BLOOD SAMPLES

It is critical to confirm that the sample of blood obtained is fetal in origin and to be aware of any contamination with either amniotic fluid or maternal blood. The mean corpuscular volume of fetal red cells is much larger than that of the adult, so one can make this distinction by comparing the red cell size distribution of the aspirated sample to that of the mother. These parameters are not very sensitive in detecting small degrees of sample contamination, since they are only reliable with more than 5% maternal blood and 20% amniotic fluid contamination. A blood smear with Giemsa stain; human chorionic gonadotropin B-subunit (B-hCG) analysis; coagulation factors II, V, VII, and IX assays; and red cell (I/i) antigen determination can be performed to detect very small degrees of contamination. When assessing fetal hematologic parameters it is essential that they be compared with reference values for that specific gestational age.

## RISKS AND COMPLICATIONS

Despite these drawbacks the fetal loss rate related to fetal blood sampling appears to be relatively low. The exact risk of fetal blood sampling cannot be assessed at this time; however, it appears to be between 1% and 2%, which is not very much higher than that with amniocentesis (Table 23-2).

The most common complication of fetal blood sampling is transient fetal bradycardia. Since prolonged bradycardia is a potentially serious complications, PUBS should be performed in an area where immediate operative delivery is possible whenever the fetus is of a viable gestational age. Fetal bleeding from the puncture site can be observed in a number of cases when the needle is removed, but this also is usually very short-lived. Severe chorioamnionitis secondary to fetal blood sampling has been reported (Table 23-3).

## FETAL SKIN BIOPSY

Some skin disorders or systemic diseases with cutaneous manifestations may now be diagnosed by such techniques as chorionic villus sampling, amniocentesis, or fetal blood sampling.

**TABLE 23-2.** Indications for Fetal Blood Sampling in the United States and Canada

| Indication | Percentage of Cases |
| --- | --- |
| Karyotype | 37.0 |
| Red cell isoimmunization | 34.0 |
| Non-immune hydrops fetalis | 6.5 |
| Fetal infections | 5.5 |
| Idiopathic thrombocytopenic purpura | 5.3 |
| Alloimmune thrombocytopenia | 2.1 |
| Hemoglobinopathies | 2.0 |
| Other | 7.6 |

Data from Ludomirski A. National PUBS Registry. Fourth International Conference, Philadelphia, 1989.

**TABLE 23-3.** Etiology of Fetal Losses After Fetal Blood Sampling

| Cause | Percentage of Loss |
|---|---|
| Chorioamnionitis | 47 |
| Rupture of membranes | 17 |
| Bleeding from puncture site | 14 |
| Fetal bradycardia | 8 |
| Thrombosis | 3 |
| Unexplained | 11 |

Data from Ludomirski A. National PUBS Registry. Fourth International Conference, Philadelphia, 1989.

Despite these advances, most primary skin disorders must be diagnosed by directly studying the fetal skin. Originally, fetal skin biopsies were performed "blindly" or by fetoscopic guidance. Recently, percutaneous insertion of the biopsy forceps under ultrasound guidance has replaced the earlier methods. Before starting the procedure, an ultrasound examination is performed to identify the best site of entry into the amniotic cavity. Because of the relatively large-bore instrument utilized, the placenta should never be punctured. In addition, the pocket selected should not contain loops of umbilical cord or fetal parts. The optimum site for fetal skin biopsy is the fetal back, buttocks, or thighs. However, for disorders of pigmentation, areas with abundant hair follicles (scalp) are preferred. Once the insertion site is selected and has been prepared aseptically, local anesthesia is injected into the maternal skin, subcutaneous tissue, and fascia. A 3- to 4-mm incision is then made with a scalpel in the skin down to the fascia, and under ultrasonic guidance a 14-gauge trocar with stylet is inserted into the amniotic cavity. The stylet is then removed and a flexible fetal skin biopsy forceps with a diameter of 1 mm is introduced through the sleeve.

Several samples of fetal skin can be taken from the same general area or from different locales. Care must be taken always to visualize the area being sampled with ultrasound because inadvertent biopsy of the amniotic sac may cause rupture of the membranes. Once adequate samples have been obtained, the instruments are removed and the skin incision is closed with a single suture. Fetal heart activity should be monitored during and after the procedure.

The loss rate due to fetal skin biopsy is not known. The main reason is that the number of fetuses requiring the procedure is extremely small. It seems reasonable to assume, however, that the risk is no greater than that of fetoscopy (2.5% to 6%), and it may be even lower, since the instruments currently being used are smaller.

Several congenital skin diseases have been diagnosed in utero by fetal tissue biopsy. In the normal fetus keratinization does not occur until 24 to 26 weeks gestation. However, prenatal diagnosis of keratinization disorders has been possible at 20 to 22 weeks by a combination of both light and electron microscopy examination. Within the group of keratinizing disorders the following have been diagnosed: lamellar ichthyosis (nonbullous congenital ichthyosiform erythroderma), epidermolytic hyperkeratosis (bullous ichthyosiform erythroderma), and harlequin syndrome. Several forms of blistering disorders have also been diagnosed in utero, such as epidermolysis bullosa letalis and some of the recessive and dominant types of epidermolysis bullosa dystrophica. Prenatal diagnosis of disorders of pigmentation, such as oculocutaneous albinism, has been possible by observing a lack of melanin synthesis in hair bulb melanocytes. This diagnosis can be made as early as 16 weeks gestation because in normal fetuses at least 50% of the melanosomes are fully pigmented at this age.

# 24.   MATERNAL PROTEIN ENZYME ANALYSES

## ALPHA-FETOPROTEIN

Alpha-fetoprotein (AFP) is the major serum protein in fetal blood early on, peaking in concentration at about 12 weeks gestation and then falling slowly for the remainder of the pregnancy. For practical purposes it can be considered feto-specific, being present in minute concentrations in nonpregnant adult serum ($< 0.5$ to $2.0$ ng/mL).

Although helpful to some women, the overall diagnostic effectiveness of amniotic fluid AFP testing to the general pregnancy population has been severely restricted; only 3% to 5% of the annual births affected by open neural tube defects occur in families known to be at high risk. Realizing this to be the case, a number of investigators have turned their attention to measuring AFP in maternal serum, to learn whether open neural tube defects might be associated with higher AFP levels in that compartment as well. Pregnancies identified by the MSAFP screening process as being at high risk would then become candidates for amniocentesis, in a similar fashion to pregnancies identified as being at high risk because of a positive family history.

### DEVELOPING ACETYLCHOLINESTERASE TESTING IN AMNIOTIC FLUID AS A SECOND DIAGNOSTIC TEST

Although analysis of AFP in amniotic fluid has proved highly sensitive, false-positive results have occurred occasionally, and the search has therefore continued for additional biochemical products that might serve as markers for open neural tube defects and that might be more specific. Acetylcholinesterase (AChE) was found to be such a marker, and its introduction as a second diagnostic test, along with AFP, has significantly improved the laboratory's ability to distinguish affected from unaffected pregnancies (Fig. 24-1). AChE cannot be measured, however, in maternal serum.

### THE DISCOVERY THAT LOWER MSAFP LEVELS ARE ASSOCIATED WITH FETAL TRISOMY 21

AFP screening and diagnostic protocols for detecting open neural tube defects were well established by 1984, when a new and unexpected association was

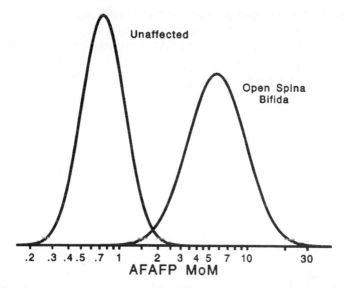

**FIGURE 24-1.** Amniotic fluid alpha-fetoprotein (AFAFP) distributions in singleton, unaffected pregnancies and in pregnancies affected by open spina bifida, during the second trimester. AFAFP measurements are expressed as multiples of the unaffected population median (MoM) on a logarithmic scale. Distributions of AFAFP values are log Gaussian for both of the populations, and a small degree of overlap is present, forming the basis for defining detection and false-positive rates at various AFAFP cut-offs. The odds of being affected, given a positive AFAFP measurement, can also be estimated using these distributions and the individual's prior risk.

discovered between lower MSAFP levels and certain autosomal trisomies (trisomy 21, trisomy 18). This discovery, prompted by a query from a patient whose MSAFP value was low and who subsequently gave birth to an infant with trisomy 18, was rapidly confirmed, and over the succeeding years, interpretation of low MSAFP values became incorporated into the routine of most MSAFP screening programs in the United States. Prior to MSAFP screening, no method existed of identifying a high-risk group for trisomy 21 among younger women (other than the unusual circumstance of a known balanced translocation).

## OTHER FETOPLACENTAL BIOCHEMICAL PRODUCTS THAT ARE ALTERED WITH TRISOMY 21

The relatively low sensitivity of MSAFP as a screening test for trisomy 21 stimulated a search for other possible biochemical markers in maternal blood, and human chorionic gonadotropin (hCG) and unconjugated estriol (uE3) were subsequently found to occur in different concentrations from unaffected pregnancies, when trisomy 21 was present in the fetus. A subsequent study analyzed the extent of interdependence of these new markers with AFP, concluding that there was a high degree of independence and that the three markers together could identify 60% of all pregnancies affected by trisomy 21 at a screening cut-off that selected 5% of the screened population for amniocentesis.

## ALPHA-FETOPROTEIN IN AMNIOTIC FLUID AS A DIAGNOSTIC MARKER FOR FETAL OPEN NEURAL TUBE DEFECTS AND OTHER FETAL DISORDERS

### WHY AFP IS UNIQUELY SUITED TO SERVE AS A MARKER FOR OPEN FETAL DEFECTS

Some researchers have selected AFP as a likely candidate to indicate the presence of an open fetal defect, because AFP was produced almost solely by the fetus. They have reasoned that AFP might transudate into amniotic fluid from the open fetal lesion and that it might prove to be a more sensitive marker than a protein shared by both fetus and mother. The bulk of amniotic fluid protein is now known to be maternally derived, and no other major serum protein has been found helpful in identifying open fetal defects.

### THE ORIGIN OF NORMAL BACKGROUND LEVELS OF AFP IN AMNIOTIC FLUID

AFP is normally present in amniotic fluid during the second trimester, as a result of leakage through the fetal kidney into fetal urine. For this reason it became necessary to define normal ranges for each gestational week during the second trimester, during which time AFP normally decreases steadily in concentration in a similar pattern to the AFP concentration in fetal serum.

### SENSITIVITY AND SPECIFICITY OF AFP MEASUREMENT IN AMNIOTIC FLUID TO DETECT OPEN NEURAL TUBE DEFECTS

In a study carried out in the United Kingdom, the 20 collaborating laboratories each had their own AFP standards; therefore, it became necessary for the study organizers to convert each contributing center's AFP measurements into multiples of its own unaffected population's median (MoM) as a first step toward a combined analysis. Using this approach, it became possible to define distributions of AFP concentrations in both unaffected and affected pregnancies. In the relationship between amniotic fluid AFP values in unaffected pregnancies and pregnancies affected with open spina bifida, there is a small degree of overlap. A stepwise cut-off was then defined, based on gestational age, that allowed 99.5% of anencephaly cases and 98% of open spina bifida cases to be identified at a false-positive rate of approximately 7 out of 1000 amniotic fluid samples analyzed. With this information it became possible to estimate the likelihood of an amniotic fluid AFP elevation being a true positive, and it became clear that the likelihood depended heavily on the woman's prior risk of having an affected pregnancy.

### REASONS FOR FALSELY ELEVATED AFP MEASUREMENTS IN AMNIOTIC FLUID

Most false positive AFP elevations in amniotic fluid could be traced to fetal blood contamination related to the procedure. If the amniotic fluid sample were visibly bloodstained and if the blood could be documented as fetal in origin (either by Kleihauer-Betke analysis or by counterelectrophoresis to detect hemoglobin F), then any accompanying AFP elevation would need to be viewed as a false positive until proved otherwise. Unexplained AFP elevations do occasionally occur in amniotic fluid, even in the absence of blood contamination. Appreciation of the less-than-absolute ability of AFP measurements to diagnose open fetal defects had led prenatal diagnostic laboratories to emphasize interpreting positive test results to patients in relative terms.

## OTHER FETAL DISORDERS ASSOCIATED WITH AFP ELEVATIONS IN AMNIOTIC FLUID

A variety of other fetal disorders are now known to be associated with AFP elevations in amniotic fluid, among them open ventral wall defects (omphalocele and gastroschisis), congenital nephrosis, and a severely distressed or recently dead fetus. These can be factored into the interpretation of an elevated AFP measurement, depending on their local prevalence. Congenital nephrosis, an autosomal recessive disorder, is rare in most of the world but occurs frequently in Finland, where it figures prominently among the fetal disorders diagnosed prenatally. In the United States open ventral wall defects are the second most common major open fetal malformation identified by AFP elevations in amniotic fluid, occurring at an approximate rate of 3 per 10,000 second trimester pregnancies.

## ACETYLCHOLINESTERASE (AChE) IN AMNIOTIC FLUID AS A DIAGNOSTIC MARKER FOR FETAL OPEN NEURAL TUBE DEFECTS AND OTHER FETAL DISORDERS

In one study, the assay relied on first separating AChE from other cholinesterases in amniotic fluid and then developing the gel with a substrate that allowed the AChE enzyme band to be magnified for easy visibility. This qualitative assay provided a clear definition between affected and unaffected pregnancies, in that a discrete band was visible in amniotic fluid in the presence of open neural tube defects, whereas no band could be seen in unaffected pregnancies. This analytic system not only proved highly sensitive for detecting open neural tube defects (99% of anencephaly cases, 98% of open spina bifida cases with positive AFP results), but also was found negative in 9 out of 10 cases where the amniotic fluid AFP measurement was falsely elevated.

## AFP LEVELS IN MATERNAL SERUM IN RELATION TO FETAL OPEN NEURAL TUBE DEFECTS AND OTHER FETAL DISORDERS

### DEFINING REFERENCE RANGES FOR MSAFP DURING THE SECOND TRIMESTER

The discovery that maternal serum alpha-fetoprotein (MSAFP) levels were higher in association with fetal open neural tube defects than with unaffected singleton pregnancies in the second trimester led to a multicenter study in the United Kingdom aimed at testing the feasibility of using this biochemical marker for screening or diagnostic purposes. MSAFP concentrations rise steadily throughout the second trimester in unaffected singleton pregnancies (by approximately 15% per week), and so it was necessary for each participating center to establish normative data against which MSAFP measurements from affected pregnancies could be compared. Because of this relationship between MSAFP concentration and gestational age, it is important to ensure accuracy of dating. Any laboratory carrying out MSAFP screening needs to be capable of demonstrating a rise in MSAFP values similar to that displayed in Figure 24-2. The higher AFP levels in maternal blood found in association with pregnancy are contributed from the fetus. There is no evidence that maternal production of AFP is altered.

## CONDITIONS OTHER THAN OPEN FETAL DEFECTS ASSOCIATED WITH MSAFP ELEVATIONS

A variety of conditions in pregnancy could result in higher MSAFP levels, among them multiple gestations (twin pregnancies had MSAFP levels twice as high, on average, as singletons; triplets, three times as high; and so on) and fetal death, which often are associated with very increased MSAFP levels. Higher MSAFP levels were also found to be associated with increased risk for preterm delivery and intrauterine growth retardation, once multiple gestation, fetal death, and

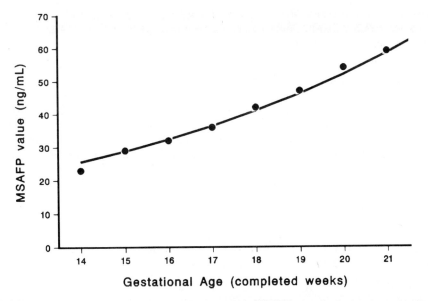

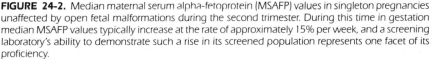

**FIGURE 24-2.** Median maternal serum alpha-fetoprotein (MSAFP) values in singleton pregnancies unaffected by open fetal malformations during the second trimester. During this time in gestation median MSAFP values typically increase at the rate of approximately 15% per week, and a screening laboratory's ability to demonstrate such a rise in its screened population represents one facet of its proficiency.

open fetal malformations had been ruled out. This all indicated that an elevated MSAFP measurement was relatively nonspecific in relation to open fetal defects and might be suitable as a screening, but not as a diagnostic, test.

## THE USE OF MULTIPLES OF THE MEDIAN TO NORMALIZE MSAFP MEASUREMENT

In analyzing the multicenter study, Wald and Cuckle began by converting data from all the centers into multiples of the unaffected populations' median (MoM).* At the time of the study, large differences in assay standards existed between the contributing centers, meaning that an MSAFP level of 40 ng/mL as measured in one center might be measured as 75 ng/mL in a second center. Although both of these measurements eventually were found correct when analyzed according to the normative data for their respective laboratories, it was impossible to compare them without using a conversion factor. The median was chosen as a reference point for each laboratory's unaffected population data, because it was the most stable and reliable measure of the midpoint, being less subject to the influence of occasional outlying measurements than the mean. This conversion also allowed the midpoint value for each gestational week to be designated as 1.0 MoM, thereby avoiding the confusion that might arise from having to consider different within-laboratory differences in mass unit values for each gestational week. Unifying the midreference point for each laboratory meant that it was now possible to establish the median for twin pregnancies (2.0 multiples of the singleton unaffected population median), for pregnancies affected with open spina bifida (3.8 MoM), for pregnancies associated with anencephaly (7.7 MoM), and for a number of other well-defined disorders whose MSAFP values differed in distribution from the singleton, unaffected pregnancies. Being able to define the distributions of MSAFP values in MoM as well as the midpoints meant that the extent of overlap between unaffected and affected populations could also be analyzed, meaning that both collective and individual odds could be estimated for a pregnancy with a given fetal disorder.

## ESTIMATING INDIVIDUAL AND COLLECTIVE ODDS FOR OPEN SPINA BIFIDA, BASED ON THE MSAFP MEASUREMENT

The ability to estimate individual and collective odds for a lesion such as open spina bifida provided a rational basis for decision making that allowed the background population risk to be combined with MSAFP measurements as a means of deciding a reasonable cut-off for high-risk classification. For example, the first U.K. collaborative study demonstrated that 3.4% of screened pregnancies from the general population and 85% of open spina bifida pregnancies were associated with MSAFP values at, or above, 2.5 MoM. The birth prevalence of open spina bifida at that time was approximately 2 in 1000. Given this information, it was

---

* Wald and Cuckle. Maternal serum alpha-fetoprotein measurement in antenatal screening for ancephaly and spina bifida in early pregnancy. Report of the UK Collaborative Study on alpha-fetoprotein in relation to neural tube defects. Lancet 1977;1:1323.

possible to estimate that for every 10,000 pregnancies screened, 340 would initially be classified as at high risk and 17 of those (1 in 19) actually would be affected with open spina bifida. In the United States, where the birth prevalence of open spina bifida was 1 per 1000, 1 in 38 of the pregnancies initially classified as at high risk would be affected by open spina bifida. It also became possible to assign individual risk estimates for open spina bifida based on the woman's initial MSAFP value. To accomplish this, a line was first drawn vertically from the point on the baseline where the woman's MSAFP value was located to intersect the two curves (one curve representing the distribution of the unaffected population, and the other representing that of the open spina bifida population). Measurements were then made of the distance from baseline to unaffected curve intersection and from baseline to open spina bifida curve intersection (Fig. 24-3). These two measurements were expressed as a ratio of affected to unaffected, called the likelihood ratio. If the height of the affected were four times that of the unaffected, the likelihood ratio would be 4. This ratio could then be multiplied by the rate in the general population to determine the woman's new risk based on her MSAFP value. If the background risk were 1 in 1000, this would be multiplied by 4 to produce a new risk of 4 in 1000.

## REPEATING THE MSAFP MEASUREMENT AFTER AN INITIALLY ELEVATED RESULT: THE CONCEPT OF REGRESSION TO THE MEAN

The midpoints of the unaffected singleton population and the open spina bifida population are widely separated (1.0 MoM for unaffected, 3.8 MoM for open spina

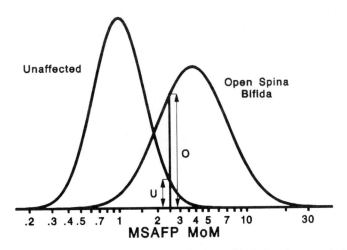

**FIGURE 24-3.** Estimating a pregnant woman's individual odds during the second trimester for carrying a fetus affected by open spina bifida, once her maternal serum alpha-fetoprotein (MSAFP) value has been determined. The distributions of MSAFP values for unaffected and affected populations are expressed as multiples of the median (MoM). In this example, the woman's MSAFP level is 2.5 MoM, and the measurements from that point on the baseline to intersection with the unaffected and affected curves are 1.0 and 4.0 units, respectively, producing a likelihood ratio of 4:1. Based on her MSAFP level, the woman's individual odds for a pregnancy affected by open spina bifida are now four times as great as those in the general population.

bifida), and MSAFP measurements above the cut-offs used by most centers (2.0 to 2.5 MoM) often are located between the central points of the two populations. A repeat MSAFP measurement, in such cases, is highly likely to move in one direction for unaffected pregnancies (lower) and in another if the pregnancy is affected with open spina bifida (higher). Other major open fetal malformations associated with MSAFP elevations also have MSAFP MoM midpoints widely separated from the unaffected population (e.g., anencephaly, open ventral wall defects), and the principle of regression to the mean applies in those cases as well.

Repeating MSAFP measurements following an initial elevation has proved helpful to many screening programs as a way to sort out falsely positive screening results. A repeat MSAFP measurement that falls within the normal range does not, however, exclude the possibility of an open fetal malformation; it only reduces its likelihood, and this is a particularly important aspect of the screening process to explain to the patient.

## WHY REPEATING THE MSAFP MEASUREMENT AFTER AN INITIAL LOW VALUE IS CONTRAINDICATED

When screening for Down syndrome using MSAFP measurements was first introduced, it seemed natural to call for repeat testing after an initial positive test result. Unfortunately, the MSAFP distributions of the unaffected singleton and Down syndrome populations overlap considerably, and the midpoints are close together. For that reason nearly all the MSAFP measurements labeled as positive fall away from the two medians in the same direction. The tendency to regress, therefore, is in the same direction, whether or not the pregnancy is associated with Down syndrome (Fig. 24-4). The net effect of repeating is to decrease the sensitivity of the screening test, and a number of cases of Down syndrome are known to have been missed using this type of approach. It is now generally recommended that repeat MSAFP testing not be done when screening for Down syndrome.

## LIMITATIONS OF SENSITIVITY OF MSAFP SCREENING TO DETECT OPEN FETAL DEFECTS

Among the major open fetal malformations detected by MSAFP screening, anencephaly is the most readily detected, being associated with MSAFP values above the screening cut-off in more than 90% of cases. Gastroschisis is also readily detected, and MSAFP screening sensitivity for that condition approaches that for anencephaly. Open spina bifida is associated with MSAFP values that more often overlap with the unaffected population, and screening sensitivity for detecting that condition is approximately 75%. A smaller proportion of omphalocele cases is detected than of open spina bifida (about 60%). The reasons for not identifying a greater proportion of cases through screening are not always correctly perceived.

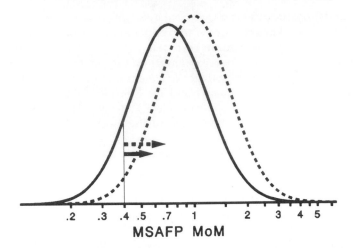

**MSAFP MoM**

**FIGURE 24-4.** The effect of repeating the maternal serum alpha-fetoprotein (MSAFP) measurement when the initial value falls below the screening cut-off for detecting Down syndrome. In this example, the woman's initial MSAFP value falls at 0.4 multiples of the median (MoM). At age 28 or greater, this places her in a high-risk category for having a fetus affected with Down syndrome. The MSAFP value falls considerably below the center points of both the unaffected (MSAFP = 1.0 MoM) population distribution and the population distribution for Down syndrome (MSAFP = 0.75 MoM). The line drawn vertically from 0.4 MoM indicates that the woman's individual odds for having an affected pregnancy are about three times that of unscreened pregnancies of the same age. When a second serum sample is obtained and measured for AFP, there will be a tendency for the value to be higher, regardless of whether the pregnancy is affected with Down syndrome. The net effect of using repeat measurements will be to reduce both Down syndrome detection and false positives equally. This is also an example of regression to the mean.

## IMPROVED GESTATIONAL DATING AND BIPARIETAL DIAMETER MEASUREMENTS AS WAYS TO IMPROVE SCREENING SENSITIVITY

Certain steps can be undertaken by both physician and laboratory that will lead to some improvement in both the sensitivity and specificity of the screening process. The first of these has to do with gestational dating. Most pregnancies are still dated from the first day of the last menstrual period (LMP) at the time in gestation when MSAFP testing is performed, and the original estimates for both sensitivity and specificity were made using LMP dates. Even when LMP dates are carefully obtained, they are incorrect by more than 2 weeks about 20% of the time. Furthermore, there is a tendency to think that a pregnancy is further advanced than it really is. This diminishes screening sensitivity, on the one hand, and yields false-positive screening results, on the other, because MSAFP measurements normally rise by about 15% per week during the second trimester, and normative data are based on this rise.

A brief ultrasound study would correct the dates of pregnancies further advanced than predicted by LMP and would also identify twins, thereby reducing false-positive screening results. Cases of anencephaly would also be identified at that point. Systematically using BPD measurements would reduce screening program costs and avoid unnecessary anxiety for many women.

## THE RELATIONSHIP BETWEEN A WOMAN'S WEIGHT AND HER MSAFP CONCENTRATION

The AFP concentration in the mother's blood is partly dependent on her weight: the larger the woman, the lower the average MSAFP concentration, presumably because of a dilution effect from the larger vascular compartment.

## A WOMAN'S RACE IN RELATION TO HER MSAFP CONCENTRATION

Black women have, on average, MSAFP screening measurements that are 15% higher than those of white women. In mixed population screening where this is not taken into account, an inappropriately high proportion of black pregnant women will be identified as having positive screening results and will be sent on for further diagnostic procedures.

## INSULIN-DEPENDENT DIABETES AND MSAFP CONCENTRATION

A more occasional variable that influences MSAFP measurements is maternal insulin-dependent diabetes, which is associated with 20% lower MSAFP values, on average, than the unaffected singleton population. Women with insulin-dependent diabetes also are at greater risk for having pregnancies affected by open neural tube defects. No MSAFP differences have been observed in gestational diabetes. It is not presently known whether insulin-dependent diabetic women with pregnancies associated with open spina bifida also have lower average MSAFP values, but this is not a critical point, since correcting MSAFP values in diabetic pregnancies will always increase screening sensitivity. Adjusting MSAFP measurements in diabetic women is now carried out routinely in most screening centers.

## THE BIOLOGY OF AFP AS IT RELATES TO SCREENING AND DIAGNOSTIC TESTING

### AFP PRODUCTION AND CIRCULATION IN FETAL AND MATERNAL COMPARTMENTS

Alpha-fetoprotein is the major circulating fetal protein early in pregnancy, reaching a peak concentration of approximately 3000 mg/L at 12 weeks gestation and then slowly falling in concentration. AFP is thought to be the fetal albumin equivalent, and its molecular structure is similar to that of albumin, even though antibodies raised against AFP have virtually no cross-reactivity with albumin. This latter characteristic is critical in allowing a variety of antibody-based assays to be developed for measuring AFP in amniotic fluid, maternal serum, and other body fluids as well (all of which also contain very high concentrations of albumin). For practical purposes, AFP can be thought of as feto-specific (the circulating level in nonpregnant adults is up to 2 µg/L).

### NORMAL TRANSPORT OF AFP INTO AMNIOTIC FLUID AND MATERNAL SERUM

Normally, AFP levels are relatively high in amniotic fluid during the second trimester, because of sieving through the fetal kidney (about 20 mg/L at 14 weeks gestation, and falling at a constant rate thereafter). The steady fall in concentration coincides with the increasing amniotic fluid volume, and it is necessary to establish a reference range for amniotic fluid AFP that takes gestational age into account. Fetal AFP normally appears in the maternal circulation via two routes: transplacental and transamniotic. About 70% of the fetal contribution of AFP to the maternal circulation has been estimated to be transplacental; the rest is estimated to be transamniotic under normal conditions.

## NORMAL PATTERNS OF AFP CONCENTRATIONS IN AMNIOTIC FLUID AND MATERNAL SERUM

Normally, median levels of MSAFP rise steadily at the rate of about 15% per week during the second trimester, at a time when both amniotic fluid and fetal serum levels are falling. This paradox has not been explained experimentally, but one possible explanation is that the placenta is growing rapidly during this time and provides a larger surface area for both transplacental and transamniotic diffusion.

## TRANSPORT OF AFP INTO AMNIOTIC FLUID AND MATERNAL SERUM IN THE PRESENCE OF FETAL MALFORMATIONS

Understanding this transfer process helps us to appreciate why maternal serum AFP measurements are less sensitive and specific for detecting open fetal malformations. When open spina bifida is present in the fetus, AFP leaks directly from the exposed surface into the amniotic fluid, leading to levels raised sufficiently that the lesion can be detected 97% of the time. The same mechanism operates with anencephaly, where the lesion is usually larger and leaks even higher amounts of AFP (leading to 99% detection).

The increased concentrations of AFP in amniotic fluid are reflected in maternal serum, because of diffusion across the amnion. But the amnion is a barrier with some variability in sieving characteristics. Furthermore, the transplacental contribution is not likely to be increased in the presence of fetal lesions and stands as a constant background source of AFP that may interfere with the signal being provided by the transamniotic AFP.

## ABNORMAL TRANSPORT OF AFP WITH IMPENDING OR PREEXISTING FETAL DEATH

When a fetus has died just prior to MSAFP screening, the amniotic fluid contains higher than normal concentrations of AFP, and MSAFP levels are also elevated. It is likely that these higher AFP levels result from a general breakdown in the normal fetal tissue barriers to diffusion and filtration. MSAFP levels are also elevated in some instances when the fetus is viable at the time of MSAFP screening but dies subsequently, in some cases several weeks later. Recognizing that elevated MSAFP measurements indicate a high risk for subsequent fetal death after other conditions have been ruled out, many clinicians have increased surveillance of such pregnancies, but no strategy has yet been found successful in preventing those deaths. Risk of fetal death is approximately six times higher with MSAFP elevation than when the MSAFP measurement is not elevated.

## ABNORMAL TRANSPORT OF AFP IN CASES OF FALSE POSITIVES

Fetal blood is often a problem when either amniotic fluid or maternal serum AFP levels are being measured. If, during amniocentesis, the fetal circulation is inadvertently breached, the fetal blood in the amniotic fluid sample will carry high concentrations of AFP with it and can produce false-positive test results. Fetal blood in the maternal circulation is a second and frequent source of false-positive test results, this time for the MSAFP screening test. Fetal blood can enter the maternal circulation through a placental hemorrhage (the usual source) or may enter in conjunction with a procedure, such as amniocentesis.

## ABNORMAL TRANSPORT OF AFP INTO MATERNAL SERUM AND RISK FOR LOW BIRTH WEIGHT

Elevated MSAFP values in conjunction with normal amniotic fluid AFP values also signal a high risk for low birth-weight outcomes, some due to prematurity and others to intrauterine growth retardation. This is a further example of the nonspecificity of MSAFP as a screening test but also demonstrates that even false-positive screening results (in relation to open fetal malformations) are providing additional information about high-risk pregnancies. Just as with fetal deaths, no management protocol has been discovered that reduces risk of low birth weight. This risk is increased between three and four times over the risk in pregnancies with normal MSAFP measurements.

## VAGINAL BLEEDING AND ABNORMAL TRANSPORT OF AFP INTO MATERNAL SERUM

Vaginal bleeding during pregnancy is associated with higher risk for fetal morbidity and mortality and is associated with placental hemorrhage. When the presence or absence of vaginal bleeding is considered in relation to MSAFP measurements, it is found to be an independent risk factor for both low birth weight and fetal death. It is therefore helpful to know if a woman with an elevated MSAFP measurement also has vaginal bleeding; when both risk factors are present, the risk for fetal death is considerably higher.

## AN UNEXPLAINED ASSOCIATION BETWEEN MSAFP ELEVATIONS AND OLIGOHYDRAMNIOS

Oligohydramnios is another condition found occasionally in association with elevated MSAFP measurements. In some instances the reason for oligohydramnios becomes apparent with the ultrasound study, including conditions such as urinary tract anomalies and extrauterine pregnancies. Whether or not an explanation is found, the prognosis for viability of the pregnancy is poor, with the survival rate being estimated at less than 20%.

## TRANSPORT OF AFP INTO MATERNAL SERUM IN ASSOCIATION WITH TWINS

Twin pregnancies are associated with MSAFP values that are, on average, twice as high as those of singleton pregnancies, and if a cut-off for MSAFP screening is set at 2.0 MoM, half of the twin pregnancies will fall above that cut-off. Most centers simply double their singleton cut-off, a policy that is both reasonable and easy to remember. Screening sensitivity for open fetal malformations in twins is reduced at any given cut-off, however, because in most instances only one of the twins is affected when an open fetal lesion is present in the pregnancy. Other risk factors, such as fetal death and low birth weight, can also be roughly estimated, using the two times higher cut-off.

## MSAFP LEVELS IN ASSOCIATION WITH FETAL DOWN SYNDROME AND OTHER CONDITIONS

### VERY LOW MSAFP LEVELS IN RELATION TO FETAL DEATH AND MISDATED PREGNANCY

When the screened pregnancies were dated by LMP, between 50% and 75% of the very low MSAFP values could be explained subsequently by correcting the dates via ultrasound. Also found in association with very low MSAFP measurements were fetal deaths that had occurred a long time prior to the blood sample being obtained. In such cases the AFP had simply undergone autolysis. Miscellaneous other conditions were also discovered when very low MSAFP values were followed up, including molar pregnancy and nonpregnancy.

### COMBINING LOW MSAFP MEASUREMENTS WITH WOMEN'S AGE TO SCREEN FOR TRISOMY 21

The potential significance of low MSAFP values changed in 1984, when Merkatz and colleagues reported that MSAFP values were lower in pregnancies where the chromosomal constitution of the fetus was trisomy 21 (Down syndrome) or trisomy 18 (Edwards' syndrome). Over 5% of all pregnancies annually occur in women aged 35 and older, and approximately 20% of the cases of Down syndrome are born to those women. The remaining 80% of the births of Down's syndrome babies are to women younger than age 35, and it was estimated that 20% of the cases of Down syndrome could be identified in that younger population by using a combination of MSAFP and age-related risk.

Cord blood levels of AFP were also lower, on average, when the baby suffered from Down syndrome. This all suggested that fetal liver AFP production or disposition was altered with Down syndrome. A recent analysis of second trimester fetal blood AFP levels failed to identify lower concentrations when Down syndrome was present.

## A MULTICENTER FIELD TRIAL TO DETERMINE THE EFFICACY OF MSAFP SCREENING FOR FETAL TRISOMY 21

During the 14-month enrollment period for a New England study, 77,273 pregnancies were screened with MSAFP measurements by eight centers. Out of that number, 4.7% were initially classified as being at high risk for Down syndrome, and 2.7% of the pregnancies remained at high risk after gestational dates had been confirmed. Seventy-six percent of these high-risk women elected to have amniocentesis, and 18 fetuses with Down syndrome and 4 fetuses with trisomy 18 were identified in this group. One fetus with Down syndrome was identified per 89 amniocenteses performed (approximately 1 per 150 amniocenteses performed in women aged 35 and older is associated with Down syndrome), and an additional three Down syndrome births were identified from among the women who refused amniocentesis. It was estimated that approximately 25% of the fetal Down syndrome cases could be identified in younger pregnant women, and the study concluded that this type of screening was feasible.

## ADDITIONAL BIOCHEMICAL MARKERS OF POTENTIAL VALUE IN SCREENING FOR TRISOMY 21

More recently, two additional biochemical products in a pregnant woman's blood, human chorionic gonadotropin (hCG) and unconjugated estriol (uE3), have been identified as potential screening markers for Down syndrome during the second trimester. Unconjugated estriol is synthesized in three steps: production of dehydroepiandrosterone (DHEAs) in the fetal adrenal, conversion of DHEAs to 16αOH-DHEAs in the fetal liver, and conversion of 16αOH-DHEAs to uE3 in the placenta. Unconjugated estriol is then released into the maternal serum circulation and excreted. Using a combination of these three tests, it may be possible to raise the sensitivity for detecting fetal Down syndrome to approximately 60%, while keeping the false-positive rate similar to that for AFP alone.

# PART VIII. METHODS OF EVALUATION OF FETAL DEVELOPMENT AND WELL-BEING

## 25. PRENATAL DIAGNOSIS OF DEVIANT FETAL GROWTH

Fetal growth is a fundamental characteristic of the continuity of life and fetal well-being. Cell divisions, cell hyperplasia, and cell hypertrophy are the cornerstones of fetal growth. It has been suggested that early in pregnancy, growth of fetal organs takes place first by cell hyperplasia or cell division, then by cell hypertrophy, and finally by the cessation of hyperplasia, after which growth continues by cellular hypertrophy alone. In this chapter we will discuss the two extreme types of deviant fetal growth—diminished (intrauterine growth retardation) and accelerated (macrosomia). In addition, prenatal diagnosis of these conditions will be discussed. (For a more thorough discussion of this topic, please see Chapter 44 in Reece EA, Hobbins JC, Mahoney MJ, and Petrie RH, eds. Medicine of the fetus and mother. J.B. Lippincott, 1992.)

### INTRAUTERINE GROWTH RETARDATION

### ETIOLOGY AND DEFINITION

Intrauterine growth retardation (IUGR) is an abnormality of fetal growth and development that affects 3% to 7% of all deliveries, depending on the diagnostic criteria used. The growth-retarded fetus is at greater risk for mortality and morbidity. It is estimated that perinatal mortality is 5 to 10 times higher in the growth-retarded neonate than in the neonate who is sized appropriately for gestational age.

There are several causes of IUGR. These may be conceptually divided into three main categories: maternal, fetal, and uteroplacental (Table 25-1). It should be stressed, however, that in almost one-half of the cases of IUGR, the etiology is unknown. Furthermore, it has been found that the single most important maternal clinical risk factor is a previous history of IUGR. Therefore, suspicion of IUGR should not be based only on the existence of clinical risk factors during the index pregnancy.

One point of confusion and disagreement is the criteria that are used to define IUGR. Intrauterine growth retardation has been defined variously as an infant whose birth weight is below the 3rd, 5th, and 10th percentile for gestational age or

**TABLE 25-1.** Risk Factors of Intrauterine Growth Retardation

**Maternal Risk Factors**
Alcohol
Smoking
Drugs
  Steroids
  Propranolol
  Dilantin
  Coumadin
  Heroin
Anemia
Malnutrition
Prepregnancy weight < 50 kg
Cyanotic heart disease
Chronic hypertension
Pregnancy-induced hypertension
Diabetes mellitus (with vasculopathy)
Connective tissues disease

**Fetal Risk Factors**
Genetic disorders (eg, dwarf syndromes)
Chromosomal abnormalities (eg, trisomies 13, 18, 21)
Congenital anomalies (eg, gastroschisis)
Fetal infection (eg, viral, protozoan)

**Uterine and Placental Risk Factors**
Müllerian anomalies (eg, septate uterus)
Placental insufficiency due to:
  Infarctions
  Infection
  Chorioangioma
  Multifetal pregnancy
  Circumvallate placenta
  Previa
  Focal abruption
  Marginal insertion of the cord

whose birth weight is more than 2 standard deviations below the mean for gestational age.

The ponderal index is determined in the neonate by the following formula:

ponderal index = birth weight × 100/(crown-heel length).

The ponderal index may identify a neonate who has a small amount of soft tissue clinically evident by loss of subcutaneous tissue and muscle mass, even though the birth weight is normal for gestational age. Neonates with a ponderal index below the 10th percentile for gestational age are probably suffering from malnutrition in utero. Unfortunately, there is presently no practical method to evaluate ponderal index in utero. Hence, the most commonly used definition of IUGR is a fetal weight below the 10th percentile for gestational age.

Another index, the crown-heel length, has been used to evaluate neonatal size. However, prediction from femur length measurement (FL) has been found to be too imprecise to be useful.

One unresolved problem concerns which growth curve should be used. Discrepancies between different birth-weight charts from different geographic areas underscore the need for generating birth-weight curves from the population to which they will be applied.

## CLASSIFICATION OF IUGR

Clinically, three categories of IUGR may be recognized. Each of them reflects the time of onset of the pathologic process.

### Type 1 or Symmetrical IUGR

Type 1 IUGR refers to the infant with decreased growth potential. This type of IUGR begins early in gestation, and the entire fetus is proportionally small for gestational age. Head and abdominal circumferences, length, and weight are all below the 10th percentile for gestational age. However, these infants have a normal ponderal index.

Type 1 IUGR is a result of growth inhibition early in gestation. This early stage of embryonic-fetal development is characterized by active mitosis from 4 to 20 weeks gestation and is called the hyperplastic stage. Any pathologic process during this stage may lead to a reduced number of cells in the fetus. Symmetric IUGR accounts for 20% to 30% of growth-retarded fetuses. This condition may result from the inhibition of mitosis, as is seen in intrauterine infection (e.g., herpes simplex, rubella, cytomegalovirus, toxoplasmosis), chromosomal disorders, and congenital malformations. It should be remembered, however, that symmetrically small fetuses may be constitutionally small and suffer from no abnormality at all.

In general, type 1 IUGR is associated with a poor prognosis; this is in direct relation to the pathologic condition that causes it. Weiner and Williamson (1989) showed that in the absence of an identifiable maternal factor and sonographically detected abnormality, approximately 25% of fetuses evaluated for severe, early-onset growth retardation have aneuploidy.* Therefore, the performance of percutaneous umbilical blood sampling is strongly recommended to search for karyotypic abnormality.

### Type 2 or Asymmetrical IUGR

This term refers to the neonate with restricted growth, and is most frequently due to uteroplacental insufficiency. Type 2 IUGR is a result of a later growth insult than type 1 and usually occurs after 28 weeks gestation. Normal fetal growth is characterized by a process of hypertrophy in the late second trimester. In this hypertrophic stage, there is a rapid increase in cell size and formation of fat, muscle, bone, and other tissues. In this phase, the process of hyperplasia is decreased.

The symmetrically growth-retarded fetuses have a near-normal total number of cells, but these cells are decreased in size. Asymmetrical IUGR fetuses have low ponderal indices with below-average infant weight but normal head circumference (HC) and fetal length. In these cases of asymmetrical IUGR, fetal growth is

---

*Weiner CP, Williamson RA. Evaluation of severe retardation using cordocentesis-hematologic and metabolic alterations by etiology. Obstet Gynecol 1989;73:225.

normal until late in the second trimester or early in the third, when head growth remains normal while abdominal growth slows (brain-sparing effect). This asymmetry is a result of a fetal compensatory mechanism that responds to a state of poor placental perfusion. Redistribution of fetal cardiac output occurs with increased flow to the brain, heart, and adrenals, and decreased glycogen storage and liver mass. However, if placental insufficiency is aggravated during late pregnancy, the head growth may be flattened and its size may drop below the normal growth curve.

It is estimated that 70% to 80% of growth-retarded fetuses are type 2 IUGR. This form of IUGR is frequently associated with maternal diseases such as chronic hypertension, renal disease, diabetes mellitus with vasculopathy, and others (see Table 25-1).

## Intermediate IUGR

Indeterminate IUGR refers to growth retardation that is a combination of types 1 and 2 IUGR. The insult to fetal growth in intermediate IUGR most probably occurs during the middle phase of fetal growth—that of hyperplasia and hypertrophy—which corresponds to 20 to 28 weeks gestation. At this stage, there is a decrease in mitotic rate and a progressive overall increase in cell size.

This form of IUGR is estimated at being responsible for 5% to 10% of all growth-retarded fetuses. Chronic hypertension, lupus nephritis, or other maternal vascular diseases that are severe in nature and that begin early in the second trimester may result in an intermediate IUGR with symmetrical growth and no significant brain-sparing effect.

## ULTRASONIC MEASUREMENTS USED IN THE DIAGNOSIS OF IUGR

The intrauterine detection of IUGR is possible in approximately 30% of affected pregnancies. Ultrasonography offers an objective, reliable, and effective means of identifying retarded intrauterine fetal growth. However, in order to make a proper diagnosis and appropriately manage the growth-retarded fetus, it is crucial to determine the gestational age as accurately as possible.

Pregnancy dating has traditionally been based on historical and clinical clues. The certain date of a patient's last menstrual period had been regarded as the most reliable method of estimating a fetus's gestational age. However, it is estimated that 20% to 40% of pregnant women fail to recall the exact date of their last menstrual period.

Therefore, ultrasonography may be of help in dating a pregnancy. In the first trimester, crown-rump length measurement allows for an estimation of gestational age with a range of 4.7 days at the 95% confidence level. Between 12 to 24 weeks gestation, the biparietal diameter (BPD) measurement provides reliable estimates comparable to that of the first trimester crown-rump measurement. Beyond 28 to 30 weeks gestation, there is a progressive increase in BPD variations, and the establishment of accurate gestational age is less satisfactory. The FL correlates with gestational age, particularly during 14 to 22 weeks gestation, with a range of 6.7 days at the 95% confidence level. Accurate antenatal diagnosis of IUGR may prevent the high perinatal morbidity and mortality associated with this condition and permits appropriate management and obstetrical intervention when fetal compromise is evident. Most authorities believe that whenever IUGR is diagnosed after 37 weeks gestation, delivery is indicated in order to decrease the risk of fetal death. The following sections review several sonographic parameters that may be used in the diagnosis of IUGR.

## BIPARIETAL DIAMETER

Nomograms of BPD or HC are available to provide calculated estimates of weekly increments for the size of the fetal head (Tables 25-2, 25-3). When comparing the observed increase in BPD with the expected rate of growth, the physician should be able to identify the growth-retarded fetus whose head is affected in the growth curtailment. However, single and serial BPD measurements alone are considered to be of poor value by most authors in the detection rates of IUGR, with reported accuracy rates ranging from 43% to 82%.

It seems clear that BPD alone cannot be used as a good predictor of IUGR. This is not surprising, because almost two-thirds of IUGR cases are of the asymmetric type, with normal growth of the head until late in pregnancy as a consequence of the brain-sparing process. Therefore, BPD in asymmetric IUGR may be normal until late in gestation. In addition, distortion of the fetal head shape (e.g., dolichocephaly, or in breech presentation) may lead to a falsely small BPD. Thus, when utilized singly, BPD determinations fail to identify about 20% to 50% of IUGR infants and cannot be used as the only parameter in screening for IUGR.

**TABLE 25-2.** Gestational Age from the BPD

| BPD (mm) | Percentile | | | BPD (mm) | Percentile | | |
|---|---|---|---|---|---|---|---|
| | 5th | 50th | 95th | | 5th | 50th | 95th |
| 11 | 7 + 2 | 10 + 2 | 13 + 3 | 41 | 14 + 4 | 17 + 5 | 20 + 5 |
| 13 | 7 + 5 | 10 + 5 | 13 + 5 | 43 | 15 + 1 | 18 + 2 | 21 + 2 |
| 15 | 8 + 1 | 11 + 1 | 14 + 1 | 45 | 15 + 6 | 18 + 6 | 21 + 6 |
| 17 | 8 + 4 | 11 + 4 | 14 + 4 | 47 | 16 + 3 | 19 + 3 | 22 + 4 |
| 19 | 9 | 12 | 15 | 49 | 17 | 20 + 1 | 23 + 1 |
| 21 | 9 + 3 | 12 + 3 | 15 + 3 | 51 | 17 + 5 | 20 + 5 | 23 + 6 |
| 23 | 9 + 6 | 12 + 6 | 16 | 53 | 18 + 2 | 21 + 3 | 24 + 3 |
| 25 | 10 + 2 | 13 + 3 | 16 + 3 | 55 | 19 | 22 | 25 + 1 |
| 27 | 10 + 6 | 13 + 6 | 17 | 57 | 19 + 5 | 22 + 5 | 25 + 6 |
| 29 | 11 + 2 | 14 + 3 | 17 + 3 | 59 | 20 + 3 | 23 + 3 | 26 + 3 |
| 31 | 11 + 6 | 14 + 6 | 18 | 61 | 21 + 1 | 24 + 1 | 27 + 1 |
| 33 | 12 + 3 | 15 + 3 | 18 + 3 | 63 | 21 + 6 | 24 + 6 | 27 + 6 |
| 35 | 12 + 6 | 16 | 19 | 65 | 22 + 4 | 25 + 4 | 28 + 5 |
| 37 | 13 + 3 | 16 + 4 | 19 + 4 | 67 | 23 + 2 | 26 + 2 | 29 + 3 |
| 39 | 14 | 17 + 1 | 20 + 1 | | | | |

(Modified with permission from Jeanty P, Romero R. Obstetrical Ultrasound. New York: McGraw-Hill, 1984.)

**TABLE 25-3.** Gestational Age from the Head Circumference

| HC (mm) | Percentile | | | HC (mm) | Percentile | | |
|---|---|---|---|---|---|---|---|
|  | 5th | 50th | 95th |  | 5th | 50th | 95th |
| 65 | 9 + 1 | 11 | 12 + 5 | 210 | 20 + 2 | 22 | 23 + 5 |
| 75 | 9 + 6 | 11 + 4 | 13 + 2 | 220 | 21 + 1 | 22 + 6 | 24 + 5 |
| 85 | 10 + 3 | 12 + 1 | 14 | 230 | 22 + 1 | 23 + 6 | 25 + 4 |
| 95 | 11 + 1 | 12 + 6 | 14 + 4 | 240 | 23 + 1 | 24 + 6 | 26 + 4 |
| 105 | 11 + 5 | 13 + 4 | 15 + 2 | 250 | 24 + 1 | 25 + 6 | 27 + 4 |
| 115 | 12 + 3 | 14 + 1 | 16 | 260 | 25 + 1 | 26 + 6 | 28 + 5 |
| 125 | 13 + 1 | 14 + 6 | 16 + 5 | 270 | 26 + 1 | 28 | 29 + 5 |
| 135 | 13 + 6 | 15 + 5 | 17 + 3 | 280 | 27 + 2 | 29 | 30 + 6 |
| 145 | 14 + 5 | 16 + 3 | 18 + 1 | 290 | 28 + 3 | 30 + 1 | 31 + 6 |
| 155 | 15 + 3 | 17 + 2 | 19 | 300 | 29 + 4 | 31 + 2 | 33 |
| 165 | 16 + 2 | 18 | 19 + 6 | 310 | 30 + 5 | 32 + 3 | 34 + 1 |
| 175 | 17 + 1 | 18 + 6 | 20 + 4 | 320 | 31 + 6 | 33 + 4 | 35 + 2 |
| 185 | 18 | 19 + 5 | 21 + 3 | 330 | 33 | 34 + 6 | 36 + 4 |
| 195 | 18 + 6 | 20 + 4 | 22 + 3 | 340 | 34 + 2 | 36 | 37 + 5 |

(Modified with permission from Jeanty P, Romero R. Obstetrical Ultrasound. New York: McGraw-Hill, 1984.)

## TRANSVERSE CEREBELLAR DIAMETER

The cerebellum can be easily visualized as early as the first trimester as a butterfly-shaped figure in the posterior fossa of the fetal head, behind the thalami and in front of the echolucent cisterna magna. The transverse cerebellar diameter (TCD) in millimeters has been shown to correlate with gestational age in weeks up to 24 weeks. Above 24 weeks gestation, the growth curves turn upward, and this uniform correlation no longer exists. Goldstein and colleagues have constructed a nomogram of the TCD throughout pregnancy (Table 25-4).

Researchers subsequently evaluated the TCD measurement in IUGR fetuses. They reported that TCD measurement was not significantly affected by retarded fetal growth, and therefore the TCD could be used as a reliable predictor of gestational age even in cases of IUGR. This parameter is particularly useful because it is a standard against which other parameters can be compared. Duchatel and colleagues (1989) have corroborated these findings in their report of 12 cases of IUGR below the 3rd percentile in which the TCD remained unaltered.[†] Other investigators have provided additional support for the usefulness of the TCD by constructing a nomogram of the ratio between TCD and abdominal circumference (AC) ratio. In a small series, these investigators have shown that this ratio permits the identification of IUGR by demonstrating the fairly consistent growth of the TCD relative to the decrease in AC in cases of IUGR. In yet another study by Hill and colleagues (1990), the TCD was found to be within 2 standard deviations in only 40% of IUGR cases, and in 60% of cases, the TCD was greater

[†] Duchatel F, Mennesson B, Berseneff H, Owry JF. Antenatal echographic measurement of the fetal cerebellum. Significance in the evaluation of fetal development. J de Gynecologi, Obstetrique et Biologie de la Reproduction 1989;18:879.

**TABLE 25-4.** A Nomogram of the Transverse Cerebellar Diameter, Biparietal Diameter, and Head Circumference According to Percentile Distribution

| Gestational Age (wk) | Cerebellum (mm) | | | | |
|---|---|---|---|---|---|
| | 10 | 25 | 50 | 75 | 90 |
| 15 | 10 | 12 | 14 | 15 | 16 |
| 16 | 14 | 16 | 16 | 16 | 17 |
| 17 | 16 | 17 | 17 | 18 | 18 |
| 18 | 17 | 18 | 18 | 19 | 19 |
| 19 | 18 | 18 | 19 | 19 | 22 |
| 20 | 18 | 19 | 20 | 20 | 22 |
| 21 | 19 | 20 | 22 | 23 | 24 |
| 22 | 21 | 23 | 23 | 24 | 24 |
| 23 | 22 | 23 | 24 | 25 | 26 |
| 24 | 22 | 24 | 25 | 27 | 28 |
| 25 | 23 | 21.5 | 28 | 28 | 29 |
| 26 | 25 | 28 | 29 | 30 | 32 |
| 27 | 26 | 28.5 | 30 | 31 | 32 |
| 28 | 27 | 30 | 31 | 32 | 34 |
| 29 | 29 | 32 | 34 | 36 | 38 |
| 30 | 31 | 32 | 35 | 37 | 40 |
| 31 | 32 | 35 | 38 | 39 | 43 |
| 32 | 33 | 36 | 38 | 40 | 42 |
| 33 | 32 | 36 | 40 | 43 | 44 |
| 34 | 33 | 38 | 40 | 41 | 44 |
| 35 | 31 | 37 | 40.5 | 43 | 47 |
| 36 | 36 | 29 | 43 | 52 | 55 |
| 37 | 37 | 37 | 45 | 52 | 55 |
| 38 | 40 | 40 | 48.5 | 52 | 55 |
| 39 | 52 | 52 | 52 | 55 | 55 |

Modified from Goldstein I, Reece EA, Pilu G, Bovicelli L, Hobbins JC. Cerebellar measurements with ultrasonography in the evaluation of fetal growth and development. Am J Obstet Gynecol 1987;156:1065.

than 2 standard deviations below the mean.[‡] The results of this paper are at variance with the three reports discussed earlier. The majority of data available would suggest that the use of the TCD is extremely valuable when gestational age is unknown or IUGR is suspected. The accuracy of the TCD can be enhanced by using biometric ratios, especially FL:AC, as well as amniotic fluid volume and the presence or absence of fetal ossification centers.

## Abdominal Circumference

The abdominal circumference (AC) has been reported to be the best fetal biometric parameter that correlates with fetal weight and is the most sensitive parameter for detecting IUGR. Warsof and colleagues studied the effectiveness of three ultra-

[‡] Hill LM, Guzick D, Rivello D, Hixson J, Peterson C. The transverse cerebellar diameter cannot be used to assess gestational age in the small for gestational age fetus. Obstet Gynecol 1990;75:329.

sonic growth parameters—BPD, HC, and AC—to detect IUGR in a large group of obstetric populations.[§] They demonstrated that AC measurements are more predictive of IUGR than BPD or HC, singly or in combination. In this study, it was shown that screening at 34 weeks gestation for IUGR results in a sensitivity of approximately 70% and a positive predictive value of 50%. However, sensitivity was maximized by using the 25th rather than 10th percentile measurement to determine a positive result.

Others have found results that further demonstrate that AC is the single best predictor of IUGR, with accuracy that may reach 96% of cases. In fact, in contrast to the BPD measurement, AC is smaller in both symmetric and asymmetric types of IUGR, and therefore its measurement has higher sensitivity. Animal studies have shown that the liver is the most affected organ in IUGR. Since the liver is the largest intra-abdominal organ, assessment of the AC at the level of the liver is actually an indirect indication of the nutritional status of the fetus.

Unfortunately, AC has more intraobserver and interobserver variation than either BPD or FL. Furthermore, AC variability may result from fetal breathing movements, compression, or position of the fetus. To obtain the proper AC, the section should be round and at the level of the fetal stomach and the portal umbilical vein (or the bifurcation of the main portal vein into the right and left branches). Normal values of AC are presented in Table 25-5.

## Long Bones
The FL is another important parameter in evaluating fetal growth (Table 25-6). Long bones other than the femur can be equally useful in the assessment of gestational age (Table 25-7). It has been demonstrated by several authors that there is a linear relationship between FL specifically and long bones in general and crown-heel length of a newborn.

## Body Proportionality
Indices of body proportionality that have been studied and found clinically useful in the diagnosis of IUGR include the HC:AC ratio (Table 25-8) and the FL to AC ratio.

**Head Circumference: Abdominal Circumference Ratio.** Although the ratio of HC to AC has been shown to have a sensitivity of approximately 70% in detecting asymmetric IUGR, its use is limited by its high false-positive rate in screening a general population.

Further limitations of this technique are its inability to detect symmetric growth retardation and the need for accurate knowledge of gestational age in order to make the diagnosis of IUGR. It is therefore believed that the value of the HC:AC ratio lies in the assessment of proportionality, and thus it may assist the clinician to classify IUGR as symmetrical or asymmetrical. Obviously, an elevated ratio suggests asymmetrical IUGR.

**Femur Length: Abdominal Circumference Ratio.** The ratio of FL to AC is the equivalent of the postnatal ponderal index and has been proposed as a useful method in detecting asymmetrical IUGR. This ratio has the advantage of being

§ Warsof SL, Cooper DJ, Little D, et al. Routine ultrasound screening for antenatal detection of intrauterine growth retardation. Obstet Gynecol 1986;67:33.

**TABLE 25-5.** Normal Values for the Abdominal Circumference

| Week Number | 5th | Jeanty 50th Percentile | 95th | Deter 50th Percentile |
|---|---|---|---|---|
| 12 | 35 | 57 | 80 | 63 |
| 13 | 45 | 67 | 90 | 74 |
| 14 | 55 | 77 | 100 | 84 |
| 15 | 65 | 88 | 110 | 95 |
| 16 | 76 | 98 | 120 | 106 |
| 17 | 86 | 109 | 131 | 117 |
| 18 | 97 | 119 | 142 | 128 |
| 19 | 108 | 130 | 152 | 139 |
| 20 | 119 | 141 | 163 | 150 |
| 21 | 129 | 152 | 174 | 161 |
| 22 | 140 | 163 | 185 | 172 |
| 23 | 151 | 173 | 196 | 183 |
| 24 | 162 | 184 | 206 | 194 |
| 25 | 172 | 195 | 217 | 205 |
| 26 | 183 | 205 | 227 | 216 |
| 27 | 193 | 215 | 238 | 227 |
| 28 | 206 | 225 | 248 | 238 |
| 29 | 213 | 235 | 257 | 249 |
| 30 | 222 | 244 | 267 | 260 |
| 31 | 231 | 254 | 276 | 271 |
| 32 | 240 | 262 | 285 | 282 |
| 33 | 248 | 271 | 293 | 293 |
| 34 | 256 | 279 | 301 | 304 |
| 35 | 264 | 286 | 309 | 315 |
| 36 | 271 | 293 | 316 | 326 |
| 37 | 278 | 300 | 322 | 337 |
| 38 | 283 | 306 | 328 | 348 |
| 39 | 289 | 311 | 333 | 359 |
| 40 | 294 | 316 | 338 | 370 |

Geirrson RT, Patel NB, Christie AD. Efficiency of intrauterine volume, fetal abdominal area and biparietal diameter measurements with ultrasound in screening for small-for-dates babies. Br J Obstet Gynaecol 1985;92:929.

age-independent and thus may help in the diagnosis of IUGR when gestational age is unknown. In fact, FL:AC ratios have a constant value of 22% ± 2% after 21 weeks gestation.

### Estimated Fetal Weight

Several formulas that use multiple ultrasonic parameters are used to estimate fetal weight. The most widely used formula is that of Shepard and colleagues (1982), in which estimated fetal weight (EFw) is derived from the BPD and AC.[||] This equation predicts fetal weight with an accuracy of 15% to 20%.

[||]Shepard MJ, Richards VA, Berkowitz RL, et al. An evaluation of two equations for predicting fetal weight by ultrasound. Am J Obstet Gynecol 1982;142:47.

**TABLE 25-6.** Gestational Age Estimated from the Femur Length

| Femur Length (mm) | Percentile | | | Femur Length (mm) | Percentile | | |
|---|---|---|---|---|---|---|---|
| | 5th | 50th | 95th | | 5th | 50th | 95th |
| 10 | 10 + 3 | 12 + 4 | 14 + 6 | 46 | 23 + 1 | 25 + 3 | 27 + 4 |
| 12 | 11 + 1 | 13 + 2 | 15 + 4 | 48 | 24 | 26 + 1 | 28 + 3 |
| 14 | 11 + 5 | 13 + 6 | 16 + 1 | 50 | 24 + 6 | 27 | 29 + 1 |
| 16 | 12 + 3 | 14 + 4 | 16 + 6 | 52 | 25 + 4 | 27 + 6 | 30 |
| 18 | 13 | 15 + 1 | 17 + 3 | 54 | 26 + 3 | 28 + 4 | 30 + 6 |
| 20 | 13 + 5 | 15 + 6 | 18 + 1 | 56 | 27 + 2 | 29 + 4 | 31 + 5 |
| 22 | 14 + 3 | 16 + 4 | 18 + 6 | 58 | 28 + 1 | 30 + 2 | 32 + 4 |
| 24 | 15 + 1 | 17 + 2 | 19 + 4 | 60 | 28 + 6 | 31 + 1 | 33 + 2 |
| 26 | 15 + 6 | 18 | 20 + 1 | 62 | 29 + 6 | 32 | 34 + 1 |
| 28 | 16 + 4 | 18 + 5 | 20 + 6 | 64 | 30 + 5 | 32 + 6 | 35 + 1 |
| 30 | 17 + 1 | 19 + 3 | 21 + 4 | 66 | 31 + 4 | 33 + 5 | 35 + 6 |
| 32 | 17 + 6 | 20 + 1 | 22 + 2 | 68 | 32 + 3 | 34 + 4 | 36 + 6 |
| 34 | 18 + 5 | 20 + 6 | 23 + 1 | 70 | 33 + 2 | 35 + 4 | 37 + 5 |
| 36 | 19 + 3 | 21 + 4 | 23 + 6 | 72 | 34 + 1 | 36 + 3 | 38 + 4 |
| 38 | 20 + 1 | 22 + 3 | 24 + 4 | 74 | 35 + 1 | 37 + 2 | 39 + 4 |
| 40 | 20 + 6 | 23 + 1 | 25 + 2 | 76 | 36 | 38 + 1 | 40 + 3 |
| 42 | 21 + 5 | 23 + 6 | 26 + 1 | 78 | 36 + 6 | 39 + 1 | 41 + 2 |
| 44 | 22 + 4 | 24 + 5 | 26 + 6 | 80 | 37 + 6 | 40 | 42 + 1 |

(Modified with permission from Jeanty P, Romero R. Obstetrical Ultrasound. New York: McGraw-Hill, 1984.)

Ott and Doyle (1984) reported accurate predictions of IUGR in 90% of cases in a high-risk population when EFw was determined by BPD and AC.[*] The use of this formula may introduce errors that are related to the variations in BPD which usually occur as a result of changes in head shape in the last weeks of pregnancy, in malpresentation, and in pregnancies complicated by spontaneous rupture of membranes. Biparietal diameter may be inaccurate if there is dolichocephaly or brachycephaly. We therefore strongly recommend that the physician calculate the cephalic index in each case. If the cephalic index is abnormal (< 75% or > 80%), one should not rely on estimated weight formulas that include the BPD.

## MACROSOMIA

The etiology of fetal macrosomia is believed to be multifactorial. Although this condition is often associated with diabetes mellitus in pregnancy, especially in women without vasculopathy, macrosomia may also occur in nondiabetics. Fetal macrosomia is defined either as an EFw > 4000 g at term or EFw > 90th percentile for gestational age.

[*] Ott WJ, Doyle S. Ultrasonic diagnosis of altered fetal growth by use of a normal ultrasonic fetal weight curve. Obstet Gynecol 1984;63:201.

**TABLE 25-7.** Gestational Age as Obtained from the Long Bones in Weeks and Days

| Bone Length (mm) | Humerus Percentile 50th | Ulna Percentile 50th | Tibia Percentile 50th |
|---|---|---|---|
| 10 | 12 + 4 | 13 + 1 | 13 + 3 |
| 12 | 13 + 1 | 13 + 6 | 14 + 1 |
| 14 | 13 + 6 | 14 + 4 | 14 + 6 |
| 16 | 14 + 4 | 15 + 3 | 15 + 4 |
| 18 | 15 + 1 | 16 + 1 | 16 + 1 |
| 20 | 15 + 6 | 16 + 6 | 17 |
| 22 | 16 + 5 | 17 + 5 | 17 + 6 |
| 24 | 17 + 3 | 18 + 4 | 18 + 4 |
| 26 | 18 + 1 | 19 + 3 | 19 + 2 |
| 28 | 19 | 20 + 2 | 20 + 1 |
| 30 | 19 + 6 | 21 + 1 | 21 |
| 32 | 20 + 5 | 22 + 1 | 21 + 6 |
| 34 | 21 + 4 | 23 + 1 | 22 + 4 |
| 36 | 22 + 4 | 24 + 1 | 23 + 4 |
| 38 | 23 + 3 | 25 + 1 | 24 + 3 |
| 40 | 24 + 2 | 26 + 1 | 25 + 2 |
| 42 | 25 + 2 | 27 + 1 | 26 + 1 |
| 44 | 26 + 1 | 28 + 2 | 27 + 1 |
| 46 | 27 + 1 | 29 + 3 | 28 |
| 48 | 28 + 1 | 30 + 4 | 29 |
| 50 | 29 + 2 | 31 + 4 | 29 + 6 |
| 52 | 30 + 2 | 32 + 6 | 30 + 6 |
| 54 | 31 + 3 | 34 | 31 + 6 |
| 56 | 32 + 4 | 35 + 1 | 32 + 6 |
| 58 | 33 + 4 | 36 + 3 | 33 + 6 |
| 60 | 34 + 6 | 37 + 5 | 34 + 6 |
| 62 | 35 + 6 | 39 | 35 + 6 |
| 64 | 37 + 1 | 40 + 2 | 37 |
| 66 | 38 + 2 | | 38 |
| 68 | 39 + 4 | | 39 + 1 |

(Modified with permission from Jeanty P, Rodesch F, Delbeke D, et al. Estimation of gestational age from measurements of fetal long bones. J Ultrasound Med 1984;3:75.)

Macrosomic infants and their mothers are at increased risk for intrapartum injury, and perinatal mortality is more common among these fetuses. The principal causes of injury include shoulder dystocia, fractures, and neurologic damage.

Accurate prenatal diagnosis of fetal macrosomia would permit fetuses to be delivered by cesarean section, thus obviating these complications. On the other hand, liberal cesarean section may expose the mother to unnecessary operative risks.

Prenatal diagnosis of macrosomic fetuses is often difficult because < 40% of such infants are born to mothers with identifiable risk factors for macrosomia.

**TABLE 25-8.** Head Circumference/Abdominal Circumference
Ratio Compared with Gestational Age

| Gestational Age (wk) | Head Circumference | | |
|---|---|---|---|
| | − 2SD | Mean | + 2SD |
| 14 | 1.085 | 1.230 | 1.375 |
| 15 | 1.080 | 1.225 | 1.365 |
| 16 | 1.075 | 1.215 | 1.350 |
| 17 | 1.070 | 1.205 | 1.340 |
| 18 | 1.065 | 1.195 | 1.330 |
| 19 | 1.060 | 1.185 | 1.320 |
| 20 | 1.055 | 1.178 | 1.305 |
| 21 | 1.050 | 1.177 | 1.295 |
| 22 | 1.045 | 1.165 | 1.285 |
| 23 | 1.040 | 1.155 | 1.275 |
| 24 | 1.030 | 1.145 | 1.265 |
| 25 | 1.025 | 1.135 | 1.255 |
| 26 | 1.050 | 1.125 | 1.245 |
| 27 | 1.010 | 1.120 | 1.235 |
| 28 | 1.000 | 1.110 | 1.225 |
| 29 | 0.999 | 1.095 | 1.215 |
| 30 | 0.975 | 1.085 | 1.200 |
| 31 | 0.965 | 1.075 | 1.190 |
| 32 | 0.945 | 1.060 | 1.175 |
| 33 | 0.935 | 1.045 | 1.163 |
| 34 | 0.925 | 1.030 | 1.150 |
| 35 | 0.915 | 1.020 | 1.135 |
| 36 | 0.910 | 1.005 | 1.120 |
| 37 | 0.905 | 0.995 | 1.100 |
| 38 | 0.900 | 0.980 | 1.085 |
| 39 | 0.896 | 0.970 | 1.065 |
| 40 | 0.895 | 0.965 | 1.046 |
| 41 | 0.894 | 0.960 | 10.250 |

From Campbell S, Metreweli C, eds. Practical abdominal ultrasound. Chicago; Year Book Medical Publishers, 1978.

A number of sonographic parameters have been used in an attempt to diagnose altered fetal growth, including the BPD, HC, HC:AC or HC:thoracic circumference ratio, the macrosomic index, and the EFw. Tamura and colleagues (1986)** showed that the EFw determined by Shepard and colleagues (1982), when greater than the 90th percentile, correctly predicted macrosomia at birth in 74% of cases. When both the AC and the EFw exceeded the 90th percentiles, macrosomia was correctly diagnosed in 88.8% of pregnant women with diabetes mellitus. The BPD and HC percentiles were significantly less predictive of macrosomia.

** Tamura RK, Sabbagha RE, Depp R, Dooley SL, Socol ML. Diabetic macrosomia: accuracy of third trimester ultrasound. Obstet Gynecol 1986;67:828.

## SUMMARY

Although the etiology of IUGR is variable, prenatal diagnosis is possible using a variety of biometric parameters. When the gestational age is certain, IUGR is diagnosed if sonographic predictors of gestational age reflect an age significantly reduced from the expected, or an EFw less than the 10th percentile. Adjunctive indices which can enhance the prenatal diagnosis include reduced amniotic fluid volume, early third trimester grade 3 placenta, abnormal Doppler waveform analysis, and abnormal biometric ratios.

When the gestational age is unknown or uncertain, it is necessary to differentiate between the IUGR fetus and the normally grown fetus identified at an inaccurate gestational age. The transverse cerebellum is a useful parameter for estimating gestational age even in IUGR fetuses and can be a parameter against which other biometric indices are compared. Biometric ratios, especially FL:AC, may also be useful adjuncts in the prenatal diagnosis of IUGR.

The prenatal diagnosis of macrosomia is best accomplished by the use of EFw. However, a certain amount of caution should be exercised in light of the fact that a margin of error exists with this method of weight estimation. EFw is reported to be accurate within 10% of the actual birth weight 85% of the time. In the remaining 15%, EFw is less accurate, and the error can range from 15% to 20% of the actual birth weight.

# 26. DOPPLER ULTRASONOGRAPHY AND FETAL WELL-BEING

Doppler ultrasound provides a noninvasive clinical tool to assess blood flow in pregnancy.

## DOPPLER INSTRUMENTATION

When an ultrasound beam strikes a blood vessel, the moving column of red blood cells scatters and reflects the ultrasound beam with a new frequency. The change in frequency or Doppler frequency shift (incident frequency − reflected frequency) is proportional to the velocity of the red blood cell scatterers. This change in frequency may be displayed and used to calculate blood flow.

Depending upon the method of processing, the information about blood flow may be nondirectional or directional. Two types of Doppler systems are in use—continuous wave and pulsed. They differ in a number of ways. Continuous-wave systems are continuously emitting from one crystal and receiving through another. They are relatively simple, cheap, and portable. The reflected echoes from any moving structure within the ultrasound beam are detected, so that there is no spatial resolution. Positioning the transducer and line of sight of the ultrasound beam is more readily done. In the pulsed system, a short burst of the ultrasound wave is transmitted, and the crystal then acts as a receiver. A range gate circuit allows recording only at a specified time after the pulse emission, so the Doppler shift detected originates from a fixed depth. This type of processing may be referred to as setting the sample volume to a known depth. These Doppler velocimeters may exist as stand-alone items, but are also built into ultrasound imaging systems. Integration with an imaging facility provides the ability to steer the ultrasound beam and, for pulsed Doppler systems, to locate the sample volume precisely over the vessel to be studied.

With medical equipment and vascular studies, the Doppler shift frequency usually falls in the audible range; therefore, the simplest display of the Doppler frequency shift is an audio signal. The method of choice is spectral analysis. If the vessel is totally insonated, the frequency spectrum represents all the different velocities across its lumen. The process of spectral analysis is carried out by a spectrum analyzer and is therefore also subject to the possibility of frequency aliasing if too fast a sampling rate is required. Equipment usually carries out the spectral analysis sufficiently quickly (less than 10 msec per spectrum) so that it is available in real time. A recent development is to display the frequency and direction of blood flow by color coding superimposed on the real-time ultrasound two-dimensional image ("color flow mapping").

Because blood flow velocity is directly proportional to Doppler frequency shift, the information made available to the clinician by the Doppler instrumentation is a blood flow velocity waveform (FVW). The envelope of this wave is the maximum flow velocity. Beneath this is a frequency distribution, representing the various velocities of blood flow in the vessel under study. Both instantaneous and temporal mean flow velocities can be determined from this. If the angle between the ultrasound beam and vessel is known, then velocity can be calculated absolutely. This requires the use of pulsed Doppler systems. Volume blood flow may be determined as the product of mean velocity and vessel area.

## THE BLOOD FLOW VELOCITY WAVEFORM

Blood flow is pulsatile. With each contraction of the heart, a pressure pulse or wave propagates down the aorta and its branches with an initial wave speed of 5 m/sec. This creates a time-varying pressure gradient between neighboring points along the arterial tree. Blood flows ahead of this pressure gradient from high to low pressure. The blood flow is also pulsatile—the flow velocity waveform. Doppler ultrasound systems record this flow velocity waveform. Early in systole the pressure and flow waveforms are in phase, but this breaks down later in systole because of the arrival of waves reflected from points of branching along the arterial tree and the periphery. The flow velocity wave travels more slowly than the pressure wave, and its amplitude decreases as it moves away from the heart. In the ascending aorta following the opening of the aortic valve, blood flow velocity increases to a peak and then falls. After closure of the aortic valve, the blood is close to stationary for the remainder of the cardiac cycle.

The pressure and flow waveforms are influenced by the cardiac contraction, physical properties of the arterial walls and the blood within, and outflow impedance from the arterial tree. Traditionally, blood flow is described in terms of pressure and flow. Resistance has been defined as the ratio of mean pressure difference (or pressure head) across a vascular bed to mean flow through it. Resistance may also be conceptualized as how difficult it is to force blood through the circulation. Changes in resistance in clinical physiology are more often than not due to changes in the caliber of small blood vessels. It also depends on the distensibility of the arterial walls and blood viscosity. Impedance takes into consideration the pulsatile nature of blood flow, being the ratio of pulsatile pressure to pulsatile flow. Various indices derived from the FVW pattern have been defined to assess "resistance."

The shape of the waveform envelope can be considered a characteristic of the vascular site. Waveforms recorded from arteries supplying low-impedance vascular beds (e.g., internal carotid, umbilical, and uterine artery in pregnancy) exhibit relatively high forward velocities throughout diastole. A triphasic waveform shape, where there is a period of reverse flow in diastole, is characteristic of sites with high distal impedance. The peripheral impedance, the vessel wall elasticity, the degree and geometry of any proximal stenoses, and the condition of the upstream pump all affect the waveform. All of these factors are important, all can be affected in the disease state being investigated, and none can be independently eliminated or controlled in clinical practice. Even in normal, presumably healthy subjects, blood flow patterns at a site with complicated geometry such as the carotid bifurcation are very complex.

The fetal circulation is uniquely suited to Doppler waveform analysis by simple empirical indices. This is because of the absence of degenerative arterial disease. The indices used in the fetal circulation have been directed toward assessing downstream resistance. Three are in common usage. All of these are highly correlated. Coefficients in excess of 0.9 have been demonstrated when the indices are compared. This means that the indices are all providing the same information.

## THE UMBILICAL CIRCULATION

The umbilical cord is ideal for Doppler studies. The two umbilical arteries travel along this cord without branching or changes in lumen diameter. Studies of the umbilical artery flow velocity waveform using the indices of resistance have been carried out to assess the downstream vascular bed—the fetal placenta.

## NORMAL PREGNANCY

Blood flow through the umbilical circulation increases throughout pregnancy and represents some 40% of combined ventricular output of the fetus. Blood flow to the placenta appears to be the result of the balance between resistance to other fetal vascular beds and the placenta. The umbilical circulation is a low-resistance vascular bed, which is reflected in the pattern of the umbilical artery FVW. Throughout pregnancy, the increase in umbilical blood flow is achieved by a decrease in resistance. Gestational age is an important influence in determining the normality of the umbilical FVW. There is a weak relationship between FHR and waveform index over the physiological range of heart rates. The correction suggested is very small in comparison to the difference between normal and abnormal waveform patterns.

Fetal breathing movements do alter the flow velocity waveform. Behavioral states do not influence the FVW pattern or indices of resistance in the umbilical circulation. This is in contrast to the aortic waveform. There has been debate about variations in the umbilical FVW along the length of the cord. Close to the fetus, a higher value may be obtained for the systolic: diastolic ratio. There is a transition from the typical aortic to umbilical waveform. At the placental end, the resistance indices have been reported lower than the values recorded from free-floating loops of cord. This difference is very small in comparison to differences between normal and abnormal pregnancy. In recording the umbilical FVW, it is necessary to review a sequence of 10 to 20 cycles to confirm that variations due to fetal activity are absent.

## MODELS AND EXPERIMENTAL STUDIES OF THE UMBILICAL CIRCULATION TO AID FVW INTERPRETATION

Two quite different approaches have been taken to establish models of the umbilical placental circulation for the study and understanding of the blood FVW. The placental vasculature has been modeled as a lumped electrical circuit equivalent, and animal preparations have been used in experimental studies.

Two groups have suggested that a lumped electrical circuit equivalent could be used to model the umbilical placental circulation. This approach has been used extensively in modeling blood flow in other circulations.

This approach is simple and attractive. The only assumption is that each artery can indeed be represented by a resistor and capacitor. Using this model, it can be shown that the pulsatility index (PI) of the FVW is proportional to the pulsatility of the pressure waveform and the resistance of the umbilical placental villus vascular tree.

$$PI = (P^1/P^0)(1 + R_2/R_1)$$

where
$P^1$ = peak systolic pressure
$P^0$ = mean pressure
$R_2$ = resistance of umbilical placental vascular bed
$R_1$ = resistance of main umbilical artery

Assuming a diffuse vascular pathology, it can be shown that the FVW index of resistance increases as the fraction (q) of terminal arterial vessels obliterated increases. This increase is not linear.

It is not until some 50% to 60% of the vessels have been obliterated that the PI is increased beyond the "normal range." Thereafter it rises rapidly. It highlights the presence of extensive disease before Doppler detection is possible, and emphasizes the reserve capacity of the placenta.

This model of the placental circulation was used to examine the influence of growth (more vascular channels) of the placenta on PI. A major difference was shown between the response of a large and a small vascular bed to superimposed vascular obliteration. The same fraction obliteration (q) produced a much greater increase in PI when the placenta was small. It follows from this prediction that a large, late third trimester placental vascular bed can accommodate a considerably greater obliteration with minimal change in resistance index in comparison to a smaller, second trimester placenta. This parallels recent clinical reports indicating that Doppler studies have a low sensitivity in predicting fetal compromise in postdate pregnancies. Doppler umbilical studies are a far more sensitive test for the detection of placental vascular pathology earlier in pregnancy.

In ovine pregnancy, the Doppler indices have been demonstrated to be a measure of resistance in the umbilical circulation. Embolization of the umbilical cotyledon circulation increases the resistance of the peripheral vascular bed. This causes a rise in the umbilical systolic:diastolic ratio and a rise in calculated vascular resistance (Fig. 26-1).

## PATHOPHYSIOLOGY OF ABNORMAL UMBILICAL DOPPLER FVW

In normal pregnancy, placental growth continues throughout. The overall increase in placental size is associated with an increase in the number of tertiary stem villi and, therefore, total small arterial channels. The normal decrease in the umbilical artery FVW indices of resistance is consistent with this. The abnormal umbilical Doppler FVW waveform is characterized by decreasing diastolic flow velocities relative to the systolic peak and, in extreme cases, by absent or even reversal of blood flow in diastole.

A histological study was performed to correlate the umbilical artery FVW pattern with the "resistance" vessels in the umbilical placental vascular tree in pregnancies classified according to whether the antenatal umbilical Doppler studies were normal or abnormal. The modal tertiary villus small arterial vessel count was significantly less in the group with the abnormal umbilical artery FVW.

Placental lesion of vascular sclerosis, with obliteration of the small muscular arteries of the tertiary stem villi, could be expected to cause an increase in flow resistance in the umbilical placenta. This lesion in the fetal placenta could best be described as "umbilical placental insufficiency."

**FIGURE 26–1.** The three indices of downstream resistance in common clinical use for the analysis of arterial flow velocity waveforms.

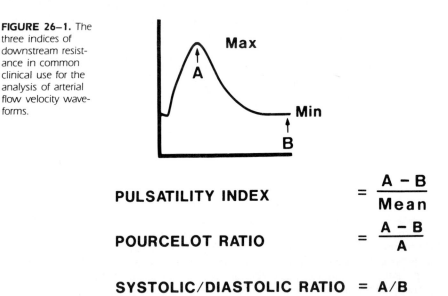

$$\text{PULSATILITY INDEX} = \frac{A - B}{\text{Mean}}$$

$$\text{POURCELOT RATIO} = \frac{A - B}{A}$$

$$\text{SYSTOLIC/DIASTOLIC RATIO} = A/B$$

The origin of the umbilical placental vascular obliteration remains to be determined. It is attractive to implicate the vasoactive prostaglandins, prostacyclin and thromboxane. Thromboxane-mediated vasoconstriction and, ultimately, vessel obliteration could well account for the increase in Doppler resistance index. Further support for a role for thromboxane has been provided by the demonstration that fetuses in whom the umbilical Doppler study is abnormal have a significantly lower platelet count than controls.

## CLINICAL CORRELATES OF ABNORMAL UMBILICAL DOPPLER FVW IN HIGH-RISK PREGNANCY

The abnormal umbilical artery Doppler FVW is characterized by a pattern of reduced, absent, or even reversed diastolic flow velocities relative to the systolic peak velocity (Fig. 26-2). In this situation, the indices of resistance are increased.

Analyzing the umbilical artery FVW with the various indices of resistance does not indicate a fetal condition, but rather the presence of a vascular lesion in the placenta—umbilical placental insufficiency. The fetal effects consequent upon this vascular lesion are the clinical correlates. Poor fetal outcome, particularly in terms of birth of an infant small for gestational age (SGA), is the major clinical association reported (Table 26-1).

The most abnormal studies (highest systolic:diastolic ratio group) have had the greatest incidence of fetal growth failure as indexed by the centile birth weight. Both fetal and neonatal deaths were highest in this group. The requirement for neonatal level 3 nursery care and the duration of stay also correlated with the antenatal Doppler result.

Fetal outcome in the group suggests the possibility of grading fetal risk by the degree of waveform abnormality. Despite this, the umbilical waveform detects a placental vascular lesion. An effect on fetal condition in this truly "at risk" group should be sought using the other fetal tests before delivery. Some fetuses in the high and extreme groups have a good outcome.

Among fetuses born small for gestational age, an abnormal Doppler umbilical study predicted those more likely to require early delivery and neonatal intensive care and those with the highest mortality. The trend of umbilical Doppler results proved a very useful measure of neonatal morbidity in those patients with serial studies. A decreasing systolic:diastolic ratio was associated with a good outcome. Such a result suggests continuing placental growth.

## UMBILICAL DOPPLER FVW AND SPECIFIC PREGNANCY COMPLICATIONS

### Hypertensive Disease of Pregnancy
Hypertensive disease of pregnancy may be associated with abnormal umbilical FVWs. Those pregnancies with an abnormal Doppler study were most likely to be associated with fetal compromise. The abnormal umbilical study may precede the hypertension.

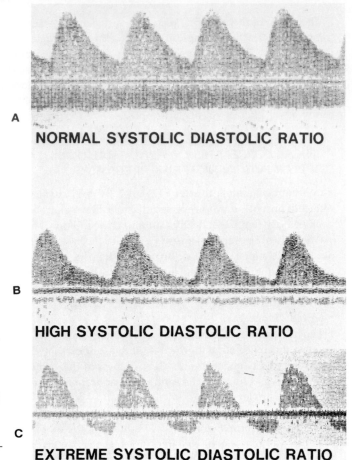

A

**NORMAL SYSTOLIC DIASTOLIC RATIO**

B

**FIGURE 26–2.** Examples of (**A**) a normal umbilical artery waveform, (**B**) a waveform in which the systolic diastolic ratio is high, and (**C**) an extremely abnormal waveform, in which the diastolic flow velocities are reversed.

**HIGH SYSTOLIC DIASTOLIC RATIO**

C

**EXTREME SYSTOLIC DIASTOLIC RATIO**

**TABLE 26-1.** Results of the Last Study Prior to Delivery in a Group of 53 Small-for-Gestational-Age Fetuses

|  | Umbilical Artery Waveforms | |
|---|---|---|
|  | Normal | Abnormal |
| No. of fetuses | 19 | 34 |
| Mean gestational age at delivery | 37.6 | 34.6 |
| Admission to neonatal intensive care | 3 | 23 |
| Neonatal deaths | 0 | 7 |

Data from Trudinger BJ, Cook CM, Giles WB, Ng S, Fong E, Connelly A, Wilcox W. Fetal umbilical artery velocity waveforms and subsequent neonatal outcome. Br J Obstet Gynaecol 1991;98:378.

## Diabetes Mellitus

Normal studies are recorded from the macrosomic fetus continuing to grow, but cessation of growth, even if the fetus is macrosomic (i.e., earlier in pregnancy the growth stimulus had been excessive), is associated with the development of a high resistance pattern in the umbilical artery waveform (Fig. 26-3). Mothers with vascular disease affecting the small vessels of the uterus may have a fetus that is small, and here growth cessation is associated with abnormal umbilical FVW studies.

## Multiple Pregnancy

The umbilical recordings must be matched against real-time observation of the fetal heart to ensure the identity of the fetus being studied. The great value of Doppler studies in twin pregnancy management lies in the early recognition of an abnormal Doppler finding in the fetus at risk. An abnormal Doppler study identified patients who could be followed by a program of intensive fetal surveillance. Although a consistent Doppler picture in the case of twin transfusion syndrome has been disputed, it is possible to suspect this diagnosis. Discordance in ultrasound measures of fetal size, cord diameter, and amniotic fluid volume between the members of the twin pair exists, yet similar umbilical waveforms for the two fetuses are recorded.

## Isoimmunization and Fetal Anemia

The systolic:diastolic ratio has been reported low in association with fetal anemia. Fetal transfusion in utero has been observed to increase toward normal the low systolic:diastolic ratio index of resistance in the umbilical placental circulation.

## Lupus Obstetric Syndrome

Fetal deterioration is predicted by the development of an abnormal umbilical artery waveform. Frequent studies, at least weekly in the third trimester, are recommended because fetal demise may occur over a short time.

## Major Fetal Anomaly

Major fetal anomaly is not consistently associated with an abnormal umbilical artery waveform. The systolic:diastolic ratio has been reported high in association with fetuses with trisomy 13, 18, and 21.

## Postdate Pregnancy

It appears that the Doppler studies of the umbilical artery FVW do not predict fetal compromise in postdate pregnancy. On the basis of mathematical modeling of the placental vascular tree, we have shown that the larger the placental size, the greater the fraction of the vascular tree that needs to be obliterated to cause a detectable increase in the systolic:diastolic ratio. This, combined with a greater susceptibility of the mature fetus to the effects of hypoxemia, could account for the poor Doppler predictive value.

# UMBILICAL VEIN VOLUME FLOW STUDIES

Doppler ultrasound measurement of volume flow in the umbilical circulation is possible by recording from the umbilical vein as it traverses the fetal liver.

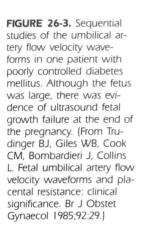

**FIGURE 26-3.** Sequential studies of the umbilical artery flow velocity waveforms in one patient with poorly controlled diabetes mellitus. Although the fetus was large, there was evidence of ultrasound fetal growth failure at the end of the pregnancy. (From Trudinger BJ, Giles WB, Cook CM, Bombardieri J, Collins L. Fetal umbilical artery flow velocity waveforms and placental resistance: clinical significance. Br J Obstet Gynaecol 1985;92:29.)

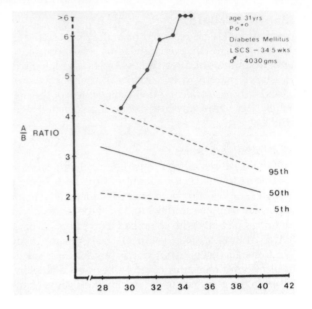

Studies in high-risk pregnancy suggest that a reduced umbilical vein flow is associated with growth retardation. The application of measures of umbilical vein volume flow to obstetric practice has been limited by the need for a detailed technique, by measurement errors, and by complex equipment.

## THE RELATIONSHIP OF UMBILICAL DOPPLER TO FETAL WELFARE TESTS

Tests of fetal welfare exist to identify the potentially compromised fetus (sometimes termed the "at-risk" fetus) and to quantitate fetal condition. The recognition of imminent fetal demise (i.e., the fetus in a terminal state) may be too late to prevent damage or loss of potential. The umbilical Doppler study recognizes a vascular pathology in the fetal placenta that may lead to a fetal effect.

Several comparative studies have demonstrated a greater sensitivity (the proportion of abnormal outcomes identified by the test) for umbilical Doppler in comparison to nonstressed FHR monitoring in recognizing the SGA fetus. The association of an abnormal nonstressed FHR test with an abnormal Doppler study selects a group with a very high risk of morbidity.

Although sonographic biometry was a more sensitive technique for identifying the small fetus, the umbilical artery systolic:diastolic ratio was noted to be abnormal at a significantly earlier gestation when serial studies were available.

Good fetal outcome has been reported in the ultrasonically small fetus with a normal umbilical Doppler study. Among a group of fetuses clinically suspected of being SGA, Doppler umbilical studies identified the fetus at risk of adverse perinatal outcome in comparison to ultrasonic abdominal circumference, which better identified the small size only.

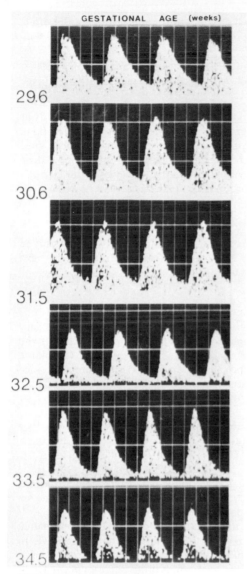

GESTATIONAL    AGE    (weeks)

29.6

30.6

31.5

32.5

33.5

34.5

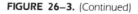

**FIGURE 26–3.** (Continued)

## CLINICAL STRATEGIES

The approach of the obstetrician to fetal compromise progresses through a sequence of steps, which can be summarized as:

1. Recognition of high-risk pregnancy on the basis of clinical history and examination, supported by the ancillary aids of maternal–fetal movement counting and fundal height measurement (Is it a high-risk pregnancy?)
2. Confirmation of fetal risk by identifying the placental vascular lesion with Doppler ultrasound studies of the umbilical artery FVW (Is there a placental pathology threatening the fetus?)

3. Determination of the extent to which the fetus is affected using the direct fetal assessments of biophysical profile, ultrasound growth, and FHR monitoring (How sick is the fetus?)
4. Therapy aimed at improving the intrauterine environment by treating mother or fetus, and delivery if the risk to the fetus of intrauterine death or damage exceeds that of delivery

The above scheme involves the use of the Doppler umbilical waveform study as a discriminator or doorway test to determine which fetuses are truly at risk and in need of intensive fetal surveillance. Doppler umbilical studies have also been used to guide specific therapies aimed at reversing the placental lesion. Low-dose aspirin provides a means of treatment of placental insufficiency if the Doppler diagnosis can be made early and before marked fetal effect.

## OTHER FETAL DOPPLER STUDIES

Within the fetal body, the aortic and cerebral circulations are the two most studied vascular trees, although reports of FVW in the renal and external iliac arteries have been made.

## FETAL AORTA

A pulsed Doppler system integrated with a real-time B-mode image is necessary to record from the fetal aorta. The most common site used for recording is the midthoracic part of the descending aorta (above the diaphragm). The fetal aortic blood FVW has been analyzed using the same indices of downstream resistance described in the assessment of umbilical artery FVW.

### Normal Pregnancy
The pulsatility index of the maximum velocity waveform in the thoracic aorta does not change with gestation.

### High-Risk Pregnancy
Studies of aortic FVW have been evaluated as predictors of fetal growth retardation and fetal distress. It was demonstrated that the most abnormal waveforms were seen in fetuses exhibiting perinatal morbidity.

The likely explanation for the change in the aortic FVW seen in these pregnancy complications is the increase in downstream flow resistance in the placenta. There is no evidence to suggest that the use of aortic FVWs provides additional predictive value over that of the umbilical artery waveform. A quite different approach to analysis of the aortic flow velocity waveform has determined the peak mean velocity of the aortic waveform and demonstrated its correlation with hypoxemia, hypercarbia, hyperlactemia, and acidemia as determined from fetal blood obtained at cordocentesis.

## FETAL CEREBRAL CIRCULATION

The combined use of duplex B-mode imaging and pulsed Doppler ultrasound has made possible the recording of FVWs from the fetal internal carotid artery and the individual arteries of the human fetal cerebral circulation.

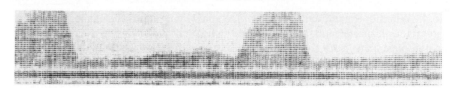

**FIGURE 26–4.** An abnormal pregnancy with a high resistance pattern, uteroplacental bed, arterial flow velocity waveform.

### Normal Pregnancy

The waveform of the fetal internal carotid artery is a typical low-resistance pattern.

### High-Risk Pregnancy

Intrauterine fetal growth retardation may be associated with a fetal internal carotid FVW pulsatility index lower than normal. The presence of a normal fetal carotid FVW and a high-resistance umbilical FVW was suggested to indicate the maintenance of normal cerebral flow. Later, with a deteriorating fetal condition, cerebral vasodilation occurs. This effect is adaptive to maintain cerebral oxygen supply consequent on the occurrence of fetal hypoxia and hypercarbia.

## MATERNAL UTERINE CIRCULATION

Both pulsed and continuous-wave ultrasound have been used to record flow velocity waveforms from the uterine circulation. Pulsed Doppler systems allow simultaneous imaging and recording from the main internal iliac artery, as well as from branches of the uterine artery in the myometrium. Color Doppler systems allow the main uterine artery to be imaged. The signal recorded from the site of placental implantation is a lower resistance pattern in comparison to the nonplacental site. Problems of vessel identification limit studies with continuous-wave ultrasound systems to the myometrial segments of the uterine artery, either within the placental bed or away from it.

The same indices of downstream resistance are used to assess flow velocity waveforms of uteroplacental arteries. Attention has also been focused on the presence of an early diastolic "notch," which has been suggested to be due to increased downstream resistance.

## NORMAL PREGNANCY

A decrease in resistance in uterine artery branches causes higher end-diastolic flow velocities, and this can be detected in early pregnancy. After 20 weeks of gestation, there is little change in the waveform of the uteroplacental arteries throughout the remainder of the pregnancy. There is no direct evidence linking the trophoblast invasion of the spiral arteries with uterine blood flow or flow velocity waveform changes, although this was commonly assumed to be so.

## HIGH-RISK PREGNANCY

Both severe growth retardation and maternal hypertension may be associated with uteroplacental waveforms demonstrating a high systolic:diastolic ratio (Fig.

26-4). Whether the reduction of uteroplacental circulation is the cause or effect of pregnancy hypertension remains an open question. Based on the hypothesis that trophoblast invasion of the spiral arteries causes the change in the uterine waveforms during the first half of pregnancy, and that this invasion is less developed in pregnancy hypertension, studies have also been evaluated for screening in early pregnancy.

# 27. FETAL BIOPHYSICAL PROFILE SCORING: APPLICATIONS IN HIGH-RISK OBSTETRICS

Traditional methods of fetal risk assessment were limited until recently to relatively nonspecific clinical methods or to monitoring of a single fetal biophysical variable, the fetal heart rate. Since fetal disease encompasses a spectrum of conditions—including acute and chronic asphyxia of diverse etiologies, as well as functional and/or structural developmental anomalies—it is not surprising that clinical examination of the gravid uterus and heart rate monitoring alone may not provide a completely accurate prediction of impending fetal trouble.

An understanding of the fetal biophysical response to hypoxemia and acidemia (asphyxia) is essential to interpreting the fetal biophysical profile score (BPS). In the animal models fetal hypoxemia, usually induced by maternal isocapnic hypoxemia, results in a profound alteration in CNS-regulated fetal biophysical activities. Thus, the fetus, like its extrauterine counterpart, responds to central hypoxemia by an alteration in its movement, tone, breathing, and heart rate patterns. Specifically, hypoxemia in the fetal lamb or monkey model causes profound reduction or even cessation of breathing movements; in the fetal lamb model it causes a significant and sustained reduction in fetal limb movements. Direct experimental confirmation of a response similar to hypoxemia in the human fetus obviously falls outside accepted ethics, but indirect evidence from observation of fetuses whose mothers are hypoxemic from disease or of fetuses whose mothers smoke suggests that the human fetus may react similarly. The mechanism by which fetal hypoxemia causes a change in biophysical activities is not known but is presumed to be the result of hypoxemia-induced central nervous system cellular dysfunction. The corollary of this hypothesis is of major importance: in the presence of normal fetal biophysical activities, CNS tissue is functional and is therefore not hypoxemic. Fetal aortic body chemoreceptor responses to arterial hypoxemia create a second and important set of recognizable fetal adaptations. (For a more thorough discussion of these topics, please see Chapter 47 in Reece EA, Hobbins JC, Mahoney MJ, and Petrie RH, eds. Medicine of the fetus & mother. J.B. Lippincott, 1992.)

Fetal biophysical responses to asphyxia may then be divided into two general categories (Fig. 27-1). These are (1) acute or immediate responses (i.e., a change in

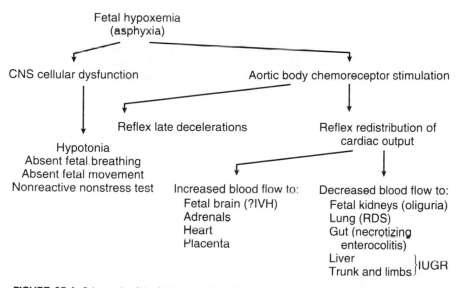

**FIGURE 27-1.** Schematic of the fetal biophysical effects of hypoxemia on the fetus. The conditions in parentheses refer to neonatal sequelae of fetal asphyxia. (CNS, central nervous system; IUGR, intrauterine growth retardation; IVH, intraventricular hemorrhage; RDS, respiratory distress syndrome.)

or a loss of CNS-regulated activities) and (2) chronic responses (i.e., a reduction in amniotic fluid production [oligohydramnios], impaired fetal growth, and an increased probability of neonatal complication). In a given fetus the mix of these acute and chronic biophysical markers of asphyxial disease will vary with the severity, the repetitive frequency, and the chronicity of the asphyxial process. From practical clinical experience it is well recognized that human fetal asphyxial insults present as a wide spectrum, ranging from acute catastrophic asphyxia (as seen with massive sudden placental abruption) to progressive indolent asphyxia (as seen in the growth-retarded fetus in the hypertensive mother). It is further recognized that in the human the superimposed effect of uterine contraction on the failing uteroplacental unit is an obvious and major compounding factor. Experimental animal models to study fetal asphyxia commonly use maternal hypoxemia as the initiating event, but in the pregnant woman maternal hypoxemia is a rare cause of fetal disease. In the compromised human fetus the nature of the asphyxial insult is most certainly different than it is in the experimental animal model. In the human fetus the degree of fetal asphyxia varies with both the severity and progression of uteroplacental failure and with the frequency, intensity, and duration of urine contraction. Further, the CNS and reflex responses of the fetus will vary with the extent of hypoxemia. Thus, in human pregnancy a wide range of fetal biophysical response may be expected. With mild to moderate chronic uteroplacental failure fetal hypoxemia may occur only during uterine contraction with normal fetal oxygen tension between contractions. If the contractions are widely spaced in time or vary widely in intensity, then the only cumulative fetal effect may be the aortic arch chemoreceptor redistribution reflex, leading to oligohydramnios. The postmature human fetus presenting with oligohydramnios but normal CNS-regulated biophysical variables is the most common clinical example of this phenomenon. With mild to moderate uteroplacental failure and frequent and intense uterine contractions or, in severe uteroplacental failure, with or without uterine contraction, fetal hypoxemia may be severe and prolonged and result in both CNS depression (loss of acute biophysical variable) and intense aortic body chemoreceptor stimulation (oligohydramnios). In clinical practice the dysmature IUGR fetus most closely approximates this model. Acute onset of severe uteroplacental failure produces yet another clinical picture. Serial studies of the rate of decrease of amniotic fluid volume in fetuses destined to develop oligohydramnios indicate the time for progression from normal fluid to marginal fluid (largest pocket < 2 cm) to be on average 9 days, and that to decreased fluid (largest pocket < 1 cm) to be 11 days (Fig. 27-2). Therefore, with acute onset of fetal asphyxia the CNS-regulated variables may be absent while amniotic fluid volume may still be normal. Left untreated, many of these fetuses will die before there is sufficient time to develop a measurable change in amniotic fluid volume. Finally, in some clinical conditions a pathologic increase in amniotic fluid volume may occur coincidentally with an exaggerated risk of fetal asphyxia. These fetuses may also present with a loss of CNS-regulated biophysical variables alone. (The diabetic and alloisoimmunized pregnancies are good examples.)

## FETAL BIOPHYSICAL PROFILE SCORING: THE METHOD

At Women's Hospital of the University of Manitoba, fetal biophysical profile scoring is used only in referred patients with recognized high-risk factors; indications for testing among the first 12,620 referred high-risk patients have been reported. The gestational age at which testing is begun has been arbitrarily set at the minimal gestational age at which intervention would be considered should an abnormal result be encountered. Over the years since the inception of the program, the lower limit of fetal age for testing has fallen. At present, initial testing is begun as early as 26 weeks. At each testing, in addition to the fetal BPS, fetal morphometric data are obtained (biparietal diameter, femur length, abdominal circumference), an anatomical screen for structural or functional anomaly is done, and the placenta and umbilical cord are assessed. The fetal BPS is obtained by components. The uterine cavity is scanned to identify the largest pocket of amniotic fluid and the largest vertical or near vertical axis of the fluid pocket is measured and recorded. In patients with normal amniotic fluid the presence of loops of umbilical cord with the fluid pocket does not influence the measurement. However, when oligohydramnios is present, some additional care is exercised in selecting a cord-free fluid pocket, since approximation of the umbilical vein due to looping of the cord can give a false impression of the actual size of the fluid pocket. The fetus is then scanned in a longitudinal plane such that the fetal face, forelimbs, and particularly hand(s) and thorax are visualized. On achieving the proper scan plane the time is noted and observation is continued until either normal activity is seen or 30 consecutive minutes of scanning have elapsed. Attention is paid to the presence or absence of three discrete biophysical variables:

1. *Fetal breathing movements* are defined by initial inward movement of the thorax with descent of the diaphragm and abdominal contents, followed by a

return to the original position. Recognition of both the thoracic and abdominal component of fetal breathing is important so that extrinsic chest wall movement, which may occur with fetal movements, is not misinterpreted as representing fetal breathing. Fetal "hiccups" are interpreted as a variant of normal fetal breathing. At present the rate and pattern of the breathing movements are not considered clinically significant except in extreme cases. Fetal breathing movements are said to be normal when at least 30 seconds of breathing activity have been observed.

2. *Fetal movements* are defined as single movements or clusters of activity involving the limbs or the fetal body. In our method isolated hand and arm movements are considered to represent normal movements. Fetal movements are considered as normal if at least three episodes are observed in the study period. At present other movements (e.g., facial grimace, thumb sucking, tongue extension, swallowing, and eye movement), although easily seen, are not included in our criteria for normal movement.

3. The definition of *fetal tone* has changed as the imaging quality of ultrasound equipment has improved. In our initial reports we described tone as normal when at least one fetal movement characterized by limb or trunk extension with return to flexion was observed. With the more sophisticated ultrasound equipment we have refined the definition of fetal tone. At present, normal fetal tone is defined as at least one episode of opening of the hand with finger and thumb extension with a return to closed fist formation. In the absence of any hand movement fetal tone is still recorded as normal if the hand remains in fist formation for the entire 30-minute observation period. Abnormal fetal tone is defined by the fetal hand remaining in an open position with fingers and thumb extended despite the presence or absence of fetal movements.

Each of the four variables of the BPS is coded as normal or abnormal according to fixed criteria and is then assigned an arbitrary score of 2 if normal and 0 if abnormal (Table 27-1). In the original and early prospective clinical studies of the method, nonstress test results were also included, yielding a maximal score of 10 (five variables). Subsequently, we modified the method by selective use of the nonstress test; at the time of writing, it is our policy to perform a nonstress test only when one or more of the ultrasound-monitored variables are abnormal. The modification has caused no change in our negative predictive accuracy and has limited the use of the nonstress test to less than 5% of tests.

Clinical management is based on the test score result as interpreted against obstetrical factors (e.g., favorability of the cervix for induction), the extent and progression of maternal disease, and other fetal factors—including the presence or absence of anomalies and, in selected cases, confirmation of pulmonary maturity by amniotic fluid phospholipid profile (Table 27-2).

The fetal BPS provides an accurate estimate of the risk of fetal death in the immediate future. When this risk is low, as with a normal score, intervention is indicated only for obstetrical or maternal factors. Thus, in the postdates pregnancy with a favorable cervix (obstetrical factor), we would induce labor regardless of the test score. In contrast, in the postdates fetus with an unfavorable cervix and a normal score, we would delay induction and rely on serial fetal assessment.

**TABLE 27-1.** Biophysical Profile Scoring: Technique and Interpretation

| Biophysical Variable | Normal (Score = 2) | Abnormal (Score = 0) |
|---|---|---|
| Fetal breathing movements | ≥1 episode of ≥30 sec in 30 min | Absent or no episode of ≥30 sec in 30 min |
| Gross body movements | ≥3 discrete body-limb movements in 30 min (episodes of active continuous movement considered) | ≤ 2 episodes of body/limb movements in 30 min as single movement |
| Fetal tone | ≥1 episode of active extension with return to flexion of fetal limb(s) or trunk. Opening and closing of hand considered normal tone | Either slow extension with return to partial flexion movement of limb in full extension or absent fetal movement |
| Reactive fetal heart rate | ≥2 episodes of acceleration of ≥15 bpm and of >15 sec associated with fetal movement in 20 min | >2 episodes of acceleration fetal heart rate or acceleration of <15 bpm in 20 min |
| Qualitative amniotic fluid volume | ≥1 pocket of fluid measuring 2 cm in vertical axis | Either no pockets or largest pocket <2 cm in vertical axis |

**TABLE 27-2.** Recommended Clinical Management by Fetal Biophysical Profile Score

| Test Score | Interpretations | Recommended Management |
|---|---|---|
| 10/10 | No evidence of distress | No intervention. |
| 8/10 (NST-not done)* | | Serial testing as per protocol. |
| 8/10 (N-AFV)† | | |
| 8/10 (ABN-AFV)† | No evidence of acute asphyxia; chronic asphyxia likely | Deliver if gestational age >36 weeks. If <36 weeks serial testing. Deliver if BPS <6. |
| 6/10 (N-AFV) | Acute asphyxia possible | If gestational age >34 weeks, deliver. If <34 weeks repeat test within 24 hours; delivery for repeat score <6. |
| 6/10 (ABN-AFV) | Acute asphyxia possible; chronic asphyxia likely | Deliver if gestational age >26 weeks. |
| 4/10 (N-AFV) | Acute asphyxia likely | If gestational age >32 weeks, deliver. If <32 weeks repeat test same day; repeat test <6 deliver. |
| 4/10 (ABN-AFV) | Acute asphyxia likely; chronic asphyxia likely | Deliver if gestational age >26 weeks. |
| 0/10 | Acute/chronic asphyxia | Deliver if gestational age >26 weeks |

* Socol ML, Manning FA, Murata Y, et al. Maternal smoking causes fetal hypoxemia: experimental evidence. Am J. Obstet. Gynecol. 1982;142:214.
† Normal (N) and abnormal (ABN) amniotic fluid volume (AFV), from Manning FA, Wyn-Puch E, Boddy K. Effect of cigarette smoking on fetal breathing movements in normal pregnancies. Br Med J 1975;1:552.

When an abnormal score or oligohydramnios is encountered, we would induce labor regardless of the cervical state. With serious maternal disease (e.g., pre-eclampsia), we would intervene despite a normal fetal biophysical score if the maternal condition was deteriorating. However, in the same patient with severe but stable disease, we would use a normal test score result to delay intervention until the fetal maturity was certain and the cervix was favorable for induction. Oligohydramnios in the presence of a normal fetus, with functioning renal tissue (as evidenced by fetal bladder emptying and filling) and with intact membranes, is always considered an indication for induction, despite the presence of normal movement, breathing, tone, and heart rate reactivity. This approach is based on an extensive review of the relationship of ultrasound-defined oligohydramnios to perinatal mortality, and the subsequent prospective study indicating that inter-vention for oligohydramnios can improve perinatal outcome. In the mature fetus with an equivocal test but normal fluid (score 6 of 10) we advocate delivery; when the cervix is not favorable for induction, repeat testing is undertaken within 24 hours. If subsequent testing is normal, as it will be in 75% of all cases, no intervention for fetal indication is contemplated. If the repeat test remains equivo-cal, or becomes abnormal, intervention for fetal indications is indicated. In the fetus with an abnormal score (<4 of 10), we would always advocate immediate intervention unless there are recognized, and remedial, compounding factors. Such factors might include a history of fetal trauma, an intrauterine condition for which treatment is possible (e.g., rhesus isoimmunization), maternal drug effects on the fetus (e.g., recent narcotic or sedative administration), or a gestational age (<26 weeks) that renders extreme fetal immaturity certain.

## FETAL BIOPHYSICAL PROFILE SCORING: CLINICAL RESULTS

### PERINATAL OUTCOME: BLINDED STUDY

The concept of fetal biophysical profile scoring was first tested in a prospective blind study of 216 referred high-risk patients. In these patients, a fetal BPS was obtained within 1 week of delivery and, in more instances (52%), it was obtained within 2 days of delivery. The mean gestational age at the time of delivery was 38.7 weeks ±0.2 SEM (range of 30 to 44 weeks). Fetal biophysical profile scores were not revealed before delivery and therefore did not influence perinatal outcome. A relationship was noted between the last fetal biophysical score and perinatal outcome, as measured by the 5-minute Apgar score, fetal distress in labor, and perinatal mortality. The incidence of low 5-minute Apgar score (<7) varied inver-sely with the profile score of 0. A similar increased relationship between the last fetal BPS and the incidence of fetal distress in labor was noted. Perinatal mortality increased progressively as the score decreased; the perinatal mortality with a score of 10 was 1, and increased to 600 per 1000 when the score before delivery was 0.

### PERINATAL MORTALITY: CLINICAL STUDY

The results of seven published series are given in Table 27-3. These collective data strongly suggest that the application of fetal biophysical profile scoring to the high-risk pregnant population results in a dramatic improvement in perinatal mortality rates.

**TABLE 27-3.** The Relationship of Biophysical Profile Scoring to Perinatal Death

| Author | No. of Patients | No. of Tests | Perinatal Mortality (per 1000) Corrected* | False-Negative Rate (per 1000) | False-Positive Rate (%) |
|---|---|---|---|---|---|
| Manning et al (1985) | 12620 | 26257 | 24 (1.9) | 8 (0.6) | — |
| Baskett et al (1987) | 4184 | 9624 | 13 (3.1) | 4 (1.0) | 71.8 |
| Platt et al (1983) | 286 | 1112 | 2 (7.0) | 2 (7.0) | 71.4 |
| Shime et al (1984) | 274 | 274 | 0 | 0 | 100.0 |
| Schifrin et al (1981) | 158 | 240 | 2 (12.7) | 1 (6.3) | 42.6 |
| Vintzileos et al (1983) | 150 | 342 | 4 (26.6) | 0 | 60.0 |
| Golde et al (1984) | 107 | 459 | 0 | 0 | 75.0 |
| Total | 23780 | 54337 | 59 (2.27) | 18 (0.77) | 42.6–100 |

* Lethal anomalies excluded.

## PERINATAL MORBIDITY: CLINICAL STUDY

In our most recent study, the relationship between the last test score and individual perinatal outcome variables fell into three general categories. First, a highly significant *inverse linear* correlation was observed for five variables. These were fetal distress, admission to a neonatal intensive care unit, intrauterine growth retardation, 5-minute Apgar score of ≤7, and cord pH of ≤7.20 (see Fig. 27-2). Combinations of these variables also exhibited the same highly significant inverse linear correlation with test score. The second relationship was observed between the last test score and perinatal mortality both in total and by components; this relationship was *inverse and exponential* and demonstrated a highly significant correlation (Fig. 27-3). The third relationship (or *lack thereof*) was that between the last test score and the incidence of meconium staining of amniotic fluid and the incidence of major anomaly (Fig. 27-4). The incidence of meconium staining rose significantly between the last normal score and the equivocal score but then remained essentially unchanged for deteriorating test scores (see Fig. 27-4). In contrast, the incidence of major anomaly was similar for all last test scores except for the very abnormal score (BPS = 0), where a significant increase is recorded (see Fig. 27-4). The explanation for these observed relationships is intriguing and may offer considerable insight into the nature of fetal compromise and the characteristics of fetal adaptive responses.

The effect of hypoxemia on the human fetus may be expected to vary according to the characteristics of the hypoxemia and the fetal response. From both serendipitous observation in the human fetus and experimental observation of the animal fetus it is known that hypoxemia abolishes CNS-generated acute biophysical activities and that the duration of abolition of activities exceeds the duration of hypoxemia, often by a considerable margin. Variation in sensitivity of discrete CNS signal sources to graded hypoxemia is suspected but as of yet incompletely characterized. Oligohydramnios is also a consequence of hypoxemia, but it evolves more slowly and is due to different mechanisms. In the human, fetal hypoxemia, at least in the evolving stages, is unlikely to be sustained; rather, it is likely to be intermittent, the modulation of episodes that result from superimposed reduction

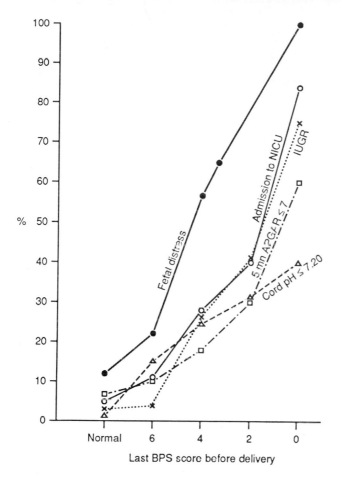

**FIGURE 27-2.** The relationship between any perinatal morbidity and the presence of fetal distress, admission to NICU, IUGR, 5-minute Apgar < 7, and umbilical vein pH < 7.20, either alone or in any combination. A highly significant inverse linear correlation is observed. In contrast, no relationship was observed between meconium staining of amniotic fluid and the presence of a major anomaly.

of perfusion of the failing uteroplacental unit induced by spontaneous uterine contraction. According to this hypothesis, changes in measured fetal biophysical variables and the net effect, a change in the fetal BPS, indicate the cumulative effect of episodes of hypoxemia.

Clinical application of these data requires consideration of other obstetrical and maternal factors in addition to the test of fetal well-being. The object is not to treat the test score but to interpret test score data within the overall clinical context. In our experience it is in this context that the test scoring method has been most valuable. We would consider, for example, a score of 6 of 10 to be indicative of compromise and an indication for delivery in the mature fetus. In contrast, in the very immature fetus (<28 weeks gestation) repeat testing may be in order before intervention is recommended. Although the correlation between adverse perinatal outcome and mortality is well defined in this study, it is equally apparent that the converse of positive predictive accuracy (i.e., the false-positive rate) is directly related to test scoring. We note that almost 40% of fetuses with the last score of 6 exhibited none of the markers of fetal compromise, whereas no fetuses with a

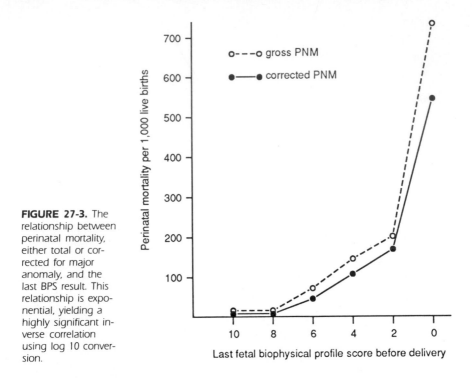

**FIGURE 27-3.** The relationship between perinatal mortality, either total or corrected for major anomaly, and the last BPS result. This relationship is exponential, yielding a highly significant inverse correlation using log 10 conversion.

score of 0 demonstrated absence of perinatal disease. Furthermore, whereas fetal hypoxemia appears to be one cause of suppression of fetal biophysical variables, it cannot be the only cause. Rhythmic variation in the frequency of biophysical activities is known to occur in the fetus. Since the study was interventional in design, it offers only incomplete information regarding the natural progression of the abnormal or equivocal score. Nonetheless, we are aware of several cases in which a score of 6 reverted to a score of normal on repeat testing and was not associated with adverse outcome. This occurrence was less frequent with a score of 4 or 2 and has not occurred with a score of 0.

## DISEASE-SPECIFIC TESTING: BPS

### THE DIABETIC PREGNANCY

Ultrasound-based fetal assessment using the BPS is well suited for fetal surveillance in the diabetic pregnancy. It is notable that no deaths among structurally normal fetuses occurred within the prescribed testing intervals. This is consistent with previous observations that a normal BPS conveys a low risk of stillbirth. The reported rate is 0.65 per 1000 among 19,221 high-risk patients. Recently, we have observed a fetal death in a well-controlled insulin-dependent diabetic within 7 days of a last normal BPS. It may well be that such nonasphyxial ("acute metabolic") fetal deaths will escape detection by BPS, because of their rapid progression. Despite this recent setback, it is clear that accurate intervention in the few

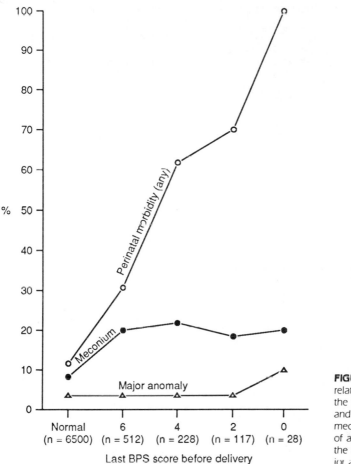

**FIGURE 27-4.** The relationship between the last test score and the incidence of meconium staining of amniotic fluid and the incidence of major anomaly.

who required it and a confident conservative approach in the majority led to significant clinical advantages for both mother and infant.

## THE POSTDATES PREGNANCY: THE ROLE OF ULTRASOUND

The appropriate management of the obstetric patient whose gestation has exceeded 42 completed weeks (postmaturity or postdates syndrome) remains one of the most difficult problems in modern perinatal medicine. The perinatal risks of the postdates syndrome are well established; perinatal mortality doubles for each additional week after the 42nd week.

Johnson and colleagues (1986) have applied this method, using a standard protocol, to 307 postdates pregnancies (Fig. 27-5). In those fetuses with normal biophysical activities and normal amniotic fluid volume ($n = 211$) who were managed according to protocol, there were no perinatal deaths or fetal distress,

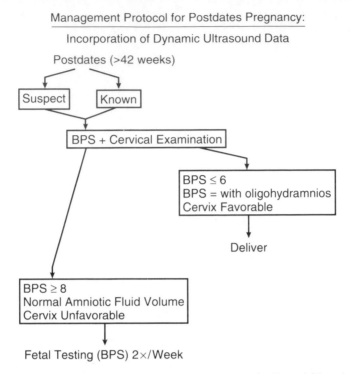

Management Protocol for Postdates Pregnancy:

Incorporation of Dynamic Ultrasound Data

**FIGURE 27-5.** A management protocol for postdates pregnancy (> 42 weeks) based on clinical assessment of the cervix and fetal assessment by the fetal biophysical profile scoring method. The experience with this protocol in 243 postdates pregnancies has been reported recently. (Data from Johnson JM, Harman CR, Lange IR, et al. Biophysical profile scoring in the management of the post term pregnancy: an analysis of 307 patients. Am J Obstet Gynecol 1986;154:269.)

low Apgar scores were infrequent (3.31% and 1.89%, respectively), and subsequent neonatal morbidity was unusual (1.9%). In contrast, in those fetuses exhibiting an abnormal BPS or oligohydramnios ($n = 32$), fetal distress (22%), low Apgar scores (12.5%), and neonatal morbidity (19%) were all substantially and significantly increased. When considered collectively, neonatal morbidity ranged from 3.7% when the fetal BPS was normal to 18.7% when the score was abnormal. These data indicate that fetal biophysical profile scoring facilitates differentiation of the normal noncompromised fetus from the compromised fetus within a population of postdates pregnancies. Accurate recognition of fetal risk, in turn, combined with maternal obstetric assessment (including cervical findings), allows for a rational and selective approach to patient care. The potential beneficial impact of such a selective approach in reducing maternal morbidity is clear. In the Johnson study some of this benefit was realized. The cesarean section rates for patients with a normal fetus managed conservatively and those with a normal fetus delivered because of favorable cervical findings were similar (15% and 13%, respectively) and were not increased as compared to the population at large (16.5%). In contrast, both were sharply and significantly lower than the cesarean section rate observed in patients induced in a nonselective manner on the basis of gestational age alone (42%). Perinatal mortality was absent, morbidity was low, and intervention rates were reduced, at least as compared with those observed among patients with nonselective intervention based on gestational age alone. Based on these findings, it may no longer be reasonable to elect routine delivery of all patients at or beyond 42 completed weeks of gestation. In view of the proved reliability of fetal assessment methods and the potential risk of nondiscriminative intervention, selective patient care appears to be the method of choice.

## MANAGEMENT OF IUGR: INTEGRATION OF ULTRASOUND DATA

The algorithm for diagnosis and management of IUGR is complex and subject to variation by preference and experience. The patient enters the diagnostic point from a variety of routes, most notably by either clinical suspicion of IUGR or recognition of suggestive signs in the course of ultrasound examination for other purposes. At initial assessment both morphometric and functional data are considered. The determination of IUGR at the outset is almost always based on the fetal morphometric data. Nonderived morphometric indices (e.g., abdominal circumference) are recommended over derived indices (e.g., fetal weight estimate) since the risk of compounding error is eliminated. Morphometric index ratios such as the head-to-abdomen ratio against gestational age are not of any real clinical value.

If at first visit in a patient with known dates or at repeat visits in a patient with unknown dates the selected growth variable is below the lower limit ascribed (5th percentile), a diagnosis of IUGR is established and efforts are directed toward determining etiology, severity, and prognosis. In such fetuses ultrasound assessment should be done at a frequent interval (at least weekly) and conservative management should be continued, provided fetal growth is demonstrated and functional signs remain normal. Intervention in such fetuses may take place when fetal maturity is affirmed and delivery may be instituted with minimal difficulty. In the fetus with proved major anomaly a decision toward total conservative management with a view to absolute minimization of maternal risk is the usual role. In our center either a confirmed abnormal BPS (<4) or the isolated observation of oligohydramnios by defined criteria (<2 cm largest vertical pocket), or both, in an IUGR fetus of at least 25 weeks gestation are considered an indication for prompt delivery regardless of gestational age. In our center umbilical artery velocimetry and intrafetal proportion are used not to precipitate intervention but to guide the frequency of fetal surveillance. In the presence of a distinctly abnormal pulsatility index or absent diastolic flow, fetal well-being surveillance should be intensified. The use of reverse diastolic flow to prompt delivery in the IUGR fetus remains undefined at present, but it seems likely that with further experience this finding will also be used to precipitate immediate delivery. In the dysmature IUGR fetus, as well as other types, it has been our policy to continue conservative management only until fetal maturity is confirmed and delivery can be accomplished with minimal maternal risk. This method of management has been applied now to more than 1200 proved IUGR fetuses, yielding a corrected perinatal mortality (anomaly exclusion) of 12.5 per 1000, a very significant reduction from the expected rate among IUGR fetuses (60 to 80 deaths per 1000).

## OTHER CONSIDERATIONS

### COMPARISON WITH OTHER METHODS

The comparative accuracy and clinical applicability of fetal biophysical profile scoring and the nonstress test has been an area of investigation. These comparative data suggest that fetal biophysical profile scoring may be a more accurate method for identification of the fetus at risk for asphyxia.

### LIMITATIONS OF THE METHOD

The subjective or semiqualitative nature of some of the measurements (e.g., tone, qualitative amniotic fluid volume) is a potential source of difficulty, although in practice this is more theoretical than real. The observation of fetal tone rarely is a cause for disagreement among experienced observers. Decreased amniotic fluid is more subject to observer interpretation, but the limitations here apply more to the inexperienced observer. Measurement of an amniotic fluid pocket of 2.1 cm, for example, is not incompatible with the diagnosis of oligohydramnios by two experienced observers. Overreliance on marginal measurements of fluid in providing reassurance suggests a degree of scientific precision that is impossible to justify by the very nature of the imaging process.

---

# 28. ANTEPARTUM FETAL HEART RATE MONITORING

---

The controversy regarding which mode of antepartum testing is most prognostic continues. Regardless of this, antepartum testing for the at-risk fetus has become the standard of care in the United States. Newer techniques are being used more extensively to replace or augment the traditional NST and contraction stress test (CST). The current clinical armamentarium of antepartum surveillance techniques includes fetal movement counts, nonstress testing, contraction stress testing, fetal "stimulation" studies that augment nonstress testing, the biophysical profile, ultrasound-determined amniotic fluid volume status, Doppler ultrasound, and fetal acid-base status via funicentesis. (For a more thorough discussion of this topic, please see Chapter 48 in Reece EA, Hobbins JC, Mahoney MJ, and Petrie RH, eds. Medicine of the Fetus & Mother. J.B. Lippincott, 1992.)

### DEMOGRAPHIC IDENTIFICATION OF INFANTS AT RISK

Currently, fetal death after 20 weeks gestation occurs in about 1% of all pregnancies. In 50% of cases, antepartum risk factors are present; of these, 25% to 70% are amenable to prenatal modification. The purpose of identifying epidemiologic risk factors for fetal death is to begin antepartum evaluation and risk-appropriate interventions in view of reducing perinatal morbidity and mortality. Table 28-1 reflects a compilation of the major indications for antepartum testing.

The concept of uteroplacental insufficiency underlies the basis for selection of individuals who are candidates for improvement in obstetric performance by the application of antepartum surveillance techniques. Uteroplacental insufficiency implies inadequate nutritive and respiratory exchange due to decreased uterine blood flow or decreased placental surface area. Various maternal and fetal conditions predispose to uteroplacental compromise. Fetuses at risk should be observed in utero until it is believed that maximum benefit from the intrauterine environment has been achieved and that extrauterine life is superior to continued gestation.

One of the newer indications for the application of antepartum surveillance techniques is elevation of maternal serum alpha-fetoprotein (MSAFP). Data suggest that elevations of midtrimester MSAFP in the absence of a malformed fetus are associated with low birth weight and increased perinatal loss due to prematurity and intrauterine growth retardation. These associations appear to be stronger when MSAFP is elevated on two occasions and when the magnitude of MSAFP elevation is high. The pathophysiologic explanation of this phenomenon may be due to midtrimester placental abnormalities in the form of chronic villitis, placental infarction, or intervillous thrombosis.

**TABLE 28-1.** Indications for Antepartum Surveillance

Hypertensive disorders
  Chronic hypertension
  Mild preeclampsia
Insulin-dependent diabetes mellitus
Chronic renal disease
Collagen vascular disorders
Maternal cyanotic heart disease
Hemoglobinopathies (SS, SC, S-Thal)
Decreased maternal perception of fetal movements
Elevated maternal serum AFP with normal amniotic fluid AFP
Certain medications/drugs (indomethacin, methadone)
Third trimester bleeding
Placenta previa
Preterm rupture of membranes
Suspected oligohydramnios
Intrauterine growth retardation
Post dates pregnancy (>42 weeks)
Isoimmunization
Multiple gestation
Previous unexplained fetal demise
Selected fetal anomalies
Other medical complications
Other obstetric complications

## TECHNIQUES OF SURVEILLANCE

### FETAL MOVEMENT COUNTS

Systematic assessment of fetal movements has been advocated as a method of antepartum surveillance because it is inexpensive, noninvasive, carries no contraindications, and is a reliable mode of fetal surveillance. The observation of fetal activity in utero gives indirect evidence of an intact central nervous system.

Some findings have indicated that the number of fetal movements per day increases rapidly until about midgestation, then increases steadily and is maintained at 12 to 60 movements per hour until term. There is not, as is commonly believed, a sharp diminution in fetal activity in the days preceding delivery.

Diurnal and shorter periodic variations in fetal activity have been described by several authors who have monitored fetal activity for prolonged periods of time. Fetuses demonstrate alternating periods of activity with periods of inactivity that tend to be characteristic for that gestation. The longest period of lack of gross body movements in a group of fetuses in good health with normal obstetric outcome was 75 minutes.

Tobacco and certain depressant medications may acutely diminish fetal motor activity. There appears to be no relationship between maternal meals or activity and the pattern of fetal activity.

Fetal movements can be quantitated by tocodynamometry, direct ultrasound techniques, or maternal assessment and tabulation. Maternal perception of fetal movements correlates well with real-time observations of fetal activity. It has been demonstrated that maternally perceived movements are visible ultrasonically, and 55% to 88% of major ultrasonically visualized movements are perceived by the mother. Certain variability in women's sensitivity to fetal movements is to be expected. Small fetus movements may be below the threshold for maternal perception, but can be detected with real-time and Doppler ultrasound which makes fetal "kick counting" prone to false-positive results.

The technique of fetal kick counting by the gravida is not complicated. Women at 26 or greater weeks gestation are asked to count fetal movements for an hour, 2 hours after a meal, while positioned in the left lateral recumbent position. The minimum number of fetal movements thought to be reassuring varies among investigators from ten per 2 hours to four per 12 hours. Another frequently used method to assess fetal activity is to count the time necessary to achieve ten fetal movements. Fetal kick counting allows the gravida to participate in monitoring for fetal well-being and ensures at least 1 hour per day of optimal uterine perfusion in the left lateral decubitus position. Women are instructed to contact their physician if ten movements are not experienced in 2 hours.

Maternal assessment of fetal movements appears to be an effective screening test when the minimum number of fetal movements that triggers the "alarm" is not set too low. A scheme of daily kick counting also augments other forms of antepartum testing by providing day-to-day assessment of fetal condition. As with other forms of antepartum surveillance, a reassuring test has better predictive value than an abnormal one. Therefore, with our present level of understanding, abnormal kick counts should be followed with other antepartum assessment techniques.

## THE NONSTRESS TEST

The nonstress test (NST) is predicated on the normal neurologic development and central control of the fetal heart. Specifically, fine-tuning of baseline heart rate and expression of accelerative patterns is dependent on the normal integration of central nervous system activity and maturing sensitivity to endogenous neurotransmitters. Baseline fetal heart rate is the product of sympathetic and parasympathetic influences. Stimulation of sympathetic nerves located in the heart releases norepinephrine, causing increased cardiac rate and contractility. Parasympathetic stimulation via the vagus nerve causes reflex slowing of conduction at the sinoatrial and atrioventricular nodes, thus decelerating fetal heart rate. *Variability* of fetal heart rate is probably more dependent on parasympathetic than sympathetic on input. Fetal heart rate decreases with advancing gestation, indicating progressive maturation of tonic, parasympathetic expression.

An expression of maturation of the normal central nervous system is the coordinated association of fetal activity and acceleration of the fetal heart rate. Nonperiodic fetal heart rate accelerations appear to be mediated by a transient decrease in parasympathetic tone or a transient increase in sympathetic tone. Numerous studies have validated the association between movement-related fetal heart rate accelerations and successful perinatal outcome.

In the pathological condition, lack of fetal heart rate accelerations can be a manifestation of fetal hypoxia. During hypoxemia, the fetus redistributes blood flow preferentially toward the brain stem, cerebral cortex, coronary arteries, and adrenals. Some researchers have demonstrated in chronically instrumented animals that loss of heart rate accelerations occurs when fetal arterial pH drops significantly from baseline levels. Gestational age has considerable influence on the result of the nonstressed cardiotocogram. The ratio of fetal heart rate accelerations with fetal movements to fetal movements increases linearly after 25 weeks, from 20%, to 65% at 40 weeks. Therefore, with advancing gestational age, a greater number of reactive NSTs are encountered (Table 28-2). After 32 weeks, the vast majority (90% to 99%) of NSTs in normal fetuses should be reactive. These findings have caused some investigators to question the current criteria for reactivity at gestational ages prior to 30 to 32 weeks.

Certainly, fetal state is an important determinant of fetal heart rate variability and accelerations. Timor-Tritsch and coworkers, in 1978, described comparable

**TABLE 28-2.** The Influence of Gestational Age on Fetal Heart Rate Reactivity

| Gestation (wk) | Total No. of Nonstress Tests | Reactive Nonstress Tests | | Nonreactive Nonstress Tests | |
|---|---|---|---|---|---|
| | | n | % | n | % |
| 23–27 | 36 | 6 | 16.7 | 30 | 83.3 |
| 28–32 | 32 | 21 | 65.6 | 11 | 34.4 |
| 33–37 | 42 | 38 | 90.5 | 4 | 9.5 |
| 38–42 | 18 | 17 | 94.4 | 1 | 5.6 |

From Smith CV, Phelan JP, Paul RH. A prospective analysis of the influence of gestational age on the baseline fetal heart rate and reactivity in a low-risk population. Am J Obstet Gynecol 1985;153:780.

epochs of quiet sleep, active sleep, and transitional periods clustered into longer time periods representing behavioral states.* In quiet states, fetal movements and fetal heart rate accelerations are largely absent and have a mean duration of 22.8 minutes. In studies of fetuses during the last 10 weeks of gestation, there is evidence that fetal movements, breathing, heart rate, and heart rate variability are governed by nonrandom repeat patterns. One must be certain that errors in the assessment of a fetus's overall pattern are not incurred by ignoring inherent periodicities. One could easily observe a fetus for less than an hour, during a sleep cycle, and make inaccurate inferences as to the overall behavioral activity of that fetus. The time between two fetal heart rate accelerations of ten beats per minute for 6 seconds in healthy term fetuses may be as long as 37 minutes. Thus, current arbitrary cut-offs of 20 or 40 minutes for NST durations ignore inherent fetal biorhythms.

Besides hypoxia, fetal state, and gestational age, other factors impact on the presence or absence of antepartum fetal heart rate accelerations. Moderate maternal exercise appears to increase fetal heart rate baseline, but does not decrease NST reactivity. Smoking, conversely, is associated with decreased NST reactivity. Phenobarbital has been demonstrated to result in a greater number of nonreactive nonstress tests. Propranolol has also been implicated in the genesis of a nonreactive NST. Lack of accelerations may therefore be a reflection of normal fetal sleep-wake cyclicity, external influences, or hypoxia.

The NST is accomplished in a noninvasive manner and carries no specific contraindications; it is performed with the woman in left lateral tilt position with her head elevated 15 to 20 degrees. Blood pressure is assessed before the NST and at every 15 minutes of testing. All attempts are made to avoid supine hypotension. In general, fetal heart rate tracings are recorded using phonocardiographic or Doppler-derived techniques. Uterine activity is recorded using a strain gauge secured to the maternal abdomen by means of an elastic strap. The mother is asked to record fetal movements via a hand-held "event marker," and the results are then displayed on the tocodynamometric channel of the fetal monitor. Fetal movements can thus be related to fetal heart rate accelerations.

Technical difficulties in obtaining adequate fetal heart rate tracings may be encountered in the presence of morbid maternal obesity, excessive fetal activity, polyhydramnios, or fetal hiccoughs. Maternal hypotension or discomfort may also hamper attempts at fetal monitoring.

The NST is interpreted as reactive or nonreactive. The standard of practice adopted by the American College of Obstetricians and Gynecologists as of 1987 is to define a reactive test by the occurrence of two accelerations of at least 15 beats per minute sustained for at least 15 seconds, within a 20-minute period. Failure to meet reactive criteria within a 40-minute period constitutes a nonreactive or abnormal test.

The predictive value of a negative test is uniformly high in reviews of the literature, with a range of 72% to 100%. Overall, a reactive NST predicts a good perinatal outcome (absence of intrapartum fetal distress, mortality, neonatal depression, or complications) in 95% of cases.

---

* Timor-tritsch IE, Dierker LJ, Hertz RH, Deagan NC, Rosen MG. Studies of antepartum behavioral state in the human fetus at term. Am J Obstet Gynecol 1978;132:524.

False-positive NST results continue to be a source of diagnostic error in the interpretation of this form of surveillance. The predictive value of a positive test remains low at 11.5% to 86%, but is below 40% in most studies. Although excellent specificity is achieved with a reactive NST, the nonreactive NST would result in a large number of unnecessary interventions if used as the only measure of fetal well-being. Given our present level of understanding, a nonreactive NST must be confirmed with other tests of fetal well-being, such as the CST or biophysical profile. Several acceptable options for follow-up of the nonreactive NST exist: CST, biophysical profile, or stimulation of the monitored fetus.

False-negative nonstress test results fortunately occur infrequently. They are reported to be 0% to 2% for perinatal mortality and 1% to 15% for the occurrence of fetal distress in labor. In a review by Phelan and coworkers (1982) of 1564 women who delivered within 7 days of a reactive NST, there were four fetal deaths, for a rate of 0.26%.[†] These deaths were due to cord accidents and abruptio placentae. Among postdate patients, however, the majority of fetal deaths occur within 3 to 5 days of testing. Investigators have therefore questioned the reliability of once-weekly nonstress testing in the postdate population, in favor of increased frequency of testing and assessment of amniotic fluid volume. When variable decelerations are noted during the NST in a postdate patient, delivery should be accomplished.

Boehm and colleagues (1986) demonstrated a significant reduction in perinatal mortality when nonstress tests were performed twice weekly in a high-risk population.[‡] His study was retrospective in nature, using a historical comparison group. However, the stillbirth rate following a reactive NST fell from 6.1/1000 to 1.9/1000 after institution of twice-weekly NSTs. Schneider and associates (1988) noted that the stillbirth rate at Columbia University was lower within 4 days of a normal antepartum fetal heart rate test (0.027%), compared with a test interval of 5 to 7 days (0.11%).[§] These studies question the current concept of once-weekly, instead of twice-weekly, nonstress testing.

When interpreting NST monitor strips, attention should also be directed toward other unusual fetal heart rate features. At times, variable decelerations or bradycardia may be noted. The presence of these decelerative patterns has been demonstrated to be associated with fetal death, intrauterine growth retardation, and neonatal mortality. Furthermore, there is a higher incidence of fetal distress in labor, low Apgar scores, neonatal intensive care unit admissions, and nuchal cord location. The presence of fetal heart rate accelerations concomitant with variable decelerations is more likely to indicate a favorable perinatal outcome. Fetal bradycardia in the antepartum period may be due to supine hypotension or spontaneous uterine hyperstimulation. In the absence of explanatory conditions and fetal heart rate reactivity, the presence of repetitive variable decelerations should give cause to deliver the term fetus. The preterm fetus under similar conditions

---

[†] Phelan JP, Cromartie AD, Smith CV. The nostress test: the false negative test. Am J Obstet Gynecol 1982;142:293.

[‡] Boehm FH, Salyer S, Shah DM, Vaughan WK. Improved outcome of twice weekly nonstress testing. Obstet Gynecol 1986;67:566.

[§] Schneider EP, Hutson JM, Petrie RH. An assessment of the first decade's experience with antepartum fetal heart rate testing. Am J Perinatol 1988;5:134.

should have management individualized with regard to the risk of prematurity versus the risk of continued gestation. Whenever variable decelerations (whether moderate or prolonged) are found on NST, search should ensue for nuchal cord or oligohydramnios.

### Modifications of the Nonstress Test

Becasue of the relative lack of predictive value for a nonreactive NST, several investigators have tried to modify the NST in favor of greater selectivity. Extending the diagnostic window for the occurrence of one acceleration of 15 beats per minute for 15 seconds decreased the false-positive rate from 19.5% to 5%. Greater positive predictive value is possible by increasing the length of the NST to 90 minutes or 120 minutes. When 120 minutes was allowed to elapse in order to achieve five accelerations in 20 minutes, the predictive value of a nonreactive test was increased to 85.7% and the negative predictive value for a reactive NST was 98.5%. Given that fetal activity is episodic, it is reasonable to expect that extension of the testing time would eliminate some false-positive results due to quiet sleep states of the normoxemic fetus.

## FETAL STIMULATION TESTS

Several investigators have aspired to decrease the incidence of false-positive tests by attempting to stimulate the fetus toward a reactive pattern. The intent of such fetal stimulation devices is to awaken a sleeping, healthy fetus and thereby distinguish it from the fetus in jeopardy.

Manual manipulation of the fetus does not appear to improve the incidence of nonreactive results. Maternal administration of neither orange juice nor glucose results in a decreased incidence of nonreactive tests or a reduction in testing time. Despite experimental evidence of futility, both dispensing orange juice and pushing the mother's abdomen continue to be performed.

## CONTRACTION STRESS TEST

The CST is a test of fetal well-being that involves evaluation of the fetal heart rate response to uterine contractions. In effect, the fetal respiratory or oxygen reserve is assessed. When a fetus with adequate reserve is subjected to the stress of relative circulatory stasis in the intervillous space caused by uterine contractions, no ominous heart rate pattern will develop. That is, late decelerations will not be seen. Conversely, if fetal respiratory reserves are inadequate, as in the case of uteroplacental insufficiency, uterine contractions may cause fetal oxygen levels to drop to a critical level. Hypoxia stimulates fetal carotid chemoreceptors with resultant alpha-adrenergic response. The peripheral vasoconstriction and sudden hypertension produced via this reflex stimulate baroreceptors, which results in vagal-mediated bradycardia, manifested as late decelerations. This mechanism of late decelerations produced through the reflex arc occurs even in the absence of fetal acidemia. If left unchecked, chronic hypoxic stress will lead to fetal reliance on anaerobic metabolism and acidosis. The second mechanism of late decelerations occurs in the already acidotic fetus who suffers direct myocardial depression.

In general, exogenous oxytocin is used to evoke uterine contractions and is known as the oxytocin challenge test (OCT). The CST rationale and technique are explained to the patient at or prior to the first testing session. Blood pressure is measured prior to initiation of the study and every 15 minutes throughout. In semi-Fowler position, on a bed or in a recliner, the gravida has tocodynamometer and Doppler transducers applied, as in the procedure for the NST. A baseline 20-minute recording of fetal heart rate and uterine activity is accomplished. If three spontaneous contractions occur in 10 minutes, oxytocin is withheld and the procedure is considered completed. Failing a spontaneous CST, oxytocin is administered through a free-flowing intravenous line at a keep-open rate, beginning with an infusion rate of 0.5 mIU/hour. The rate is doubled every 20 minutes until three contractions in 10 minutes are achieved. When criteria for adequate uterine frequency are reached, the oxytocin is discontinued. The patient is instructed to record fetal movements by depressing a button, which represents an "event" on the uterine activity channel. At our institutions, the OCT is performed on labor and delivery, because this study follows one or more nonreassuring fetal surveillance examinations.

Nipple stimulation, rather than oxytocin, may be used to induce uterine activity. The technique of Huddelston is described. The gravida is instructed to gently stroke one nipple, through her clothes, with the palmar surface of her fingers for 2 minutes. After a rest period of 5 minutes, stimulation for 2 minutes is resumed. The stimulation-rest cycle is repeated until adequate contractions are achieved. Mothers are instructed to cease breast stimulation at the onset of uterine activity until the frequency of contractions can be assessed. The use of this methodology resulted in a 2% hyperstimulation rate, with no failed tests in 345 trials. Regardless of the method employed to evoke uterine contractions, the patient is monitored until uterine contractions diminish to pretest frequency and any late decelerations resolve.

Interpretation of the CST according to Freeman's criteria is outlined in Table 28-3. Each tracing is evaluated for the presence or absence of late decelerations associated with contractions and the presence or absence of fetal heart rate accelerations. It appears that late decelerations associated with 50% of uterine contractions would satisfy most authorities. A CST is said to be suspicious if late

**TABLE 28-3.** Interpretation of the Contraction Stress Test

| Interpretation | Criteria |
| --- | --- |
| Nonreactive | No acceleration of at least 15 bpm in amplitude or of 15-second duration during test |
| Reactive | Any acceleration $\geq$15 bpm for $\geq$15 seconds during test |
| Negative | No late deceleration with a contraction frequency of at least 3 per 10 min |
| Positive | Consistent, persistent late decelerations, regardless of contraction frequency, in the absence of uterine hyperstimulation |
| Equivocal | |
| Suspicious | Nonpersistent late decelerations |
| Hyperstimulation | Fetal heart rate deceleration in the presence of uterine activity exceeding 5 per 10 minutes or duration >90 seconds |

decelerations occur in association with uterine contractions but are neither consistent nor persistent. Therefore, a suspicious CST is defined by late decelerations occurring with fewer than 50% of contractions. An unsatisfactory CST occurs in the presence of insufficient tracing of fetal heart rate or inability to achieve the critical uterine contractile pattern of three contractions in 10 minutes. If late decelerations persistently accompany contractions, it is not necessary to achieve three contractions in 10 minutes to assign a positive test result.

A negative, reactive contraction stress test is thought to signify adequate placental respiratory reserve. The incidence of antepartum fetal deaths within 1 week of study per negative CST is 0.2% to 0.7%. Proponents of the CST recommend subsequent examinations weekly in the presence of a stable maternal condition. The exception is insulin-dependent diabetes, in which some type of testing should occur twice weekly.

The object of the CST, as with other forms of antepartum testing, is to prevent perinatal mortality. It is effective in this regard, but it is not a perfect test. In one study, the perinatal mortality rate was 114/1000, compared to 31/1000 in the negative CST group. Sixty-seven percent of the positive tests were falsely positive and 17% of the negative tests were falsely negative with respect to the occurrence of late decelerations in labor. Specificity of the CST is reportedly variable, but is over 90% in half of the studies reviewed by Thacker.[||]

The incidence of false-negative CSTs is 0% to 8% with respect to perinatal mortality in a recent large review. False-positive results are particularly problematic in the overall assessment of the efficacy and reliability of contraction stress testing. Review of the literature reveals the incidence of false-positive results to be greater than 50% in 19 of 30 studies. Unfortunately, intervention based on a false-positive test result could result in unnecessary morbidity due to prematurity. Therefore, unless several surveillance techniques (generally NST or CST and biophysical profile) reveal fetal compromise, attempts should be made to ascertain fetal maturity.

As an alternative to the use of oxytocin, the CST can be performed via nipple stimulation to invoke uterine contractions. Nipple stimulation results in release of endogenous oxytocin. Failure to achieve uterine activity meeting the criteria for an adequate CST occurs in 0% to 31% of reported series requiring follow-up with the classic OCT. Several investigators report predictability to be similar to the classic OCT or to spontaneously occurring CSTs, but with considerable savings in time. In a prospective, randomized trial, some researchers found the nipple-stimulation CST not to save time overall when the time necessary to perform OCT following a failed test was taken into account.

Contraindications to the contraction stress test are described in Table 28-4. Disadvantages of the oxytocin challenge CST include the following:

1. The procedure is invasive, requiring peripheral access, unless spontaneous contractions or a nipple-stimulation CST is performed.
2. The time taken to achieve the desired contraction pattern may be considerable—90 to 120 minutes.

[||] Thacker SB, Berkelman RL. Assessing the diagnostic accuracy and efficacy of elected antepartum fetal surveillance techniques. Obstet Gynecol Surv 1986;41:121.

**TABLE 28-4.** Contraindications to the Contraction Stress Test

Classical cesarean section scar (or previous myomectomy)
Placenta previa
Premature rupture of membranes
Preterm labor in current gestation
Multiple gestation
Incompetent cervix

3. The occurrence of equivocal results may further add to the time necessary to achieve a prognostic test.
4. The cost is greater than that of other testing techniques that do not require intravenous access and constant attendance of personnel capable of administering an OCT.

These reasons, and the rise in popularity of ultrasonic methods of biophysical assessment, have kept the CST as a secondary method of antepartum surveillance in many institutions. When the advantages and disadvantages of the NST and CST are compared, it appears that the NST is more suitable for large-scale screening.

## ANTEPARTUM TESTING TECHNIQUE COMPARISONS

It should be considered that the primary goal of both methods of antepartum heart rate testing is the timely termination of pregnancy in order to prevent perinatal mortality. In fact, to this end, both the CST and the NST have low rates of false-negative results.

As previously outlined, the NST measures fetal well-being by assessment of functional and neurologic integration of the parasympathetic and sympathetic nervous system as predicted by fetal heart rate. The CST evaluates the functional respiratory reserve of the fetus by classification of fetal heart rate response to reduced intervillous space blood flow caused by uterine contractions. In general, these two tests of antepartum surveillance are considered to be interchangeable. In fact, each test evaluates different, yet overlapping, aspects of fetal condition.

There have been only a few randomized trials that assess the efficacy of the NST, and none for the CST. The total number of patients in these studies is not high enough to achieve the statistical power to make meaningful negative conclusions. The nonstress test and the contraction stress test have been found to be of similar predictive value in the identification of an unhealthy fetus.

Correlation between a reactive NST and a negative CST is excellent (99.4%), but between a nonreactive NST and a positive CST is poor (24.9%). Although this suggests that the CST is a better indicator of morbidity, this is only true in the presence of a nonreactive NST.

The limitations of antepartum heart rate testing must also be recognized. The brain stem rather than the cerebral cortex controls fetal heart rate modulation. A fetus with cortical damage is capable of normal antepartum heart rate testing, yet will not have normal neurological development. An infant who has suffered in utero compromise but has an intact brain stem may not show alterations in antepartum testing.

## CONGENITAL ANOMALIES

A proportion of fetuses with congenital malformations display aberrations in antepartum heart rate testing and abnormal fetal activity profiles. As many as 51% demonstrate abnormal fetal heart rate tracings in the antepartum period or during labor. An abnormal NST or CST is associated with a lethal anomaly in 2.54% of cases, whereas the general population incidence of anomalies is about 1%. Indeed, fetuses identified as having persistently abnormal NSTs should undergo ultrasonic anatomic survey, most conveniently performed at the time of biophysical profile.

## SUMMARY

Current forms of antepartum heart rate testing are conspicuously more successful in correctly identifying the fetus who is normal than in identifying the fetus in jeopardy. There is no consensus regarding the best antepartum routine to evaluate fetal well-being. The biophysical tests outlined have different end points that must be considered, and measure somewhat different aspects of uteroplacental function. It is inappropriately believed by some clinicians that a reassuring antepartum heart rate test is a 1-week life insurance policy for the fetus. It should be remembered that the obstetric and metabolic stability of the mother is tantamount to a successful outcome, even in the face of a normal test.

# 29. INTRAPARTUM SURVEILLANCE FOR FETAL OXYGEN DEPRIVATION

## THE REASON FOR INTRAPARTUM FETAL SURVEILLANCE

The principal reason to monitor the fetus during labor is to evaluate the fetal oxygenation status. A number of causes for fetal/newborn morbidity and mortality may be evident at birth. The only cause for fetal/newborn morbidity and mortality that has a potentially remediable origin during the labor process is fetal oxygen deprivation. If fetal oxygen deprivation can be identified sufficiently early, before neurological damage has occurred, the fetus may be appropriately managed in utero or removed from the uterus prior to the occurrence of permanent neurological loss. If operative intervention is delayed beyond a critical point, fetal oxygen deprivation may lead to permanent neurological damage or even death. Recent studies have demonstrated that remediable fetal oxygen deprivation-induced neurological damage occurring during labor is considerably less common than prior expectations had calculated.

When fetal oxygen deprivation occurs and the Kreb's cycle does not produce sufficient ATP, then a nonoxidative process is employed to produce ATP. The Embden-Meyerhof pathway produces smaller amounts of ATP, and the by-products are pyruvic and lactic acid. Pyruvic acid is rapidly converted into lactic acid. Lactic acid in sufficiently great concentration will cause brain cell damage.

As it is currently understood, fetal oxygen deprivation is a function of an inadequate supply of oxygen delivered to the fetus as a result of blood flow from the maternal circulation to the placenta and the intervillous space. Uteroplacental insufficiency may have its clinical cause in problems such as maternal hypotension, maternal hypertension, uterine hyperactivity, severe forms of anemia, and so on. Because the umbilical cord has no rigid protective support, it is possible to interrupt blood flow and the delivery of oxygen to the fetus by umbilical cord compression. On occasion cord compression may produce sufficient oxygen deprivation to necessitate an early delivery.

The form of intrapartum fetal oxygen deprivation which the obstetrician is currently equipped to recognize and manage is acute fetal oxygen deprivation due to alterations in uteroplacental or fetal-placental blood flow delivery of oxygen to the fetus. The manner in which this occurs is relatively simple. The intramyometrial pressure rises during a uterine contraction, as a function of that contraction. If this elevation in pressure becomes greater than the pressure responsible for providing blood flow to the placenta, then a decrease in flow occurs.

An infant that is markedly depressed at birth, as evidenced by very low Apgar scores, marked fetal metabolic acidosis, seizure activity shortly after birth, and evidence of other neonatal organ system insult or damage, can point to intrapartum fetal oxygen deprivation of the acute type.

## SURVEILLANCE TECHNIQUES
## FOR FETAL OXYGEN DEPRIVATION

The principal screening surveillance technique for the intrapartum evaluation of the fetal oxygenation state is *fetal heart rate monitoring*. With normal fetal heart rate data, most investigators consider that it is safe to allow labor to continue toward completion and delivery.

*Intermittent fetal heart rate monitoring* is currently performed by three different methods. The first is the use of a Doppler/ultrasound device that is hand-held with a transducer placed over the gravid abdomen. In a similar technique, a stethoscope is placed over the gravid abdomen and the actual heart tones are obtained. The third technique involves the intermittent use of continuous electronic fetal heart rate monitor (either external or internal) to detect, instantaneously calculate, and automatically record the fetal heart rate on graphic tracing.

The technique for the evaluation of fetal oxygenation can be used in almost all low-risk labors, as well as most appropriately selected high-risk pregnancy labors. A stethoscope (fetoscope) or a hand-held Doppler device is used to listen to the fetal heart tones for evaluation. The recommended procedure for intermittent fetal heart rate monitoring as outlined by NAACOG is given below:

Palpate the maternal abdomen to identify the fetal presentation and position (Leopold's maneuvers).

Place the bell of the fetoscope or Doppler device over the area of maximum intensity of the fetal heart sounds (usually over the fetal back).

Place a finger over the maternal radial pulse to differentiate maternal–fetal heart rate.

Palpate for uterine contractions using the period of fetal heart rate auscultation to clarify relationship between fetal heart rate and uterine contractions.

Count fetal heart rate during a uterine contraction and for 30 seconds thereafter to identify fetal response.

Count fetal heart rate between uterine contractions for at least 30 to 60 seconds to identify average baseline rate.

If distinct differences are made between counts, recounts for longer periods are appropriate to clarify the presence of possible periodic fetal heart rate changes such as abrupt versus gradual changes.

To clarify accelerations, recounts for multiple brief periods of 5 to 10 seconds may be particularly helpful.

The frequency of fetal heart rate determinations varies depending on the probability of fetal oxygen deprivation (high risk versus low risk). It is recommended that for low-risk patients the fetal heart rate should be determined at least every hour in the latent phase of labor, every 30 minutes in the active phase of labor, and every 15 minutes during the second stage of labor. When monitoring high-risk patients, it is recommended that the fetal heart rate be determined every 30 minutes during the first stage of labor and in latent labor, every 15 minutes in active phase labor, and every 5 minutes during the second stage of labor.

When using intermittent Doppler/stethoscopic fetal heart rate monitoring, traditionally reassuring rates have varied from 110 to 120 beats per minute at the lower range and 150 to 160 beats per minute at the upper range. It is normal to note the presence of fetal heart rate accelerations in the absence of decelerations following contractions. The fetal rate of 100 to 119 beats per minute in the absence of other nonreassuring fetal heart rate data is generally not associated with fetal compromise. Nonreassuring fetal heart rate data include a baseline fetal heart rate of less than 100 beats per minute; fetal heart rate of less than 100 beats per minute 30 seconds after a contraction or an unexplained fetal baseline tachycardia greater than 160 beats per minute, especially if the patient is at risk and tachycardia persisting through three or more contractions in spite of corrective measures (it should be noted that a moderate bradycardia of 80 to 100 beats per minute may be associated with fetal head compression and not necessarily associated with non-reassuring patterns).

When it is ascertained that an abnormality may exist, the use of additional methods of evaluation for potential fetal oxygenation are employed and include external continuous fetal cardiotocography, internal continuous fetal cardiotocography, fetal scalp blood sampling for acid–base determinations, or fetal stimulatory data that correlate fetal heart rate accelerations to acid–base data to gain commentary regarding fetal acid–base status. This often includes umbilical cord arterial and venous respiratory blood gas determinations at delivery.

*Continuous electronic fetal heart rate monitoring* is performed by two methods. External continuous fetal heart rate monitoring is carried out extra-amniotically from transducers that are placed on the gravid abdomen overlying the fetal heart. Currently, the most commonly used technique is that of a Doppler/ultrasound device that detects one of four cardiac events (aortic opening, aortic closing, mitral opening, or mitral closing); with each beat of the fetal heart, the cardiotachometer instantaneously calculates and causes the rate to be recorded on a graph.

Once the cervix dilates to 1 to 2 cm and the chorioamnion is or has been ruptured, one may apply an electrode to the fetal presenting part for the collection of fetal electrocardiographic signals and place an intrauterine pressure catheter for the collection of uterine activity data in the form of intra-amniotic pressures. The value of internal continuous electronic monitoring over external continuous fetal heart rate monitoring and intermittent fetal heart rate monitoring is that, with an electrode attached to the fetal presenting part and with an intrauterine pressure catheter positioned, precise information regarding fetal heart rate and uterine activity is available on a continuous basis. With external monitoring, some degree of variation in rate may occur due to nonpredictability in the selection of one of the four cardiac events (aortic opening, aortic closing, mitral opening, and mitral closing). At the same time, when a tocodynamometer is used to detect uterine activity, precision relating to quantitation of uterine activity in terms of frequency, duration, and amplitude of a contraction is lost, whereas the use of intrauterine pressure to represent uterine contractions is a continuous and quantitatively precise database for evaluation.

Using internal monitoring, the "R" wave from the fetal ECG is obtained and the temporal interval between each "R-R" interval is measured in milliseconds. A calculation for rate is made based on the assumption that the "R-R" interval would be uniform for a whole minute. Each "R-R" interval's rate is individually recorded. For a rate of 120 beats per minute, the "R-R" interval is 500 milliseconds. Instantaneously calculated fetal heart rate and intrauterine pressure are recorded on graph paper that moves uniformly at a given speed. Usually the graph paper speed is 3 cm/min, although 1 cm/min may be used to save paper. Vertical scaling is from 30 to 240 beats per minute and covers a 7-cm vertical distance and from 0 to 100 mmHg over a 4-cm vertical distance. Generally, wider vertical lines occur once every minute.

The *baseline rate* is that rate in between contractions and represents persistent periods for an interval of 10 minutes or greater of heart rate at a given level. Fetal heart rate above 160 beats per minute is classified as a baseline tachycardia, and rates below 120 beats per minute are classified as fetal bradycardia. It is generally thought that rates between 120 and 160 beats per minute are in the normal range; however, rates of 90 to 180 beats per minute are not uncommon or necessarily abnormal in the absence of other abnormal fetal heart rate markers. Persistent fetal bradycardia or tachycardia is slightly more likely to be associated with some degree of fetal oxygen deprivation than a normal rate. Other conditions may cause a fetal tachycardia or a fetal bradycardia. These include maternal fever, fetal infection, maternal thyrotoxicosis, fetal anemia, and fetal tachyrhythmias that cause fetal tachycardia. A fetal bradycardia may be observed in patients managed with pharmacologic agents such as beta blockers (e.g., propranolol), in the fetus with cephalic presentation in a posterior position, and in the fetus with a congenital heart block. In instances in which the mother receives certain drugs such as beta-sympathomimetic tocolytic agents or vagolytic agents such as scopolamine or atropine, a fetal tachycardia may be observed. In instances where the mother has systemic lupus erythematosus, an antibody may be produced that crosses the placenta and damages the fetal heart's conduction system, causing a congenital heart block.

A *sinusoidal fetal heart rate* occurs infrequently, but may be of considerable clinical importance. This baseline rate is usually within the normal range of 120 to 160 beats per minute. There usually is an absence of short-term variability. The rate is relatively smooth and has a somewhat undulating pattern of uniform, long-term variability with an aptitude of 5 to 20 beats per minute that resembles a sine wave. A sinusoidal fetal heart rate is often noted with fetal anemia, particularly with Rh isoimmunization. The sinusoidal-like heart rate can be seen following the administration of narcotic analgesic and related agents. The presence of a persistent nonpharmacologically induced fetal sinusoidal heart rate is generally thought to represent potential fetal oxygen deprivation. To allow labor to continue, it is necessary to obtain information regarding fetal anemia and fetal acid-base status.

*Fetal heart rate variability* in the form of normal beat-to-beat heart rate variability is perhaps the most reliable indicator of fetal well-being that is available to the obstetrician. Normal fetal heart rate variability recorded on a graph represents one of the best indicators of intact integration between the nervous system of the fetus and the fetal cardiovascular system. Although the loss of fetal heart rate variability potentially may suggest fetal hypoxia, other factors may be responsible, including fetal sleep state, pharmacologic agents that depress the central nervous system, a fetal tachycardia greater than 180 beats per minute, and anomalies of the heart and central nervous system. It is possible for a fetus of a gestational age of 28 or more weeks to demonstrate normal fetal heart rate variability. Without other significant markers of potential fetal oxygen deprivation, a reduction or loss of fetal heart rate variability represents a potential of less than 2% for a significant degree of fetal oxygen deprivation.

*Periodic heart rate* or *fetal heart rate patterns* are transient alterations in the fetal heart rate associated with uterine contractions. These may be transient increases or transient decreases in heart rate, which are referred to as accelerations or decelerations. Generally, these transient changes are temporally related to the onset of a contraction and return to baseline heart rate prior to the onset of the next contraction. An *acceleration* in the fetal heart rate may occur at any time, but is frequently associated with a contraction and may be seen with a breech presentation. Generally, the acceleration is thought to represent early or mild cord compression and is a sympathetic nervous system response. The fetal heart rate acceleration is perhaps the single best indicator of adequate fetal oxygenation and generally is thought to represent a healthy fetus.

There are four forms of fetal heart decelerations that may be noted during the course of labor. *Early deceleration* is generally thought to be secondary to fetal head compression as the head moves through the dilating cervix and the bony pelvis. Early deceleration is termed such inasmuch as deceleration begins as the contraction begins, and it represents an inverted mirror image of the uterine contraction, reaching its greatest point of deceleration as the acme of the contraction is reached and returning to baseline as the contraction is terminated. Early deceleration is mediated by the vagus nerve with the release of acetylcholine at the sinoatrial node. It does not fall below 110 to 100 beats per minute. Classical early deceleration has been demonstrated by a number of studies to be completely innocuous

**TABLE 29-1.** Principles of Grading Variable and Late Decelerations

| Criteria of Grading | Mild | Moderate | Severe |
|---|---|---|---|
| Variable deceleration; level to which FHR drops and duration of deceleration | <30 sec duration, regardless of level >80 bpm, regardless of duration 70–80 bpm, <60 sec | <70 bpm, >30–<60 sec 70–80 bpm, >60 sec | <70 bpm, >60 sec |
| Late deceleration; amplitude of drop in FHR | <15 bpm | 15–45 bpm | >45 bpm |

bpm, beats per minute; FHR, fetal heart rate.
From Kubli FW, Hon EH, Khazin AF, et al. Observations on heart rate and pH in the human fetus during labor. Am J Obstet Gynecol 1969;104:1190

and does not represent any degree of fetal oxygen deprivation or acidosis (see Tables 29-1, 29-2, and 29-3).

*Variable deceleration* may begin before, at the onset of, or following the onset of a uterine contraction. On occasion, it may be seen independent of a uterine contraction. Variable deceleration usually drops many beats per minute in absolute rate within a few fetal heartbeats. It is occasionally referred to as the V or W shape deceleration because of this sudden drop and often a sudden return to baseline. It is somewhat jagged, irregular, or sawtoothed in nature and may last from just a few seconds to a minute or more. The criteria for grading the severity of variable deceleration are given in Table 29-1. Mild variable deceleration is usually innocuous. Repetitive and severe variable deceleration, particularly if it is prolonged, when associated with rising baseline heart rate, loss of beat-to-beat variability, and loss of acceleration prior to the deceleration, may herald the onset of significant fetal oxygen deprivation. This pattern is thought to be mediated by the vagus nerve through the barochemoreceptors when the umbilical cord is compressed,

**TABLE 29-2.** Relationship Between Qualitative Periodic Fetal Heart Rate Changes and Mean Fetal pH

| Pattern | Kubli (1969)* | Beard (1971)† | Tejani (1975)‡ |
|---|---|---|---|
| Normal | 7.30 ± 0.04 | 7.34 ± 0.06 | 7.33 ± 0.01 |
| Accelerations | | 7.34 ± 0.03 | 7.34 ± 0.01 |
| Early decelerations | 7.30 ± 0.04 | 7.33 ± 0.05 | 7.33 ± 0.01 |
| Variable decelerations (all) | | 7.31 ± 0.05 | 7.30 ± 0.01 |
| Moderate | 7.26 ± 0.04 | | |
| Severe | 7.15 ± 0.07 | | |
| Late decelerations (all) | | 7.28 | 7.29 ± 0.01 |
| Moderate | 7.21 ± 0.05 | | |
| Severe | 7.12 ± 0.07 | | |

* From Kubli FW, Hon EH, Khazin AF, et al. Observations on heart rate and pH in the human fetus during labor. Am J Obstet Gynecol 1969;104:1190.
† From Beard RW, Filshie GM, Knight CA, et al. The significance of the changes in the continuous fetal heart rate in the first stage of labor. Br J Obstet Gynaecol 1971;78:865.
‡ From Tejani N, et al. Obstet Gynaecol 1975;46:392 and Obstet Gynecol 1976;48:460.

**TABLE 29-3.** Relationship of Fetal Heart Rate Pattern, Fetal Acid-Base, 5-Minute Apgar Score, and Umbilical Acid-Base

| Pattern | 5-Minute Fetal Scalp Blood pH | Apgar Scores ≥ 7 (%) | Umbilical pH ≥ 7.25 (%) |
|---|---|---|---|
| Normal tracing | 7.33 ± 0.01 | 92 | 91 |
| Accelerations | 7.34 ± 0.01 | 91 | 97 |
| Early decelerations | 7.33 ± 0.01 | 92 | 93 |
| Variable decelerations | 7.30 ± 0.01 | 78 | 77 |
| Late decelerations | 7.29 ± 0.01 | 63 | 66 |

Correlation of fetal heart rate–uterine contraction patterns with fetal scalp blood pH (1975).
Data from Tejani N, et al. Obstet Gynecol 1975;46:392, and Correlation of fetal heart rate patterns and fetal pH with neonatal outcome. Obstet Gynecol 1976;48:460.

causing fetal peripheral vascular resistance with a fall in fetal $pO_2$ and a rise in $pCO_2$. To be significant, the fetal heart rate usually falls below 90 beats per minute. Variable deceleration is the most common periodic pattern noted during the course of labor. As the umbilical cord is compressed, via the vagus nerve, acetylcholine is released at the sinoatrial node, causing a parasympathetic response or fall in fetal heart rate commensurate with the degree of cord compression, as long as the fetal heart rate does not fall below 80 beats per minute or the duration of the deceleration is not too long. It is uncommon for cord compression, even when repetitive, to be of major clinical significance; however, with moderate and severe variable decelerations, significant reduction in umbilical blood flow may occur with the accumulation of significant amounts of carbon dioxide in the fetal compartment, thus causing a respiratory acidosis (Tables 29-2 through 29-4). When the decelerations become severe, repetitive, or prolonged in duration, fetal oxygen deprivation, resulting in a metabolic acidosis, may occur. When this occurs and there is potential for significant fetal oxygen deprivation, a delay in recovery of the fetal heart rate to the baseline level may be noticed. When this is seen, steps should be taken to correct this pattern by alteration of maternal position, amnioinfusion, or use of a tocolytic agent to remove the stress of uterine activity.

**TABLE 29-4.** Fetal Scalp Capillary Blood Base Deficit Correlation (Collected Within 30 Minutes Prior to Delivery) With Fetal Heart Rate Patterns

| Fetal Heart Rate Pattern | Mean (mEq/L) ± SE | Range (mEq/L) |
|---|---|---|
| Normal | 6.98 ± 0.16 | 0.3–15.5 |
| Early decelerations | 6.97 ± 0.44 | 1.0–13.4 |
| Mild variable decelerations | 7.84 ± 0.19 | 2.0–13.4 |
| Moderate variable decelerations | 8.98 ± 0.44 | 2.5–21 |
| Severe variable decelerations | 10.44 ± 0.93 | 2.5–15.7 |
| Mild late decelerations | 9.29 ± 0.49 | 2.0–15.5 |
| Moderate late decelerations | 10.79 ± 0.43 | 4.8–16.8 |
| Severe late decelerations | 12.88 ± 0.77 | 10.1–18.8 |

Adapted from Hon EH, Khazin A. Observation of fetal heart rate and fetal biochemistry I. Base deficit. Am J Obstet Gynecol 1969;105:721, with permission.

Below 60 beats per minute, nodal control of the fetal heart may be lost. At the depth of a severe variable deceleration, a transient "cardiac arrest" for a few seconds may be noted. This is uncommon and, although it may be tempting to treat the finding with a vagolytic pharmacologic agent such as atropine, this should not be done because it only clouds the marker and does not improve fetal oxygenation. Management should follow the standard management for severe variable deceleration. This brief "cardiac arrest," even if repetitive, does not require an early instrument-assisted delivery or cesarean section. Fetal death or damage is almost never encountered.

*Late decelerations* are transient slowings of the fetal heart rate that are noted to occur after the onset of the contraction or late in the contraction phase of uterine activity. The deceleration reaches its lowest point following the acme of the contraction, and it returns to baseline well after the contraction is over. In many instances, the late deceleration will appear very much as an early deceleration that is delayed in onset. For this pattern to become clinically significant, it must be repetitive in nature. Most investigators believe that there is no such entity as a single late deceleration and that this pattern must be seen following three or more contractions to be called a late deceleration pattern. When the late deceleration is first noted, the deceleration may represent a reflex vagally mediated response, which is associated with normal heart rate variability. It has been noted that late decelerations develop from fetal myocardial hypoxia, trigger a chemoreceptor response, and cause transient fetal hypotension, thereby stimulating fetal barore-ceptors. The degree of potential fetal oxygenation deprivation for a deceleration pattern is related to the duration and depth of the deceleration, as well as the interval from the onset of the contraction to the onset of the deceleration. The shorter the interval from onset of contractions to onset of the deceleration, the greater is the likelihood of a greater degree of oxygenation deprivation. The same is true for the deceleration's duration and depth. The longer a deceleration pattern persists, the greater the likelihood of significant fetal oxygenation deprivation.

Late decelerations may indicate that uteroplacental insufficiency with decreased intervillous exchange between the mother and the fetus may exist, with persistent or intermittent fetal oxygen deprivation. The criteria for grading the severity of late deceleration are given in Table 29-1. Fetal oxygenation may be impaired as the uterine contraction peaks, thus limiting intervillous space blood flow. Poorly oxygenated blood ultimately reaches the fetus—thus the late timing of the fetal heart rate deceleration (see Tables 29-2 through 29-4). Late decelerations are noted with placental abruption, excessive uterine activity of either a spontaneous or oxytocin-induced nature, maternal hypotension, anemia, or ketoacidosis. Mild, repetitive late decelerations of only five to ten beats per minute may indicate a significant potential for fetal oxygen deprivation such that metabolic acidosis and neurologic damage may result. When the clinician notes the pattern of recurrent repetitive late deceleration, the pattern must be corrected by the usual common steps, inasmuch as up to 35% to 40% of these fetuses may have significant fetal oxygen deprivation. The temporal interval between the onset of fetal heart rate data that may indicate the potential for significant fetal oxygen deprivation and actual damage is unknown, but the interval probably ranges from approximately 0.5 to 2.0 hours. The customary correction plan consists of improvement of maternal hypotension, appropriate repositioning of the patient, administration of maternal oxygen, or reduction of the intensity and duration of uterine contractions with a tocolytic agent. For labor to continue with the presence of repetitive late decelerations, normal acid-base values must be obtained at a regular interval of every 15 to 20 minutes or commentary from fetal stimulation for evaluation of fetal well-being with the presence of fetal accelerations. The continuation of labor in the presence of repetitive late deceleration and a reassuring acid-base or fetal stimulatory test is most commonly carried out in the active phase of labor, when a delivery process is not too distant. This situation is most often applicable to a multipara whose delivery is expected quite shortly. It has been demonstrated that the cesarean section rate in this situation can be significantly lowered with the use of dual fetal surveillance with fetal heart rate and commentary regarding acid-base status.

*Prolonged deceleration occurs* infrequently and unexpectedly. Usually, the fetal heart rate will fall below 80 beats per minute and the deceleration can last for several minutes, in the manner of a prolonged variable or reflex deceleration. These sudden, prolonged decelerations can be related to uterine activity, fetal manipulation, conduction anesthesia with hypotension, supine hypotension, and a maternal respiratory arrest secondary to intravenous narcotic use. Although the mechanism for the deceleration is usually a reflex mechanism, as with a variable deceleration pattern, if there is no demonstrable, readily apparent, and correctable cause for the sudden prolonged deceleration, the fetal heart rate following recovery should be observed carefully. When a second or third sudden prolonged deceleration occurs, the patient may be moved to an operating room for corrective measures such as would be performed with a severe variable deceleration pattern, including maternal evaluation of blood pressure, repositioning, oxygenation, and so forth. The possibility of a prolapsed cord should be investigated. Intravenous fluid may be increased and oxygen may be given to the mother. If delivery is not too far distant, substantiation of a satisfactory fetal acid–base commentary may allow the labor to continue. If this pattern repeats with evidence of fetal oxygen deprivation by acid-base determinations, particularly when associated with the rising fetal base excess and a falling pH, an early vaginal delivery or an operative delivery may be prudent.

*Mixed deceleration.* Often this is a combination of late and variable decelerations, but on occasion there may be combinations of early and late or early and variable decelerations. In some instances, there may be combinations of accelerations and decelerations. When this mixed pattern deceleration is noted to be repetitive in nature, the labor should be managed according to the most ominous aspect of the mixed or combined pattern of deceleration.

*Fetal acid-base evaluation* by fetal scalp capillary blood sampling for fetal acidosis was used to monitor the well-being of the known high-risk fetus before continuous fetal cardiotocography was introduced in the late 1960s and early 1970s. Fetal acid-base monitoring represents an intermittent commentary regarding the acid-base status or well-being of the fetus. A 2-mm scalpel is used to make a single "stab-like" incision into the scalp or skin. Approximately 40 $\mu$L of blood (about 2 inches in the capillary tube) is needed to obtain a complete set of respiratory blood gases, including pH, $pO_2$, $pCO_2$, bicarbonate, and base excess. Following the collection, the incisional site is inspected and pressure from a forceps-held swab is applied through three contractions. The site is subsequently inspected through a contraction, and if there is no bleeding, the cone is removed. Using modern equipment and with minimal training, labor suite personnel can perform these analyses.

When the technique was introduced, at first Doppler- and stethoscopic-determined alterations in fetal heart rate were followed up by the collection of fetal blood for pH determinations. When there was no alteration in the intermittent form of fetal heart rate monitoring, fetal capillary blood samples were collected randomly during high-risk labors as a dual intermittent surveillance system, especially when chronic fetal oxygen deprivation could be present. Currently, determinations of the fetal acid-base status represent the most precise information that the obstetrician has available for the diagnosis of the loss of fetal health. A transient fall in fetal pH may be secondary to acute umbilical cord compression, leading to the accumulation of carbon dioxide with a resultant fetal respiratory acidosis. Of greater importance is fetal oxygen deprivation, which is due to impaired fetal oxygen-carbon dioxide exchange in the intervillous space. When there is fetal oxygen deprivation sufficient to cause use of the anaerobic (Embden-Meyerhof) pathway for energy production, lactic acid will be accumulated and the fetal pH level will fall. If sufficient fetal oxygen deprivation and acidosis develop, neurological damage or death may result. There is a close relationship between fetal capillary blood gas values that are collected just prior to birth and umbilical cord arterial values collected at birth.

Recent studies have demonstrated that it is uncommon to find significant fetal neurological damage until a pH range of less than 7.10 is noted, and it is possible that the value may be as low as 7.00. Normal umbilical cord blood and fetal capillary pH and respiratory gas values are given in Tables 29-2 through 29-8. Fetal

**TABLE 29-5.** One-Minute Apgar Score (355 Patients)

|  | Apgar Score | |
| --- | --- | --- |
| Fetal pH | 1-6 | 7-10 |
| ≥7.20 | 10.4% (false normal) | 64.4% |
| ≤7.19 | 17.6% | 7.6% (false abnormal) |

From Hutson JM, Bowe ET, Petrie RH: The reliability of fetal acid-base determinations for prediction of normal Apgar scores: a reappraisal using the 5-minute score. Society of Perinatal Obstetricians Abstracts 1982:99, with permission.

**TABLE 29-6.** Five-Minute Apgar Score (355 Patients)

|  | Apgar Score | |
| --- | --- | --- |
| Fetal pH | 1–6 | 7–10 |
| ≥7.20 | 1.7% (false normal) | — |
| ≤7.19 | — | — |

From Hutson JM, Bowe ET, Petrie RH: The reliability of fetal acid-base determinations for prediction of normal Apgar scores: a reappraisal using the 5-minute score. Society of Perinatal Obstetricians Abstracts 1982:99, with permission.

**TABLE 29-7.** Fetal Capillary Blood Respiratory Gas Values

| Normal | Respiratory Acidosis | Metabolic Acidosis |
| --- | --- | --- |
| pH 7.25–7.40 | Decreased | Decreased |
| $pO_2$ | Usually stable | Decreased |
| $PCO_2$ | Increased | Usually stable |
| Base deficit 0–12 | Usually stable | Increased |

**TABLE 29-8.** Normal Umbilical Cord Acid-Base Values

| | pH | $pO_2$ | $PCO_2$ | Base Excess |
| --- | --- | --- | --- | --- |
| Umbilical arterial | 7.242 (7.10–7.37) | 16.6 (6.8–33.4) | 49.9 (37.2–59.5) | −6.8 (−3.2——13.6) |
| Umbilical venous | 7.312 (7.20–7.42) | 28.9 (16.5–42.0) | 39.1 (33–49.8) | −5.5 (2.7——8.6) |

Adapted from Wible JL, Petrie RH, Koons A, et al. The clinical use of umbilical cord acid-base determinations in perinatal surveillance and management. Cl in Perinatology 1982;9:387, with permission.

capillary scalp pH values will normally fall in early labor, from approximately 7.35 to 7.25 at delivery. In clinical practice, it has been determined that serial pH determinations correlate best with the clinical setting and are probably of greater significance than an absolute value of one or two determinations of pH. Fetal heart rate variability provides important commentary on the severity of periodic patterns that may herald potential fetal oxygen deprivation.

A *base excess* (deficit) value is an indicator of fetal buffer reserves that are present to neutralize H+ ions or fixed acids. The base excess/deficit value can be clinically useful as an indicator of impending loss of fetal well-being when fetal pH values are satisfactory but the fetal heart rate pattern is the cause for concern (Table 29-4). The longer the fetus is exposed to recurrent stress, the more likely it is that its acid-base status will suddenly deteriorate. Recently, fetal stimulation for evoking a fetal heart rate acceleration or comparison to pH/buffer evaluation has become somewhat widely used as commentary regarding fetal acid-base status. This allows use of fetal acid-base status without the actual collection of fetal blood for determinations of pH and respiratory gases by a machine. A number of stimuli, including injections of cold sterile water through an intrauterine pressure catheter, pain from the pinching of the fetal scalp, physical movement of the fetus, or a noise as in a vibroacoustic stimulation of the fetal auditory system, have gained popularity in recent years.

Recent investigators have studied the use of an evoked fetal heart rate acceleration during fetal scalp sampling as a stimulation at the time of the collection of fetal capillary blood. It was observed that, during the fetal capillary blood collecting process, when the scalp was stimulated an acceleration of 15 beats per minute with an excursion away from baseline for 15 seconds or greater was almost always indicative of a pH value of 7.22 or greater. Conversely, the absence of a fetal heart acceleration when the fetus was stimulated is not absolutely predictive of a fetus who is acidotic; although some of the fetuses will be acidotic, the remainder will have a normal acid-base status. An acceleration in response to fetal scalp stimulation generally is accepted as a sufficient acid-base commentary to allow labor to continue. As long as an abnormal fetal heart rate is noted, normal acid-base commentary or acid-base determinations performed at intervals of every 15 to 20 minutes have been reliable to safely continue labor (see Tables 29-5 and 29-6). When this intermittent form of acid-base commentary is to be used over a prolonged period of time, it is probably prudent to collect a sample of fetal capillary blood, as well as a sample of free-flowing maternal venous blood, occasionally to substantiate a satisfactory acid-base status, inasmuch as fetal stimulation and correlation to accelerations for acid-base commentary is a relatively recent innovation.

Some investigators have used vibroacoustic stimulation during labor to bring about a fetal heart rate acceleration. An artificial larynx (AT&T, Parsippany, NJ 07054) that generates 81 decibels of mixed noise and vibration can be placed on the maternal abdomen, approximately one-third the distance from the symphysis pubis to the xiphoid process, to stimulate the fetus. Stimulation intervals of from 2 to 5 seconds are commonly used. Such a stimulation may evoke a fetal heart rate acceleration. With such fetal heart rate accelerations, generally the fetus is in good condition from the physiologic and acid-base status. When using the internal form of fetal heart rate monitoring, a 5-second vibroacoustic stimulation to the fetus that results in either a 10-beats-per-minute acceleration with a 10-second excursion away from baseline or a 15-beats-per-minute acceleration with a 15-second excursion away from baseline is correlated with a mean pH of 7.29 ± 0.07.

Umbilical cord pH and respiratory blood gas values are frequently used at birth to compare intrapartum fetal heart rate data with acid-base status and newborn condition (see Table 29-8). These values frequently help identify the degree of fetal/newborn oxygenation at delivery. Following the delivery, 10 cm to 30 cm of a doubly clamped segment of the umbilical cord is obtained, and using two preheparinized small syringes, samples of umbilical cord blood from the artery and vein are collected separately. The blood samples are analyzed for pH and respiratory gases and correlated to both newborn conditions and fetal heart rate data during labor. By placing the umbilical cord segment or the blood samples on ice, one may delay the actual determination by a half-hour or more but still obtain reliable determinations. Many obstetricians now include umbilical artery and vein pH and respiratory gases as an integral part of the delivery process.

*Uterine activity evaluation* is an exceedingly important part of intrapartum fetal surveillance. Many clinicians believe that manual palpation of the uterus for contractions or tocodynametric or external uterine monitoring is sufficient to carry out a successful intrapartum fetal surveillance protocol. Often this is the case; nevertheless, a careful evaluation of uterine activity that can be quantitated and evaluated may be critical in the high-resolution protocol. The early detection of dysfunctional labor secondary to inadequate uterine activity, although not totally dependent on internal quantitated monitoring of uterine activity, certainly is benefited by it. The early detection of a placental abruption can be very rewarding in some instances, and the evaluation of uterine activity for the establishment of the effects of drugs on labor and uterine activity, or progress in labor is equally rewarding. It is the use of uterine activity data for the proper identification of periodic patterns that is critically important. In many instances, the fetal heart rate data may be good and clear, but uterine activity surveillance, using an external form of fetal monitoring, is of such poor quality that the true identity of fetal heart rate changes cannot be easily appreciated. For this reason, the use of an intrauterine pressure catheter to evaluate uterine activity is recommended. Although many people believe that the presence of a foreign body such as an intrauterine pressure catheter is a cause of infection, the data do not support this.

## FETAL INTRAPARTUM MANAGEMENT

On occasion, when uterine activity is excessive, causing an immediate fetal heart rate abnormality, such as with significant variable decelerations, the temporary use of a tocolytic agent such as intravenous magnesium sulfate by an intravenous injection of 4 to 6 g over a 15- to 20-minute interval or 0.25 to 0.5 mg of terbutaline subcutaneously may reduce uterine activity sufficiently to allow the fetus to recover and then return to a productive labor.

In conditions where reduced amniotic fluid is a potential, such as labor with a premature fetus, intrauterine growth retardation, prolonged gestation, pregnancy-induced hypertension, and even diabetes mellitus, the use of an *amnioinfusion* to buffer the umbilical cord can be of considerable help, especially with significant cord compression in a premature fetus. The use of amnioinfusion in gestations complicated by meconium has been demonstrated to be of benefit. Some have found that amnioinfusion for the elimination of meconium is safe, simple, and effective. Amnioinfusion has been demonstrated to significantly reduce the thickness of meconium, the incidence of neonatal acidemia, and the incidence of significant meconium below the vocal cords at delivery. A number of protocols are used for amnioinfusion. Miyazaki (1983)* and Nageotte (1985, 1990)† have advocated the use of amnioinfusion for cord compression, and they use 0.5 to 1 L of normal saline infused at 150 to 200 mL/hour as long as the decelerative pattern persists. Once the pattern has been ameliorated, a maintenance infusion of 10 to 20 mL/hour is used. Until recently, amnioinfusion required warming of the saline solution to body temperature prior to infusion; recently, however, it has been reported that saline at room temperature has been found to be as effective as fluid warmed to body temperature.

## POTENTIAL PROBLEMS OF FETAL SURVEILLANCE

The critics of continuous fetal heart rate monitoring point out that this technique has caused the cesarean section rate to soar for obstetrically unwarranted reasons. There is no doubt that increased surveillance of the fetus has caused the cesarean section rate to rise to some degree; however, the impact of the increased attention

---

* Miyazaki FS, Taylor NA. Saline amnioinfusion for relief of variable or prolonged decelerations. Am J Obstet Gynecol 1983;146:670.

† Nageotte MP, Bertucci L, Towers CV, Lagrew DC, Mondanlou H. Prophylactic amnioinfusion in pregnancies complicated by oligohydramnios or thick meconium: a prospective study. Society of Perinatal Obstetricians, Tenth Annual Meeting, Houston [abstracts] 1990, page 78. Nageotte MP, Freeman RK, Sarite TJ, Dorchester W. Prophylactic intrapartum amnioinfusion in patients with preterm premature rupture of membranes. Am J Obstet Gynecol 1985;153:557.

paid to intrapartum fetal surveillance by the legal system is impossible to evaluate. There is no doubt that in programs where dual surveillance systems are used, the incidence of cesarean sections for fetal distress has actually declined.

The use of fetal stimulation to obtain a fetal heart rate acceleration as a marker of fetal acid-base status without collecting fetal capillary blood is being used with increasing frequency. This form of fetal surveillance would appear to be without problem, except for the possibility of not being able to identify the fetus with good acid-base status who does not respond with an acceleration.

Some obstetricians are somewhat uncomfortable following a patient with repetitive heart rate indicators of potential fetal oxygen deprivation in the presence of normal fetal acid-base evaluation. In an obstetrical unit that routinely uses acid-base determinations as a secondary surveillance system, especially when base excess is used, dual fetal surveillance is rarely found to be a problem. With repetitive stress, a normal acid-base status can deteriorate over a period of time; thus, it is important that as long as the fetal heart rate pattern is suggestive of potential fetal oxygen deprivation, commentary regarding acid base status is necessary every 15 to 20 minutes. In this particular instance, the use of fetal capillary blood pH and base excess will be more reassuring than pH alone. Base excess will enable the obstetrician to determine when the fetal buffer reserves are being exhausted, to be shortly followed by a deterioration in the pH values.

On occasion, the obstetrician will be required to monitor a multiple gestation in labor. Many commercial monitors now have the ability to monitor two fetuses on one unit. It is possible, by using two monitors, to evaluate up to three fetuses concomitantly. If internal monitoring is being used for the first fetus, a sterile tubing can be run from the dome of the strain gauge of the first monitor to the dome of the strain gauge on the second monitor. With appropriate filling of the tube connecting the two domes, intrauterine pressure can be available on both monitors for the proper evaluation of heart rate data in relation to uterine contractions. In the high-risk multiple gestation, some maternal-fetal medicine specialists believe that if one is unable to adequately monitor a fetus during labor, a delivery by cesarean section may be in order.

# 30.  AMNIOTIC FLUID ASSESSMENT AND SIGNIFICANCE OF CONTAMINANTS

## PHYSIOLOGIC ASPECTS OF AMNIOTIC FLUID

The amniotic sac is created approximately 12 days after fertilization, as follows: A cleft enclosed in the primitive amnion is found adjacent to the embryonic plate. It rapidly enlarges and fuses to the body stock. When it fuses with the chorion, the amniotic sac is created. Once formed, this sac fills with a colorless liquid, presumably from maternal plasma. This is the amniotic fluid.

With advancing gestation, the composition of the amniotic fluid changes. In the first half of pregnancy, the amniotic fluid is isotonic and similar to maternal plasma, but the amniotic fluid contains less protein concentration than maternal plasma and is devoid of particulate matter. By 20 weeks gestation, the osmolality and concentration of sodium and urea are similar to maternal serum concentrations. In the second half of pregnancy, the composition changes with increases in particulate matter. In particular, desquamated fetal cells, lanugo and scalp hair, and vernix caseosa increase in the latter half of pregnancy. While this is occurring, the osmolality of the amniotic fluid decreases. In effect, the amniotic fluid becomes hypotonic. In comparison with the first half of pregnancy, there is a 20 to 30 mOsm, or 10%, decrease with advancing gestation. Moreover, the osmolality of the amniotic fluid is approximately 92% of that of the maternal serum.

In many respects, amniotic fluid represents extracellular fluid, with a composition similar to fetal urine. The kidney, with its importance in urine production, appears to be the major contributor to the changes in the amniotic fluid in the latter half of pregnancy. For instance, there are noticeable increases in urea, creatinine, and uric acid. By 24 weeks gestation, the concentration of these urinary by-products is two to three times higher than fetal plasma; this change represents a 70% to 250% increase in the concentration of these compounds. Electrolyte changes similarly occur in the latter half of pregnancy. The amniotic fluid concentrations of sodium, potassium, and chloride are usually 20% to 33% less than the fetal and maternal plasma levels. In fact, the amniotic fluid sodium level is 92% of that of maternal serum.

Amniotic fluid protein increases progressively during the first 6 months of pregnancy. From 32 weeks to term, there is a progressive decline in the amniotic fluid protein concentration.

With the changes in amniotic fluid content, the amniotic fluid volume changes dramatically during pregnancy. These changes are frequently related to the mechanisms responsible for amniotic fluid production. For example, in the first half of pregnancy, the amniotic fluid volume is proportional to the increases in fetal weight. It is during this time that the fetal skin is highly permeable to water and sodium and can transport urea. By 25 weeks gestation, the skin becomes keratinized and becomes impermeable to the fluid in the uterine cavity.

In contrast to the first half of pregnancy, amniotic fluid regulation involves the complex interaction between fetal swallowing, tracheal fluid production, and urination. For example, although the role of fetal swallowing in controlling amniotic fluid volume is undefined, fetal swallowing does play a dominant role when the amniotic fluid volume is normal. Using radioactively labeled red blood cells, Pritchard (1965) was able to determine the impact of fetal swallowing during pregnancy.* From 16 weeks until term, he showed that the fetus swallowed 7 to 20 mL/per hour. This amounted to over 500 mL over a 24-hour period, equivalent to half the amniotic fluid volume in the term gestation.

It is estimated that at term, 50 to 80 mL of fluid per hour are generated. The true origin of the fetal tracheal fluid is less clear as to whether it represents previously swallowed or "aspirated" amniotic fluid or the respiratory tree's contribution to the amniotic fluid volume. However, tracheal fluid does play an important role in

---

* Pritchard JA. Deglutition by normal and anencephalic fetuses. Obstet Gynecol 19565; 25:289.

amniotic fluid volume dynamics, and may be a critical factor in the evolution of polyhydramnios.

In the latter half of pregnancy, fetal urine production is estimated to be 500 mL per day, and constitutes the major source of amniotic fluid. According to Pritchard, urine flow (output) equals swallowing (input), or 500 mL per day.

In the postdate period, fetal urine production declines and probably accounts for the reductions in amniotic fluid volume that are frequently observed.

## TECHNIQUES TO ASSESS AMNIOTIC FLUID VOLUME

With the introduction of ultrasonography, invasive techniques to assess amniotic fluid volume were no longer necessary. Instead, an array of ultrasound techniques were developed to estimate the amniotic fluid volume (Table 30-1).

With real-time ultrasound, a total intrauterine image could not be readily accomplished in a single view. As a consequence, newer techniques to assess the amniotic fluid volume were sought. In 1987, Phelan and associates described the amniotic fluid index. This technique for assessing amniotic fluid volume is illustrated in Figure 30-1. Using the umbilicus as one reference point, the uterus is divided into upper and lower halves. The linea nigra is then used to divide the uterus into right and left halves. The transducer is then placed on the maternal abdomen along the longitudinal axis of the mother, with the transducer perpendicular to the floor. The vertical diameter of the largest pocket in each quadrant is measured. The numbers obtained from each quadrant are summed. This summation represents the amniotic fluid index in centimeters for that patient.

In low-risk pregnancies, the mean amniotic fluid index was 16.2 ± 5.3 cm. As part of their investigation, these investigators established definitions for oligo- and polyhydramnios. Oligohydramnios was defined as an amniotic fluid index ≤5.0 cm, and polyhydramnios was considered whenever the amniotic fluid index was in excess of 25.0 cm.

Subsequent work has demonstrated that the amniotic fluid index is simple, easy to perform, and reproducible, and provides a semiquantitative measurement of the amniotic fluid volume. Recent evidence also suggests that 1 cm is approximately equal to 50 mL of amniotic fluid. The amniotic fluid index has the advantage that it can be correlated with changes in amniotic fluid volume during pregnancy. These findings suggest that it may be clinically useful for following the amniotic fluid volume in patients with premature rupture of the membranes or who are on amniotic fluid volume reduction therapy with indomethacin.

**TABLE 30-1.** Techniques to Assess Amniotic Fluid Volume During Pregnancy

|  | Technique |
| --- | --- |
| Gohari | Total intrauterine volume |
| Manning | "One-centimeter rule"* |
| Chamberlain | "Two-centimeter rule"* |
| Crowley | "Three-centimeter rule"* |
| Phelan | Amniotic fluid index |

*Vertical diameter of the largest pocket.

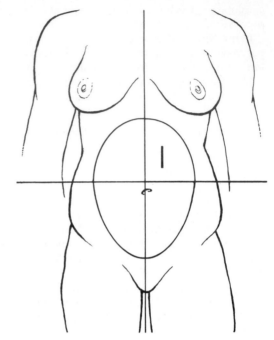

**FIGURE 30-1.** The uterus is divided into four quadrants. The linea nigra divides the uterus into right and left halves; the umbilicus divides the uterus into upper and lower halves. (From Phelan JP, Smith CV, Broussard P, et al. Amniotic fluid volume assessment using the four-quadrant technique in the pregnancy between 36 and 42 weeks. J Reprod Med 1987;32:540.)

## AMNIOTIC FLUID VOLUME DISORDERS

### POLYHYDRAMNIOS

Polyhydramnios is the pathologic accumulation of amniotic fluid. It is associated with a high maternal and perinatal morbidity and mortality. Quantitatively, polyhydramnios is considered whenever the amniotic fluid volume is in excess of 2000 mL, or when the amniotic fluid index is in excess of 25 cm. Under these circumstances, the incidence of polyhydramnios in a general population ranges from 0.2% to 1.6%.

To determine a cause for the polyhydramnios depends to a large extent on its severity. For example, Hill and associates (1987) found the cause to be apparent in 17% of patients with mild polyhydramnios and in 91% of those with moderate or severe polyhydramnios.[†] When a basis for the polyhydramnios can be found, the diagnosis usually falls into the following categories: fetal malformations and genetic disorders, diabetes mellitus, Rh sensitization, and congenital infections. A targeted ultrasound evaluation focusing on the more commonly identified fetal malformations is necessary (Table 30-2).

Commonly, polyhydramnios is associated with some impairment of the fetal swallowing mechanism. In the case of central nervous system abnormalities, the

[†] Hill, Breckle R, Thomas RL, Fries JK. Polyhydramnios: ultrasonically detected prevalence and neonatal outcome. Obstet Gynecol 1987;69:21.

**TABLE 30-2.** Fetal Malformations Commonly Associated with Polyhydramnios

Central nervous system
  Anencephaly
  Hydrocephaly
  Encephalocele
Gastrointestinal
  Gastroschisis
  Omphalocele
  Tracheo-esophageal fistula
  Duodenal atresia
Respiratory tract
  Pulmonary hypoplasia
  Chylothorax

From Phelan JP, Martin GI. Polyhydramnios: fetal and neonatal implications. Clin Perinatol 1989;16:987.

pathophysiologic mechanism may also be related to transudation of fluid across the fetal meninges or the lack of antidiuretic hormone and resultant polyuria.

In contrast, gastrointestinal tract abnormalities are not associated with an inability of the fetus to swallow, but are frequently due to an obstructive process, such as duodenal atresia. Moreover, the closer the obstruction is to the oropharynx, the greater is the likelihood of a pathologic accumulation of amniotic fluid. In the case of an omphalocele or gastroschisis, the polyhydramnios is believed to be due to transudation of fluid. Impaired swallowing in chromosomal errors such as trisomies 13 and 18 might also contribute.

Amniotic fluid also plays a direct role in pulmonary development and contributes in part to lung growth. In the fetal lungs, the flow of tracheal fluid is bidirectional. If there is an interruption of this exchange process across the surface area of the lungs, polyhydramnios can occur, as in conditions such as pulmonary hypoplasia.

In addition to fetal structural malformations, chromosomal and genetic abnormalities are also increased in polyhydramnic patients. In fact, the incidence of chromosomal abnormalities may approach 35%. The most common chromosomal abnormalities involve the trisomies 13, 18, and 21. Neuromuscular disorders may also be manifested clinically as polyhydramnios.

In the absence of a sonographic abnormality, the evaluation should also include screening tests for toxoplasmosis and cytomegalovirus, diabetes mellitus, and Rh sensitization. If these evaluations are negative, amniotic fluid volume reduction with prostaglandin synthetase inhibitors would seem reasonable.

## OLIGOHYDRAMNIOS

Oligohydramnios, little or scant amniotic fluid, is considered whenever the amniotic fluid volume is less than 400 mL or when there is an amniotic fluid index ≤5.0 cm. Multiple causes (Table 30-3) and consequences (Table 30-4) for this condition have been identified. The clinical focus will depend to a large extent on the trimester of pregnancy. For example, the finding of second trimester oligohydramnios should alert the clinician to the possibility of urinary tract malformations or preterm premature rupture of the membranes, whereas third trimester

**TABLE 30-3.** Clinical Conditions Commonly Associated with Oligohydramnios

| |
|---|
| Intrauterine growth retardation |
| Urinary tract malformations |
| Ruptured membranes |
| Postdate pregnancy |

**TABLE 30-4.** Potential Consequences of Oligohydramnios

| |
|---|
| Umbilical cord compression |
| Meconium-stained amniotic fluid |
| Fetal demise |
| Deformation syndrome |
| Pulmonary hypoplasia |
| Maternal/neonatal infection |

**TABLE 30-5.** Urinary Tract Malformations Associated with Oligohydramnios

| |
|---|
| Renal agenesis |
| Dysplastic kidneys |
| Polycystic kidney |
| Uteropelvic obstruction |
| Posterior urethral valve |

From King JC. Oligohydramnios In: Charles D, Glover DD, eds. Current therapy in obstetrics. Philadelphia: BC Decker, 1988:46.

oligohydramnios should alert the clinician to the possibility of intrauterine growth retardation or postdate pregnancy. In the latter circumstance, the estimated incidence of oligohydramnios is 20%.

Second trimester oligohydramnios is associated with a poor prognosis for the fetus. For example, of 34 pregnancies without premature rupture of the membranes, 9 (27%) fetuses had congenital malformations, 11 (32%) fetuses died in utero, and 6 (18%) had an entirely normal outcome.[‡] In contrast, patients with premature rupture of the membranes remote from term are more likely to have a favorable outcome.

Prolonged exposure to oligohydramnios can lead to the deformation syndrome, such as cranial, facial, or skeletal abnormalities, or pulmonary hypoplasia. Of patients with oligohydramnios, 10% to 15% will develop the deformation syndrome, and 17% are at risk for pulmonary hypoplasia.

Of patients with oligohydramnios unrelated to premature rupture of the membranes, urinary tract malformations are the most common abnormality (Table 30-5). As part of the evaluation, if possible, amniocentesis to assess the fetal chromosomal complement is also helpful in the subsequent management of these pregnancies.

[‡] Mercer LJ, Brocon LG. Fetal outcome with oligohydramnios in the second trimerster. Obstet Gynecol 1986;67:840.

Third trimester oligohydramnios should alert the clinician to these aforementioned possibilities, but should also give rise to the clinical suspicion of intrauterine growth retardation or a postdate pregnancy. The finding of oligohydramnios in the third trimester is associated with increased incidence of cord compression, with variable fetal heart rate decelerations, meconium-stained amniotic fluid, nonreactivity, and adverse perinatal outcome. Unlike the patient with premature rupture of the membranes, this kind of oligohydramnios is probably related to fetal compromise and associated with a less favorable outcome for the fetus. In the case of third trimester oligohydramnios, ultrasound evaluation will often need to be complemented by fetal heart rate monitoring to determine the extent of fetal compromise. Because of the potential for fetal compromise, these patients ought to be considered for delivery.

## CLINICAL APPLICATIONS

### ANTEPARTUM FETAL SURVEILLANCE

An outgrowth of amniotic fluid volume assessment is its implementation in the area of antepartum fetal surveillance (Table 30-6). Its present use is in combination with current fetal heart rate techniques, such as the nonstress test or contraction stress test. One study demonstrated not only an inverse relationship between pregnancy outcome and the amniotic fluid index, but also that this risk, although lessened by the presence of a reactive nonstress test, was significantly greater in the low amniotic fluid index group. Thus, patients undergoing testing for whatever indication will have an assessment of immediate (nonstress test) and previous (amniotic fluid index) fetal condition at each visit.

If the nonstress test (NST) is reactive and the amniotic fluid index is in excess of 5 cm, the patient is retested in 1 week or sooner, depending on the indication for testing. For example, patients with a history of diabetes mellitus, postdate pregnancy, and intrauterine growth retardation are tested twice weekly. All other patients are tested once a week, unless circumstances dictate earlier retesting. Those patients who manifest a nonreactive NST complete the remaining portions of the fetal biophysical profile (Table 30-7). If the fetal biophysical profile score is considered normal, the patient is retested at her usual testing interval. If the fetus has a score of 6, the test is considered suspicious and a repeat test is recommended within 12 to 24 hours. If, however, the patient manifests a fetal biophysical profile score of 4 or less, she is considered for delivery. In the term and postterm fetus, the indications for intervention include the presence of oligohydramnios (amniotic fluid index ≤5 cm), a fetal heart rate bradycardia, or a fetal biophysical profile score of ≤4. With term fetuses who exhibit a fetal heart rate deceleration during the NST and have a normal amniotic fluid index (>5 cm), repeat testing within 3 to

**TABLE 30-6.** Clinical Application of Amniotic Fluid Volume Assessment

Antepartum fetal surveillance
Fetal admission test
Premature rupture of the membranes
Amnioinfusion
Polyhydramnios

**TABLE 30-7.** Biophysical Profile Scoring System as Modified by the Use of the Amniotic Fluid Index for a 30-Minute Observation Period

| Component | Points |
|---|---|
| Nonstress–Reactive | 2 |
| Fetal breathing movements | 2 |
| Fetal movement | 2 |
| Fetal tone | 2 |
| Amniotic fluid index >5 cm | 2 |

4 days is recommended. If, at the time of repeat testing in the term fetus, the fetal heart rate deceleration pattern persists, consideration should be given for delivery by a trial of labor. In the postdate pregnancy, the fetus who exhibits a fetal heart rate deceleration is at significant risk for perinatal morbidity and mortality. As a consequence, induction of labor with oxytocin and continuous fetal surveillance during labor should be considered in order to reduce the morbidity associated with this fetal heart rate pattern. With this combination approach, perinatal morbidity and mortality can be significantly reduced.

## FETAL ADMISSION TEST

Third world countries have used the fetal admission test to reallocate risk status in labor. For example, patients with normal fetal surveillance test results are allocated to auscultation rather than continuous fetal monitoring. However, those patients with an abnormal admission test (a nonreactive fetal heart rate pattern with or without decelerations) undergo continuous fetal surveillance.

Although fetal heart rate patterns have been the basis for the fetal admission test, amniotic fluid volume assessment also appears to be a reasonable consideration. For example, a normal amniotic fluid volume in the nonlaboring patient is associated with a favorable fetal outcome. Similar results are seen in patients with normal amniotic fluid volume on admission to labor and delivery. More research is needed to confirm these observations.

## PRETERM PREMATURE RUPTURE OF THE MEMBRANES

Preterm premature rupture of the membranes affects 6% of all patients and is responsible for 30% of preterm deliveries. Ultrasound assessment of amniotic fluid volume appears to be helpful in predicting subsequent duration of pregnancy, identifying patients at risk for intrauterine infection and the potential selective use of amniocentesis, and in the antepartum assessment of fetal well-being.

Either on admission or subsequently, the assessment of amniotic fluid can serve as an indicator of potential underlying amnionitis. A low amniotic fluid volume or nonreactive fetal heart rate pattern has been shown to be associated with a 67% probability of intrauterine infection. Thus, patients with abnormal fetal surveillance tests on or subsequent to admission would appear to be candidates for amniocentesis to determine the presence of fetal infection.

With combined fetal surveillance testing with the NST and amniotic fluid index

**TABLE 30-8.** Potential Complications Associated with Polyhydramnios

| |
|---|
| Premature labor |
| Placental abruption |
| Puerperal hemorrhage |
| Perinatal mortality |
| Maternal respiratory difficulties |

done on a daily or less frequent basis, one can clinically monitor the changes in fetal status. For example, changes such as variable decelerations or a declining amniotic fluid index may represent a sign of early fetal infection. Late manifestations of an underlying fetal infection appear to be a loss of fetal movement and tone. Thus, with heightened scrutiny of fetal condition, intrauterine infection or impending fetal distress can be detected earlier.

Fetal assessment in the patient with preterm premature rupture of the membranes is similar to assessment in the patient with intact membranes. The key difference is that in the patient with preterm premature rupture of the membranes, the goal is to avoid, when possible, preterm delivery. If fetal heart rate decelerations or oligohydramnios (amniotic fluid index ≤5 cm) are observed, the patient is referred to labor and delivery for continuous electronic fetal monitoring. There, the patient is monitored to determine the extent or frequency of an abnormal fetal heart rate pattern or evidence of infection. Criteria for delivery are not well delineated. There does not appear to be a bright line to dictate the appropriate time of delivery in these circumstances. Thus, clinical judgment remains the mainstay of subsequent management.

## AMNIOINFUSION

Ultrasound assessment of the amniotic fluid volume may be used to determine candidates for amnioinfusion. The lower the amniotic fluid volume, the greater the likelihood of umbilical cord compression producing fetal heart rate decelerations.

Thus, many patients who present with repetitive variable decelerations during labor undergo cesarean delivery to remedy the fetal situation. However, restoration of the amniotic fluid volume with saline amnioinfusion has been shown to be effective in reducing the requirement for cesarean delivery for patients with this intrapartum fetal heart rate abnormality. In those series published to date, the overall cesarean delivery rate for fetal distress was reduced 87% in patients undergoing saline amnioinfusion.

In an effort to better identify those patients at risk for intrapartum fetal distress, Strong infused saline in a group of patients with sonographic evidence of oligohydramnios (amniotic fluid index ≤5 cm).[§] In the Strong series, the group receiving amnioinfusion had significantly lower rates of meconium passage, severe variable decelerations, end-stage bradycardias, and operative deliveries for fetal distress. Moreover, higher umbilical arterial blood pH values were also observed in the infusion group. The amniotic fluid index was kept in excess of 8 cm. At this level, significantly lower risk of an adverse perinatal outcome was observed.

[§] Strong TH, Hetzlre G, Sarno AP, Paul RH. Prophylactic intrapartum amnioinfusion: a randomized clincial trial. Am J Obstet Gynecol 1990;162:1370.

## POLYHYDRAMNIOS—VOLUME REDUCTION

Ultrasound is helpful in confirming polyhydramnios and determining the cause for the extra-amniotic fluid. Uncorrected polyhydramnios can be associated with a number of obstetrical complications (Table 30-8). Theoretically, these risks could be reduced with volume reduction.

Amniocentesis or prostaglandin inhibitors are the techniques commonly used for this purpose. The use of repeated amniocentesis to reduce the amniotic fluid volume is fraught with tremendous difficulty. For example, the amniotic fluid volume appears to turn over every 2.9 hours. As a consequence, any effort to reduce the amniotic fluid volume with amniocentesis would require placement of a catheter to permit amniotic fluid drainage or repeated amniocentesis. Either approach is associated with considerable discomfort for the patient and exposes the patient to a greater risk of infection or decompression-related complications, such as abruption.

Prostaglandin synthetase inhibitors have been suggested as an alternative to reduce the amniotic fluid volume. Indomethacin at a dose of 25 mg orally every 6 hours appears to operate by decreasing fetal urinary output or the amnion-chorion production of amniotic fluid. While patients are on indomethacin therapy, the amniotic fluid volume should be monitored frequently. The amniotic fluid index seems to be ideally designed to assist in the clinical management of these patients.

# PART IX. MATERNAL BIOLOGIC ADAPTATIONS TO PREGNANCY

## 31. MATERNAL BIOLOGIC ADAPTATIONS TO PREGNANCY

Remarkable anatomic and physiologic changes begin to occur in the female shortly after conception. The maternal-fetal interaction is the prime basis for these alterations, and it is necessary to have a thorough understanding of these changes in order to properly interpret normality and pathology during the gestation. Indeed, many of the biological adaptations could be considered major disease states if pregnancy were not present.

### THE REPRODUCTIVE TRACT

### THE UTERUS

Because the fetus, placenta, and amniotic fluid must grow and function within the uterus, it is necessary for the uterus to undergo some dramatic changes. The uterus in the nonpregnant state weighs approximately 40 to 70 g, depending on parity. The majority of uterine growth occurs as a result of myometrial cellular hypertrophy, although some hyperplasia is seen, particularly in the first trimester. The nonpregnant myometrial cell of 50 to 90 μm in length reaches 500 to 800 μm by term. By term, the uterine weight approaches 1200 g.

In the first trimester, uterine wall thickness increases, only to become thinner as the conceptual mass increases. In addition, the uterus becomes softer in pregnancy. Initially, the uterus maintains its pear shape. It becomes more spherical by 12 to 16 weeks gestation, and then becomes ovoid as length increases more than width. Another important change occurs in the isthmus of the uterus. By 12 weeks of gestation, this area has elongated to become part of the uterine cavity. Finally, this portion of the lower uterine segment becomes relatively thin, with decreased myometrial cellular content.

The uterus is known to contract in both the nonpregnant and pregnant state. Early in gestation, the uterus is relaxed, with sporadic contractions occurring. As term approaches, the frequency of these contractions increases.

In parallel fashion to the increase in uterine growth is a progressive increase in uterine perfusion. Although various approaches to indirect measurements in the human have been made, all with potential errors, uterine blood flow values in the range of 500 to 700 mL/min have been estimated in late gestation. The blood flow per gram of uterus and contents is probably relatively constant. At least 80% of the blood flow is to the placental implantation site, thus providing for the increased oxygen and nutrient needs of the developing fetal tissues.

## THE CERVIX

The cervix undergoes increased softening during pregnancy. This is due to a marked increase in vascularity, a change in connective tissue with decreased association of collagen fibers, edema, and a marked proliferation of the endocervical glands. These glands produce thick, tenacious mucus that obstructs the canal.

The explanation of parturition must include an understanding of the ripening process of the cervix, which permits the cervix to be withdrawn in back of the presenting part at term, after previously being an obstruction to the conceptus for many months. Although the exact etiologic mechanisms of cervical ripening remain to be defined, near term there is an increase in hyaluronic acid and increased collagen dissociation. It is thought that relaxin and arachidonic acid metabolites play a role in this ripening process.

## THE VAGINA

Increased vascularity lends a bluish purple color to the vaginal mucosa, the so-called Chadwick's sign of early pregnancy. In addition, there is a marked thickening of the vaginal mucosa, hypertrophy of the underlying smooth muscle, and a general loosening of the abundant surrounding connective tissue. All of these changes facilitate marked distensibility of the vaginal canal prior to parturition. The vaginal mucosa is rich in glycogen, and increased vaginal secretions (and cervical secretions) result in a more pronounced white, somewhat thick, acidotic discharge.

## THE ADNEXA

A significant change in the ovaries is that ovulation ceases and the corpus luteum of pregnancy persists with production of progesterone and maintenance of early pregnancy for the first 5 weeks after conception. The corpus luteum also secretes relaxin throughout pregnancy.

## THE CARDIOVASCULAR SYSTEM

### PLASMA VOLUME

Plasma volume rises progressively throughout pregnancy, beginning at approximately 6 to 8 weeks of gestation and tapering off at about 30 to 32 weeks of gestation. The normal primigravid woman can expect a total increase in plasma volume of about 40% to 50%. Women carrying multiple pregnancies have proportionally higher increases in plasma volume.

### RED CELL VOLUME

Total red cell volume increases by about 20% to 30% during normal gestation, depending on the use of iron supplementation. This increase in red cells progresses steadily between the end of the first trimester and term. The disproportionately larger increase in plasma volume relative to red cell volume results in a significant drop in maternal hematocrit, which is evident at the beginning of the third trimester. Red cell volume decreases dramatically at delivery as a result of blood loss, and the return to normal, nonpregnant blood volumes is accomplished by 3 weeks after delivery.

### PERIPARTUM CHANGES IN BLOOD VOLUME

Vaginal delivery of a singleton infant at term is associated with an average blood loss of 500 mL, and uncomplicated cesarean delivery results in an average blood loss of 1000 mL. The normal gravida with a prepartum hemoglobin of at least 12 g/dL can tolerate the loss of 1000 mL of blood without a significant fall in hemoglobin concentration. A significant drop in hemoglobin or hematocrit by 5 days after delivery is indicative of either inappropriate total blood volume expansion during pregnancy or increased total blood loss at the time of delivery.

The massive increase in total blood volume that occurs during pregnancy serves several purposes in the protection of both the maternal and fetal condition. The reserves in intravascular volume manifested by term offer some maternal protection against prepartum hemorrhage, as well as from late pregnancy hypotension, when an increased proportion of blood volume is entrapped by the lower extremities. The disproportionate increase in plasma volume over red cell volume results in a decrease in viscosity and, subsequently, a decreased resistance to blood flow. This mechanism allows the maternal increase in cardiac output to occur with a smaller proportionate increase in cardiac work. Much of the increased cardiac output of normal pregnancy is distributed to the skin, to allow for heat loss, and to the kidneys, to allow for excretion of both maternal and fetal metabolic waste. These excretory functions depend on an increase in plasma volume rather than red cell volume. The increase in red cell volume during pregnancy approximates the increase in oxygen requirement to support both maternal cardiovascular function and fetal growth.

## ANATOMIC CHANGES OF THE HEART AND GREAT VESSELS

Myocardial hypertrophy begins at the end of the first trimester. Myocardial contractility is also increased during gestation. The progressive upward displacement of the diaphragm, along with a small amount of benign pericardial effusion during pregnancy, increases the width of the cardiac silhouette on chest radiograph, making the diagnosis of cardiomegaly by nonpregnant standards inappropriate.

Several significant auscultatory changes are also evident during pregnancy. The first heart sound becomes louder and develops an exaggerated split between the mitral and tricuspid valvular closures. The second heart sound remains essentially unchanged. An audible third heart sound is present in close to 90% of gravidas by midgestation, and a fourth heart sound is audible in fewer than 5%, and is an indication of pathologic cardiac function. The ubiquitous systolic ejection murmur of pregnancy is best heard along the left lateral sternal border.

The increased blood volume and blood flow through the great vessels result in the anatomically prominent appearance of both the pulmonary artery and its vasculature on chest radiograph during pregnancy.

## CARDIAC OUTPUT

Cardiac output rises 30% to 50% during normal pregnancy, with the majority of this change occurring in the late first trimester, and a small but continued rise until approximately 32 weeks of gestation. Increased stroke volume is the predominant factor in the rise during the first half of pregnancy. Heart rate rises progressively throughout pregnancy and is responsible for the continued rise of cardiac output through most of the second half of gestation. Assumption of the standing position results in a significant drop in cardiac output.

The peripartum period represents a time of acute hemodynamic stress for the gravid patient. Maternal cardiac output in late labor is additionally increased by approximately 13% over the resting output. This additional increase in cardiac output is thought to be primarily due to a further increase in stroke volume. At the peak of uterine contractions, further increase in cardiac output by one third above the baseline value for labor occurs. The anxiety and pain associated with labor may produce increased catecholamine release and tachycardia, creating an additional slight increase in cardiac output. It is clear that these mechanisms will contribute to the potential rapid deterioration of the gravida with even minimal underlying cardiac dysfunction in the face of active labor, because pulmonary artery wedge pressure will be increased acutely during uterine contractions and may contribute to the development of pulmonary edema in these patients.

The choice of anesthetic for labor and delivery also affects cardiac output. The initiation of epidural anesthesia results in a 37% increase in cardiac output over baseline, whereas the induction of general anesthesia results in a 26% increase in cardiac output. The massive increases in cardiac output associated with normal pregnancy, labor, and delivery abate rapidly postpartum, as evidenced by a 25% decrease in cardiac output when measured 2 weeks postpartum.

## BLOOD PRESSURE

As with other cardiovascular hemodynamic parameters in pregnancy, the position in which blood pressure is measured is of critical importance. Although the maximal fall of systolic blood pressure during pregnancy is approximately 12 mmHg, diastolic pressures fall between 10 and 20 mmHg, resulting in an increased pulse pressure. Diastolic blood pressures higher than 90 mmHg at any time during pregnancy represent abnormal values. It has been postulated that diastolic blood pressures greater than 80 mmHg in the second half of pregnancy are not normal and may represent latent hypertension.

## DISTRIBUTION OF INCREASED CARDIAC OUTPUT

The increase in cardiac output observed during normal gestation is distributed among several maternal organ systems. The low-resistance uteroplacental circulation manifests a tenfold increase in blood flow. Figure 31-1 graphically represents the redistribution of maternal cardiac output during pregnancy.

## SUMMARY

Normal maternal physiologic adaptation to pregnancy results in a hyperdynamic state characterized by elevations in cardiac output, heart rate, and stroke volume,

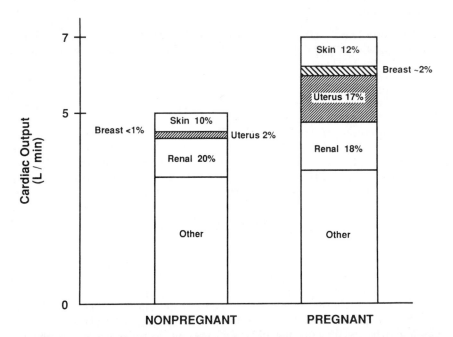

**FIGURE 31-1.** Distribution of maternal cardiac output in the nonpregnant and term pregnant state. Note that although the percentage of renal, skin, and breast blood flow does not increase, the absolute blood flow to these organs increases during pregnancy because of the large increase in cardiac output.

accompanied by significant decreases in systemic vascular resistance and mean arterial pressure. These hemodynamic changes maintain stroke work within a normal range, are evident by the end of the first trimester of pregnancy, and are clearly out of proportion to the needs of the growing fetus at that time.

## HEMOSTASIS DURING PREGNANCY

The normal physiological adaptation to pregnancy is marked by an increase in the hepatic production of coagulation factors. The dramatic increase in the production of fibrinogen results in an increase in fibrin, which is subsequently deposited in the vessel walls of the uteroplacental circulation. These changes are accompanied by a significant depression in fibrinolysis. Teleologically, one supposes that these changes, in combination with the increased blood volume of pregnancy, serve to protect the gravida from the potential catastrophe of severe postpartum hemorrhage. These mechanisms render pregnancy a hypercoagulable state.

The generation of prostacyclin by the vascular endothelium allows platelet adhesion, but prevents pathologic aggregation and thrombus formation. The disruption of the normal production and function of prostacyclin within vessels in diseases such as preeclampsia, hemolytic uremic syndrome, and thrombocytopenic purpura will make the vascular environment conducive to thrombus formation.

A recent review of all information on platelet counts during normal pregnancy would suggest that, if anything, there is a slight decrease in platelet count as normal pregnancy progresses toward term. There is also evidence of increased turnover of platelets, as well as low-grade platelet activation during pregnancy. It is generally accepted that the normal physiologic adaptation to pregnancy includes a chronic, low-grade intravascular coagulation within the uteroplacental vasculature.

## INTRINSIC/EXTRINSIC CASCADE CHANGES

Both activated partial thromboplastin time (aPTT) and prothrombin time (PT) have been reported to be reduced in pregnant women when compared with nonpregnant controls. The aPTT and PT are direct measures of the functionality of both the intrinsic and extrinsic mechanisms of coagulation. These two pathways merge to a final pathway following the activation of factor X. The intrinsic pathway evolves slowly, requiring approximately 5 to 20 minutes to result in visible fibrin formation. However, the lipoprotein thromboplastin, which is present in all tissues, markedly accelerates the rate at which blood clots. Thromboplastin is present in high concentrations in lung, brain, and placenta. Placental thromboplastin activation will produce the formation of fibrin within 12 seconds by bypassing the intrinsic pathway of coagulation. During pregnancy, there are increases in factors VII, VIII, X, and plasma fibrinogen, from the end of the first trimester.

Mechanisms are also in place that normally limit clot formation at the site of vascular injury in order to prevent generalized thrombosis. Antithrombin III (AT III), synthesized in the liver, is the major physiologic inhibitor of coagulation factors II, IX, X, XI, XII, and thrombin. To date, there is no information to indicate that pregnancy produces an alteration in AT III levels. Peripartum alterations of

AT III concentrations have been reported to be decreased at delivery and increased in the postpartum period, potentially increasing puerperal thrombosis development. Familial AT III deficiency results in an increased risk of thrombosis. The protein C-thrombomodulin-protein S system also exerts natural anticoagulant activity. Factors X and XIII are inactivated by protein C, which is a vitamin K–dependent substance also produced in the liver. Familial inherited deficiency of protein C or protein S results in increased risk of thromboembolic disease. Limited information is currently available on longitudinal measurements of this system throughout pregnancy, although the data available seem to indicate small fluctuations within the normal nonpregnant range throughout pregnancy.

## FIBRINOLYSIS

The physiologic adaptation to normal pregnancy includes a decrease in plasma fibrinolytic activity that persists through the process of parturition and then returns rapidly to normal within a short time after delivery of the placenta. The placental production of fibrinolytic inhibitors is responsible for this rapid alteration.

In summary, hemostatic changes in normal pregnancy are characterized by an ongoing, low-grade activation of the coagulant system. The deposition of fibrin has been documented in the uteroplacental vasculature (both spiral arteries and intervillous space). The smooth muscle and elastic lamina of the spiral arteries are eroded by the trophoblast and replaced partially by fibrin. These anatomic changes allow for increased vessel diameter, which accommodates the tenfold increase in uteroplacental blood flow by producing a decreased vascular resistance in the uteroplacental circulation. Increased levels of coagulation factors and fibrinogen allow the normal gravida to successfully coagulate the placental separation site at delivery. These changes result in a hypercoagulable state during normal pregnancy that places even the normal gravida at increased risk for thromboembolic disease during pregnancy and the puerperium.

## THE RESPIRATORY SYSTEM

### ANATOMICAL/MECHANICAL CHANGES

During pregnancy, the configuration of the thorax changes before there is any increase in uterine size that could exert a mechanical pressure. The level of the diaphragm rises by approximately 4 cm, the transverse diameter of the thorax increases by 2 cm, and the thoracic circumference increases by approximately 6 cm. The actual excursion of the diaphragm, despite the enlarging conceptual mass, is increased by 1.5 cm.

The upper airway also participates in the increased vascularity of pregnancy, leading to mucosal hyperemia and edema. The result is increased nasal stuffiness, and nasal bleeding is not rare.

### LUNG VOLUMES

Although the basic respiratory rate is unchanged during pregnancy, some rather major changes occur in various components of ventilation. The resting tidal volume is increased by approximately 40%, with a similar rise in minute ventilation. These changes occur in the first trimester, and they remain essentially unchanged for the remainder of gestation.

The residual volume (both the expiratory reserve volume and the residual volume) is decreased by approximately 20%. The effective alveolar ventilation is increased even further. The vital capacity is essentially not changed. Due to the decrease in functional residual volume, the total lung volume is decreased about 5%.

## PULMONARY FUNCTION

There is no significant change during gestation in large airway resistance. Oxygen consumption during pregnancy is increased by approximately 20%. The partial pressure of arterial oxygen ($PaO_2$) is minimally changed, and the arteriovenous oxygen difference decreased. Due to the increase in minute ventilation, the partial pressure of arterial carbon dioxide ($PaCO_2$) falls to approximately 30 mmHg very early in gestation. This decrease in $PaCO_2$ is compensated by an equivalent increase in renal excretion of bicarbonate and a resultant decrease in plasma bicarbonate concentration.

The increase in ventilation and the resultant decrease in $PaCO_2$ is due to progesterone, in part acting on the central respiratory center. In addition, carbonic anhydrase in red cells, which facilitates carbon dioxide transfer, is increased in pregnant patients and in patients receiving oral contraceptives. Despite, if anything, an improvement in ventilation during gestation, at least half of pregnant women experience a sense of breathlessness or dyspnea. The basis of this symptom has not been delineated.

## THE URINARY SYSTEM

### ANATOMIC ALTERATIONS

Both kidneys increase in overall size during pregnancy, increasing in length by 1 to 1.5 cm. In addition, there is a dilatation of the renal pelvis, and the calyceal system as well as the ureters above the pelvic brim. The portion of the ureters below the pelvic brim is rarely dilated. The ureters frequently elongate, become more tortuous, and may be displaced laterally.

The increase in dead space of the collecting systems may predispose to urinary tract infection, and alters interpretation of functional evaluation of the urinary system and intravenous pyelography. Urodynamic studies have shown that bladder pressure is doubled from the first trimester to late pregnancy, indicating a reduction in bladder capacity and increased demand on the ability of the urethra to close. A compensatory feature is that the absolute and functional lengths of the urethra are increased at the end of pregnancy by approximately 20%, along with a similar percentage increase in intraurethral closure pressure. These latter features tend to counteract the possibility of stress incontinence, which has been reported to be present to some degree in two-thirds of pregnant women.

## RENAL FUNCTION

Increases in effective renal plasma flow of approximately 50% over nonpregnant flow rates are present by midpregnancy and remain elevated until late pregnancy. The glomerular filtration rate (GFR) also increases in the first trimester. Creatinine clearances in the pregnant patient in midpregnancy approximate 140 to 160 mL/min, and near term approximate 120 mL/min. Serum creatinine concentrations approximate 0.7 mg/dL by the end of the first trimester and 0.5 to 0.6 mg/dL by midgestation. Blood urea nitrogen concentrations approximate 8 to 9 mg/dL by midgestation. Serum uric acid concentrations decrease by at least 25% in the first trimester, only to rise back to normal, nonpregnant levels by midpregnancy, reaching similar nonpregnant concentrations by term.

There is an overall net retention of approximately 1000 mEq of sodium distributed among the maternal extracellular space and the fetus. This positive sodium balance occurs gradually over the gestation. Increased tubular reabsorption is promoted by the increase in plasma aldosterone as well as other hormones, such as estrogen, deoxycortisone, and placental lactogen. Plasma osmolality, as a result of water retention in slight excess of solute, is reduced to approximately 280 mOsm/L, beginning in the first trimester. Although one would expect this decrease to promote a diuresis, this does not occur, probably because of a resetting of osmotic control thresholds. All three components of the renin-angiotensin-aldosterone system are elevated in pregnancy, beginning in the first trimester.

A number of nutritional substrates are also affected by the increase in glomerular filtration. At least 10% of an unselected obstetrical population may have random glucosuria, but less than 1% of these have abnormal glucose tolerance tests. There is a very slight increase of urinary albumin excretion of 7 to 18 ng/24 hours. Aminoaciduria also occurs in pregnancy.

## ORAL/ESOPHAGEAL/GASTROINTESTINAL SYSTEM

Nausea and vomiting occur early and are suggestive signs of early pregnancy. The basis for the increase in the first trimester of nausea and emesis, which typically occurs in the morning and tends to abate during the day, is unknown. It has been postulated that chorionic gonadotropins may play a role. Most women experience an increase in appetite by the end of the first trimester, and although quantitation is lacking, pica, defined as an abnormal craving for unnatural foods, is reportedly increased.

## ORAL CAVITY

The gingiva become softer and hyperemic during pregnancy, with the result that gingival bleeding increases in frequency. A specific pregnancy-related lesion, the epulis of pregnancy, may occur at any time. This is a localized vascular growth that is frequently pedunculated and is benign. It will usually regress after delivery, but may need excision for excessive bleeding.

The production of saliva is probably unchanged during gestation. Excessive salivation or ptyalism is an uncommon complication of pregnancy that can lead to loss of 2 liters of saliva a day. The cause is unknown.

Although some have suggested that tooth disease is increased, there is no evidence that the incidence or progression of dental caries is altered by the presence of gestation.

## ESOPHAGUS AND STOMACH

There is an increased potential for gastric reflux and esophagitis, giving rise to a high incidence of heartburn (pyrosis) experienced by pregnant women. The reported increased incidence of hiatus hernia during pregnancy could also contribute to the symptom of heartburn.

The stomach also has decreased tone and motility, which leads to delayed gastric emptying. Acid secretion is higher in the last trimester than in nonpregnant women. These features also predispose the pregnant patient to regurgitation and aspiration during inhalation anesthesia used for delivery.

## INTESTINES

There is decreased tone and motility of the small and large bowel, with resultant decreased transit times. There is approximately a 60% increase in water absorption in the large bowel which, combined with the decreased tone, leads to a high incidence of constipation during pregnancy. Constipation and increased circulating blood volume and venodilatation result in higher rates of hemorrhoidal formation.

## LIVER AND GALLBLADDER

### THE LIVER

Normal pregnancy is frequently associated with tests of hepatic function that would be considered abnormal results from the nonpregnant woman (Table 31-1). The bromosulfophthalein (BSP) test, when performed in pregnancy, shows reduced clearance of the injected dye. Various hepatic enzymes and proteins synthesized in the liver are also altered in pregnancy, and partially summarized in Table 30-1. The rise in alkaline phosphatase is due in part to placental production of a heat-stable isoenzyme, which can account for up to two-thirds of the enzyme activity. Serum albumin and total protein concentrations decrease in pregnancy. Serum albumin concentration is approximately 25% to 30% lower in pregnancy, or about 3 g/dL. There is a slight increase in the alpha and beta fractions of globulins, and an overall decrease in albumin/globulin. Serum concentrations of fibrinogen increase by approximately 50%, and clotting factors VII, VIII, IX, and X are elevated. Levels of prothrombin are unchanged. There is also a major increase in the serum concentrations of various lipids. Serum cholesterol concentrations rise linearly throughout gestation until near term, when they have approximately doubled.

### THE GALLBLADDER

Both fasting and residual gallbladder volumes are increased in mid- and late pregnancy to twice that observed in nonpregnant women. Because the decreased

**TABLE 31-1.** Changes in Liver Function Evaluations in Pregnancy

| | |
|---|---|
| Alkaline phosphatase | ↑ 2× |
| Alanine aminotransferase (SGPT) | ↔ |
| Albumin | ↓ 20% |
| Albumin/globulin | ↓ |
| Aspartate aminotransferase (SGOT) | ↔ |
| α and β globulin | sl ↑ |
| Bilirubin | → |
| Bromosulphalein clearance | sl ↓ |
| Ceruloplasmin | ↑ 2× |
| Cholesterol | ↑ 2× |
| Prothrombin | → |
| Fibrinogen | ↑ 50% |

motility in pregnancy would predispose to stone formation, it is thought that repetitive pregnancy may increase the probability of cholelithiasis.

## THE ENDOCRINE SYSTEM

### PANCREATIC FUNCTION AND CARBOHYDRATE METABOLISM

Normal pregnancy is characterized by hyperplasia of the insulin-producing beta cells. Fasting blood glucose in normal pregnancy decreases by 10% to 20% in the first trimester, long before fetal demands are significant. This fasting hypoglycemia is a result of pancreatic beta cell hyperplasia, increased insulin secretion, and an increased peripheral glucose usage. As pregnancy progresses and the growing fetus has greater nutrient demands, maternal glucose stores are mobilized and hepatic glycogenolysis occurs. Increasing insulin resistance during pregnancy is mediated by ever-increasing placental production of human placental lactogen and, to a lesser extent, prolactin and cortisol. In contradistinction to fasting hypoglycemia, postprandial glucose levels in normal pregnancy are elevated to approximately 130 to 140 mg/dL, probably because of the effect of placentally produced anti-insulin hormones.

Plasma concentrations of glucose in the postabsorptive state decrease as pregnancy advances. This is due to an increase in placental uptake of glucose. Gluconeogenesis seems to be limited in pregnancy as the major substrate, alanine, is increasingly taken up by the placenta.

Insulin resistance is part of the normal physiologic adaptation to pregnancy. During the first half of pregnancy, increased insulin levels allow excess maternal calories to be directed to lipid stores and tissue glycogen, while blood glucose levels remains low. However, in the second half of pregnancy, as the placenta produces increasing amounts of human placental lactogen and other anti-insulin hormones, the insulin response is blunted at the postreceptor level, increasing maternal circulatory glucose, which is then available for transfer to the fetus. Insulin degradation is unaltered during normal pregnancy.

Inpaired glucose tolerance during normal pregnancy is the result of both increasing insulin resistance *and* a relative paucity of circulating insulin. Most normal pregnant women are able to increase their insulin secretion appropriately to counteract the physiologically produced insulin resistance. However, gestational diabetes can result in those women with limited ability to secrete insulin.

## MATERNAL-PLACENTAL-FETAL TRANSFER OF NUTRIENTS

Glucose is transported to the fetus by carrier-mediated diffusion, which equilibrates fetal blood glucose levels with maternal levels. Fetal concentrations of most amino acids are higher than those of maternal concentrations, and are maintained against a concentration gradient within the placenta. There is rapid transfer of the essential branched-chain neutral amino acids across the placenta, while straight-chained amino acids such as alanine and glycine are slowly transferred. There is essentially no transport of the acidic amino acids glutamate and aspartate, whose fetal requirements need to be satisfied by fetal synthesis. The placenta is responsible for the de novo synthesis of nonessential amino acids, which are then transported to the fetus. Free fatty acids cross the placenta by gradient-dependent diffusion and are used by the fetus.

The increase of human placental lactogen in the second half of pregnancy also stimulates lipolysis, which subsequently allows for the availability and transfer of increased amounts of both glucose and amino acids to the fetus during the period of maximal fetal growth.

## THYROID FUNCTION

The thyroid gland undergoes noticeable enlargement during normal gestation. In parts of the world where there may be iodine deficiency in the diet, the thyroid gland must hypertrophy in order to respond to the normal demands of pregnancy for increased thyroid hormone. In parts of the world where dietary intake of iodine is high, this compensatory hypertrophy of the thyroid gland does not occur and the incidence of goiter is no higher than in the nonpregnant female population.

The secretion of thyroid-binding globulin (TBG) by the liver is doubled by the 12th week of pregnancy. Despite the increase in the total concentrations of both $T_4$ and $T_3$, the amounts of circulating free (unbound) hormone are not significantly increased over the nonpregnant state. Mean plasma concentrations of $T_4$ during pregnancy range from 9 to 16 mg/dL, as compared with 5 to 12 mg/dL in the nonpregnant woman.

Thyroid-stimulating hormone (TSH) is produced by the pituitary gland. Chorionic thyrotropin has been identified as a second thyroid-stimulating substance that is produced by the placenta and transported to the maternal circulation. Placental production of human chorionic gonadotrophin (hCG) also results in stimulation of maternal thyroid activity, particularly in women with pregnancies complicated by hydatidiform mole.

## FETAL-MATERNAL THYROID FUNCTION INTERACTION

Because of the relative inability of TSH, $T_4$, and $T_3$ to cross the placenta, thyroid function in mother and fetus remain independently regulated (Fig. 31-2). Maternal TRH is the only thyroid-related hormone that crosses the placenta in signifi-

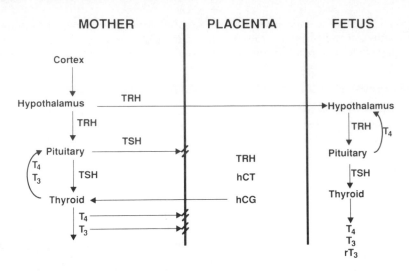

**FIGURE 31-2.** Maternal–placental–fetal thyroid hormone interactions. Note that thyrotrophin-releasing hormone (TRH) is synthesized in the placenta to some degree, and is the only hormone capable of crossing the placenta from mother to fetus. (hCT, human chorionic thyrotrophin; hCG, human chorionic gonadotrophin; $rT_3$, reverse triiodothyronine.) (Adapted from Hollingsworth DR. Endocrine disorders of pregnancy. In: Creasy RK, Resnik R, eds. Maternal-fetal medicine: principles and practice. Philadelphia, WB Saunders, 1989:998.)

cant amounts. Although the regulation of fetal thyroid function seems to be fairly independent from maternal control, the fetus is dependent on the gravida for its supply of iodine. Because iodine readily crosses the placenta, any abnormal increase in maternal ingestion may result in fetal goiter and hypothyroidism.

## PARATHYROID FUNCTION AND CALCIUM HOMEOSTASIS DURING PREGNANCY

By term, the fetus has accumulated 30 g of calcium and approximately 15 g of phosphorus. The majority of the calcium requirement for the fetus occurs in the third trimester of pregnancy, when fetal skeletal growth reaches an accelerated phase. This large demand on the part of the fetus mandates an anticipatory increase in maternal calcium absorption from early pregnancy onward, for if this did not occur, the necessary calcium would be extracted from maternal bone. Breast-feeding mothers have prolonged requirements for increased intake of calcium. Total serum calcium and phosphorus actually decrease in pregnancy. The decrease in serum calcium is accompanied by a similar decrease in serum proteins, and ionized calcium has been reported to either remain stable or rise very slightly throughout pregnancy.

Plasma levels of calcitonin are increased markedly during both pregnancy and lactation. Calcitonin acts in opposition to both parathyroid hormone and vitamin D in order to maintain skeletal calcification. PTH levels fall during the first trimester and then increase progressively until term. Plasma volume expansion, increased glomerular filtration rate, and increased transfer of calcium to the fetus collectively result in decreased maternal calcium concentrations during normal pregnancy, and may subsequently act as the trigger for increased parathyroid hormone levels. The normal adaptation to pregnancy involves the development of a mildly hyperparathyroid state, most likely in order to assist the gravida in meeting the high fetal demands for calcium.

Maternal concentrations of vitamin D during pregnancy depend on diet, exposure to sunshine, and the use of oral supplements. The activation of renal $1_\alpha$ hydroxylase activity during pregnancy results in increased concentrations of 1,25-dihydroxyvitamin $D_3$ and, eventually, increased calcium absorption. The precise initiating mechanism for this process awaits further elucidation.

The calcium-stimulated placental ATPase pump allows transfer of calcium from mother to fetus, and results in increased fetal plasma concentrations of calcium. Parathyroid tissue is present in the fetus as early as 6 weeks of gestation, and at term fetal PTH levels are decreased and calcitonin concentration increased compared with values during infancy.

The net result of pregnancy-induced changes in calcium metabolism is an increase in total maternal calcium with resultant transfer of calcium to the fetus without depleting the maternal skeleton.

## THE SKIN AND MUSCULOSKELETON

### THE SKIN

Increased pigmentation occurs in at least 90% of pregnant women to some degree. Although most patients have a mild generalized hyperpigmentation, specific areas are more involved. Melasma gravidarum (the mask of pregnancy) involves the forehead and cheeks; the bridge of the nose can be pronounced. This usually regresses after pregnancy, but can persist for months. Similar changes have been reported in nonpregnant women taking oral contraceptives. The areola of the breast, the linea alba (becomes the linea nigra), axillae, and genital skin are other areas affected.

A number of changes occur in the skin as a result of vascular dilatation and proliferation, most likely caused by the hyperestrogenic state of pregnancy. Dilatation of capillary vessels and small arteries leads to a variety of angioma. Spider angiomata are particularly common in white women, characterized by a central red elevation (central arteriole) with radiating thin vessels, most common in exposed areas of the body. Redness of the palms or palmar erythema can occur in a blotching distribution. Usually these vascular changes regress after completion of the pregnancy.

Connective tissue changes, presumably induced by estrogens, lead to the development of striae gravidarum in approximately half of all pregnancies. There is no known method of prevention, and although they become less pronounced after pregnancy, and lose coloration, they do not completely regress.

Estrogen is known to decrease the rate of hair growth. There is a transient hair loss at about 3 to 4 months after birth. However, normal growth recurs by 6 to 9 months without any therapy.

### THE MUSCULOSKELETON

Ligaments of the sacroiliac joints and pubic symphysis are reported to soften in pregnancy, leading to some separation of joints. Widening of the pubic symphysis of 3 to 4 mm can occur. In addition, there is progressive lordosis of the spine as the uterus enlarges, leading frequently to low back discomfort for the remainder of the gestation. There is accompanying flexion of the neck, and downward movement of the shoulders. This latter feature may place more traction on the ulnar and median nerves, contributing to aching and numbness. The numbness may also be due to edema increasing the carpal tunnel syndrome.

# 32.  MATERNAL NUTRITION

During the past twenty-five years, maternal nutrition has played an increasingly important role in prenatal care. Recent developments have included liberalized weight gain recommendations based on maternal pregravid weight for height, the recognition of the teratogenic effect of prenatal exposure to alcohol as the fetal alcohol syndrome, diet therapy of maternal phenylketonuria in the prenatal prevention of mental retardation, and the periconceptional use of folic acid to prevent neural tube defects. With the publication of two landmark studies in 1968, a major change occurred in the philosophy of maternal nutrition in this country. First, the Eastman and Jackson study of 25,154 pregnancies observed at the Johns Hopkins Hospital between 1954 and 1961 found that both an increase in weight gain and an increase in prepregnancy weight independently and together were associated with progressive increases in birth weight. For women of pregravid weight less than 120 pounds, they recommended liberal gains, especially during the first half of pregnancy. Preliminary analysis of 10,000 births in the Collaborative Study of Cerebral Palsy was also published in 1968. This was one of the first studies to document the influence of antepartum weight gain on infant growth and development at 1 year of age. The highest maternal weight gains (36+ pounds) were associated with higher birth weights, lower prematurity rates, and better growth and development in the infant's first year of life.

Numerous other studies since 1968 have confirmed these findings, which have improved maternal nutrition benefits for both mother and infant. A recent analysis of 3,581,000 births from the 1980 National Natality Survey reported that a low weight gain during pregnancy was associated with a lower average birth weight and a higher risk of low birth weight (<2500 g) or fetal death outcome. This study also reported that a low prepregnancy weight combined with a small weight gain was associated with a 29% incidence of low birth weight. The risk of fetal death outcome was also lowered with added weight gain, up to 35 pounds. For the gestational periods of 32–40 weeks, the risk of fetal death dropped by about half as weight gain increased from less than 16 to 26–35 pounds.

## EVALUATION OF MATERNAL NUTRITION
### CRITERIA FOR REFERRAL AND ADMISSION

Although every woman should have the opportunity to have a thorough nutritional evaluation by a nutritionist or registered dietitian specially trained in maternal nutrition, this is not always practical or feasible. When resources are limited, antepartum patients should be screened during the first prenatal visits and those women with a history of a previous low-birth-weight infant or who currently have a pregnancy with intrauterine growth retardation or SGA should be referred to nutrition counseling (Table 32-1). Other indications for referral include maternal pregravid weight 20% or more above ideal weight for her height or excessive weight gain during pregnancy (7 pounds or more per month); 10% or more below ideal weight for height or inadequate weight gain during pregnancy (less than 2 pounds per month after the first trimester); or excessive vomiting, sufficient to cause weight loss or ketonuria. Additional indications for nutrition counseling include the possibility of diet-related anemias (iron deficiency, pica, or vegetarianism), any medical problems that existed before conception, and gestational diabetes, lactose intolerance, alcoholism, or drug use. In some instances the nutrition-related problems during pregnancy become so severe as to retard fetal growth and seriously threaten maternal health and well-being. In these cases the antepartum patient should be admitted for intensive hydration, elemental alimentation, and monitoring of her own health status and that of her unborn child. Guidelines for admission for maternal malnutrition are given in Table 32-2.

## PREGRAVID WEIGHT

The two strongest predictors of infant birth weight, after length of gestation, are maternal pregravid weight and gestational weight gain. In view of the findings of the Collaborative Study of Cerebral Palsy, the findings of the 1980 National Natality Survey, and the most current recommendations from the National Academy of Sciences, pregravid weight should be average for height, or even higher to

**TABLE 32-1.** Criteria for Referral for Nutrition Counseling

I. Weight and/or growth problems
  A. Infant
    1. Previous low-birth-weight infant
    2. Present intrauterine growth retardation or SGA
  B. Mother
    1. Overweight
      a. Pregravid obesity (≥20% above ideal weight for height)
      b. Excessive weight gain (>7 pounds/month)
    2. Underweight
      a. Low pregravid weight (≥10% below ideal weight for height)
      b. Inadequate weight gain (<2 pounds/month after first trimester)
      c. Excessive vomiting (sufficient to cause weight loss or ketonuria)
II. Diet-related anemias
  A. Iron deficiency anemia
  B. Pica
  C. Vegetarian
III. Medical problems
  A. Gestational diabetes
  B. Lactose intolerance
  C. Alcoholism
  D. Drug use

**TABLE 32-2.** Guidelines for Admission for Maternal Malnutrition

1. *Weight loss* of 10% or more of pregravid weight during the first trimester
2. *Inadequate net weight gain* (less than 10 pounds) by 30 weeks gestation
3. *Hyperemesis gravidarum:* as defined by meeting two of the following criteria:
   a. Inability to retain any solid or liquid food
   b. Abnormal electrolytes (especially chlorides); acidosis
   c. Acetonuria
   d. Weight loss or no gain by 12 weeks gestation or later
   e. Failure of drug therapy
3. *Discrepancy between size and dates* of 2 weeks or more at 20 weeks gestation or later
   with weight loss or failure to gain

include a margin of safety for variations in weight gain during gestation. Those women at either extreme, underweight or overweight, before conception are at increased risk for prematurity or low birth weight, as well as other complications. Underweight is defined as 10% or more below a standard or ideal weight for height, or a body mass index [BMI = weight (kg)/height (m2)] < 19.8; overweight is 20% or more above standard weight for height, or a BMI > 26.0. Optimal range for pregnancy, therefore, is ideal or standard to about 15% above, or a BMI of 19.8–26.0 (Table 32-3).

## OBSTETRICAL HISTORY

Research has shown that there is a tendency to repeat low-birth-weight and small-for-gestational-age (SGA) deliveries in subsequent births. The relative risk of a second birth also being SGA was found to be 3.4; similar results were found for

**TABLE 32-3.** Ideal and Deviations of Pregravid Weight for Height

| Height | Ideal | Underweight (<10%) | Normal Range (−9% to +19%) | Optimal Range (ideal to +15%) |
|--------|-------|--------------------|-----------------------------|-------------------------------|
| 4'9"   | 104   | 94                 | 95–124                      | 104–120                       |
| 4'10"  | 107   | 96                 | 97–127                      | 107–123                       |
| 4'11"  | 110   | 99                 | 100–131                     | 110–127                       |
| 5'0"   | 113   | 102                | 103–135                     | 113–130                       |
| 5'1"   | 116   | 104                | 105–138                     | 116–133                       |
| 5'2"   | 118   | 106                | 107–141                     | 118–136                       |
| 5'3"   | 123   | 111                | 112–147                     | 123–141                       |
| 5'4"   | 128   | 115                | 116–153                     | 128–147                       |
| 5'5"   | 132   | 119                | 120–157                     | 132–152                       |
| 5'6"   | 136   | 122                | 123–162                     | 136–156                       |
| 5'7"   | 140   | 126                | 127–167                     | 140–161                       |
| 5'8"   | 144   | 130                | 131–172                     | 144–166                       |
| 5'9"   | 148   | 133                | 134–177                     | 148–170                       |
| 5'10"  | 152   | 137                | 138–181                     | 152–175                       |

Adapted from Luke B, Johnson TRB, and Petrie RH. Clinical maternal-fetal nutrition. Boston: Little, Brown, 1993.

**TABLE 32-4.** Summary of RDAs for Women Ages 24 and Older, Changes from Nonpregnant to Pregnant, and Food Sources

| Nutrient | Nonpregnant | Pregnant | Percent Increase | Dietary Sources |
|---|---|---|---|---|
| Folic acid | 180 mcg | 400 mcg | + 122 | Leafy vegetables, liver |
| Vitamin D | 5 μg | 10 μg | + 100 | Fortified dairy products |
| Iron | 15 mg | 30 mg | + 100 | Meats, eggs, grains |
| Calcium | 800 mg | 1200 mg | + 50 | Dairy products |
| Phosphorus | 800 mg | 1200 mg | + 50 | Meats |
| Pyridoxine | 1.6 mg | 2.2 mg | + 38 | Meats, liver, enriched grains |
| Thiamin | 1.1 mg | 1.5 mg | + 36 | Enriched grains, pork |
| Zinc | 12 mg | 15 mg | + 25 | Meats, seafood, eggs |
| Riboflavin | 1.3 mg | 1.6 mg | + 23 | Meats, liver, enriched grains |
| Protein | 50 g | 60 g | + 20 | Meats, fish, poultry, dairy |
| Iodine | 150 mcg | 175 mcg | + 17 | Iodized salt, seafood |
| Vitamin C | 60 mg | 70 mg | + 17 | Citrus fruits, tomatoes |
| Energy | 2200 kcal | 2500 kcal | + 14 | Proteins, fats, carbohydrates |
| Magnesium | 280 mg | 320 mg | + 14 | Seafood, legumes, grains |
| Niacin | 15 mg | 17 mg | + 13 | Meats, nuts, legumes |
| Vitamin B-12 | 2.0 mcg | 2.2 mcg | + 10 | Animal proteins |
| Vitamin A | 800 μg | 800 μg | 0 | Dark green, yellow, or orange fruits and vegetables, liver |

repeat low-birth-weight or preterm deliveries. Other research has shown that the recurrence rate of fetal growth retardation was nearly 50%. Stein and Susser (1984) suggest that the "most widespread environmental cause of IUGR (intrauterine growth retardation) is probably maternal undernutrition."* The nutritional status of a woman both before and during pregnancy is therefore an important influence on both the adequacy of intrauterine growth and the length of gestation.

## DIETARY RECOMMENDATIONS

### THE RDAS AND RINS

Table 32-4 lists the recommended dietary allowances (RDAs) for non-pregnant and pregnant adolescents and adult women, developed by the Food and Nutrition Board of the National Research Council, and the recommended intakes of nutrients (RINs), formulated by the Food and Agriculture Organization. The RDAs suggest higher protein; calcium; iron; vitamins A, $B_{12}$, D, C; and thiamine than the RINs, whereas the RINs suggest generally more calories for females 19 years of age and younger. The RDAs provide the most current standard for the United States for prescribing a balanced diet during gestation and will be the basis of this section.

Table 32-4 also gives a summary of the changes in RDAs for women aged 24 years and older from the nonpregnant to the pregnant state, as well as food

---

*Stein ZA, Susser M. Intrauterine growth retardation: epidemiological issues and public health significance. Semin Perinatol 1984;8:5.

sources for each nutrient. Contrary to popular belief, nutrient requirements generally do not double during gestation. As shown in Table 32-4, only iron, folic acid, and vitamin D requirements increase 100% over nonpregnant requirements, whereas other nutrients, such as calcium, phosphorus, thiamine, and vitamin $B_6$, increase between 33% and 50%. Requirements for protein, zinc, and riboflavin increase about 20% to 25%, whereas those for energy, magnesium, iodine, niacin, and vitamins A, $B_{12}$, and C increase by 17% or less.

## CALORIC INTAKE AND PATTERN OF GAIN

As recommended in the National Academy of Sciences 1990 report on nutrition during pregnancy, caloric intake should be based on the pregnant woman's pregravid weight and best rate of weight gain to achieve the optimal total gestational weight gain. For women who begin pregnancy within the optimal weight range for height (BMI 19.8–26.0), a good total gestational gain would be 25–35 pounds. This weight should be gained at the rate of about 3.5 pounds during the first trimester and about 1 pound per week for the second and third trimesters. For women who are overweight when they begin pregnancy (20% or more above ideal, or BMI > 26.0), the total gestational weight gain should be about 15–25 pounds, at the rate of about 2 pounds during the first trimester and about two-thirds of a pound per week during the second and third trimesters. For women who begin pregnancy underweight (10% or more under ideal, or BMI < 19.8), the total gain should be about 28–40 pounds, depending on the severity of their pregravid weight deficit. For these women, much of the initial weight gain goes to correcting their own weight, with little remaining for the developing fetus. Research has shown that only after the mother's own weight has been brought up to within a normal range for her height can any additional nutrients be effectively utilized for normal growth of the fetus. For this reason weight gain for the underweight woman should be about 5 pounds during the first trimester and slightly more than a pound per week during the second and third trimesters.

## SPECIAL CONSIDERATIONS

### ALCOHOL USE DURING PREGNANCY

The adverse effects of maternal alcohol use on the developing fetus have been known empirically since ancient times. It was not until 1968 that a formal description appeared in the scientific literature when Lemoine and associates (1968) reported a set of abnormalities that were consistently observed in children born to alcoholic women: prenatal growth deficiency, an unusual facies, psychomotor retardation (IQ 70), and a 25% incidence of congenital anomalies (especially cleft palate and cardiac malformations).[†] This pattern of abnormalities was also reported by other investigators, and in 1973, Jones and Smith designated this pattern of altered growth and dysmorphogenesis the fetal alcohol syndrome (FAS). Since Jones and Smith's original description of the characteristic features of

---

[†] Lemoine P, Harrousseau H, Borteyru JP, Menuet J. Les enfants de parents alcooliques: observé. A propos de 127 cas. Triest Medical 1968;25:476.

FAS, many other clinicians and investigators have added their cases and additional clinical findings. It has been estimated that the worldwide incidence of FAS is 1.9 per 1000 live births (full characteristics), and of fetal alcohol effects 2.5–5 per 1000 live births (partial characteristics). Among alcoholic women, the incidence of FAS is estimated at 25 per 1000 live births, whereas fetal alcohol effects are estimated at 90 per 1000. It is the leading cause of mental retardation in the Western world, surpassing Down's syndrome and cerebral palsy. Many experimental animal models (including primates) demonstrating the teratogenicity of alcohol have been developed and have shown a clear dose–response effect between maternal alcohol consumption and fetal risk. Central to the characterization of this syndrome is retarded and deviant growth, manifested in nearly every organ system in proportion to timing and amount of alcohol exposure in utero. These effects may be the result of direct or indirect consequences of alcohol metabolism. Both alcohol and its major metabolite, acetaldehyde, readily cross the placenta, and both can be directly teratogenic. Both alcohol and acetaldehyde have been shown to impair nucleic acid and protein synthesis directly in vitro.

Metabolism of alcohol is very different for the mother than it is for the developing fetus. Because alcohol is both water and lipid soluble, it passes readily through all biological membranes, equilibrating rapidly throughout the entire water volume of the maternal-placental-fetal unit. The amniotic fluid acts as a reservoir for unchanged alcohol and acetaldehyde and because the fetus lacks the necessary enzymes to degrade these substances, it is exposed to them long after they have been cleared from the maternal system. It has also been suggested that alcohol or acetaldehyde may be toxic to the placenta as well as to the fetus, and that ethanol-associated placentotoxicity could result in "selective" fetal malnutrition, independent of maternal nutritional status.

Maternal undernutrition and/or malnutrition often accompanies alcohol abuse, potentiating its effects. For example, protein malnutrition is known to exacerbate alcohol's hepatotoxicity, and alcohol itself impairs the absorption, utilization, and metabolism of nutrients. Poor nutritional status of the mother, plus the toxic effects of alcohol, may be more detrimental to the developing fetus than either factor alone. In addition, impairment of placental transport of amino acids by alcohol may result in transient or chronic deprivation of essential amino acids, resulting in intrauterine growth retardation, as well as potentially compounding any toxic effects of ethanol in embryogenesis. Reduced placental transfer of zinc and folic acid have also been demonstrated in animal models of alchol-induced teratogenesis.

In addition to the nutritional implications of alcohol abuse, there are a wide variety of other indirect ways in which alcohol can impair fetal development. Alcohol-related hypothermia, dehydration, fetal hypoxia and acidosis, placental pathology and dysfunction, and endocrine disturbances have all been shown to occur with increasing maternal alcohol intake. Genetic factors, including individual variation in the metabolism of alcohol, as well as the possibility of paternal influence on the susceptibility of the fetus to alcohol's teratogenic actions, may also be important in the expression of this disorder.

## MATERNAL PHENYLKETONURIA

Phenylketonuria (PKU) was the first metabolic disorder to be screened for on a national basis. Newborns were screened for this genetic disorder of amino acid metabolism starting in 1961 and treated with diet therapy until 6 years of age. After this age, many of the affected individuals were lost to medical follow-up because further treatment was unnecessary. As a result of this screening and treatment program, many of these individuals are now of childbearing age, and affected females pose a special problem during their pregnancies, that of screening for and treating maternal PKU to prevent the development of mental retardation in utero. The unique clinical challenge today is to develop an approach that will ensure assure an improved course and outcome for women with PKU.

It has been known for many years that excess maternal phenylalanine levels have a teratogenic effect on the developing fetus. During pregnancy there is a positive gradient of phenylalanine from mother to fetus. Maternal blood phenylalanine levels above 20 mg/dL during pregnancy are associated with a 90% incidence of mental retardation, microcephaly, congenital heart defects, and low birth weight among the surviving offspring; maternal blood phenylalanine levels below 16 mg/dL result in a 20% incidence of these adverse outcomes. Spontaneous abortion is also more common among women with PKU, thought to be due to the possible toxic effects of high levels of phenylalanine or its related metabolites on the fetus. It has been estimated that if each woman with PKU were to have two offspring, within one generation the prevalence of mental retardation related to PKU could rebound to the level present in the population before the advent of mass screening and treatment of this disorder.

Clinical studies have found that initiation of dietary therapy prior to conception results in the most favorable outcomes. Specific dietary guidelines have been developed to provide adequate prenatal nutrition while restricting dietary phenylalanine sufficiently to lower and maintain blood phenylalanine levels in the range of 2–8 mg/dL.

## FOLIC ACID AND NEURAL TUBE DEFECTS

Neural tube defects (NTDs) include the congenital anomalies of spina bifida, anencephaly, and encephalocele. Each year approximately 400,000 children with NTDs are born worldwide, including 4000 in the United States. The risk of NTD is 2% to 3%, but the risk of recurrence is much higher. NTDs are thought to result from an interaction between genetics and the prenatal environment, specifically micronutrient metabolism. Folate is the single nutrient most strongly implicated in studies of NTDs. Data from animal studies indicate that NTDs can result from altered folate metabolism. Data from clinical studies suggest that maternal folate metabolism may be abnormal in those who give birth to infants with NTDs, although findings are conflicting. Lower red cell folate levels, but not serum folate levels were reported in women with affected infants compared to controls. These finding suggest that NTDs may be associated with altered folate metabolism, but not necessarily a lower dietary intake of folate.

During the past decade several large studies have attempted to clarify the role of the periconceptional use of folate in reducing the risk of NTDs. The most recent study, conducted by the British Medical Research Council Vitamin Study Group, demonstrated a 71% reduction in recurrence of NTDs with periconceptional (1 to 3 months before conception to 6 weeks of gestation) use of 4 mg folic acid. Based on these and other findings, the Centers for Disease Control recommended in

August, 1991, that women who have had a previous pregnancy which resulted in an infant or fetus with an NTD be given 4 mg of folic acid (as a separate supplement, not as part of a multivitamin) beginning at least 4 weeks before conception and through the first 3 months of pregnancy. However, the Centers for Disease Control cautioned that this dose of folic acid is ten times the pregnancy RDA and 20 times the nonpregnant RDA for folic acid. The use of folic acid at this dosage may complicate the diagnosis of vitamin $B_{12}$ deficiency because it may mask megaloblastic anemia while neurologic manifestations progress.

## MULTIPLE BIRTHS

Multiple births increased in the 1980s, mainly because women were delaying childbirth and older women have a higher incidence of twins, and because of the increased use of fertility drugs and in vitro fertilization.

There are no current standardized dietary recommendations for the woman with a multiple gestation. A recent monograph on twins recommended that the maternal caloric intake be increased an additional 300 kcal/day above the recommendations for singleton pregnancies, for a projected total weight gain of about 48 pounds. Recent research indicates that both higher maternal pregravid weight for height and greater rates of gestational gain and total weight gain augment intrauterine growth in twins and increase length of gestation. Recent studies on term twin births suggest that higher pregravid weight and gains of about 45 pounds are associated with better birth weights.

## CONCLUSION

Technological advances during the twentieth century will continue to push back the limits of viability. In future decades the nutrition–fertility link will be expanded at the opposite end of the spectrum, and nutrition in utero will emerge as a powerful tool with which to augment growth, development, and vitality. Careful evaluation and aggressive therapy will help ensure the most positive outcomes during gestation as a foundation of childhood health.

# PART X. MATERNAL DISEASES COMPLICATING PREGNANCY

## 33. TRAUMA, SHOCK, AND CRITICAL CARE OBSTETRICS

### DEFINITION OF SHOCK

"Shock is a condition in which circulation fails to meet the nutritional needs of the cell and fails to remove metabolic wastes." This condition may result from hypovolemia (absolute or relative) or cardiac dysfunction. When the circulating blood volume is less than the capacity of its vascular bed, hypotension with diminished tissue perfusion results, leading to cellular hypoxia and, ultimately, cell death. Depending on the duration and severity of the insult, irreversible organ damage or even death of the individual may ensue.

### ETIOLOGY OF SHOCK

Shock in the obstetric patient may be categorized as either hypovolemic, septic, neurogenic, or cardiogenic. Although these etiologies are different, they often can share common pathophysiologic pathways and ultimately lead to hypoperfusion at the tissue and cellular levels. This decreased perfusion, secondary to hypovolemia or cardiac pump failure, leads to hypoxia and acidosis, which results in the clinical shock picture.

### GENERAL SUPPORTIVE MEASURES

#### INITIAL TREATMENT

Several important initial steps should be performed when the diagnosis of shock is made in the obstetric patient. Placement of two large-bore intravenous lines, preferably 16-gauge, for rapid expansion of intravascular volume is the first step. One liter of normal saline or lactated Ringer's solution should be infused over the first 15 minutes while other measures are taken. An indwelling catheter is placed for hourly determination of urine output. An arterial line allows continuous measurement of systemic blood pressure, as well as easy access for laboratory investigations. Oxygen should be administered via nasal prongs or face mask at 6 to 8 L/min and the $F_IO_2$ adjusted according to arterial blood gas results. If the ability to maintain an adequate tidal volume or arterial oxygenation is impaired or

 E. Albert Reece, John C. Hobbins, Maurice, J. Mahoney and Roy H. Petrie (Eds). *Handbook of Medicine of the Fetus & Mother.* Copyright © 1995 by J.B. Lippincott Company

if the airway is obstructed, endotracheal intubation with positive pressure ventilation may be required.

Initial laboratory investigation should include blood type and cross-match, complete blood count, platelets, prothrombin time, partial thromboplastin time, fibrinogen, electrolytes, blood urea nitrogen and creatinine, and arterial blood gases. Urine postcatheterization should be sent for analysis and microscopic evaluation. When the patient is stabilized, cultures from blood, urine, sputum, amniotic fluid, endometrial cavity, and stool are taken, as indicated, if sepsis is suspected.

## VOLUME REPLACEMENT

Standard dextran with a molecular weight averaging 75,000 may initiate intravascular coagulation. Low-molecular-weight dextran, with a molecular weight averaging 40,000, carries a smaller risk of initiating disseminated intravascular coagulopathy (DIC), but also has less tendency to pull fluid into the intravascular space. A 1984 American College of Obstetricians and Gynecologists technical bulletin entitled "Hemorrhagic Shock" recommends avoidance of dextran because of its anticoagulant effects and risks of anaphylaxis.

If initial crystalloid therapy does not result in the desired clinical improvement, the administration of colloids for further volume expansion should be strongly considered.

In the case of hemorrhagic hypovolemic shock and in cases of disseminated intravascular coagulation, blood component therapy will be indicated, mostly by laboratory parameters. An obvious exception is profuse hemorrhagic shock, for which immediate blood components—specifically, packed red blood cells—are indicated. It must be remembered that, grossly, the degree of hemorrhage is often underestimated by as much as 50%.

Packed red blood cells (PRBC) are administered through an 18-gauge or larger intravenous line in order to increase blood volume and oxygen-carrying capacity to the tissues. The term *massive blood replacement* is used when one total volume is replaced over a 24-hour period.

The use of fresh-frozen plasma (FFP) is now under scrutiny and requires specific indications: replacement of isolated factor deficiencies, reversal of warfarin effect with active bleeding or requiring emergency surgery, antithrombin-III deficiency, immunodeficiencies, thrombotic thrombocytopenia purpura, and massive blood transfusion in cases in which factor deficiencies are presumed to be the sole or principal derangement. Because pathologic hemorrhage in the patient receiving massive transfusion is usually due to thrombocytopenia rather than depletion of coagulation factors, empiric administration of FFP should be allowed only in those patients in whom factor deficiencies are presumed to be the sole or principal derangement.

Platelet transfusion should be performed when the platelet count falls below 20,000/$\mu$L, or below 50,000/$\mu$L in preparation of a surgical procedure or in the face of active bleeding.

Cryoprecipitate should be administered instead of FFP when the calculated coagulation factor defect based on blood fibrinogen levels may result in volume overload.

## INOTROPIC AGENTS

If adequate intravascular volume replacement is not successful in supporting blood pressure (i.e., a systolic blood pressure of at least 80 mmHg), an advanced stage of shock should be suspected and inotropic therapy instituted. Dopamine is considered the first-line inotropic agent.

## VASOPRESSOR AGENTS

If blood pressure does not respond to inotropic therapy, a peripheral vasoconstrictor should be started to maintain systemic vascular resistance (Table 33-1). Phenylephrine, an $\alpha$-adrenergic agonist, may be initiated at 1 to 5 $\mu$g/kg/min. Norepinephrine, a mixed alpha and beta agonist with powerful vasoconstrictive properties, may be added to provide generalized vasoconstriction and increased systemic vascular resistance. This agent should be used only in situations where blood pressure is dangerously low despite other therapy, because perfusion to vital organs, such as the kidneys and lungs, may be reduced by the vasoconstriction.

Caution must be exercised with use of these agents in gravid patients. The primary goal is stabilization of the mother; however, consideration must be given to the fetus. In pregnant ewes subjected to spinal hypotension, dopamine administered in sufficient doses to maintain blood pressure resulted in further diminishment of uterine blood flow and increased uterine vascular resistance in comparison to controls.

## INVASIVE MONITORING

The uses of the Swan-Ganz catheter have become increasingly important in managing critically ill patients. Many clinical indications exist for use of the Swan-Ganz catheter, some of which are unique to obstetrics (Table 33-2).

The pulmonary artery catheter provides a direct means of measuring central venous pressure, pulmonary capillary wedge pressure, cardiac output, systemic vascular resistance, and mixed venous oxygen saturation, and may be used to initiate atrioventricular pacing and fluid challenge.

Upon insertion of the Swan-Ganz catheter, advancement to the right side of the heart demonstrates characteristic pressure tracings through the right atrium, right

**TABLE 33-1.** Vasopressor Agents

| Vasopressor Agent | Mechanism of Action | Dosage |
|---|---|---|
| Phenylephrine (Neo-Synephrine) | $\alpha$-adrenergic increased SVR | 1–5 $\mu$g/kg/min |
| Norepinephrine (Levarterenol) | Mixed adrenergic alpha and beta generalized vasoconstriction, increased SVR | 1–4 $\mu$g/min |

Modified from Lee W, Clark SL, Cotton DB, et al. Septic shock during pregnancy. Am J Obstet Gynecol 1988;159:410.

**TABLE 33-2.** Indications for Pulmonary Artery Catheterization During Pregnancy

1. Massive blood loss with large transfusion requirements, particularly in the face of oliguria or pulmonary edema
2. Septic shock, especially when accompanied by hypotension or oliguria, required volume resuscitation or vasopressor therapy
3. Cardiac failure or pulmonary edema of uncertain etiology
4. Severe pregnancy-induced hypertension complicated by pulmonary edema, oliguria unresponsive to initial fluid challenge, or severe hypertension refractory to conventional therapy (hydralazine)
5. Labor and delivery in patients with significant cardiovascular disease (New York Heart Association Functional Class III and IV patients)
6. Intraoperative cardiovascular decompensation (eg, pulmonary hypertension with shunting secondary to amniotic fluid embolism)
7. During peripartum period in patients with severe preeclampsia and structural cardiac defects
8. Thyroid storm with evidence of high output failure
9. Diabetic ketoacidosis with severe hypovolemia and oliguria

ventricle, pulmonary artery, and pulmonary capillary wedge positions. From these waveforms, specific hemodynamic and ventilatory parameters can be determined (Table 33-3). Cardiac output may then be used to construct a ventricular function curve. Hemodynamic subsets of ventricular function can be evaluated by plotting stroke index against left ventricular filling pressure. A knowledge of pulmonary capillary wedge pressure, pulmonary artery diastolic-wedge gradient, and the AV-02 difference make it possible to ascertain the precise etiology of cardiopulmonary compromise.

After placement of the Swan-Ganz catheter, a chest x-ray should be obtained to rule out pneumothorax and to confirm the catheter's position. Complications of Swan-Ganz catheter placement range from 0.4% to 9.9%.

**TABLE 33-3.** Hemodynamic and Ventilatory Parameters

| | Nonpregnant | Pregnant |
|---|---|---|
| Central venous pressure (mmHg) | 1–7 | Unchanged |
| Pulmonary capillary wedge pressure (mmHg) | 6–12 | Unchanged |
| Mean pulmonary artery pressure (mmHg) | 9–16 | Unchanged |
| Systemic vascular resistance (dynes·sec·cm⁵) | 800–1200 | Decreased 25% |
| Pulmonary vascular resistance (dynes·sec·cm⁵) | 20–120 | Decreased 25% |
| Cardiac output (L/min) | 4–7 | Increased 30% to 45% |
| Arterial pO₂ (mmHg) | 90–95 | 104–108 |
| Arterial pCO₂ (mmHg) | 38–40 | 27–32 |
| Arterial pH | 7.35–7.40 | 7.40–7.45 |
| Oxygen consumption (mL/min) | 173–311 | 249–331 |

From Kirshon B, Cotton DB. Invasive hemodynamic monitoring in the obstetric patient. Clin Obstet Gynecol 1987;30:579.

## SPECIFIC ETIOLOGIES AND THEIR DIAGNOSES, PATHOPHYSIOLOGIES, AND TREATMENTS

### HYPOVOLEMIC SHOCK

Hypovolemia may result from hemorrhage or solely from loss of intravascular fluids. The causes of hemorrhage in obstetrics are numerous. The most common cause of hemorrhage is uterine atony following delivery of the placenta.

Treatment of hemorrhagic shock involves correcting the initiating process as well as instituting general supportive measures, as previously discussed in this chapter. If medical therapy is unsuccessful, surgical procedures, such as uterine artery ligation, internal iliac artery ligation, and emergency hysterectomy, are required. Over the years, uterine atony and placenta accreta have replaced uteroplacental apoplexy (Couvelaire uterus) and simple dehiscence of a uterine scar as major indications for hysterectomy at the time of cesarean section. Other modalities, such as percutaneous transcatheter hypogastric artery embolization and the use of the gravity suit, may have their place in certain situations but are not without their own risks.

Response to therapy is reflected by hemodynamic parameters and laboratory values. Blood products should be administered after identifying the underlying disorder by laboratory indices. While quantitative laboratory tests are pending, the clot observation test may be performed by drawing maternal venous blood into a clean, dry test tube and observing for clot formation.

### UTERINE ATONY

Uterine atony, occurring in one of 20 deliveries, is the most common cause of postpartum hemorrhage.

The diagnosis is made following delivery of the placenta when excessive bleeding is noted per vaginam. The uterine fundus is boggy. Examination of the birth canal reveals no lacerations that may account for bleeding. The uterine cavity should be explored to rule out retained placenta, retained blood clots, and disruption of the uterine wall. Initial management includes bimanual fundal massage and administration of oxytocin (Pitocin, Syntocinon), 20 to 30 U/L at a rapid intravenous rate or via intramyometrial injection. Methylergonovine maleate (Methergine), 0.2 mg, may be given intramuscularly but should be avoided in hypertensive patients.

### PLACENTA PREVIA

Placenta previa may be classified as marginal, partial, or total, depending on the relationship of the placenta to the internal os of the cervix. The overall incidence near term is 1 in 200 pregnancies.

The major hazards associated with placenta previa are profound maternal hemorrhage and shock, with significant perinatal morbidity and mortality.

Diagnosis is best made by ultrasound, which may also be useful in predicting, during the early second trimester, which patients will be at risk for total placenta previa at term. If the diagnosis based on ultrasound is in question, a double set-up examination should be performed, with preparations made for blood transfusion and cesarean section.

Placenta previa is also associated with placenta accreta, increta, and percreta, especially in the presence of a previous cesarean section.

## PLACENTA ACCRETA, INCRETA, AND PERCRETA

When Nitabuch's membrane is deficient and trophoblastic tissue attaches directly to the myometrium, placenta accreta is said to occur. If the trophoblast invades the myometrium or penetrates the myometrium, placenta increta and placenta percreta exist.

Rare cases of invasion into extrauterine structures, such as the bladder, requiring bladder resection and massive transfusion, have been reported in the literature.

## ABRUPTIO PLACENTAE

Abruptio placentae is estimated to occur in 1 of 120 deliveries. The exact etiology is unknown, but associated conditions include hypertensive disorders, parity, and history of previous abruption.

Another possible risk factor for abruption is cocaine abuse during pregnancy. Cocaine can cause placental vasoconstriction, decreased blood flow to the fetus, and increased uterine contractility.

Initial treatment includes placement of large-bore intravenous access, oxygen supplementation, type and cross-match for red blood cells, hematologic and coagulation laboratory studies, fetal heart rate monitoring, maternal urinary output via indwelling catheter, and amniotomy with use of oxytocin in selective cases. Simultaneous correction of anemia and coagulation defects should be instituted. The decision about whether to allow vaginal delivery or to proceed with cesarean section with a live fetus has been somewhat facilitated by the advent of electronic fetal monitoring.

## ECTOPIC PREGNANCY

Ectopic pregnancy continues to play a major role in maternal morbidity and mortality in the United States. The incidence is said to be 1 per 100 pregnancies. Over the last 30 years, a steady rise has occurred in the ectopic rate, with a fall in the death-to-case rate.

Acute salpingitis is probably the most important factor associated with ectopic pregnancy. Other factors, such as tubal surgery and adhesion formation, intrauterine device use, and history of infertility, have been identified as causative agents.

The usual symptoms associated with ectopic pregnancy include abdominal pain, amenorrhea or irregular vaginal bleeding, pregnancy symptoms, and sometimes syncope and shoulder pain secondary to intraperitoneal bleeding. Common signs include adnexal tenderness, adnexal mass, slightly enlarged uterus, and, in patients who have sustained significant blood loss, tachycardia and hypotension.

## TRAUMA

For the purpose of categorization, trauma may be described as obstetric-related or non-obstetric-related. Obstetric trauma may occur spontaneously, as with laceration of the lower genital tract during the second stage of labor, spontaneous uterine rupture, and spontaneous rupture of the liver, which may occur in patients with pregnancy-induced hypertension. Obstetric trauma may also occur as a result of surgical procedures (e.g., during episiotomy, forceps operations, cesarean section, dilatation and curettage, and induced abortion). Non-obstetric-related trauma may, for practical purposes, be subdivided into blunt trauma, as occurs during a fall or motor vehicle accident, and penetrating trauma, such as that sustained from gunshot and stab wounds.

The pathophysiologic significance of trauma is usually related to hypovolemia; however, tissue damage and necrosis may play an integral role in the pathophysiologic process as well.

## SPONTANEOUS OBSTETRIC TRAUMA

### Uterine Rupture

Spontaneous rupture of the gravid uterus still carries a significant maternal and fetal mortality rate. The incidence is approximately 1 in 2000 deliveries.

Conditions associated with uterine rupture include use of oxytocin, cephalopelvic disproportion, grand multiparity, and abruption. Some older studies identified previous cesarean section scars to be the most important etiologic factor.

The most common clinical presentation is that of mild vaginal bleeding, shock, and lower abdominal pain. In some instances, the area from which fetal heart tones can be observed will be shifted. Sometimes, acute bradycardia is noted.

Treatment of uterine rupture should be individualized. Abdominal hysterectomy is no longer advocated in all cases. If the fetus is still undelivered or if uterine bleeding is felt to be secondary to a uterine or cervical defect, prompt laparotomy is indicated. In many cases, the diagnosis is made only at the time of repeat cesarean section. If the patient desires future childbearing and surgical repair is possible, hysterectomy should be avoided. In cases in which the tear extends either laterally into the broad ligament or in which damage is extensive, hysterectomy is indicated for control of blood loss. Sometimes, removal of the adnexa on the involved side is required to control broad-ligament bleeding. If a defect is found at the time of postpartum examination but no bleeding is noted and the patient is otherwise stable, close observation without laparotomy may be warranted.

### Spontaneous Hepatic Rupture

The patient, often diagnosed with preeclampsia, develops epigastric or right upper quadrant pain associated with nausea and vomiting. Occasionally, upper abdominal tenderness is present on examination. If subcapsular hepatic hemorrhage has extended beyond Glisson's capsule and intraperitoneal bleeding occurs, signs and symptoms of shock follow.

Laboratory values may show evidence of a falling hematocrit, elevated liver enzymes and serum bilirubin, and developing coagulopathy.

The diagnosis is often made on clinical grounds; however, paracentesis, liver scan, ultrasonography, and computed tomography may be helpful in establishing the diagnosis.

Expedient exploratory laparotomy is mandated for a patient in shock with evidence of intraperitoneal bleeding, since delay in laparotomy has been associated with increased mortality. Packing the liver and adequate drainage are recommended. Death is usually secondary to massive, uncontrollable hemorrhage. In cases where bleeding was controlled by hepatic artery ligation or lobectomy, death usually followed postoperatively secondary to hepatic failure and multisystem organ failure. It is postulated that the preexisting hepatic damage may not allow sufficient hepatic reserve following arterial occlusion or partial liver resection to sustain life.

## SURGICAL OBSTETRIC TRAUMA

### Legal Abortion
If unusual postabortal bleeding does not resolve, diagnostic laparoscopy or exploratory laparotomy should be performed without delay.

Laparoscopy or laparotomy is performed in a patient in whom persistent bleeding is suspected or cannot be ruled out, damage to intraperitoneal organs is suspected, or pain is felt to be excessive or worsening.

## NONOBSTETRIC TRAUMA

The incidence of accidental injury during pregnancy is estimated to be 6% to 7%. In most cases, injury is minimal and is not associated with a significant increase in perinatal mortality.

### Blunt Trauma
Simple falls that do not result in loss of consciousness or bruises are unlikely to produce significant injury to the mother or the fetus. We recommend some type of fetal assessment (NST or biophysical profile) to provide reassurance to a concerned mother and her physician. Maternal Rh status should be checked and the Kleihauer-Betke test should be considered. Clotting studies are indicated if placental abruption is suspected.

Serious falls are associated with multiple bone fractures and internal injury. Diagnostic peritoneal lavage for blunt trauma in pregnant women has been found to be both safe and accurate in diagnosing intra-abdominal injuries. Physical examination of the abdomen is felt to be less reliable in the pregnant patient.

Pelvic fractures are usually associated with motor vehicle accidents. Serious complications are related to urologic and vascular damage. Retroperitoneal hemorrhage may be massive, resulting from minor pelvic fractures with minimal bony displacement. Nonexpanding retroperitoneal hematomas found at laparotomy should probably be left alone to prevent further hemorrhage. The most common site of fracture occurs through the anterior half of the pelvic ring, at the horizontal pubic rami. Fewer than 10% of patients with pelvic fractures require cesarean section secondary to pelvic deformity.

### Penetrating Trauma
The gravid uterus becomes the most frequently injured organ in cases of penetrating abdominal trauma. As the uterus expands, the bowel is compartmentalized into the upper abdomen. Because of the physical forces involved, gunshot wounds

carry a substantially higher mortality rate than stab wounds. In all cases of gunshot wounds to the abdomen, exploratory laparotomy should be performed to determine the extent of visceral injury. However, exploratory laparotomy is not a reason to perform a cesarean section. Maternal indications for delivery include severely compromised maternal cardiovascular status and obstruction of the operating field by the gravid uterus that limits surgical exposure of damaged vital structures. Fetal indications for delivery include fetal hemorrhage and distress and intra-amniotic infection. Such factors as suspected fetal injury and fetal distress must be balanced against those of fetal maturity. Even if labor has begun, some authors feel that vaginal delivery following exploratory laparotomy is preferable to hysterotomy.

Stab wounds of the abdomen are somewhat more complicated in management. Determination of whether the peritoneal cavity has been violated can be difficult. Fistulograms using Hypaque and peritoneal lavage have been promoted in the management of stab wounds. Stab wounds only require surgical repair in about one-half of reported cases. As with gunshot wounds, if the wound is confined to the lower abdomen, the uterus usually sustains most injuries, whereas other viscera are spared. Because of a high incidence of upper abdominal wounds, treatment and consideration for exploratory laparotomy should be individualized.

## ACQUIRED COAGULOPATHY

Acquired coagulation defects in pregnancy are not uncommon.

## RETAINED DEAD FETUS SYNDROME

With the advent of ultrasonography, improved methods of labor induction, and aggressive management, the retained dead fetus syndrome is rarely encountered in obstetric practice today.

The cause of coagulopathy is postulated to be the release of tissue thromboplastin from the fetus or placenta, activating the extrinsic pathway and resulting in DIC and secondary activation of the fibrinolytic system.

The patient may present in a compensated or decompensated hemostatic state, as manifested by clinical evidence of bleeding and laboratory studies. Coagulation screening of all patients with intrauterine fetal demise should be done prior to delivery of the fetus in order to detect a potentially lethal coagulopathy. Laboratory studies should include a complete blood count, platelet count, fibrinogen, fibrin split products, prothrombin time, and partial thromboplastin time.

If the patient is found to have DIC and is in labor, fibrinogen is replaced by administration of cryoprecipitate, as the volume of fresh-frozen plasma may be excessive and result in volume overload. If the patient is not in labor, heparin may be administered by continuous intravenous infusion until fibrinogen levels rise to between 200 and 300 mg/dL and platelets are greater than 60,000/$\mu$L. Heparin is then discontinued and induction of labor is instituted 6 hours after discontinuation of heparin.

## AMNIOTIC FLUID EMBOLISM AND DIC

The clinical diagnosis of amniotic fluid embolism is rare, estimated to be 1 in 20,000 to 1 in 80,000 deliveries. Of great significance is an overall mortality rate of approximately 80%.

Risk factors include advanced maternal age, multiparity, vigorous uterine contractions, meconium presence in amniotic fluid, large fetal size, and fetal demise. Fetal death prior to the acute episode occurs in 40% of cases, and abruptio placentae may accompany 50% of cases.

Passage of amniotic fluid into the maternal vasculature results in cardiopulmonary compromise mimicking pulmonary hypertension and cor pulmonale. Later, DIC results from the coagulant activity of amniotic fluid. Microemboli may pass through the pulmonary capillary bed and into the systemic vessels.

The patient classically develops chills, restlessness, dyspnea, cyanosis, nausea, vomiting, altered mental status, and then hypotension and tachycardia. Cardiorespiratory arrest follows.

Treatment includes cardiovascular resuscitation, respiratory support, and correction of the abnormal coagulation state. Intravenous heparin has been reported in the treatment of amniotic fluid embolism, but is not in widespread use. Inotropic support is warranted in the face of left ventricular failure and pulmonary edema.

## PREGNANCY-INDUCED HYPERTENSION

Delivery of the products of conception is the only known treatment for patients with preeclampsia and HELLP syndrome. Replacement of fluids, blood products, and other supportive measures are instituted as indicated.

## TRAUMA AND DIC

DIC may result from trauma in several ways. Massive crushing injuries cause release of substances, probably from damaged tissue, into the circulation, activating the coagulation cascade. Massive hemorrhage from injury may result in depletion of coagulation factors. Trauma to the uterus may result in abruption or amniotic fluid embolism, which are both known to cause DIC. Treatment includes replacement of blood and coagulation products, general supportive care, and measures directed to correcting the inciting factors.

## INHERITED COAGULOPATHIES

Hereditary disorders of coagulation occur in approximately 1 to 2 per 10,000 persons and therefore are rarely encountered in obstetric practice. A deficiency of any factor in the intrinsic, extrinsic, or common pathways of blood coagulation may result in a clotting disorder.

Screening tests include platelet count, prothrombin time (PT), partial thromboplastin time (PTT), bleeding time, thrombin clotting time (TCT), and clot stability test.

## ANAPHYLACTIC SHOCK

Anaphylactic reactions may be fatal in as many as 10% of cases. Obstetric patients are especially at risk, as they will, at some point during pregnancy, probably receive some form of pharmacologic therapy. Antibiotics, nonsteroidal anti-inflammatory agents, narcotics, local anesthetics, iodinated radiocontrast agents, hormones, blood products, colloid solutions, and antivenoms are all known to have the potential to cause anaphylactic reactions. Few reports exist in the current obstetric literature regarding this subject.

Clinical manifestations may be mild to severe (Table 33-4). Life-threatening events include airway obstruction and cardiovascular collapse.

The first priority of management is ventilation, oxygenation, and external cardiac massage, which, in general, is followed by the subcutaneous administration of epinephrine in 0.2-mg increments up to a total dose of 1.0 mg. In obstetric patients, ephedrine, 25 to 50 mg by IV push, has been recommended because other vasoactive agents carry detrimental uteroplacental effects. However, failure to achieve clinical response with ephedrine should not contraindicate the use of other, more potent agents, such as epinephrine, dopamine, norepinephrine, and isoproterenol, in patients with unresponsive shock.

## SEPTIC SHOCK

Septic shock is rare in obstetrics; however, it is one of the most frequent causes of maternal mortality in the United States. Many infections may result in septic shock in obstetric patients, but endometritis, chorioamnionitis, and pyelonephritis are the most common causes. Before legalization of abortion, septic shock resulting from criminal abortion was common.

Diagnosis requires identification of the source of infection. This source is usually found to be the genital or urinary tract in obstetric patients. Clinical signs include fever, tachycardia, warm-flushed or cool-clammy skin, and tenderness elicited over the affected tissues. Routine laboratory evaluation of patients with suspected septic shock include complete blood count (CBC) with differential, platelets, coagulation studies, electrolytes, BUN, creatinine, lactate, urinalysis,

**TABLE 33-4.** Clinical Spectrum of Anaphylactic Reactions

| Mild | Moderate | Severe |
|---|---|---|
| Local erythema/itching | Dizziness | Hypotension/cyanosis |
| Pruritus/urticaria | Generalized skin reactions | Angioedema |
| Coryza | Hoarseness | Stridor/wheezes |
| Nausea/vomiting | Swelling of lips/tongue | Cardiac arrhythmias |
| Diarrhea | Tachypnea | Syncope/seizures |
| Conjunctival suffusion | Tachycardia | Altered mental status |
| Anxiety | Increasing respiratory distress and anxiety | Shock Cardiopulmonary arrest |

From Carlson RW, Bowles AL, Haupt MT. Anaphylactic, anaphylactoid, and related forms of shock. Crit Care Clin 1986;2:347.

and arterial blood gases. Laboratory evidence of infection may include leukocytosis on peripheral blood smear, pyuria and bacteriuria on urinalysis, and blood gas aberrations, such as a metabolic acidosis with compensatory respiratory alkalosis. In some patients, evidence of coagulopathy is manifested by abnormalities in platelet count, fibrinogen, prothrombin time, partial thromboplastin time, and the presence of fibrin-split products.

Cultures should be obtained in all patients from the urine, blood, and, if possible, the amniotic fluid or the endometrium. The technique of endometrial culture may affect bacteriologic findings. Other specific sources, such as stool, wound, and sputum, are cultured as indicated. Lumbar puncture should be considered in patients with altered mental status.

Chest x-ray should be obtained to rule out infiltrates, evidence of pulmonary edema, and adult respiratory distress syndrome (ARDS). Abdominal x-rays should be obtained to rule out free air under the diaphragm or a foreign body.

Treatment of septic shock requires general supportive measures, including restoration of intravascular volume and often inotropic support (see the section on general supportive measures). Adequate oxygenation is essential. Antibiotic therapy for sepsis should be tailored directly to the suspected source guided by information obtained by gram stain.

## SEPTIC ABORTION

Treatment includes general supportive measures, antibiotics, and removal of the infected necrotic tissue. Broad coverage with an aminoglycoside, clindamycin, and penicillin or ampicillin is recommended because the infection is usually of a mixed aerobic–anaerobic type. Dilatation and curettage is performed to remove the infectious nidus in the uterus. Antibiotic therapy and evacuation of uterine contents will successfully control approximately 95% of all cases. If the infection has progressed beyond the endometrium and is not responsive to conservative therapy, exploratory laparotomy, hysterectomy, and possibly removal of the adnexa are required.

## CHORIOAMNIONITIS

The diagnosis is usually made on clinical grounds based on evidence of leakage of fluid from the vagina, fever, maternal or fetal tachycardia, leukocytosis, uterine tenderness, and foul-smelling amniotic fluid. Gram stain of amniotic fluid obtained by transabdominal amniocentesis or through intrauterine pressure catheters may be helpful.

Treatment consists of hydration, administration of parenteral antibiotics, and prompt delivery of the fetus. Diagnosis-to-delivery time limits should not be set. Vaginal delivery is preferable to cesarean section in the presence of chorioamnionitis except when the maternal condition deteriorates, fetal distress ensues, or the usual obstetric indications for cesarean section are present.

## PYELONEPHRITIS

Septic shock occurs in 1.3% to 3% of patients hospitalized for acute pyelonephritis. Cunningham and others reported four cases of respiratory insufficiency with multisystem derangement associated with pyelonephritis in pregnancy, thought to be secondary to endotoxin effects.

Treatment of pyelonephritis necessitates early administration of an antibiotic to which the organism is susceptible. If urosepsis is suspected, broad-spectrum coverage is recommended. The choice of antibiotics should be based on known bacterial drug resistance at each individual hospital. Because of a high incidence of *E. coli* resistance to ampicillin, therapy at our institution is begun with cefazolin, 1 g intravenously every 8 hours. If severe infection or urosepsis is suspected, we provide wider coverage by administering an aminoglycoside plus ampicillin. Hydration with crystalloid solutions is another crucial aspect of therapy. After the patient has been afebrile for 24 hours, intravenous antibiotics are discontinued and an oral antibiotic to which the organism is known to be sensitive is started.

## APPENDICITIS

Appendicitis is the most common nonobstetric indication for exploratory laparotomy in the obstetric patient. The incidence of appendicitis is 1 per 1500 deliveries.

The classic signs and symptoms of appendicitis are present less frequently in the pregnant patient. Rebound tenderness and rectal tenderness are common early in pregnancy, but become less frequent as pregnancy advances. Localization of abdominal tenderness may change as gestation progresses.

Useful laboratory values include leukocytosis in the range of 10,000 to 15,000/μL, with a quarter of patients having a WBC count of less than 10,000/μL and a quarter of patients having a WBC count greater than 15,000/μL. Urinalysis may reveal pyuria without bacteriuria. Urinalysis is normal in 91% of cases.

Treatment is surgical. Exploratory laparotomy is performed through an incision that will allow access to other suspect anatomical regions, since diagnostic accuracy is around 75% at best.

## TOXIC SHOCK SYNDROME

Toxic shock syndrome (TSS) has been reported to occur in association with vaginal delivery, spontaneous abortion, cesarean section, and mastitis. The exact incidence of nonmenstrual TSS is unknown. Mortality may be as high as 5%.

TSS is defined by a fever greater than 102°F, diffuse macular erythrodermal rash with desquamation, hypotension, and evidence of multiple organ system involvement caused by systemic absorption of exotoxin produced by certain strains of *Staphylococcus aureus*. Vasodilation and egress of intravascular fluid and serum proteins into the extravascular compartment result in oliguria, hypotension, edema, low central venous pressure, hypoproteinuria, and hypoalbuminemia.

Initial clinical management requires aggressive fluid replacement to correct systemic hypotension. Invasive monitoring in an intensive care unit is necessary in many instances. Cultures should be obtained from the usual sources, such as blood and urine, as well as from the genital tract and other suspected areas (e.g., surgical wound, cutaneous lesion, or throat). β-lactamase-resistant antistaphylococcal antibiotics (oxacillin, dicloxacillin, nafcillin), first-generation parenteral cephalosporins, and aminoglycosides may be used for treatment, although they usually do not have a significant effect on the course of the acute disease.

## SUPPURATIVE PELVIC THROMBOPHLEBITIS

Septic or suppurative pelvic thrombophlebitis (SPT) describes a condition of the pelvic veins in which septic thrombosis occurs. Trauma along the surfaces of the genital tract is felt to be the inciting factor preceding thrombosis and infection. In addition to bacteremia and sepsis, thromboembolism may occur, with pulmonary infarction occurring in 45.7% of patients.

Diagnosis may be difficult and is often one of exclusion. Recently, computed tomography scan of the pelvis for detection of venous thrombosis has been proposed.

Medical therapy with broad-spectrum antibiotics (e.g., gentamicin, clindamycin, and ampicillin) for suspected endometritis is often instituted before the diagnosis of SPT is made. Institution of intravenous heparin is then begun and clinical improvement within 48 hours is anticipated. In the absence of pulmonary emboli, heparin may be continued for 10 days. Surgical therapy, which was once the mainstay, is still indicated if medical therapy is unsuccessful, if pulmonary infarction develops during medical therapy, or if the patient presents prior to therapy with pulmonary infarction.

## BURNS

Approximately 2.2 million people each year in the United States suffer burns significant enough to present for medical treatment.

Early complications of burns include severe hypovolemia secondary to fluid and electrolyte shifts resulting from vascular damage. Hypovolemia, hypotension, and shock are prevented by aggressive fluid and electrolyte replacement. Electrolytes must be monitored carefully, because sodium and potassium values may fluctuate widely.

Because experience with pregnant burn patients is limited, few specific treatment guidelines beyond electrolyte and fluid replacement, adequate ventilatory support, and antibiotic therapy have been proposed. Tocolytic therapy must be managed carefully. β-mimetic therapy may result in further electrolyte imbalance and cardiopulmonary complications. Magnesium sulfate may produce unwanted vasodilative effects. Indomethacin has been proposed as an acute temporary method of managing premature labor, which may be managed expectantly or by conventional means after the patient's condition has stabilized. As in other instances of maternal injury, maternal stability, fetal well-being, and fetal maturity must all be considered in making decisions about delivery. The route and timing of delivery should be based on obstetric indications.

## NECROTIZING FASCIITIS

Necrotizing fasciitis, a suppurative bacterial infection of the superficial and deep fasciae, is a rare but deadly complication in obstetrics. Treatment requires prompt diagnosis, wide surgical debridement of necrotic tissue, drainage, and parenteral antibiotics with emphasis on anaerobic coverage.

## CARDIOGENIC SHOCK

Cardiogenic shock may be secondary to ventricular dysfunction or extrinsic cardiac compression, both of which result in diminished cardiac output and hypoperfusion at the cellular level. Many of these processes may develop in the nonpregnant state; however, amniotic fluid embolism and peripartum cardiomyopathy are unique to the obstetric population.

## VENTRICULAR DYSFUNCTION

### BETA-ADRENERGIC AGENTS

Ventricular dysfunction, as manifested by arrhythmias, angina pectoris, pulmonary edema, or cardiovascular collapse, has been reported with the use of terbutaline, salbutamol, hexoprenaline, and ritodrine in the tocolytic therapy of premature labor. Early cessation of the tocolytic agent, close monitoring, and treatment of associated maternal arrhythmias and cardiopulmonary derangements are essential in preventing further serious complications.

## EMBOLISM

### Thrombotic Pulmonary Embolism

Treatment of thrombotic pulmonary embolism consists of cardiopulmonary support and heparin anticoagulation to prevent progressive thrombus formation. The efficacy and safety of thrombolytic agents, such as streptokinase, urokinase, and tissue plasminogen activator, remain unproven, especially in obstetrics.

## CARDIAC COMPRESSION

Extrinsic cardiac compression decreases venous return and impairs optimal pumping of the heart. Decreased cardiac output can result in shock. Tension pneumothoracardial tamponade and rupture of the diaphragm with herniation of the abdominal contents into the thoracic cavity may cause significant cardiac compression.

Placement of a chest tube will alleviate compression secondary to a tension pneumothorax. Pericardiocentesis will relieve the high intrapericardial pressure produced by cardiac tamponade. Diaphragmatic rupture with herniation of abdominal viscera is a surgical emergency.

## NEUROGENIC SHOCK

Neurogenic shock is said to occur when generalized vasodilation causes venous pooling, resulting in decreased filling of the right heart and diminished cardiac output. Neurogenic shock in obstetrics may accompany conduction anesthesia, central nervous system trauma, and puerperal uterine inversion.

## PUERPERAL UTERINE INVERSION

Shock resulting from puerperal uterine inversion traditionally has been thought to be secondary to a combination of reflex parasympathetic stimulation and acute blood loss. Although classically described as "shock out of proportion to blood loss," some authors believe that blood loss is often grossly underestimated.

Most authorities recommend that shock be corrected prior to manual replacement of the inverted uterus.

## CONDUCTION ANESTHESIA

Hypotension and shock secondary to regional anesthesia are treated by rapid fluid replacement, cardiovascular support, and ventilatory support. Placement of the patient in the Trendelenburg position and alleviating uterine aortocaval compression may be helpful. Vasopressors should be carefully used if the preceding methods are unsuccessful. Ephedrine is preferred to other vasopressors that correct hypotension at the expense of decreasing uteroplacental blood flow. Mechanical ventilatory support may be required when large doses of local anesthetics are injected into the subarachnoid space when intended for the peridural space. Hypotension may be prevented by intravenous fluid preloading, Trendelenburg positioning, and left uterine displacement. Additional caution should be taken in patients with hypertensive disorders, since greater drops in mean arterial blood pressure have been demonstrated as compared to normotensive subjects.

## COMPLICATIONS OF SHOCK

In the early 1970s, the syndrome of multisystem organ failure (MSOF) emerged. Infection is thought to be the etiology of MSOF. However, positive blood cultures were detected in only 50% of patients with established MSOF. Sepsis and organ failure are produced by any process that activates the inflammatory response, including microorganisms and necrotic tissue. Many inflammatory mediators have been identified in the pathogenesis of MSOF.

Mortality rates in MSOF are reported in a wide range. The number of organ systems involved correlates directly with mortality.

## PREVENTIVE MEASURES

In many cases, the development of shock is unforeseeable and unavoidable. However, clinical suspicion and advanced preparation may decrease the severity and subsequent morbidity and mortality of a developing event. All obstetric patients should be considered potential victims of hemorrhage. Certain patients present with conditions placing them in a high-risk category, such as placenta previa, multiple previous cesarean sections, intrauterine fetal demise near term, and pregnancy-induced hypertension. Preparation by ensuring good venous access, availability of volume expanders and blood products, anesthesia, and uterotonic agents may allow prompt and effective treatment in the event of acute blood loss, which may intercept further blood loss and prevent subsequent complications. Concern over risks of homologous blood transfusion have prompted new interest. High-risk patients, such as those with placenta previa, previous cesarean sections, and rare blood types, may benefit by avoiding transfusion reactions, antibody development, and disease transmission associated with homologous transfusion.

In general, preparedness and identification of patients at risk for shock may minimize or prevent maternal and fetal life-threatening events.

# 34.  HYPERTENSIVE DISEASES IN PREGNANCY

Approximately 10% of pregnancies are complicated by hypertension. Apart from being the most common medical complication of pregnancy, hypertensive disorders are associated with significant maternal, fetal, and neonatal morbidity and mortality. Preeclampsia accounts for 70% of hypertension in pregnancy, and chronic essential hypertension accounts for most of the remaining 30%. (For a more thorough discussion of these topics, please see Chapter 58 in Reece EA, Hobbins JC, Mahoney MJ, and Petrie RH, eds. *Medicine of the fetus and mother*. J.B. Lippincott, 1992.)

## HYPERTENSION

The American College of Obstetricians and Gynecologists Committee on Terminology defines hypertension in pregnancy as either a systolic pressure of ≥140 mmHg or an increment of ≥30 mmHg (from a baseline in the first half of pregnancy) or a diastolic pressure of ≥90 mmHg or an increment of ≥15 mmHg. The pressures or increases in pressure must be observed on at least two occasions 6 hours apart. If blood pressure in the first half of pregnancy is unknown, readings of 140/90 mmHg after 20 weeks are considered sufficiently elevated to diagnose preeclampsia. The committee also regards an increase in mean arterial blood pressure of 20 mm Hg or, if previous blood pressure is unknown, a mean arterial pressure of 105 mmHg as diagnostic of hypertension.

## PROTEINURIA

The concentration of urinary protein is highly variable. It is influenced by several factors, including contamination with vaginal secretions, blood, or bacteria; urine specific gravity and pH; exercise; and posture. Significant proteinuria is defined as >0.3 g in a 24-hour urine collection or 0.1g/L (>2+ on the dipstick), in at least two random samples collected 6 hours or more apart.

## EDEMA

Preeclampsia has been described traditionally as a triad of edema, proteinuria, and hypertension. Although excessive weight gain (>2 pounds per week in the third trimester) may be the first sign of preeclampsia, moderate edema is a feature of 80% of normotensive pregnancies. The assessment of edema is subjective. It should be considered pathologic only if it is generalized, involving the hands, face, and legs.

**344**    E. Albert Reece, John C. Hobbins, Maurice, J. Mahoney and Roy H. Petrie (Eds).
*Handbook of Medicine of the Fetus & Mother*. Copyright © 1995 by J.B. Lippincott Company

**TABLE 34-1.** Criteria for the Diagnosis of Severe Preeclampsia

1. Blood pressure ≥160 mmHg systolic or ≥110 mmHg diastolic on two occasions at least 6 hours apart with the patient at bedrest
2. Proteinuria ≥ 5 g in a 24-hour urine collection or ≥ 3+ on dipstick in at least two random clean-catch samples at least 4 hours apart
3. Oliguria (≤400 mL in 24 hours)
4. Cerebral or visual disturbances
5. Epigastric pain
6. Pulmonary edema or cyanosis

Data from Hughes EC, ed. Obstetric-gynecologic terminology. Philadelphia: FA Davis, 1972:442.

## PREECLAMPSIA

Preeclampsia is the most common hypertensive complication of pregnancy. It can be classified as mild or severe. Mild preeclampsia is diagnosed by a blood pressure of 140/90 mmHg on two occasions 6 hours apart (with or without proteinuria). According to the American College of Obstetricians and Gynecologists Committee on Terminology, severe preeclampsia is diagnosed when any one of the criteria listed in Table 34-1 is present.

## ECLAMPSIA

Eclampsia is defined as the development of convulsions or coma or both in a patient with signs and symptoms of preeclampsia. Other causes of seizures must be excluded (Table 34-2). Eclampsia may present antepartum, intrapartum, or

**TABLE 34-2.** Differential Diagnosis of Eclampsia

Cerebrovascular accidents
    Cerebrovenous thrombosis
    Cerebroarterial occlusion
    Cerebroarterial embolism
    Intracerebral hemorrhage
Hypertensive disease
    Hypertensive encephalopathy
    Pheochromocytoma
Space-occupying central nervous system lesions
    Tumor
    Abscess
Infectious disease
    Meningitis
    Encephalitis
Metabolic disease
    Hypoglycemia
    Hypocalcemia
    Water intoxication
    Epilepsy

From Villar MA, Sibai BM. Eclampsia. In: Arias F, ed. High risk pregnancy. Obstetrics and gynecology clinics of North America. Philadelphia: WB Saunders, 1988:358.

postpartum. Approximately 50% of cases occur antepartum, usually during the third trimester.

## HELLP SYNDROME

Recently, a syndrome of hemolysis, elevated liver enzymes, and low platelets was described as a variant of preeclampsia. There is considerable controversy about the definition, diagnosis, incidence, etiology, and management of HELLP syndrome. In terms of diagnosis, the most consistent finding in the literature is thrombocytopenia (platelet count $< 100,000/\mu L$).

## CHRONIC HYPERTENSION

Chronic hypertension is diagnosed if there is persistent elevation of blood pressure to at least 140/90 mmHg on two occasions more than 24 hours apart before 20 weeks gestation. Hypertension that persists for more than 42 days postpartum is also classified as chronic hypertension. Other factors that may suggest the presence of chronic hypertension include

Retinal changes on funduscopic examination
Radiologic and electrocardiographic evidence of cardiac enlargement
Compromised renal function or associated renal disease
Multiparity with a previous history of hypertensive pregnancies
Presence of hypertension more than 6 weeks postpartum

Chronic hypertension may be classified as mild or severe. Mild chronic hypertension implies a systolic blood pressure of less than 160 mmHg and a diastolic of less than 110 mmHg. Severe chronic hypertension is diagnosed if either the systolic or diastolic pressure exceeds these limits.

## SUPERIMPOSED PREECLAMPSIA

Chronic hypertension may be complicated by superimposed preeclampsia (or eclampsia). Superimposed preeclampsia is diagnosed when there is an exacerbation of hypertension (elevation of 30 mmHg systolic and 15 mmHg diastolic or 20 mmHg mean arterial pressure) and the development of proteinuria or generalized edema that was not previously apparent. About 15% to 30% of chronically hypertensive women develop this complication.

## LATENT OR TRANSIENT HYPERTENSION

Latent or transient hypertension is defined as hypertension occurring antepartum, in labor, or in the first 24 hours postpartum without generalized edema or proteinuria and with a return to normotension within 10 days of delivery.

## PATHOPHYSIOLOGY
### PREECLAMPSIA

Preeclampsia is a disorder peculiar to human pregnancy. It is principally a disease of young primigravidas and rarely presents before 20 weeks gestation. Early presentation is more likely to be associated with unrecognized renal disease, whereas onset at term or intrapartum is more often associated with transient or latent hypertension. Several risk factors have been identified as predisposing to the development of preeclampsia (Table 34-3). The pathophysiology of preeclampsia has been well described. The underlying abnormality is general arteriolar constriction and increased vascular sensitivity to pressor peptides and amines. Despite extensive investigation, the etiology of this disease is unknown.

## Proposed Etiologies

**Prostacyclin-Thromboxane Imbalance.** It has been suggested that an imbalance of prostaglandins is central to the pathophysiology of preeclampsia. Prostacyclin ($PGI_2$) is synthesized by the vascular endothelium and the renal cortex. It is a vasodilator and inhibits platelet aggregation. Thromboxane $A_2$ ($TxA_2$) is produced primarily by platelets and is a potent vasoconstrictor and aggregator of platelets.

**Immunology.** Speculation that the cause of preeclampsia may be found within the immune system has stimulated considerable interest and research over the last 10 to 15 years.

Although there is some suggestion that the humoral immune system and complement activation are involved in the preeclamptic process, there is no evidence that immunologic factors cause the condition. At present there are no data to support a role for cell-mediated immunity.

**Renin-Angiotensin-Aldosterone.** The renin-angiotensin-aldosterone system (RAAS) plays an important role in the control of vascular tone and blood pressure.

In normal pregnancy, concentrations of the components of the RAAS are increased. However, the vascular response to most pressor substances is impaired. Conversely, in preeclampsia, some of the components of the RAAS are lower than those in normal pregnancy and there is a markedly increased sensitivity to pressor peptides and catecholamines.

## ECLAMPSIA

Why some patients with symptoms of preeclampsia develop convulsions and/or coma and others do not is unknown. Several mechanisms have been suggested as predisposing factors:

**TABLE 34-3.** Risk Factors for Preeclampsia

Nulliparity
Multiple gestation
Family history of preeclampsia-eclampsia
Preexisting hypertension-renal disease
Previous preeclampsia-eclampsia
Diabetes
Nonimmune hydrops fetalis
Molar pregnancy

From Sibai BM, Moretti MM. Pregnancy induced hypertension. Contemporary Ob/Gyn 1988;31:57.

Cerebral vasospasm
Cerebral hemorrhage
Cerebral ischemia
Cerebral edema
Hypertensive encephalopathy
Metabolic encephalopathy

Most patients with eclamptic seizures have an abnormal electroencephalogram (EEG). However, EEG changes are almost always transient and resolve completely. Furthermore, they give no clue to the underlying pathophysiology. Computed tomography is also unhelpful and is rarely abnormal. Whether the newer technique of nuclear magnetic resonance imaging will prove more illuminating remains to be seen.

## CHRONIC HYPERTENSION

The most common etiology of chronic hypertension is essential hypertension. Other causes are listed in Table 34-4. Most of these other causes require specific medication in addition to antihypertensive therapy. Early diagnosis is important because, if untreated, many of these disorders are associated with significant maternal and fetal morbidity and mortality. Severe essential hypertension is characterized by end-organ damage. Total peripheral resistance continues to rise and cardiac output may begin to fall. The intravascular volume decreases further and plasma renin activity rises. These changes increase left ventricular tension and reduce myocardial contractility. Without treatment, pulmonary edema will occur.

## PREECLAMPSIA

### Management of Preeclampsia
The most effective therapy for preeclampsia is delivery of the fetus and placenta. In pregnancies at or near term where the cervix is favorable, labor should be

**TABLE 34-4.** Etiology of Chronic Hypertension

1. Renal factors
   a. Acute and chronic glomerulonephritis
   b. Acute and chronic pyelonephritis
   c. Polycystic renal disease
   d. Renovascular disease
2. Collagen disease with renal involvement
   a. Lupus erythematosus
   b. Periarteritis nodosa
   c. Scleroderma
3. Endocrine factors
   a. Diabetes with vascular involvement
   b. Thyrotoxicosis
4. Coarctation of the aorta
5. Pheochromocytoma

Data from Sibai BM. Chronic hypertension during pregnancy. In: Sciarra JJ, ed. Gynecology and obstetrics. Philadelphia: JB Lippincott, 1988.

induced. Intravenous magnesium sulfate should be administered during labor to reduce the risk of convulsions. Preeclampsia remote from term presents a much more difficult management problem. The decision of whether to intervene and deliver a preterm infant that may require prolonged intensive care or to institute expectant management is usually governed by disease severity and the length of gestation.

**Mild Preeclampsia.** Mild preeclampsia remote from term can be managed on an ambulatory basis, or the patient can be admitted to the hospital. Ambulatory management is applicable in the early stages of the disease. The patient is allowed to remain at home but advised to spend most of the day resting. The attending obstetrician must evaluate maternal and fetal well-being every second day. If there is any evidence of disease progression and or if acute hypertension develops, then prompt hospitalization is indicated.

Once a patient has been admitted to the hospital, intensive maternal and fetal monitoring should be instituted. Table 34-5 summarizes the measures used at the University of Tennessee, Memphis, to evaluate maternal and fetal well-being. The frequency of testing depends on the severity of the disease. In many cases of mild preeclampsia the disease does not progress and pregnancy can be managed conservatively until the fetus reaches maturity.

If a patient becomes normotensive after hospitalization and is remote from term with no evidence of fetal compromise, outpatient surveillance may be considered. This requires a minimum of twice-weekly maternal and fetal assessment. There is no place for conservative management if there are signs of progression to severe preeclampsia or if fetal monitoring tests become abnormal.

Conservative management of mild disease beyond term is not beneficial to the fetus, because uteroplacental blood flow is suboptimal. After 37 weeks gestation, labor should be induced as soon as the cervix is favorable.

*The Role of Antihypertensive Therapy.* Antepartum use of antihypertensive therapy for mild preeclampsia remote from term is controversial. Rubin and colleagues (1983) compared atenolol beta$_1$-selective adrenoreceptor blocking agent) against placebo in a randomized study. Some studies compared labetalol (a

---

**TABLE 34-5.** Maternal–Fetal Evaluation of Mild Preeclampsia Remote from Term

---

**Maternal Evaluation**
1. Blood pressure (four times daily)
2. Presence of generalized edema (particularly facial and abdominal edema) and/or excessive weight gain (daily)
3. Patellar reflexes (daily)
4. Symptoms of persistent occipital headache, visual symptoms, or epigastric pain (daily)
5. Urinalysis (daily) (A dipstick test will provide only a crude estimate of proteinuria. A 24-hour urine collection should be analyzed for protein and creatinine clearance—twice a week.)
6. Hematocrit and platelet count (every 2 days)
7. Serum uric acid, creatinine (twice a week)
8. Liver function tests (SGOT, LDH, serum bilirubin) (weekly)

**Fetal Evaluation**
1. Daily fetal movement records
2. Nonstress test (twice weekly)
3. Biophysical profile, if nonstress test is unreactive
4. Ultrasound assessment of fetal growth (every 2 weeks)

---

nonselective beta blocker with some alpha$_1$-blocking effects) with bedrest. These studies suggested that in mild preeclampsia, bedrest alone has little effect on blood pressure or disease progression, whereas antihypertensive therapy appeared to reduce the incidence of progression to severe disease as measured by increasing blood pressure and development of proteinuria. There was no benefit to mother or fetus apart from a reduction in hospitalization. One study compared labetalol plus hospitalization with hospitalization alone in the management of 200 mild preeclamptics remote from term. They concluded that perinatal outcome was not improved by lowering blood pressure in mild preeclampsia.

Diuretics may be harmful to both mother and fetus, and since they have no proven beneficial effect they should not be used.

**Severe Preeclampsia.** There is considerable evidence to show the deleterious effects of severe hypertension in nonpregnant humans and in experimental animals. In treating severe preeclampsia, blood pressure should be maintained below 160/110 mmHg. The most widely used antihypertensive agent in pregnancy is methyldopa. An adequate therapeutic response may be expected within 12 hours. If blood pressure cannot be controlled with a single agent, combination therapy (usually methyldopa and hydralazine) is usually effective. Intravenous hydralazine administered as a bolus of 5 mg at 15- to 20-minute intervals is the treatment of choice for acute rises in blood pressure > 160/100 mmHg. The aim is to reduce diastolic pressure gradually to the range of 90 to 100 mmHg. Intermittent therapy with hydralazine rarely produces a dramatic fall in blood pressure, but the level must be carefully and frequently monitored.

In most studies of eclampsia, 20% of women had only a minimal rise in blood pressure. Consequently, all patients who meet the blood pressure criteria for preeclampsia should be given intravenous magnesium sulfate to minimize the risk of eclampsia. In Memphis this drug is administered by a controlled continuous intravenous infusion with a loading dose of 6 g in 100 mL. Maintenance therapy is given at a rate of 2 g in 100 mL of fluid per hour. Serum magnesium levels are obtained 4 to 6 hours later, and the rate of infusion is adjusted to keep serum magnesium levels between 4.8 and 9.6 mg/dL. Treatment is continued for 24 hours postpartum. Intramuscular magnesium injections should be avoided.

Magnesium is excreted in the urine. In the therapeutic range it slows neuromuscular conduction and depresses CNS irritability. Maternal respiratory rate, deep tendon reflexes, and level of consciousness must be frequently monitored to detect magnesium toxicity. If respiratory depression does occur, 1 g of calcium gluconate should be given intravenously over 3 minutes. Magnesium sulfate may also decrease beat-to-beat variability of the fetal heart rate, and signs of neonatal hypermagnesemia have been reported after only 24 hours intravenous therapy. The mode of action of magnesium ions is uncertain and there is disagreement as to whether it has a predominantly central or peripheral effect.

Input and output should be assessed hourly, and a Foley catheter should be inserted to permit accurate measurement of urine output. The aim is to maintain urine output at 30 mL/h. If output is less than 100 mL in 4 hours, fluid input (including magnesium sulfate infusion) should be reduced accordingly. For patients in active labor, urine output often increases after 2 or 3 hours, and specific therapy is unnecessary.

Continuous epidural anesthesia has been advocated in preeclampsia and eclampsia in the belief that it not only controls pain but also aids in stabilizing blood pressure and increases renal and uterine blood flow. However, this procedure requires an arterial line and central hemodynamic monitoring (both invasive procedures), and the contracted blood volume characteristic of preeclampsia makes the risk of hypotension high. If a significant fall in blood pressure does occur following epidural anesthesia, attempts to achieve normotension by fluid loading can precipitate pulmonary edema. For these reasons, the authors would advocate the use of epidural analgesia in preeclampsia or eclampsia only if it is administered by personnel skilled in obstetric anesthesia. There should be no evidence of fetal distress, maternal platelet count should be greater than 100,000/μL, and bleeding time should be less than 12 minutes.

Blood loss at delivery in severe preeclampsia may be greater than that for a normal pregnancy. Magnesium sulfate may inhibit uterine contraction, and tolerance to blood loss is reduced by the contracted blood volume. Cross-matched blood should therefore be available in the labor and delivery area. The mode of delivery should be determined by gestational age and by fetal and maternal condition. For gestations less than 32 weeks, cesarean section is the route of choice in the absence of labor or a ripe cervix. The preterm fetus is at significant risk of intrapartum asphyxia, and the presence of severe preeclampsia increases this risk. Intrapartum electronic fetal monitoring at this gestation is often technically difficult. Furthermore, induction of labor before 32 weeks is often a prolonged process that increases the likelihood of fetal asphyxia.

Experience based on the management of 303 cases of severe preeclampsia has led the authors to conclude that the management of choice for almost all patients who are beyond 28 weeks gestation is prompt delivery. These pregnancies may be managed conservatively until fetal maturity is achieved, provided they are followed closely in a tertiary care center with daily maternal and fetal monitoring. Most will require delivery within 3 to 10 days of admission. Hence, amniocentesis should be performed for lecithin/sphingomyelin (L/S) ratio; if the fetal lung is immature, the patient should be given steroids to accelerate maturity.

The management of severe preeclampsia at less than 28 weeks gestation is a difficult problem. Figure 34-1 details the recommended management of severe midtrimester preeclampsia based on the Memphis experience.

| 25–28 Weeks ≤ Intensive Maternal–Fetal Management | 24 Weeks Termination of Pregnancy |
|---|---|
| IV magnesium sulfate for 24 hours | PGE vaginal suppository |
| Antihypertensive if diastolic BP ≥ 110 mmHg | IV magnesium sulfate |
| Daily evaluation of fetal well-being | Hydralazine if required |
| Daily evaluation of maternal status | |
| Cesarean section if there is evidence of | |
| Fetal lung maturity | |
| Fetal distress | |
| Maternal distress | |

**FIGURE 34-1.** Management of severe midtrimester preeclampsia. (From Sibai BM. Preeclampsia-eclampsia. In: Sciarra JJ, ed. Gynecology and obstetrics. Philadelphia: J.B. Lippincott, 1988, 8.)

## HELLP Syndrome

It is sometimes difficult to distinguish between HELLP syndrome and other disorders associated with liver dysfunction or hemolytic anemia (e.g., idiopathic thrombocytopenic purpura, thrombotic thrombocytopenic purpura, hemolytic uremic syndrome, gallbladder disease, and viral hepatitis). The criteria used in Memphis to diagnose HELLP syndrome are shown in Table 34-6.

**Management.** Patients with a diagnosis of HELLP syndrome should be considered as having severe preeclampsia. They should be managed as such and referred to a tertiary care center. The method of management is controversial. Some recommend immediate delivery; others favor a conservative approach in pregnancies remote from term.

## ECLAMPSIA

Eclampsia is associated with multiple organ dysfunction. Factors determining the degree of dysfunction include a delay in the treatment of preeclampsia and the presence of complicating obstetric and medical factors. Eclampsia is associated with a wide spectrum of signs and symptoms, ranging from extreme hypertension, hyperreflexia, 4+ proteinuria, and generalized edema to isolated mild hypertension. Laboratory findings also vary. Serum uric acid and creatinine are usually elevated, and creatinine clearance is reduced. Hemoconcentration reflected by an increased hematocrit and reduced plasma volume is common. Elevated liver function tests are found in 11% to 74% of eclamptic patients. HELLP syndrome complicates about 10% of eclampsia and usually occurs in long-standing disease and in patients with medical complications. Disseminated intravascular coagulopathy may develop if treatment is delayed or abruptio placentae with fetal demise has occurred (Table 34-7).

### Management

The protocol used to manage eclampsia in Memphis is outlined in Table 34-8. The first priority is to control convulsions. Magnesium sulfate is the anticonvulsant of choice. It is important to remember that the maximum dose when given over a short time should not exceed 8 g. Once convulsions have been abolished, arterial blood gas measurements and a chest radiograph should be obtained to ensure

**TABLE 34-6.** Laboratory Values used to Diagnose Hellp Syndrome

Hemolysis
  Abnormal peripheral blood smear (with burr cells and schistocytes)
  Increased bilirubin ≥ 1.2 mg/dL*
  Increased lactic dehydrogenase > 600 IU/L*
Elevated liver enzymes
  Increased SGOT ≥ 72 IU/L*
  Increased lactic dehydrogenase as above
Low platelets
  Platelet count < 100,000/μL

Data from Sibai BM, Taslimi MM, El-Nazar A, Amon E, Mabie WC, Ryan G. Maternal-perinatal outcome associated with the syndrome of hemolysis, elevated liver enzymes, and low platelets in severe preeclampsia-eclampsia. Am J Obstet Gynecol 1986;155:501.

*These values are more than four standard deviations above the mean for the Memphis population.

**TABLE 34-7.** Factors Involved in Unavoidable Eclampsia

| Factor | All Cases of Eclampsia (n = 232) | Unavoidable Eclampsia (n = 84) |
|---|---|---|
| Abrupt onset | 45 | 36 |
| Late postpartum onset | 38 | 27 |
| Convulsion of magnesium sulfate | 26 | 10* |
| Mild preeclampsia with good response† | — | 7 |
| Early onset (<21 weeks) | 6 | 4 |

*Adequate serum levels.
†Normal blood pressure after hospitalization.

**TABLE 34-8.** Authors' Protocol for Managing Eclampsia

1. Convulsions are controlled or prevented with a loading dose of 6 g magnesium sulfate in 100 mL 5% dextrose in Ringer's lactated solution, given over 15 minutes, followed by a maintenance dose of 2 g/h.
2. Serum magnesium level is obtained 4 to 6 hours later, and the rate of infusion is adjusted to maintain magnesium levels between 4.8 and 9.6 mg/dL. If serum magnesium levels are not available, the dose is adjusted according to patellar reflexes and urine output in the previous 4-hour period.
3. Diuretics, plasma volume expanders, and invasive hemodynamic monitoring are not used.
4. Induction and/or delivery is initiated within 4 hours after maternal stabilization.
5. Magnesium sulfate is continued for 24 hours after delivery or, if postpartum, 24 hours after the last convulsion. In some cases, the infusion is continued for 72 hours as needed.

adequate maternal oxygenation and exclude aspiration. Hypoxemia and acidemia should be corrected. The next step is to treat maternal hypertension. Hydralazine administered as intermittent boluses (5 to 10 mg) is a safe and effective antihypertensive in this situation.

Following stabilization of maternal condition, steps should be taken to deliver the fetus. Induction of labor with oxytocin is often successful after 32 weeks gestation. The fetal heart rate and uterine activity must be closely monitored. For gestations of less than 32 weeks, cesarean section is advocated.

Some authors have suggested that eclampsia indicates hemodynamic monitoring with Swan-Ganz catheters. Some have concluded that such intensive monitoring is rarely necessary.

## OUTCOME OF PREGNANCIES COMPLICATED BY PREECLAMPSIA OR ECLAMPSIA

For pregnancies complicated by mild preeclampsia, maternal and perinatal morbidity and mortality approach those of normotensive pregnancies. This contrasts sharply with the outcome for severe preeclampsia. Sibai and colleagues (1987) reported on 303 pregnancies complicated by severe preeclampsia.* There were 28

*Sibai BM, Spinnato JA, Watson DL, Hill GA, Anderson GD. Pregnancy outocme in 303 cases witih sever preeclampsia. Obstet Gynecol 1984;64:319.

stillbirths and 15 neonatal deaths, giving a corrected perinatal mortality rate of 135 in 1000. The severity and incidence of neonatal complications were closely related to gestational age at delivery. Maternal morbidity was common. The reported perinatal mortality for preeclampsia with HELLP syndrome ranges from 8% to 60% and maternal mortality ranges from 0% to 24%. HELLP syndrome may be complicated by acute renal failure, pulmonary edema, ascites, and hepatic rupture. There is high incidence of abruptio placentae and disseminated intravascular coagulation. Maternal mortality resulting from eclampsia is usually associated with mismanagement of a complicated case. The fetus of an eclamptic woman is particularly at risk from abruptio placentae, preterm delivery, intrauterine growth retardation, and acute hypoxia during maternal convulsions. Maternal and neonatal morbidity and mortality can be reduced by early transfer of eclamptic patients to tertiary care centers with neonatal intensive care facilities.

Patients developing severe preeclampsia or eclampsia in their first pregnancy are at increased risk of developing obstetric complications in their subsequent pregnancies. These complications include preeclampsia (incidence in subsequent pregnancies about 30%), abruptio placentae, fetal growth retardation, and premature delivery. Tables 34-9, 34-10, and 34-11 summarize the maternal and fetal outcomes of pregnancies complicated by preeclampsia or eclampsia.

## CHRONIC HYPERTENSION

Patients with hypertension secondary to renal disease, pheochromocytoma, endocrine disease, and coarctation of the aorta are relatively uncommon in pregnancy. Their management is that of the underlying disease. Most patients with chronic hypertension have essential hypertension. The presence of chronic hypertension in pregnancy increases maternal and perinatal morbidity and mortality. Most of the morbidity and mortality is related to the development of superimposed preeclampsia and abruptio placentae. Maternal and fetal risk can be reduced by proper antepartum surveillance.

Ideally, patients with chronic hypertension should be seen before conception so that full investigation and assessment of their disease can be carried out and the

**TABLE 34-9.** Maternal-Perinatal Outcome in Hospitalized Patients with Mild Preeclampsia Remote from Term

|  | Gilstrap et al. ($n = 545$) | Sibai et al. ($n = 200$) |
|---|---|---|
| Gestation ≤ 36 weeks | 373 (68.5%) | 200 (100%) |
| Significant proteinuria | 44 (8%) | 200 (100%) |
| Average pregnancy prolongation (days) | 24 | 21 |
| Mean birth weight (in grams) | 2824 | 2258 |
| Fetal growth retardation | 46 (8.4%) | 27 (13.5%) |
| Perinatal deaths | 5 (0.9%) | 1 (0.5%) |
| Abruptio placentae | 5 (1%) | 2 (1%) |
| Eclampsia | 1 (0.5%) | 0 |

From Sibai BM. Preeclampsia-eclampsia. Contemp Ob/Gyn 1988;32:109.

**TABLE 34-10.** Pregnancy Outcome in HELLP Syndrome

|  | Number | (%) |
|---|---|---|
| Maternal Outcome ($n$ = 112) |  |  |
| Abruptio placentae | 22 | 20.0 |
| DIC | 42 | 38.0 |
| Acute renal failure | 9 | 8.0 |
| Pleural effusions | 8 | 7.1 |
| Pulmonary edema | 5 | 4.5 |
| Ruptured liver hematoma | 2 | 1.8 |
| Maternal deaths | 2 | 1.8 |
| Fetal Outcome ($n$ = 114 births) |  |  |
| Perinatal deaths | 38 | 33.3 |
| Gestational age (wk) |  |  |
| ≤30 | 47 | 41.2 |
| 31–36 | 46 | 40.4 |
| ≥36 | 21 | 18.4 |
| SGA | 36 | 31.6 |

Data from Sibai BM, Taslimi MM, El-Nazer A, Amon E, Mabie WC, Ryan G. Maternal–perinatal outcome associated with the syndrome of hemolysis, elevated liver enzymes, and low platelets in severe preeclampsia–eclampsia. Am J Obstet Gynecol 1986;155:501.
DIC = disseminated intravascular coagulation.
SGA = small for gestational age.

potentially harmful effects of antihypertensive drugs can be discussed. The following evaluation should be initiated as soon as the patient attends for antepartum care:

General physical examination, including funduscopy
Measurement of blood pressure in four extremities
Effect on blood pressure of changes in physical activity and posture

Laboratory investigations should include:

Urinalysis and culture, 24 hour-urine collection for protein, electrolytes, and
    creatinine clearance
SMAC-20

**TABLE 34-11.** Maternal Complications from Eclampsia: 1977–1988

| Complication | Maternal Transfer and No Perinatal Care ($n$ = 135; % = 58) | Prenatal Care at University ($n$ = 97; % = 42) | Total ($n$ = 232; % = 100) |
|---|---|---|---|
| Abruptio placentae | 19 (14) | 4 (4) | 23 (10.0) |
| Pulmonary edema | 6 (4) | 4 (4) | 10 (4.3) |
| Cardiorespiratory arrest | 6 (4) | 2 (2) | 10 (4.3) |
| Acute renal failure | 9 (6) | 1 (1) | 8 (3.4) |
| Aspiration | 4 (3) | 1 (1) | 5 (2.1) |
| Maternal death | 1 (0.7) | 0 0 | 1 (0.4) |

In selected patients antinuclear antibodies, urine catecholamines and vanillyl-mandelic acid (VMA), chest x-ray, and electrocardiogram are indicated.

On the basis of this assessment patients are classified as either high or low risk. Some of the factors that classify the patient as high risk are:

Maternal age > 40 years
Duration of hypertension > 15 years
Blood pressure > 160/110 mmHg early in pregnancy
Diabetes (class B-F)
Cardiomyopathy
Renal disease
Connective tissue disease

Most patients are hospitalized at the time of their first prenatal visit. They are seen by a nutritionist and given dietary advice. Daily sodium intake should be restricted to 2 g. The harmful effects of smoking, stress, and caffeine on maternal blood pressure and fetal well-being are stressed and frequent rest periods are encouraged.

Patients are seen every 2 weeks up to 28 weeks and then weekly until delivery. At each visit systolic and diastolic blood pressure should be recorded and the urine tested for the presence of glucose and protein. Urine culture should be performed every trimester. Evaluation of maternal status includes serial measurements of hematocrit, serum creatinine, uric acid, creatinine clearance, and 24-hour urinary excretion of protein and sodium. Prompt hospitalization is indicated if there is an exacerbation of hypertension, development of pyelonephritis, significant proteinuria, or an elevation of uric acid. An elevation of uric acid > 6 mg/dL is often an early warning sign of superimposed preeclampsia.

Fetal evaluation includes serial ultrasound measurements of growth and antepartum fetal heart rate testing from 34 weeks. For those considered high risk, nonstress testing may commence as early as 26 weeks. Daily fetal movement counts and biophysical profiles are also used in some patients to determine the optimum time for delivery.

Antihypertensive therapy is restricted to patients with severe hypertension. Diuretics are rarely used. Low-risk pregnancies are allowed to continue to 42 weeks gestation with close monitoring. High-risk pregnancies and patients receiving antihypertensive drugs are delivered at or before 40 weeks gestation. Superimposed preeclampsia or fetal growth retardation are considered indications for delivery, regardless of gestation. If preterm delivery is contemplated, amniocentesis is performed and steroids are administered if the L/S ratio indicates that the fetal lung is immature.

## Antihypertensive Therapy

There is considerable disagreement among obstetricians worldwide about antihypertensive therapy in pregnancy, particularly about what drugs are most appropriate and at what level of blood pressure treatment should be commenced. Maternal mortality associated with chronic hypertension in pregnancy is usually due to a malignant rise in blood pressure with subsequent congestive cardiac failure or cerebrovascular accidents. There is no evidence to suggest any maternal benefits from treating mild to moderate hypertension during pregnancy. Treatment of severe hypertension, on the other hand, is associated with a reduction in maternal mortality and morbidity. Fetal and perinatal outcome are closely linked to the incidence of superimposed preeclampsia and abruption. Antihypertensive therapy does not alter the incidence of these two complications and thus confers no perinatal benefit. The drugs most commonly used in pregnancy are adrenoreceptor blocking agents, thiazide diuretics, and hydralazine.

**Adrenoreceptor Blocking Agents.** Two classes of adrenoreceptors are recognized—alpha and beta. Alpha and beta receptors are subdivided into types 1 and 2 and into presynaptic or postsynaptic, according to their location at the adrenergic nerve terminals. The action and side effects of adrenoreceptor blocking agents depend on how selective the drug is for a particular receptor type. In addition, adrenoreceptors are located peripherally and centrally. Stimulation or blockade of the receptors at different sites will produce opposite effects.

*Methyldopa.* Methyldopa is the most commonly used antihypertensive agent worldwide. It acts by stimulating central alpha$_2$ receptors. It may also be an alpha$_2$ blocker acting by a false neurotransmitter effect. The drug is given orally with a loading dose of 1 g followed by maintenance therapy of 1 to 2 g daily in four divided doses. Peak plasma levels occur within 2 hours of an oral dose, and the fall in blood pressure is maximal 4 hours after tablet ingestion. Side effects include drowsiness and a dry mouth. Hepatitis, hemolytic anemia, and a positive Coomb's test have been reported in association with long-term usage.

Adverse perinatal effects of methyldopa remain unproved, and follow-up studies on infants exposed to methyldopa in utero have shown no untoward effects at the age of 7.5 years.

A variety of beta-blocking agents have been used to treat hypertension in pregnancy. These drugs have different actions, depending on their receptor selectivity and the presence of intrinsic sympathomimetic activity. One review of their use has concluded that these agents are safe in pregnancy and in fact are associated with a better fetal outcome than either methyldopa or hydralazine.

**Thiazide Diuretics.** Although thiazide diuretics are commonly used to treat hypertension in the nonpregnant population, their role in pregnancy is highly controversial. In view of their potential detrimental effects and no proven benefits, diuretics should be avoided in pregnancy.

**Hydralazine.** Hydralazine is the drug most commonly used to control severe hypertension in pregnancy. It is usually given as intermittent injections or as a continuous infusion. Hydralazine is a potent vasodilator, with a peak hypotensive effect occurring 20 minutes after intravenous administration. Side effects include fluid retention, tachycardia, facial flushing, and headache. Chronic administration may be associated with a maternal lupus syndrome and neonatal thrombocytopenia. Oral hydralazine is a weak antihypertensive when used alone and is usually combined with methyldopa or a diuretic.

**Calcium Channel Blockers.** Calcium channel blockers have been used successfully to manage hypertension in nonpregnant patients. To date, there have been few studies relating to their use in human pregnancy. Nifedipine has been used in pregnancy both as a single agent and as a second-line drug in combination with other antihypertensives. Although these initial studies have suggested that nifedipine is an effective antihypertensive in pregnancy with few maternal side effects, further study is required to be certain of fetal safety and to determine whether this agent has any advantages over the antihypertensives in current use.

## Outcome

Chronic hypertension in pregnancy is usually associated with a good maternal and fetal outcome unless complicated by maternal renal disease or superimposed preeclampsia. Patients with mild "low-risk" chronic hypertension have a perinatal outcome similar that of the general obstetric population. Antihypertensive therapy is often not required and the pregnancy can be safely prolonged to term.

Patients with severe "high-risk" chronic hypertension have a significant risk of fetal and maternal morbidity and perinatal mortality. Outcome is closely related to the development of superimposed preeclampsia. Patients with severe chronic hypertension in early pregnancy or underlying renal disease require early referral for antenatal care, intensive fetal and maternal monitoring as described earlier, and delivery in a tertiary care center. Antihypertensive therapy is indicated and should maintain blood pressure between 140 to 150 mmHg systolic and 90 to 100 mmHg diastolic. Persistent blood pressure levels below these ranges in patients who have previously been very hypertensive may jeopardize placental perfusion.

---

# 35. CARDIAC DISEASE IN PREGNANCY

Pregnancy causes many significant alterations in the maternal cardiovascular system. The pregnant patient with normal cardiac function accommodates these physiologic changes without difficulty. However, in the presence of significant cardiac disease, pregnancy may be extremely hazardous, resulting in decompensation and even death. This chapter will focus on the interaction between structural cardiac disease and pregnancy.

## COUNSELING THE PREGNANT CARDIAC PATIENT

Counseling the pregnant cardiac patient regarding her prognosis for successful pregnancy is complicated by recent advances in medical and surgical therapy, fetal surveillance, and neonatal care. Such advances render invalid many older estimates of maternal mortality and fetal wastage.

Table 35-1 represents a synthesis of current maternal mortality estimates for various types of cardiac disease. Group I includes conditions that, with proper management, should have negligible maternal mortality (<1%). Cardiac lesions in group II carry with them a 5% to 15% risk of maternal mortality; in individual cases, and after appropriate counseling, this risk may prove acceptable to some women. Patients with cardiac lesions in group III are subject to a mortality risk exceeding 25%. In all but exceptional cases, this risk will prove unacceptable to the patient, and prevention or interruption of pregnancy should be recommended strongly.

## ATRIAL SEPTAL DEFECT

Atrial septal defect (ASD) is the most common congenital lesion seen during pregnancy and is generally asymptomatic. The hypervolemia associated with

**TABLE 35-1.** Mortality Risk Associated with Pregnancy

Group I: Mortality < 1%
  Atrial septal defect*
  Ventricular septal defect*
  Patent ductus arteriosus*
  Pulmonic-tricuspid disease
  Corrected tetralogy of Fallot
  Bioprosthetic valve
  Mitral stenosis, NYHA classes I and II
Group II: Mortality 5% to 15%
  Mitral stenosis with atrial fibrillation
  Artificial valve
  Mitral stenosis, NYHA classes III and IV
  Aortic stenosis
  Coarctation of aorta, uncomplicated
  Uncorrected tetralogy of Fallot
  Previous myocardial infarction
  Marfan syndrome with normal aorta
Group III: Mortality 25% to 50%
  Pulmonary hypertension
  Coarctation of aorta, complicated
  Marfan syndrome with aortic involvement

From Clark SL, ed. Critical care obstetrics. Oradell, NJ: Medical Economics Books, 1987.
*Uncomplicated.

pregnancy results in an increased left-to-right shunt through the ASD, and thus a significant burden is imposed on the right ventricle. Although this additional burden is tolerated well by most patients, congestive failure and death with ASD have been reported. The vast majority of patients with ASD tolerate pregnancy, labor, and delivery without complication. During labor, avoidance of fluid overload, oxygen administration, labor in the lateral recumbent position, and pain relief with epidural anesthesia, as well as prophylaxis against bacterial endocarditis, are the most important considerations (Table 35-2).

## VENTRICULAR SEPTAL DEFECT

The size of the septal defect is the most important determinant of clinical prognosis during pregnancy. Small defects are tolerated well, whereas larger defects are associated more frequently with congestive failure, arrhythmias, or the development of pulmonary hypertension. Intrapartum management considerations for patients with uncomplicated VSD or PDA are similar to those outlined for ASD.

**TABLE 35-2.** Patients at High Risk for Bacterial Endocarditis

Prosthetic heart valves (including bioprostheses)
Most congenital cardiac malformations
Surgical systemic–pulmonary shunts
Rheumatic and other acquired valvular dysfunction
Idiopathic hypertrophic subaortic stenosis (IHSS)
Previous history of bacterial endocarditis
Mitral valve prolapse with insufficiency

## PATENT DUCTUS ARTERIOSUS

As with uncomplicated ASD and VSD, most patients are asymptomatic, and PDA is generally tolerated well during pregnancy, labor, and delivery. Management considerations for patients with uncomplicated PDA, without pulmonary hypertension, are similar to those outlined under ASD.

## EISENMENGER SYNDROME

Eisenmenger syndrome develops when, in the presence of congenital left-to-right shunt, progressive pulmonary hypertension leads to shunt reversal or bidirectional shunting. Although this syndrome may occur with ASD, VSD, or PDA, the low-pressure–high-flow shunt seen as ASD is far less likely to result in pulmonary hypertension and shunt reversal than is the condition of high-pressure and high-flow symptoms seen with the VSD and PDA. Whatever the etiology, pulmonary hypertension carries a grave prognosis during pregnancy. In the presence of fixed pulmonary hypertension, such decreased right heart pressures may be insufficient to perfuse the pulmonary arterial bed. This insufficiency may result in sudden, profound hypoxemia. Such hypotension can result from hemorrhage or complications of conduction anesthesia and may result in sudden death. Avoidance of such hypotension is the principal clinical concern in the intrapartum management of patients with pulmonary hypertension of any etiology.

Maternal mortality in the presence of Eisenmenger syndrome is reported as 30% to 50%. Thromboembolic phenomena have been associated with up to 43% of all maternal deaths in Eisenmenger syndrome. However, some have reported an increased mortality associated with prophylactic peripartum heparinization. Sudden delayed postpartum death, occurring 4 to 6 weeks after delivery, also has been reported.

Because of the high mortality associated with continuing pregnancy, abortion is the preferred management of choice for the woman with pulmonary hypertension of any etiology. Dilatation and curettage in the first trimester or dilatation and evacuation in the second trimester is the method of choice. Hypertonic saline and F-series prostaglandins are contraindicated. For the patient with a continuing gestation, hospitalization for the duration of pregnancy is often appropriate. Continuous administration of oxygen, the pulmonary vasodilator of choice, is mandatory and may improve perinatal outcome. In cyanotic heart disease of any etiology, fetal outcome correlates well with maternal hematocrit, and successful pregnancy is unlikely with a hematocrit $> 65\%$. Maternal $paO_2$ should be maintained at a level of 60 to 70 mmHg or above. Third trimester fetal surveillance with antepartum testing is important because at least 30% of the fetuses will be growth retarded. Overall fetal wastage with Eisenmenger syndrome is reported to be up to 75%.

During labor, the primary concern in such patients is the avoidance of hypotension, any attempt to preload reduction (i.e., diuresis) must be undertaken with great caution, even in the face of initial fluid overload. We prefer to manage such patients on the "wet" side, maintaining a preload margin of safety against unexpected blood loss, even at the expense of some degree of pulmonary edema.

The use of epidural or intrathecal morphine sulfate, a technique devoid of effect on systemic blood pressure, has been described by some and represents perhaps the best approach to anesthetic management of these difficult patients.

Ideally, if the patient has reached a point where fetal pulmonary maturity can be documented and the cervix is favorable for induction, she would be admitted to the hospital the night prior to induction. Pulmonary artery catheterization should be performed to optimize hemodynamics prior to the initiation of labor. Because decreased cardiac output will be most hazardous for such patients, an attempt is made to maintain a high cardiac output and wedge pressure, even at the risk of incurring some pulmonary edema. A recommended therapeutic goal would be to maintain a wedge pressure in the 16- to 18-mmHg range. Any hemodynamic manipulation must be carried out with careful attention to cardiac output, blood pressure, and other maternal cardiovascular indices. A patient should labor on her side with both continuous administration of oxygen and continuous electronic fetal heart rate monitoring. Narcotic epidural anesthesia is the anesthetic method of choice for pain relief during labor and delivery and, if necessary, cesarean section. Because of the increased risk of significant blood loss and hypotension associated with operative delivery, cesarean section should be reserved exclusively for obstetric indications. Similarly, midforceps delivery is not warranted to shorten the second stage but should be reserved for standard obstetric indications only.

## COARCTATION OF THE AORTA

The most common site of coarctation is the origin of the left subclavian artery. Associated anomalies of the aorta and left heart, including VSD and PDA, are common, as are intracranial aneurysms in the circle of Willis. Coarctation is usually asymptomatic. It appears that today patients having coarctation of the aorta uncomplicated by aneurysmal dilatation or associated cardiac lesions who enter pregnancy as class I or II have a good prognosis and a minimal risk of complications or death. Even if uncorrected, uncomplicated coarctation carries with it a risk of maternal mortality of only 3% to 4%. Maternal risk is increased if preeclampsia develops. In the presence of aortic or intervertebral aneurysm, known aneurysm of the circle of Willis, or associated cardiac lesions, however, the risk of death may approach 15%; therefore, therapeutic abortion must be strongly considered.

## TETRALOGY OF FALLOT

Most cases of tetralogy of Fallot are corrected during infancy or childhood. Several published reports attest to the relatively good outcome of pregnancy in patients with corrected tetralogy of Fallot. However, in patients with an uncorrected lesion, maternal mortality ranges from 4% to 15%, with a 30% fetal mortality due to hypoxia. In patients with uncorrected VSD, the decline in SVR that accompanies pregnancy can lead to worsening of the right-to-left shunt. This condition can be aggravated further by systemic hypotension as a result of peripartum blood loss. A poor prognosis has been related to prepregnancy hematocrit exceeding 65%, history of syncope or congestive failure, electrocardiographic evidence of right ventricular strain, cardiomegaly, right ventricular pressure in excess of 120 mmHg, and peripheral oxygen saturation below 80%.

## PULMONIC STENOSIS

Pulmonic stenosis is a common congenital defect. Although obstruction can be valvular, supravalvular, or subvalvular, the degree of obstruction, rather than its site, is the principal determinant of clinical performance. A transvalvular pressure gradient exceeding 80 mmHg is considered severe and mandates surgical correction. A compilation (totaling 106 pregnancies) of three series of patients with pulmonic stenosis revealed no maternal deaths. With severe stenosis, right heart failure can occur; fortunately, this is usually less severe clinically than is the left heart failure associated with mitral or aortic valve lesions.

## PULMONIC AND TRICUSPID LESIONS

Isolated right-sided valvular lesions of rheumatic origin are uncommon; however, such lesions are seen with increased frequency in intravenous drug abusers, where they are secondary to valvular endocarditis. Pregnancy-associated hypervolemia is far less likely to be symptomatic with right-sided lesions than with those involving the mitral or aortic valves. Even following complete tricuspid valvectomy for endocarditis, pregnancy, labor, and delivery are generally well tolerated. Cautious fluid administration is the mainstay of labor and delivery management in such patients. In general, invasive hemodynamic monitoring during labor and delivery is not necessary.

## MITRAL STENOSIS

Mitral stenosis is the most common rheumatic valvular lesion encountered during pregnancy. The principal hemodynamic aberration involves ventricular diastolic filling obstruction, resulting in a relatively fixed cardiac output. Marked increases in cardiac output accompany normal pregnancy, labor, and delivery. If the pregnant patient is unable to accommodate such volume fluctuations, pulmonary edema will result.

Cardiac output in patients with mitral stenosis depends largely on two factors. First, these patients depend on adequate diastolic filling time. Thus, although in most patients tachycardia is a clinical sign of underlying hemodynamic instability, in patients with mitral stenosis, the tachycardia itself, regardless of etiology, may contribute significantly to hemodynamic decompensation. The physician should consider oral beta-blocker therapy for any patient with severe mitral stenosis who enters labor with a pulse exceeding 90 beats per minute.

A second important consideration in patients with mitral stenosis is left ventricular preload. In the presence of mitral stenosis, pulmonary capillary wedge pressure is not an accurate reflection of left ventricular filling pressures. Such patients often require high-normal or elevated pulmonary capillary wedge pressure to maintain adequate ventricular filling pressure and cardiac output. Any preload manipulation (i.e., diuresis) therefore must be undertaken with extreme caution and careful attention to maintenance of cardiac output.

Potentially dangerous intrapartum fluctuations in cardiac output can be minimized by using epidural anesthesia; however, the most hazardous time for these women appears to be the immediate postpartum period. Such patients often enter the postpartum period already operating at maximum cardiac output and cannot accommodate the volume shifts that follow delivery. In a series of patients with severe mitral stenosis, we found that a postpartum rise in wedge pressure of up to 16 mmHg could be expected in the immediate postpartum period. Because frank pulmonary edema generally does not occur with wedge pressures below 28 to 30 mmHg, it follows that the optimal predelivery wedge pressure for such patients is 14 mmHg or lower, as indicated by pulmonary artery catheterization. Such a preload may be approached by cautious intrapartum diuresis and with careful attention to the maintenance of adequate cardiac output.

In a patient with functional class II or III mitral stenosis, many of the same management considerations apply to those discussed under the section dealing with pulmonary hypertension. Bedrest and, at times, the administration of oxygen to maintain the therapeutic goal of a $PO_2$ greater than 60 mmHg are essential. Under ideal circumstances, the patient would be admitted at term with a favorable cervix. Because pulmonary artery catheterization allows the hemodynamic condition to be optimized prior to the stress of labor. The patient should labor on her side with the administration of oxygen. Epidural anesthesia will also assist in minimizing hemodynamic fluctuations during labor and delivery. Because pulmonary edema is the major concern in these patients, we recommend that diuresis be carried out in order to approach a wedge pressure of 12 to 14 mmHg.

Our experience suggests that vaginal delivery is safe even in patients with severe disease and pulmonary hypertension. Additionally, we have found it unnecessary to resort routinely to midforceps deliveries.

## MITRAL INSUFFICIENCY

This lesion generally is tolerated well during pregnancy, and congestive failure is unusual. A more significant risk is the development of atrial enlargement and fibrillation.

Congenital mitral valve prolapse is much more common during pregnancy than is rheumatic mitral insufficiency and can occur in up to 17% of young healthy women. Endocarditis prophylaxis during labor and delivery is recommended for rheumatic mitral insufficiency as well as for the more common mitral valve prolapse syndrome, if associated with regurgitation.

## AORTIC STENOSIS

There appears to be a higher maternal mortality associated with rheumatic as opposed to congenital aortic stenosis. In one recent series of pregnancies in 15 women with congenital aortic stenosis, no maternal deaths were observed. In contrast to mitral valve stenosis, aortic stenosis generally does not become hemodynamically significant until the orifice has diminished to one third or less of normal. The major problem experienced by patients with valvular aortic stenosis is maintenance of cardiac output. Because of the relative hypervolemia associated with gestation, such patients generally tolerate pregnancy well.

Delivery and pregnancy termination appear to be the times of greatest risk for patients with aortic stenosis. The maintenance of cardiac output is crucial; any factor leading to diminished venous return will cause an increase in the valvular gradient and diminished cardiac output. The literature suggests that pregnancy termination may be especially hazardous in this regard and carries a mortality of up to 40%. Hypotension resulting from blood loss, ganglionic blockade from epidural anesthesia, or supine vena caval occlusion by the pregnant uterus may result in sudden death.

The cardiovascular status of patients with aortic stenosis is complicated further by the frequent coexistence of ischemic heart disease. The overall reported mortality associated with aortic stenosis in pregnancy is 17%. Patients with shunt gradients exceeding 100 mmHg are at greatest risk. Pulmonary artery catheterization may allow precise hemodynamic assessment and control during labor and delivery. Management considerations for the patient with aortic stenosis are similar to those in women with pulmonary hypertension, in that decreases in cardiac preload and output may result in sudden death. In addition, pulmonary edema is rare in the presence of a competent mitral valve. Thus, we prefer to manage these patients on the wet side, attempting to maintain a wedge pressure of 16 to 18 mmHg during labor. Once again, midforceps or cesarean delivery should be reserved for standard obstetric indications only, assuming that continuous invasive monitoring during labor and delivery is available.

## AORTIC INSUFFICIENCY

Aortic insufficiency generally is tolerated well during pregnancy because the increased heart rate seen with advancing gestation decreases time for regurgitant flow during diastole.

## FETAL CONSIDERATIONS

Of major concern in patients with congenital heart disease is the risk of fetal congenital cardiac anomalies. Although this risk was previously felt to be on the order of 5%, recent data suggest the actual risk may be as high as 10%, or even higher in women whose congenital lesion involves ventricular outflow obstruction. In such patients, fetal echocardiography is indicated for prenatal diagnosis of congenital cardiac defects. Of special interest is the fact that affected fetuses appear to be concordant for the maternal lesion in only 50% of cases.

## PERIPARTUM CARDIOMYOPATHY

Peripartum cardiomyopathy is defined as cardiomyopathy developing in the last month of pregnancy or the first 6 months postpartum in a woman without previous cardiac disease and after exclusion of other causes of cardiac failure. It is therefore a diagnosis of exclusion that should not be made without a concerted effort to identify valvular, metabolic, infectious, or toxic causes of cardiomyopathy.

The incidence of peripartum cardiomyopathy is estimated at between 1 in 1500 and 1 in 4000 deliveries in the United States. In the United States, the peak incidence of peripartum cardiomyopathy occurs in the second postpartum month and appears most frequently among older, multiparous black females. Other suggested risk factors include twinning and pregnancy-induced hypertension. Up to 50% of patients with peripartum cardiomyopathy may manifest evidence of pulmonary or systemic embolic phenomena. Overall mortality ranges from 25% to 50%.

Therapy includes digitalization, diuretics, sodium restriction, and prolonged bedrest. In refractory cases, concomitant afterload reduction with hydralazine or nitrates may be useful. Early endomyocardial biopsy to identify a subgroup of patients who have a histologic picture of inflammatory myocarditis and who may be responsive to immunosuppressive therapy has been suggested.

A notable feature of peripartum cardiomyopathy is its tendency to recur with subsequent pregnancies. Patients whose cardiac size returned to normal within 6 to 12 months had an 11% to 14% mortality in subsequent pregnancies; those patients with persistent cardiomegaly had a 40% to 80% mortality.

## MARFAN SYNDROME

Although some authors feel pregnancy is contraindicated in any woman with documented Marfan syndrome, prognosis is best individualized and should be based on echocardiographic assessment of aortic root diameter and postvalvular dilatation. Women with an abnormal aortic valve or aortic dilatation may have up to a 50% pregnancy-associated mortality; women without these changes and having an aortic root diameter less than 40 mm have a mortality of less than 5%. In counseling women with Marfan syndrome, the genetics of this condition and the shortened maternal lifespan must be considered, in addition to the immediate maternal risk. The routine use of oral beta-blocking agents to decrease pulsatile pressure on the aortic wall has been recommended. If cesarean section is performed, retention sutures should be used because of generalized connective tissue weakness.

## MYOCARDIAL INFARCTION

Myocardial infarction in conjunction with pregnancy is rare. In a review of 68 reported cases, myocardial infarction during pregnancy was associated with a 35% mortality rate. Only 13% of patients were known to have had coronary artery disease prior to pregnancy. Two-thirds of the women suffered infarction in the third trimester; mortality for these women was 45%, compared to 23% in those suffering infarction in the first or second trimesters.

Antepartum care of women with prior myocardial infarction includes bedrest to minimize myocardial oxygen demands. In women with angina, nitrates have been used without adverse fetal effects. Delivery within 2 weeks of infarction is associated with increased mortality; therefore, if possible, attempts should be made to allow adequate convalescence prior to delivery.

## PROSTHETIC VALVES AND ANTICOAGULATION

The proper drug for anticoagulation in the patient with an artificial heart valve during pregnancy is controversial. The teratogenic effects of oral anticoagulants must be weighed against a potential increased risk of thrombosis and thromboembolism incurred by using heparin rather than warfarin. However, most physicians in the United States favor the use of heparin.

Indications for antithrombotic therapy recently were reviewed at a national conference sponsored by the American College of Chest Physicians and the National Heart, Lung, and Blood Institute. The recommendation of this committee was to treat pregnant women who have prosthetic heart valves with adjusted-dose subcutaneous heparin from conception until delivery. Sodium heparin, 8000 to 14,000 U, is injected every 8 to 12 hours to achieve an activated partial thromboplastin time of 1.5 to 2 times control 6 hours after injection.

Patients with bioprosthetic or xenograft valves usually are not treated with anticoagulants during pregnancy. This fact makes the bioprosthetic valve the ideal choice of prosthesis for young women of childbearing age.

## CARDIOVASCULAR SURGERY

There are numerous reports of cardiovascular surgery during pregnancy, most of which are favorable; they include successful correction of most types of congenital and acquired cardiac disease.

Initial reports of cardiopulmonary bypass during pregnancy were not nearly as favorable, indicating a fetal wastage of up to 33%. Initiation of cardiopulmonary bypass generally is followed by fetal bradycardia, which may be correctable by high flow rates. With the use of continuous electronic fetal heart rate monitoring, flow rate can be adjusted to avoid or correct fetal hypoperfusion and bradycardia, thus reducing fetal mortality to less than 10%. High-flow–high-pressure normothermic perfusion and continuous electronic fetal heart rate monitoring appear to be optimal for the fetus. Maternal mortality is highly dependent on the specific nature of the procedure being performed and does not appear to be increased significantly by pregnancy.

# 36. MATERNAL PULMONARY DISORDERS COMPLICATING PREGNANCY

Pregnant women are afflicted by the same respiratory ailments as nonpregnant women, but these conditions are complicated by the physiologic alterations of pregnancy. Asthma and other pulmonary diseases may first manifest during pregnancy or change their course during gestation. Respiratory illness can affect both maternal and fetal outcomes during pregnancy. Pharmacologic treatment of lung disease can be undertaken to minimize adverse effects to both mother and fetus.

## DIAGNOSTIC TECHNIQUES

### HISTORY AND PHYSICAL EXAMINATION

If the patient has been pregnant in the past, the presence of respiratory symptoms during the prior pregnancy should be noted and compared to the patient's usual respiratory symptoms when not pregnant.

Dyspnea is the most common respiratory complaint during pregnancy, with as many as 60% to 70% of previously normal women having this symptom at some time during pregnancy. The complaint usually begins in the first or second trimester but is most prevalent at term. It is not usually due to underlying lung disease but probably results from the subjective perception of hyperventilation that normally accompanies pregnancy. As the woman acclimates to this new sensation, her perception of dyspnea is reduced and the dyspnea stabilizes as the pregnancy progresses. Unlike pathologic dyspnea, symptoms do not increase with exertion.

### ARTERIAL BLOOD GASES

In a normal pregnant female, arterial blood gas measurements will usually show a compensated respiratory alkalosis due to maternal hyperventilation. The pH generally ranges from 7.40 to 7.47, and the partial pressure of arterial carbon dioxide is 25 to 32 mmHg. The partial pressure of arterial oxygen may be as high as 106 mmHg in early pregnancy, decreasing during pregnancy but remaining at 100 mmHg, or slightly higher, at term.

Calculating the oxygen content of blood requires a knowledge of the amount of oxygen dissolved in the blood, the maximum amount of oxygen able to be carried per gram of hemoglobin, the hemoglobin concentration, and the oxygen saturation of hemoglobin.

$$\text{Oxygen content} = [(\text{Hb (g/dL)} \times 1.39 \text{ mL } O_2/\text{g Hb}) \\ \times (\text{oxygen saturation})] \\ + [(0.003 \text{ mL } O_2/100 \text{ mL of blood}) \times P_{aO_2} \text{ (mmHg)}]$$

Mismatching of ventilation and perfusion is responsible for most of the defective gas exchange in pulmonary diseases. The adequacy of alveolar gas exchange can be assessed by calculating the alveolar-arterial oxygen tension gradient. Ideal alveolar oxygen tension ($P_{AO_2}$) is calculated as follows:

$$P_{AO_2} = F_{IO_2} \times (P_b - 47) - P_{ACO_2}/0.8$$

$F_{IO_2}$ = fractional percentage of inspired oxygen
$P_b$ = barometric pressure
47 = water vapor pressure
$P_{ACO_2}$ = arterial blood tension of carbon dioxide
0.8 = respiratory quotient

Since most acute lung diseases are accompanied by an increased $(A - a)O_2$ gradient, the gradient should be assessed with the pregnant patient in the upright position and should be considered abnormal if it exceeds 25 mmHg. Blood gas analysis should be accompanied by calculation of the gradient, because with the usual decreased $P_{CO_2}$ of pregnancy, a "normal" $PaO_2$ can be seen even with an abnormally increased $(A - a)O_2$ gradient (Table 36-1).

## PULMONARY FUNCTION TESTS

The enlarging fetus and the increased concentration of circulating hormones during pregnancy account for the changes in pulmonary function seen with gestation. The hyperventilation of pregnancy is characterized by an increased depth of breathing (tidal volume increases from 450 to 600 mL) and not a higher respiratory rate.

A woman with a respiratory disease that is unlikely to deteriorate during pregnancy, an $FEV_1$ greater than 1 L, and no dyspnea at rest can undertake pregnancy safely.

## RADIOGRAPHIC TESTING

If at any time during pregnancy, the health of the mother or fetus would be compromised by failure to perform a radiologic examination, the examination should be performed. Irradiation in utero may increase the risk of childhood leukemia and other malignancies by 40% to 50%. Taking into account the greatest oncogenic risk, the overall risk of any adverse effect from exposure to 1 rad is estimated to be 0.1%, a risk that is thousands of times smaller than the risks of spontaneous abortion, malformation, or genetic disease. Fetal exposure to less

**TABLE 36-1.** Pulmonary Parameters

Lung Volumes
  Tidal volume (TV): the volume of air inhaled or exhaled with each normal breath
  Residual volume (RV): the volume of air remaining in the lungs after a vital capacity maneuver
  Inspiratory reserve volume (IRV): the maximal additional volume of gas that can be inhaled after a tidal breath is inhaled
  Expiratory reserve volume (ERV): the maximal volume of gas that can be exhaled after a tidal breath is exhaled
Lung Capacities
  Total lung capacity (TLC): the volume of air in the lungs at maximal inspiration
  Vital capacity (VC): the maximum amount of air that can be exhaled after a maximal inspiration to TLC
  Inspiratory capacity (IC): the maximal volume of gas that can be inspired from the resting expiratory level
  Functional residual capacity (FRC): the volume of air remaining in the lungs after a tidal volume exhalation
  Forced vital capacity (FVC): the volume of air exhaled during a rapid forced expiration starting at full inspiration
Other Measurements Made By Spirometry
  Forced expiratory volume in one second ($FEV_1$): the volume of air expelled in one second during a forced expiration starting at full inspiration
  Minute ventilation (MV): the amount of air exhaled per minute. It is measured under resting conditions
  Peak expiratory flow rate (PEFR): the peak rate (L/min) of a forceful expiration of a vital capacity

than 5 rads is considered insufficient reason to recommend termination of a desired pregnancy.

When chest radiographs are performed in the pregnant patient, normal findings differ from those seen in nonpregnant women of childbearing age. The diaphragm may be elevated 4 cm at term, but there will be a compensatory increase in anteroposterior diameter. There is an increase in the subcostal angle from 68.5° to 103.5° from early to late pregnancy. Also, lung markings may be increased, giving a false impression of mild congestive heart failure. Postpartum pleural effusions may not be a normal occurrence.

## MATERNAL-FETAL OXYGEN EXCHANGE

In a woman with no pulmonary disease breathing room air, arterial blood typically has a $PaO_2$ of 91 mmHg and a $PCO_2$ of 36 mmHg. In the fetal umbilical vein a simultaneous blood gas would typically show a $PO_2$ of 32 mmHg and a $PCO_2$ of 50 mm. Increases in the concentration of inspired oxygen result in the expected rise in oxygen tension in the maternal arteries but not in large increases in the oxygen tension of the fetal umbilical veins. Nevertheless, even a small increase in uterine oxygen content can result in a significant increase in oxygen transfer to the fetus. This occurs because of the high maternal perfusion rate of the uterus, the enhanced avidity of fetal hemoglobin for oxygen, and the leftward shift of the fetal oxyhemoglobin dissociation curve. However, the fetus is sensitive to large shifts in oxygen delivery, caused by a fall in cardiac output, and with complete interruption of oxygen supply to the umbilical vein, the fetus has only a 2- to 4-minute oxygen reserve.

Maternal alkalosis can result in decreased fetal oxygen tensions because of reduced uterine blood flow due to hypocarbia-induced vasoconstriction of uterine arteries, because of the mechanical effects of hyperventilation causing decreased maternal venous return and because of a shift in the maternal oxyhemoglobin dissociation curve to the left, thereby impairing oxygen transfer to the fetus. In the studies of Wulf and colleagues (1972) fetal oxygen delivery was compromised when maternal pH exceeded 7.6 and $PCO_2$ was 15 mmHg, values unlikely to be reached in acute asthma.*

## ASTHMA

Asthma, or reversible narrowing of large or small airways, is the most common obstructive lung disease affecting women of childbearing age, occurring in 0.4% to 1.3% of pregnant women.

## THE EFFECT OF ASTHMA ON THE OUTCOME OF PREGNANCY

Most asthmatics experience pregnancy with few ill effects, and in general there are no striking differences between the outcome of pregnancy in asthmatics com-

---

* Wulf KH, Kunzel W, Lehmann V. Clinical aspects of gas exchange. In: Longo LD, Bartels H, eds. Respiratory gas exchange and blood flow in the placenta. Bethesda, MD: Public Health Service, 1972:505.

pared with a control population. Nevertheless, severe and inadequately managed asthma can be associated with increased maternal and fetal complications, such as enhanced maternal and fetal mortality; a slight increase in the incidence of premature births, stillbirth, low-birth-weight babies; and subsequent neurologic abnormalities in the offspring. No differences in the frequency of multiple births or congenital malformations or in the infants' Apgar scores have been seen in the children of asthmatic mothers.

## THE EFFECT OF PREGNANCY ON THE COURSE OF ASTHMA

Asthma worsens during pregnancy in slightly more than one-third of patients, improves in slightly more than one-fourth of patients, and remains unchanged in one-third of patients. The change in asthma course associated with pregnancy usually reverts to the prepregnancy course within 3 months after delivery, and the course of asthma tends to be similar in a given woman during subsequent pregnancies.

## CLINICAL PRESENTATION

Classically, two clinical patterns of asthma have been recognized. One group, the so-called extrinsic asthmatics, develops asthma at a young age, has a family history of atopy, may have other atopic manifestations (skin and nasal allergies), and has evidence of IgE-mediated responses along with blood and sputum eosinophilia. Attacks are often seasonal and precipitated by well-defined allergens. The second group, the "intrinsic asthmatics," develops asthma later in life, has no family history of asthma or atopy, has no evidence of IgE-mediated bronchospasm, uncommonly has eosinophilia, but may have severe asthma that is difficult to treat. The intrinsic asthmatic is sensitive to environmental irritants, and acute exacerbations are often triggered by viral respiratory illness. Other clinical patterns include the triad of chronic asthma, a history of nasal polyps and pansinusitis, and the development of significant reductions in airflow rates following ingestion of aspirin or nonsteroidal anti-inflammatory drugs. In these patients, bronchospasm develops within minutes to hours, and symptoms may be severe or even life-threatening. Exercise-induced asthma is another common variant and is characterized by the development of bronchospasm following discontinuation of exercise in patients who may or may not have chronic asthmatic symptoms.

An acute attack of asthma is usually heralded by the clinical triad of cough, wheezing, and dyspnea. Dyspnea may be interpreted as a tightness in the chest. Attacks often occur at night. Usually, there is a history of exposure to a specific allergen, physical exertion, a viral respiratory tract infection, or emotional excitement preceding the onset of an exacerbation, and the patient will often have a history of similar episodes in the past.

Physical examination during an exacerbation reveals audibly harsh respirations, inspiratory and expiratory wheezing with a prolonged expiratory phase, tachypnea, tachycardia, and mild systolic hypertension. The lungs are overinflated and the anterior-posterior diameter of the thorax is increased beyond that typically expected in pregnancy. With increased duration and severity of an attack, the accessory respiratory muscles become visibly active and the patient may develop a paradoxical pulse, both signs of severe respiratory compromise.

The chest radiograph during an acute attack usually shows hyperinflation of the lungs with a small, elongated heart. The chest film may be necessary to exclude complications such as pneumothorax, pneumomediastinum, cardiomegaly, pneumonia, mucoid impaction, or bronchopulmonary aspergillosis, but only when these conditions are suspected on clinical grounds.

Laboratory studies are nonspecific. A complete blood count often displays a mild to moderate eosinophilia that may be reduced or absent if the patient has been taking corticosteroids. Life-threatening risks can be avoided by careful and routine medical attention during pregnancy and by early pharmacologic intervention during an exacerbation. The clinical hallmarks of cough, wheezing, and dyspnea do not correlate in any predictable way with lung function. Thus, if the patient can perform a forced expiration, the $FEV_1$ or the peak expiratory flow rate (PEFR) should be used to assess the severity and progress of airway obstruction. Carbon dioxide retention begins to occur at an $FEV_1$ of approximately 750 mL (about 25% of the predicted value), and a PEFR of less than 100 L/min is thought to be associated with an increased risk of a potentially fatal attack. With severe asthma, accessory muscle use and pulsus paradoxicus may be seen, suggesting that the $FEV_1$ is less than 25% of normal.

## PHARMACOLOGY OF ASTHMA THERAPY

Most of the agents that are used in controlling asthma can be used safely in pregnant women when given in recommended dosages.

Beta agonists produce bronchodilation by directly stimulating $beta_2$ receptors in airway smooth muscle, whereas alpha receptor stimulation causes bronchoconstriction. $Beta_2$ receptor stimulation leads to intracellular activation of bronchial smooth muscle cell adenylate cyclase, which increases intracellular cyclic AMP (cAMP) and leads to reduced smooth muscle tone. Beta agonists also prevent the development of bronchial smooth muscle edema after exposure to mediators such as histamine. They also tend to increase mucus secretion from submucosal glands and ion transport across airway epithelium, possibly leading to enhanced mucociliary clearance.

Theophylline may function as an adenosine antagonist. Adenosine is a natural bronchoconstrictor, and theophylline is a potent inhibitor of adenosine receptors at therapeutic concentrations. In addition to causing bronchodilatation, theophylline can stimulate respiration, increase cardiac inotropy and chronotropy, stimulate diaphragmatic contraction, and cause a mild diuresis. The beneficial and undesirable effects of theophylline can be enhanced by caffeine.

Corticosteroids are transported into the target cells and conveyed to the nucleus, where they affect the DNA transcription of specific messenger RNA and subsequently of specific proteins. This sequence of events may take several hours and explains the delay in onset of most corticosteroid effects. Their actions are multiple and include vasoconstriction of the bronchial vasculature with reduction in edema formation and dilation of bronchial smooth muscle, inhibition of antibody formation, reduction in the accumulation of neutrophils and macrophages, eosinopenia, and inhibition of antigen penetration of the bronchial mucosa. In addition, they block the formation of many inflammatory mediators and increase beta-adrenergic responsiveness (thus reversing or preventing tolerance to nebulized beta agonists).

Atropine, atropine methylnitrate, and ipratropium bromide are topically active specific antagonists of muscarinic receptors. Muscarinic receptors may mediate resting bronchomotor tone, probably through tonic vagal nerve impulses. In animals cholinergic pathways may also play an important role in regulating acute bronchomotor responses by eliciting reflex bronchoconstriction via vagal pathways. Multiple controlled studies have since documented that, although muscarinic antagonists may be somewhat effective against acute challenges by agents such as sulfur dioxide, cold air, and psychogenic stress, they are less effective against antigenic challenge.

Cromolyn sodium, a prophylactic medication for asthma, was originally thought to act solely by stabilizing the mast cell membrane and thereby inhibiting the release of inflammatory mediators in response to allergen. Further research has suggested that cromolyn actually has a low potency in stabilizing human lung mast cells and that it may have effects on neurotransmission. Cromolyn sodium may also indirectly block mast cell calcium channels and the phosphorylation of a membrane protein necessary for mediator release.

## EVALUATION AND THERAPY OF THE OUTPATIENT ASTHMATIC DURING PREGNANCY

If symptoms are not well controlled, therapy is begun with beta agonist inhalation, alone or in combination with an oral theophylline preparation. If symptoms persist, the patient should be tried on a short course of oral steroids (prednisone, hydrocortisone). Corticosteroids should be given in an effective dose initially (30 to 60 mg of prednisone) and then tapered gradually over the course of approximately 4 to 7 days. A patient who requires repeated short courses of oral steroids or who requires chronic doses of steroids should probably be started on an inhaled corticosteroid in an attempt to eliminate, change to alternate day, or decrease the dose of oral corticosteroids (Table 36-2).

## THERAPY OF ACUTE ASTHMA ATTACKS

An acute attack of asthma should be aggressively managed and the patient should be evaluated carefully for possible hospital admission (Table 36-3). In approximately 10% to 15% of pregnancies complicated by asthma, the patient may require hospitalization for status asthmaticus, a condition characterized by refractory airway obstruction with failure to resolve after appropriate treatment. A quick search for a precipitating event and questioning about prior and current corticosteroid use are part of the initial history. Then examination of pulse, blood pressure, respiratory rate, pulsus paradoxus, and $FEV_1$ and/or peak expiratory flow is indicated. A pulse of more than 120/min, respiratory rate of more than 30/min, pulsus paradoxus more than 18 mmHg, peak expiratory flow less than 120 L/min, moderate to severe dyspnea, accessory muscle use, and severe wheezing at the time of presentation are all signs of potentially life-threatening disease and probably indicate a need for acute hospitalization. Additional warning signs of a fatal attack are listed in Table 36-4.

**TABLE 36-2.** Medications Relatively or Absolutely Contraindicated in the Pregnant Asthmatic

---

Antihistamines
  Brompheniramine
  Hydroxyzine
  Cyproheptadine
Tetracycline
Amobarbital
Iodide expectorants
Aspirin
Tartrazine dye
Oral and topical decongestants
  Alpha-adrenergic agonists
Antitussives
  Codeine
Mucokinetic agents
  Guaifenesin
Mucolytic agents
  Acetylcysteine

---

The most reliable guides to the severity of an attack are the blood gas tensions, especially if the patient is too distressed to perform a forced expiration. In the more severe stages of asthma, normocarbia or hypercarbia develops and arterial hypoxemia becomes more marked. Administration of oxygen is safe and is indicated to alleviate hypoxemia and minimize respiratory alkalosis. Bedside spirometry and measurement of $FEV_1/FVC$ and peak expiratory flow rate are also useful, especially when compared with previous values and when followed serially through an attack.

In an emergency setting, epinephrine (0.3 mL of 1:1000 dilution) can be given subcutaneously with serial injections leading to cumulative improvements in airway function that may persist for up to 4 hours. Subcutaneous epinephrine should be avoided in patients with marked hypertension (systolic pressure above 200 mmHg) or an irregular pulse. Acceptable alternatives to the use of epi-

**TABLE 36-3.** Prophylactic Evaluation and Management of the Outpatient Asthmatic

---

1. Take a careful history to determine the severity of asthma and to identify precipitants.
2. Discourage use of aspirin, antihistamines, decongestants, etc.
3. Optimize dosage and frequency of medications.
4. Patient counseling:
  a. Appropriate exercise with prophylactic modifications if needed
  b. Advice on how to avoid precipitants
  c. Instruction in early recognition of wheezing and need for prompt intervention
5. Take baseline PFTs including vital capacity, $FEV_1$, and PEFR with repetition as disease activity warrants.
6. Obtain serial serum theophylline levels.
7. Vaccinate against influenza in the autumn or after the first trimester
8. Immunotherapy may be continued but should not be started, nor should the dose be increased in large increments because of the risk of anaphylaxis

---

**TABLE 36-4.** Status Asthmaticus: Warning Signs of Fatal Attack

---

Previous or recurrent episodes of status asthmaticus, especially previous intubation

FVC < 1.0 L; $FEV_1$ < 0.5 L; PEFR < 100 L/min

Little or no response to bronchodilator therapy at one hour
($\Delta$ $FEV_1$ < 400 mL; $\Delta$ PEFR < 60 mL/min)

Altered consciousness

Unequivocal central cyanosis; arterial $Po_2$ < 50 mmHg

$Pco_2$ > 45 mmHg

Pulsus paradoxus

ECG abnormalities

Presence of pneumothorax or pneumomediastinum

---

From Summer WR. Status asthmaticus. Chest (Suppl) 1985;87:895.

nephrine are subcutaneous terbutaline and nebulized, inhaled beta-adrenergic agonists. If inhaled beta agonists are used, sequential inhalations can produce a greater improvement than an equivalent dose administered as a single inhalation. In an emergent setting, nebulized, inhaled beta-adrenergic agonists can be given in reduced dosages every 20 minutes for at least the first hour after presentation.

Concurrent administration of intravenous aminophylline should be started during a severe acute attack. If the patient is already taking a theophylline preparation, no loading dose is necessary; if the patient is not taking such a preparation, aminophylline 5 to 6 mg/kg (up to 400 mg) is given intravenously over 30 minutes with dosage calculations based on lean body mass. Then a continuous aminophylline infusion is given at 0.5 mg/kg/h, preferably via an infusion pump, and a theophylline blood level is checked in 10 to 12 hours to ensure that the concentration is in the safe, effective range of 5 to 14 µg/mL.

Simultaneous supportive management in the form of supplemental oxygen and intravenous fluids should be given. Oxygen is given by nasal cannula and titrated to maintain an arterial $Po_2$ ≥ 70 mmHg. Some patients with asthma may be dehydrated because of marked hyperventilation, diaphoresis, and decreased oral intake, and intravenous fluids should be used to restore normovolemia, which will aid the expectoration of sputum. Sedation to treat the anxiety associated with severe asthma is never indicated.

If the clinical examination and serial spirometries show that the patient is not responding adequately despite aggressive therapy over the course of 2 to 4 hours, if the patient has a long history of corticosteroid use for prior exacerbations, if the attack has been present for several days before the patient seeks help, or if the patient is already taking corticosteroids, then corticosteroid therapy is indicated. The recommended dose of corticosteroids for the first 24 hours of a severe attack varies between 100 and 3000 mg (average, 300 mg/24 h) of hydrocortisone or its equivalent. We recommend a regimen of 30 to 60 mg of Solu-Medrol every 4 to 6 hours as initial therapy.

It has been suggested that the elimination of peripheral eosinophilia may give some indication that adequate systemic corticosteroids are being given.

Antibiotics are used in an acute asthma attack if pneumonia is present or if bacterial respiratory infection appears to have played a precipitating role.

## THERAPY OF RESPIRATORY FAILURE DUE TO ASTHMA

Adherence to the preceding treatment program will manage most episodes of acute asthma. There remains a small population of patients who will continue to deteriorate despite aggressive, appropriate therapy. Documentation of a persistently normal or elevated arterial $PCO_2$ during an asthma attack, rather than the expected hypocarbia, warrants admission to an intensive care unit. In a patient who is near term, external fetal monitoring can be employed to ensure adequate oxygen delivery to the fetus.

Mechanical ventilation is required if, in spite of bronchodilator therapy, the patient cannot maintain a $PaO_2$ of 70 mmHg or greater with supplemental oxygen. Other grounds for early endotracheal intubation include the presence of significant mental status changes, acute respiratory acidosis, life-threatening cardiac arrhythmias, and evidence of myocardial ischemia.

## OTHER OBSTRUCTIVE LUNG DISORDERS

Severe emphysema due to $\alpha_1$-antitrypsin deficiency and cystic fibrosis (CF) can occur in women of childbearing age. Care of these patients is primarily supportive, with attention to the physiologic parameters of lung function and oxygenation discussed earlier.

A National Institutes of Health study followed 129 pregnancies in CF patients and found only 86 viable infants, leading the investigators to conclude that CF patients have greatly increased fetal wastage.[†] In the study, there were 6 spontaneous abortions, 25 therapeutic abortions, and 11 perinatal deaths. Pregnancy outcome was more closely related to the severity of maternal disease at the onset of pregnancy than to the effects of CF on pregnancy. A reasonable set of guidelines is to advise against pregnancy in any CF patient with a VC less than 50% of that predicted, hypoxemia, cor pulmonale, or pancreatic insufficiency. The absence of pancreatic insufficiency may identify a subgroup more able to tolerate pregnancy.

Bronchial drainage, antibiotic therapy, prophylactic immunization (including annual influenza vaccine administration), and optimal nutritional and psychosocial care are essential components in the care of the CF patient contemplating pregnancy.

Patients with $\alpha_1$-antitrypsin deficiency or bronchiectasis are managed using these same principles. All should be regarded as high-risk patients, and serial spirometries and blood gas analyses are indicated.

## ASPIRATION OF STOMACH CONTENTS

Mendelson's syndrome, the aspiration of low-pH liquid stomach contents into the tracheobronchial tree, with subsequent chemical pneumonitis, was first described in women undergoing labor and delivery. This syndrome is most likely to develop if aspirated material has a pH less than 2.5, but some reports suggest that respiratory dysfunction can occur even if the pH of the aspirate is higher. Other

---

[†] Cohen LF, DiSant'Agnese PA, Friedlander J. Cystic fibrosis and pregnancy: a national survey. Lancet 1980;2:842.

syndromes that can result from aspiration are bronchial obstruction by an aspirated foreign body and bacterial pneumonia from aspiration of oropharyngeal bacteria.

If the aspiration is massive, immediate clinical illness may appear, but usually there is a delay of 6 to 8 hours before the appearance of bronchospasm, tachycardia, hypotension, tachypnea, cyanosis, and frothy pink sputum production. The latter finding appears if noncardiogenic pulmonary edema and capillary leak develop. Diagnosis is facilitated by having a high index of suspicion in the postpartum patient with respiratory distress.

Treatment of acid aspiration is supportive with oxygen and mechanical ventilation if needed. If aspiration is observed, endotracheal suctioning should be performed, but saline lavage is not indicated and may even serve to spread the acid to uninvolved areas. Bronchodilators may be used to control bronchospasm, but antibiotic therapy should be withheld until the patient develops signs of infection.

Prophylaxis of aspiration should always be undertaken, with antacids given during labor to raise the gastric pH above 2.5 and thus reduce the chance of a dangerous aspiration. Adverse pulmonary reactions may result from aspirating antacid particles; thus, the use of nonparticulate agents is preferred. Recently, various combinations of oral nonparticulate antacids and $H_2$-receptor blockers have been advocated as a convenient prophylactic regimen for patients about to undergo elective or emergency cesarean section, but no particular combination appears to be clearly superior. Additional prophylactic measures include limiting oral intake to essential medications once labor has begun, nasogastric evacuation of a distended stomach, selection of regional anesthesia when possible, use of a cuffed endotracheal tube, and use of cricoid pressure during intubation.

## RESPIRATORY INFECTIONS

The upper respiratory tract infections include acute and chronic rhinitis, sinusitis, acute pharyngitis, and acute otitis media. These maladies are common in pregnant patients. Except for infections caused by the influenza viruses, they do not tend to complicate pregnancy seriously and are omitted from discussion here except to point out that treatment is modified in pregnancy. In the pregnant patient, the physician should avoid decongestants and antihistamines and should select antibiotics such as the penicillins, cephalosporins, and those erythromycins that are generally considered to be safe in pregnancy.

Acute bronchitis is characterized by upper respiratory tract symptoms, productive cough, and the absence of a significant fever. Physical examination of the chest may reveal scattered rhonchi and occasional wheezes, but there are no signs of pulmonary consolidation. Acute bronchitis is usually caused by a virus, and antibiotic treatment is not generally indicated except in patients who suffer from chronic obstructive pulmonary disease.

## BACTERIAL PNEUMONIA

Pneumonia has been reported in 0.1% to 0.84% of all pregnancies, with a mortality rate of 3.5% to 8.6%, although antibiotics and modern obstetric care seem to have improved the prognosis. *Streptococcus pneumoniae* is the most common infectious agent implicated in antepartum pneumonia, and other common bacterial pathogens include *Mycoplasma pneumonia* and *Haemophilus influenzae*. *Legionella* pneumonia and *Listeria monocytogenes* have rarely been reported to cause respiratory failure in pregnancy.

## INFLUENZA

In a review of all deaths due to influenza from 1957 through 1960, 1% to 11% occurred in pregnant patients. These deaths were concentrated late in the third trimester and early puerperium and were more likely to occur with increased maternal age. Since studies were based on the clinical diagnosis of influenza, the conclusion that pregnancy predisposes to infection or to an enhanced severity of illness is controversial.

Although influenza virus can cross the placenta, it has not been isolated from fetal blood, and transplacental passage does not appear to cause congenital defects. Although fetal abnormalities such as circulatory defects, central nervous system malformations, cleft lip, and childhood cancer have been attributed to influenza, most investigators have found that no definite influenza-induced congenital syndrome exists. Although influenza vaccination is available, it is of unproven safety in pregnancy and is recommended only during an anticipated pandemic. Since increased mortality from infections usually occurs late in pregnancy, vaccination can be delayed until the middle of the second trimester.

## VIRAL PNEUMONIA

Other life-threatening viral pneumonias can develop in the pregnant patient, including varicella pneumonia, which may accompany chickenpox and can range from a mild to a rapidly fatal illness. In pregnancy, varicella is rare, but if pneumonia develops, mortality is high, ranging from 30% to 40% in some series. In addition, varicella pneumonia has been associated with an increased incidence of premature labor. Infection in any trimester of pregnancy can be associated with infrequent, but possibly lethal, congenital anomalies. If the maternal infection occurs within 5 days of delivery, the infant is at risk of fatal disseminated infection. Despite its classification as a pregnancy risk category C drug, there are at least four case reports of acyclovir usage in pregnancy, in the third trimester, without evidence of fetal toxicity. Some authors have recommended administration of varicella-zoster immune globulin, if available, to both mother and fetus exposed to peripartum varicella.

## FUNGAL PNEUMONIA

*Cryptococcus neoformans*, *Blastomyces dermatitidis*, and *Sporothrix schenckii* have rarely been reported as causing serious respiratory infection in pregnancy. The clinical course and outcome are generally the same in pregnant and nonpregnant patients. It has been estimated that coccidioidomycosis occurs in less than 1 of every 1000 pregnancies. However, infection in pregnancy, particularly during the second and third trimesters, increases the rate of disseminated infection from 0.2% to above 20%. It has been suggested that 17-beta-estradiol has a stimulatory effect on the fungus and may be responsible for the increased risk of dissemination associated with pregnancy. The maternal mortality rate from disseminated coccidioidomycosis approaches nearly 100%, a rate approximately twice that seen in nonpregnant patients, and dissemination is associated with increased fetal prematurity and mortality.

Amphotericin B has been used to treat cryptococcosis, blastomycosis, and disseminated coccidioidomycosis in pregnancy. It crosses the placenta and can be found in both amniotic fluid and fetal blood. Although use in pregnancy has not been well studied, normal, full-term infants have been born to patients who received amphotericin B in the first trimester. Its use is associated with anemia; thus, serial hematocrits need to be followed.

## PNEUMOCYSTIS CARINII PNEUMONIA

*Pneumocystis carinii* pneumonia is the most common opportunistic infection affecting the lungs of patients with acquired immunodeficiency syndrome (AIDS). It can be confused with atypical mycobacterial infection, cryptococcosis, and histoplasmosis.

The treatment of choice in pregnant women with AIDS and *P. carinii* pneumonia is trimethoprim-sulfamethoxazole, even though trimethoprim is a folate antagonist and sulfamethoxazole is a sulfonamide. Recent studies of in utero exposure to sulfadiazine failed to show an increase in prematurity, hyperbilirubinemia, or kernicterus. Patients should be monitored for drug toxicity, such as rash, fever, neutropenia, thrombocytopenia, and hepatitis. Nausea and vomiting may occur and can exacerbate hyperemesis gravidarum.

## AMNIOTIC FLUID EMBOLISM

Although the true incidence and mortality associated with amniotic fluid embolism is difficult to establish, amniotic fluid embolism has been estimated to complicate from 1 per 8000 to 1 per 80,000 live births. This disease accounts for 11% to 13% of all maternal deaths in the United States, and fetal mortality may exceed 40%. Complications leading to maternal death include uncontrolled disseminated intravascular coagulation (DIC) and cardiorespiratory failure due to severe pulmonary hypertension and right ventricular failure. Clinically, one may see excessive bleeding, especially uterine bleeding, bronchospasm, respiratory distress, pulmonary hypertension, pulmonary edema, cyanosis, frank DIC, bradycardia, shock, and cardiovascular collapse. The differential diagnosis includes conventional causes of thromboembolic disease, toxemia of pregnancy, peripartum cardiomyopathy, Mendelson's syndrome, and fulminant pneumonia.

Amniotic fluid can enter the maternal vascular space through small endocervical veins, uterine or cervical tears, or iatrogenic uterine trauma. Tumultuous labor, use of uterine stimulants, presence of meconium in the amniotic fluid, advanced maternal age, multiparity, and intrauterine fetal death are some of the risk factors for this catastrophic event. Although most episodes occur during labor (90%), amniotic fluid embolism can occur at any time throughout pregnancy. Once access to the maternal circulation is gained, the embolus travels to the lungs, usually resulting in cardiovascular collapse. The embolized material can include amniotic fluid, fetal squames, lanugo hairs, meconium, fat, mucin, and bile. These materials can be recovered in pulmonary artery catheter aspirates, sampled as long as 3 days after the precipitating event, and sampling by this means may help establish the diagnosis. The pulmonary physiologic changes probably result from a combination of occlusive emboli, vasospasm, and possibly increased permeability pulmonary edema. Prostaglandin F2α, present in the amniotic fluid in late pregnancy, has been implicated as being at least partially responsible for the vasospastic component. Fetal lipids and mucin circulating freely in the maternal circulation may be responsible for the onset of DIC.

Treatment is supportive and includes oxygen, mechanical ventilation with or without the use of positive end-expiratory pressure (PEEP), fluid, vasopressors, reduction of uterine bleeding via mechanical massage, oxytocin infusion, and when necessary, methylergonovine maleate; blood products should be replaced as indicated. Emergency cesarean section, performed either to salvage a viable fetus or to attempt to save the mother's life, is controversial.

## VENOUS AIR EMBOLISM

Venous air embolism may account for as many as 1% of maternal deaths, with risk factors being the performance of surgery, intravenous infusions, and central venous catheter placement. However, because the venous sinuses of the uterus are particularly susceptible to the entry of air during pregnancy, air embolism can occur during normal labor, delivery of a placenta previa, criminal abortions using air, orogenital sex, and insufflation of the vagina during gynecological procedures. Maternal mortality associated with a clinically significant event exceeds 90% in untreated cases. The severity of a venous air embolism depends on the amount and rate of air entry. Small amounts of venous air may be clinically undetectable, but accidental bolus injections of 100 mL to 300 mL of air have been reported to be fatal. However, there are reports of patients surviving infusions of up to 1600 mL.

Embolization of a large bolus of venous air to the right ventricle results in mechanical obstruction to the forward flow of blood in the pulmonary artery outflow tract. In addition, the pumping action of the right ventricle acting on blood and air may produce platelet damage and fibrin formation, resulting in fibrin emboli that lodge in the pulmonary vascular bed. Maldistribution of pulmonary blood flow may result in ischemia or hyperperfusion, with the hyperperfused areas being susceptible to developing interstitial and alveolar edema. Areas that are initially ischemic may also become abnormally permeable once perfusion is restored. In animal models, the permeability pulmonary edema following venous air embolism has been related to leukocyte production and the release of toxic oxygen metabolites. Paradoxical embolization can occur if there is an atrial septal defect, resulting in arterial ischemia or occlusion.

The patient initially presents with a feeling of faintness, dizziness, fear of impending doom, dyspnea, cough, diaphoresis, and substernal chest pain. Physical examination may reveal a state of altered consciousness, cyanosis, tachypnea, wheezing, tachycardia, hypotension, elevated jugular venous pressure, gallop rhythm, and an evanescent "mill wheel" or "waterwheel" murmur heard over the precordium. Paradoxical embolism may be evidenced by bubbles in the retinal arterioles, marblelike skin (air in superficial dermal vessels), and possibly stroke or myocardial infarction. A blood gas will characteristically reveal hypoxemia, and there may be an associated metabolic acidosis. Chest radiography may occasionally demonstrate air in the right side of the heart or the main pulmonary artery, and the electrocardiogram may show signs of right heart strain, ischemia, or arrhythmia. Therapy must be instituted promptly, and the patient should be placed in the left lateral decubitus position to minimize obstruction to the right ventricular outflow tract. Administration of 100% oxygen will promote removal of nitrogen from the air bubble and result in more rapid absorption of the embolus. Nitrous oxide is highly soluble, and in a patient receiving general anesthesia, it should be discontinued, since it can increase the size of the air embolus. In the presence of cardiovascular collapse, closed chest compression and aspiration of air from the right side of the heart, via venous catheterization or transthoracic puncture, are probably warranted. Hyperbaric oxygen may be useful in the setting of cerebral venous air embolism, anticoagulation has been suggested to minimize the formation of fibrin microemboli, and mechanical ventilation may be necessary to treat permeability pulmonary edema.

## ADULT RESPIRATORY DISTRESS SYNDROME (ARDS)

Adult respiratory distress syndrome (ARDS) is the final common pathway of pathophysiologic changes occurring in the lungs as a consequence of a variety of acute bodily insults that reach the lung directly or via the vasculature (Table 36-5). Clinically, patients present with marked respiratory distress, tachypnea, hypoxemia refractory to oxygen therapy, "stiff" noncompliant lungs that require high pressures to achieve inflation, and diffuse bilateral interstitial and alveolar infiltrates on chest radiograph. The central pathophysiologic event in ARDS is injury to the alveolar-capillary membrane, either directly or via mediators delivered by the pulmonary vasculature resulting in increased vascular permeability and noncardiogenic pulmonary edema. Severe hypoxemia results from both increased shunting of unoxygenated blood and impaired ventilation and perfusion matching in the alveoli, with an arterial $Po_2$ typically less than 50 to 60 mmHg, despite an inspired oxygen concentration of 60% or more. To make the diagnosis of ARDS, chronic pulmonary disease and left heart failure (cardiogenic pulmonary edema) must be excluded, and an appropriate precipitating event should be present. Right heart catheterization is often required to demonstrate that the pulmonary capillary hydrostatic pressure is not elevated, but these data should be assessed in light of the expected decrease in colloid oncotic pressure during pregnancy and in the immediate postpartum period. Mortality in patients with ARDS continues to exceed 50%, a figure that has remained fairly constant over the last 20 years.

In the pregnant patient, ARDS can be associated with many of the factors that complicate pregnancy and delivery, including septicemia, amniotic fluid embolism, aspiration of stomach contents, eclampsia, septic abortion, pyelonephritis, air embolism, abruptio placentae, blood transfusion (with white cell agglutination in the pulmonary circulation), dead fetus syndrome (with disseminated intravascular coagulation), drug overdose (narcotics, barbiturates, aspirin), fat embolism (after long bone fracture), hemorrhagic shock, seizures, and overwhelming pneumonia.

**TABLE 36-5.** Causes of ARDS in Pregnant Women

Abruptio placentae
Air embolism
Amniotic fluid embolism
Aspiration
Bacterial pneumonia
Blood transfusion
Carcinomatosis
Dead fetus syndrome
Diabetic ketoacidosis
Drugs (narcotics, barbiturates)
Fat embolism
Fractures
Fungal and *Pneumocystis carinii* pneumonia
Head trauma
Inhaled toxin
Intra-abdominal abscess
Lung contusion
Nonthoracic trauma
Pancreatitis
Preeclampsia, eclampsia
Pyelonephritis
Seizure
Septic abortion
Septicemia
Shock
Tocolytic therapy with sympathomimetics and glucocorticoids
Tuberculosis
Uremia

## CLINICAL PRESENTATION

Clinically, the patient with ARDS of any etiology may go through four clinical stages: (1) injury, (2) apparent stability, (3) respiratory insufficiency, and (4) terminal stage. The initial injury may occur without outward clinical signs and may last for up to 6 hours. Next, the patient develops dyspnea associated with rapid shallow breathing and a persistent cough. Approximately 12 to 24 hours after injury, the chest radiograph shows bilateral infiltrates that coalesce into a diffuse haze, representing perivascular fluid accumulation, interstitial edema, and alveolar edema.

## THERAPY OF ARDS

Corticosteroids, in doses up to several grams of methylprednisone over 24 hours, have been widely used in the treatment of full-blown ARDS without a clear demonstration that they are effective. An exception is in the use of corticosteroids and mineralocorticoids to treat patients who are in shock that might be caused by

**TABLE 36-6.** Complications Associated with the Adult Respiratory Distress Syndrome

Pulmonary
  Pulmonary emboli
  Pulmonary barotrauma
  Pulmonary fibrosis
  Pulmonary complications of ventilatory and monitoring procedures
    Mechanical ventilation
      Right main stem intubation
      Alveolar hypoventilation
    Swan-Ganz catheterization
    Pulmonary infarction
    Pulmonary hemorrhage
Gastrointestinal
  Gastrointestinal hemorrhage
  Ileus
  Gastric distention
  Pneumoperitoneum
Renal
  Renal failure
  Fluid retention
Cardiac
  Arrhythmia
  Hypotension
  Low cardiac output
Infection
  Sepsis
  Nosocomial pneumonia
Hematologic
  Anemia
  Thrombocytopenia
  Disseminated intravascular coagulation
Other
  Hepatic
  Endocrine
  Neurologic
  Psychiatric

From Balk RB, Bone RC. The adult respiratory distress syndrome. Med Clin N Am 1983;67:685.

or accompanied by adrenal insufficiency. Prophylactic corticosteroid therapy for ARDS is also considered unproven and controversial. Potential adverse effects far outweigh any putative, unproven benefit. Recently, nonsteroidal anti-inflammatory drugs (NSAIDs), such as ibuprofen, meclofenamate, and indomethacin, have been studied in vitro and in animals and have shown some promise.

## MECHANICAL VENTILATION IN ARDS

Ventilator therapy should be instituted when refractory hypoxemia is present and should be considered at the earliest recognition of ARDS, to ensure fetal well-being.

If the maternal arterial oxygen saturation cannot be maintained at or above 90%, with an $FiO_2$ of 0.6 or less, then PEEP should be added. PEEP recruits atelectatic areas for gas exchange, which would otherwise collapse during expiration and which are difficult to expand due to the loss of surfactant and structural derangements. The result is an increase in systemic arterial oxygen tension and in the lung's FRC and compliance. The use of PEEP is not without pitfalls, however, since it can overdistend alveoli, thereby decreasing compliance and increasing the risk of pneumothorax. Its most important adverse effect is to decrease cardiac output by impeding venous return to the right side of the heart, particularly when the blood volume is low.

An optimal PEEP has been defined as a level that increases oxygenation without significantly reducing cardiac output, and consequently oxygen delivery.

## COMPLICATIONS OF ARDS

Therapy of ARDS requires knowledge not only of the disease process and its management, but also of associated complications. Table 36-6 lists complications resulting from intubation and mechanical ventilation and emphasizes that this severe disease can involve many organ systems in addition to the lungs. Two specific complications, pulmonary barotrauma and infection, merit special attention.

# 37.  DIABETES MELLITUS IN PREGNANCY

Diabetes mellitus is a heterogeneous disorder characterized by hyperglycemia, which is a result of relative or absolute insulin deficiency. It is estimated that diabetes mellitus affects approximately 1.5 million women of childbearing age in the United States.

## CLASSIFICATION

Recently, a new classification system has been proposed by the Diabetes Data Group of the National Institutes of Health (1986). This classification is based on etiologic factors and insulin dependency (Table 37-1).

Another classification proposed in 1949 in the *American Journal of Medicine* by White is still generally accepted and remains a useful prognostic guide.* White's classification relates the onset of diabetes, its duration, and the degree of vasculopathy to the outcome of pregnancy.

Practically speaking, women with pregnancies complicated by diabetes mellitus may be separated into one of two groups:

*Gestational diabetes.* Women with carbohydrate intolerance of variable severity, with onset or first recognition during the present pregnancy.
*Pregestational diabetes.* Women known to have diabetes before pregnancy.

Table 37-2 presents the classifications that include these two groups.

*White P. Pregnancy complicating diabetes. Am J Med 1949;7:609.

**TABLE 37-1.** Classification of Glucose Intolerance

|          | Nomenclature                                           | Old Names               |
|----------|--------------------------------------------------------|-------------------------|
| Type I   | Insulin-dependent diabetes mellitus (IDDM)             | Juvenile-onset diabetes |
| Type II  | Non-insulin-dependent diabetes mellitus                | Maturity-onset diabetes |
| Type III | Gestational diabetes or carbohydrate intolerance (GCI) |                         |
| Type IV  | Secondary diabetes                                      |                         |

Based on recommendations of the National Diabetes Data Group. Classification and diagnosis of diabetes mellitus. Washington, DC: National Institutes of Health, 1986.

## EPIDEMIOLOGY, ETIOLOGY, AND GENETICS

Since diabetes mellitus is a heterogeneous disorder rather than a single disease, the different types of diabetes should be distinguishable from each other (see Table 37-1).

Ninety percent of all pregnant diabetic patients have gestational diabetes mellitus (GDM), and insulin-dependent diabetes mellitus (IDDM, type I) and non-insulin-dependent diabetes mellitus (NIDDM, type II) account for the remaining 10%. In general, IDDM and NIDDM can be distinguished from each other using clinical criteria and/or islet-cell antibody studies (Table 27-3).

## GENETIC FACTORS IN IDDM (TYPE I)

In the past few years it has become increasingly clear that autoimmunity plays a key role in type I diabetes. It is currently believed that type I diabetes mellitus is

**TABLE 37-2.** Classification of Diabetes in Pregnancy

| Pregestational Diabetes | | | | |
|-------|-------------------|-----------------|--------------------------|-----------|
| Class | Age of Onset (year) | Duration (year) | Vascular Disease | Therapy |
| A | Any | Any | No | Diet Only |
| B | >20 | <10 | No | Insulin |
| C | 10–19 | 10–19 | No | Insulin |
| D | Before 10 | >20 | Benign retinopathy | Insulin |
| F | Any | Any | Nephropathy | Insulin |
| R | Any | Any | Proliferative retinopathy | Insulin |
| H | Any | Any | Heart disease | Insulin |

| Gestational Diabetes | | |
|-------|----------------------|---------------------------|
| Class | Fasting Glucose Level | Postprandial Glucose Level |
| A-1 | <105 mg/dL     and | <120 mg/dL |
| A-2 | >105 mg/dL     and/or | >120 mg/dL |

Based on the American College of Obstetricians and Gynecologists (ACOG), Technical Bulletin No. 92 (Chicago), May 1986, with modifications.

**TABLE 37-3.** Predominant Characteristics of IDDM and NIDDM

| Characteristics | IDDM | NIDDM |
| --- | --- | --- |
| Prevalence | 0.1–0.5% | 5–10%* |
| Weight at onset | Nonobese | Often obese |
| Age at onset | Usually young, <30 years | Usually older, >40 years |
| Seasonal variations | Yes | No |
| Insulin level | Low or absent | Variable |
| Ketosis | Most often | Unusual |
| MHC† gene associations | HLA DR$_4$, HLA DR$_3$, HLA DQ | No |
| Twin studies | 30%–50% concordance | 80–100% concordance |
| Anti-islet-cell antibodies | Positive in 70% of new IDDM or prediabetic IDDM | No |

* Prevalence in Western countries.
† MHC: Major histocompatibility complex.

actually a slow process in which insulin-secreting cells are gradually destroyed, leading to islet-cell failure and hyperglycemia. The development of type I diabetes can be divided conceptually into six stages, beginning with genetic susceptibility and ending with complete B-cell destruction (Table 37-4).

The exact mechanism of the inheritance of IDDM is not known. Formerly, it was suggested that the risk to offspring with one affected parent of inheriting diabetes was in the range of 1% to 6%. Based on recent information, it has become clear that IDDM is transmitted less frequently to the offspring of diabetic mothers than to those of diabetic fathers: 1.3% versus 6%, respectively. Family studies have shown that the estimated risk of recurrence of IDDM to offspring in a family with one already affected sibling, but with unaffected parents, is 5% to 6% (Table 37-5).

## GENETICS OF NIDDM

There are clear genetic and immunologic differences between IDDM and NIDDM. The latter is not linked with HLA, and no specific genetic markers have been found. Furthermore, NIDDM does not seem to be an autoimmune or endocrine disease. Currently available information indicates that NIDDM occurs when there is both impaired insulin secretion and insulin antagonism.

For NIDDM relatives, the empirical risk of developing the disease is much higher than it is for IDDM relatives. The risk of transmitting NIDDM to first-degree relatives is almost 15%, and as many as 30% will have impaired glucose tolerance. When both parents have type II diabetes, the chance of developing the disease is much higher, reaching 60% to 75%.

## METABOLIC CHAGNES IN NORMAL AND DIABETIC PREGNANCIES
### INSULIN SECRETION AND INSULIN RESISTANCE IN NORMAL PREGNANCY

Insulin is the major hormonal signal regulating metabolic responses to feeding and tissue use of carbohydrates; it is also the major glucose-lowering hormone. It

**TABLE 37-4.** Proposed Stages in the Pathogenesis of IDDM

| Stage and Occurrence | Comments |
| --- | --- |
| Stage I<br>  Genetic susceptibility | Most likely polygenic<br>*HLA association with IDDM*<br>Chromosome 6<br>5% of Caucasians with IDDM express HLA DR3 or DR4 or both.<br>*Non-HLA association with IDDM*<br>Immunoglobulin loci (encoded on chromosomes 2, 14) Polymorphic region 5' of the insulin gene (chromosome II)<br>T cell receptor (chromosomes 7, 14) |
| Stage II<br>  Triggering factors | Environmental factors: toxic chemicals (?); viruses such as coxsackie B, rubella, mumps; stress (?). |
| Stage III<br>  Active autoimmunity | Many immunologic abnormalities may precede overt DM by more than 9 yrs; anti-islet-cell antibodies may be present in up to 70% of pre-DM patients. |
| Stage IV<br>  Progressive loss of antibodies. | Reduction in β-cell mass, evidenced by abnormal IV GTT in ≥50% of first-degree relatives (IDDM) with islet-cell glucose-stimulated insulin secretion. |
| Stage V<br>  Early onset of overt<br>  DM | ≥10% of β-cells remain.<br>Trials of immunotherapy (i.e. steroids and cyclosporin) have been attempted. |
| Stage VI<br>  Overt DM w/complete<br>  β-cell destruction | Several years may elapse between Stages V and VI. |

DM, diabetes mellitus; GTT, glucose tolerance test.
From Hagay Z, Reece EA. Diabetes mellitus in pregnancy and periconceptional genetic counseling. Am J Perinatology 1992;9:89.

**TABLE 37-5.** Empirical Risk for Offspring of IDDM and NIDDM Developing Diabetes

| Affected Parent(s) | Empirical Risk Estimate of Offspring |
| --- | --- |
| IDDM | |
|   Diabetic mother | 1% |
|   Diabetic father | 6% |
|   Parents unaffected | Overall: 5–6% |
|     Sibling affected | |
| | No. of haplotypes shared:<br>  1 haplotype = 5%<br>  2 haplotypes = 13%<br>  No haplotypes = 2% |
|   Both parents affected | 33% |
| NIDDM | |
|   MODY | 50% |
|   Obese | 7% |
|   Nonobese | 15% |
|   Both parents affected | 60%–75% |

MODY, maturity-onset diabetes of the young.

is produced by the B cell of the pancreas and is secreted into the hepatic portal circulation, from which it reaches and acts on the liver and on other peripheral tissues (i.e., muscle and fat). Insulin suppresses endogenous glucose production by inhibition of hepatic glycogenolysis and gluconeogenesis. On the other hand, it stimulates glucose uptake and fuel storage of glycogen and triglyceride in the liver, muscle, and adipose tissue (Table 37-6).

## MATERNAL GLUCOSE HOMEOSTASIS IN THE FASTING STATE

During normal pregnancy, plasma fasting glucose levels decrease in the first few weeks of gestation, reaching a nadir by the 12th week of gestation and remaining unchanged thereafter until delivery.

## RESPONSE TO GLUCOSE LOAD

In normal pregnancy it has been shown that during late gestation, there is an increase in the 1- and 2-hour blood glucose levels after glucose tolerance testing as compared to nonpregnant controls. Moreover, postprandial glucose levels are higher in pregnancy after a standard meal.

## THE EFFECT OF PREGNANCY ON DIURNAL VARIATION OF PLASMA GLUCOSE DURING MIXED-MEAL FEEDING

The mean 24-hour glucose concentrations are significantly reduced during the second-trimester (85.6 ± 2.9 mg/dL) and the third trimester (87.3 mg/dL ± 1.7 mg/dL) compared to the postpartum control values (93.4 mg/dL ± 1.9 mg/dL). A significant elevation of the 2-hour postprandial value is clearly evident in the third trimester compared to both second-trimester and postpartum values. However, there is a progressive decrease of plasma glucose during sleeping hours from the second to the third trimester of pregnancy, and this may contribute to the decreased 24-hour glucose concentration.

**TABLE 37-6.** Summary of the Metabolic Effects of Insulin

| | |
|---|---|
| Target tissue | Enhances glucose and amino uptake |
| | Increases glycogen synthesis |
| | Converts glucose into fatty acids |
| | Inhibits glyconeogenesis |
| Muscle | Enhances glucose and amino acid uptake |
| | Increases glycogen synthesis |
| Adipose tissue | Increases glucose and amino acid transport |
| | Increases fatty acid synthesis |
| | Inhibits release of fatty acids from fat stores |
| | "Fat-sparing effect" be enhanced glucose utilization in many tissues |
| Central nervous system | Has little or no effect on uptake or metabolism of glucose |
| All tissues | Increases protein synthesis |
| | Inhibits protein catabolism |

Reprinted with permission from Brumfield C, Huddleston JF. The management of diabetic ketoacidosis in pregnancy. Clin Obstet Gynecol 1984;27(1):50.

## LIPID METABOLISM

It has been well documented that in pregnancy there is a tendency for accelerated fat mobilization and ketone body formation, particularly with prolonged periods of starvation. As mentioned previously, human placental lactogen is depressed by hyperglycemia and increased by hypoglycemia. In the fasting state, glucose levels are decreased, leading to decreased insulin levels, but are associated with increased levels of HPL. HPL increases lypolysis, so free fatty acids may serve as a source of energy for maternal metabolism to maintain an adequate supply of plasma glucose and amino acid for the fetus.

In normal pregnancy, total lipids increase in all three lipoprotein fractions (very-low-density lipoproteins, low-density lipoproteins, and high-density lipoproteins). Triglyceride and cholesterol content of the three lipoproteins are increased throughout pregnancy.

Cholesterol is increased during pregnancy, mainly due to the VLDL and LDL fractions. HDL cholesterol increases slowly until midpregnancy and then declines as pregnancy progresses.

## PROTEIN METABOLISM

The concentration of most amino acids is lower among pregnant women than among nonpregnant women. It has been suggested that this is a result of a higher transfer of amino acids to the fetus or an increase in maternal gluconeogenesis.

## PLACENTAL TRANSFER OF NUTRIENTS

The placenta is a complex organ that has an important function in the transfer of gases and nutrients between the mother and the fetus. Fetal growth is controlled by various factors and depends on the uptake of nutrients and oxygen by the placenta and on their transfer to the fetus. The availability of nutrients to the fetus depends principally on the maternal metabolic state. Placental transfer of the principal nutrients is diagrammed in Figure 37-1.

## METABOLISM IN THE DIABETIC PREGNANCY

In summary, the metabolic disturbances in diabetic pregnant patients are expressed in increased concentrations of circulating metabolic fuels, including carbohydrate, protein, and fat. This increased circulating maternal level can be transferred to the fetus and may contribute to the development of fetal macrosomia.

## GESTATIONAL DIABETES MELLITUS

### DEFINITION

Gestational diabetes mellitus is defined as carbohydrate intolerance of variable severity with onset or first recognition during the present pregnancy. This means that the glucose intolerance may have antedated the pregnancy but was not recognized by the patient or physician. Although this is infrequent, patients who

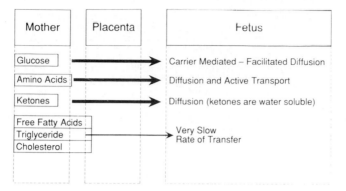

**FIGURE 37-1.** Transplacental transfer of maternal fuels to the fetus.

actually have diabetes mellitus type I or II may therefore initially be classified as having gestational diabetes.

## INCIDENCE

The incidence of gestational diabetes mellitus varies in different study populations and is estimated to occur in 3% to 5% of pregnant women.

## SCREENING FOR GESTATIONAL DIABETES

The Second International Workshop-Conference on Gestational Diabetes Mellitus recommended that all pregnant women receive screening for glucose intolerance, because selective screening based on risk factors has been found to be inadequate and ineffective. Pregnant women who have not been identified as having glucose intolerance before the 24th week of gestation should have a screening glucose challenge test between the 24th and 28th weeks consisting of 50 g oral glucose given without regard to time of the last meal or time of day. A value of plasma venous glucose of 140 mg/dL or more has been recommended as a threshold to indicate the need for a full diagnostic GTT (Table 37-7).

## DIAGNOSIS

The diagnosis of gestational diabetes is, in most cases, based on an abnormal result of an oral GTT during pregnancy. A minority of cases will be diagnosed on the basis of high fasting glucose levels during pregnancy, in which case the oral glucose tolerance test will not have to be performed. The GTT is administered under standard conditions: 100 g of glucose is given orally in at least 400 mL of water after an overnight fast of 8 to 14 hours. The patient should have at least 3 days of unrestricted diet with more than 150 g carbohydrate and should be at rest during the study. Diagnosis requires that at least two of four glucose levels of the oral GTT meet or exceed the upper limits of normal values. Whole blood and plasma glucose criteria of the oral GTT used for the diagnosis of gestational diabetes are presented in Table 37-8.

**TABLE 37-7.** Incidence of a Positive Glucose Tolerance Test Among 96 Gravidas
with 50-G, 1-Hour Screening Test Values >134 mg/dL (Plasma, Glucose Oxidase)

| Screening Test Result | Incidence of Gestational Diabetes (%) |
|---|---|
| 135–144 | 14.6 |
| 145–154 | 17.4 |
| 155–164 | 28.6 |
| 165–174 | 20.0 |
| 175–184 | 50.0 |
| >185 | 100.0 |

From Carpenter MW, Coustan DR. Criteria for screening tests for gestational diabetes. Am J Obstet Gynecol
1982;144:768. By permission.

## MANAGEMENT

Management of GDM is directed toward reducing perinatal mortality and morbidity, a goal that may be achieved by maintaining close surveillance of the mother
and fetus. Maternal surveillance includes close monitoring of glucose levels.

After the diagnosis of gestational diabetes has been made, patients receive
nutritional counseling—the mainstay of therapy in this group of patients. Since as
many as 15% to 20% of patients will have deterioration of glucose homeostasis as
gestation proceeds, it is mandatory to identify this group early and to initiate
insulin therapy. It is our practice to monitor glucose levels in gestational diabetics
once or twice weekly. If fasting plasma glucose levels are ≥105 mg/dL or 2-hour
postprandial glucose levels are ≥120 mg/dL on two or more occasions within a
2-week interval, insulin therapy is initiated.

Antenatal testing is recommended in some patients with gestational diabetes.
The gestational age at which this testing should begin and the best method of
antepartum testing have not been determined.

Because fetal macrosomia is frequent in gestational diabetes, fetal weight estimation is prudent prior to an attempted vaginal delivery. As in overt diabetes,

**TABLE 37-8.** Oral Glucose Tolerance Test (100 g) Values
for the Diagnosis of Gestational Diabetes (mg/dL)

| | O'Sullivan (1964)* | NDDG (1979)† | Carpenter and Coustan (1982)‡ |
|---|---|---|---|
| Fasting | 90 | 105 | 95 |
| 1 hour | 165 | 190 | 180 |
| 2 hours | 145 | 165 | 155 |
| 3 hours | 125 | 145 | 140 |

* O'Sullivan JB, Mahan CM. Criteria for the oral glucose tolerance test in pregnancy. Diabetes 1964;13:278.
† National Diabetes Data Group. Classification and diagnosis of diabetes mellitus and other categories of glucose
intolerance. Diabetes 1979;28:1039.
‡ Carpenter MW, Coustan DR. Criteria for screening tests for gestational diabetes. Am J Obstet Gynecol
1982;144:768.

cesarean section will be performed on most patients with estimated fetal weight of >4500 g in order to prevent shoulder dystocia and birth trauma.

In patients with estimated fetal weight between 4000 and 4500 g, management should be individualized based on the size of the pelvis and the patient's previous obstetric history.

## LONG-TERM MATERNAL OUTCOME OF GESTATIONAL DIABETES

Several investigators have shown that patients with gestational diabetes mellitus are at increased risk for developing diabetes years after pregnancy.

It is recommended, therefore, that women with GDM be followed postpartum to detect diabetes early in its course. They should be evaluated at the first postpartum visit by a fasting plasma glucose test and by a 2-hour oral GTT (30, 90, and 120 minutes) using a 75-g glucose load. The criteria of the National Diabetes Data group for the diagnosis of diabetes mellitus in nonpregnant adults include a fasting plasma glucose level of >140 mg/dL on more than one occasion, or a 75-g, 2-hour oral GTT in which the 2-hour value and at least one other value are >200 mg/dL. The criteria for the diagnosis of impaired glucose tolerance are the following: fasting plasma glucose below 140 mg/dL and 2-hour value between 140 and 200 mg/dL, and at least one other value of 200 mg/dL or more.

The risk of developing diabetes later in life in GDM is greatly influenced by body weight, with the highest rate occurring in obese patients. Therefore, obese GDM patients should be advised to control their weight.

## PREGESTATIONAL DIABETES MELLITUS

### PERICONCEPTIONAL CARE

An increasing body of evidence shows that the incidence of congenital anomalies is related to hyperglycemia in early pregnancy. One of the first goals of the prepregnancy clinic is to achieve optimum diabetic control even before the time of conception. Several studies have shown significant reduction of congenital malformations following such a prepregnancy treatment program.

### CONGENITAL ANOMALIES IN INFANTS OF DIABETIC MOTHERS

The frequency of major congenital anomalies among infants of diabetic mothers has been estimated as 6% to 10%, which represents a two- to five-fold increase over the frequency observed in the general population. Congenital malformations in fetuses of diabetic patients are now responsible for approximately 40% of all perinatal deaths, replacing respiratory distress syndrome as the leading cause of infant death. These malformations usually involve multiple organ systems (Table 37-9), with cardiac anomalies being the most common, followed by central nervous system and skeletal malformations.

#### Pathogenesis of Diabetes-Associated Congenital Anomalies

Both clinical and experimental studies are in agreement that diabetes-associated birth defects occur following disruption of developmental processes during organ-

**TABLE 37-9.** Congenital Anomalies of Infants of Diabetic Mothers

Skeletal and CNS
  Caudal regression syndrome
  Neural tube defects excluding anencephaly
  Anencephaly with or without herniation of neural elements
  Microcephaly
Cardiac
  Transposition of the great vessels with or without ventricular septal defect
  Ventricular septal defects
  Coarctation of the aorta with or without ventricular septal defect or patent ductus arteriosus
  Atrial septal defects
  Cardiomegaly
Renal anomalies
  Hydronephrosis
  Renal agenesis
  Ureteral duplication
Gastrointestinal
  Duodenal atresia
  Anorectal atresia
  Small left colon syndrome
Other
  Single umbilical artery

Reprinted by permission from Reece EA, Hobbins JC. Diabetes embryopathy, pathogenesis, prenatal diagnosis and prevention. Obstet Gynecol Surv 1986;41:325.

ogenesis and are associated with abnormal metabolism, thought to be related mostly to hyperglycemia.

### Prevention of Fetal Anomalies

Clinical studies suggest that euglycemia during organogenesis is critical in the prevention of congenital anomalies. Several investigators have recruited diabetic women before pregnancy and attempted to place them under tight glycemic control before conception. These studies have found that when greater glucose control was achieved, the malformation rate was significantly lower.

It is recommended that diabetic women contemplating pregnancy be encouraged to delay conception until satisfactory metabolic control is achieved so that embryogenesis can occur in an optimal metabolic milieu.

Glygosylated hemoglobin is expressed as a percentage of total hemoglobin and provides an integrated retrospective reflection of glycemic status over the 4 to 8 weeks preceding its determination.

It seems that the risk for delivering anomalous infants cannot be fully determined by $HbA_1$ levels, especially at low levels. It should be emphasized that diabetic embryopathy may be present even in patients with a normal $HbA_1$ level, and further evaluation is still necessary.

### Maternal Serum Alpha-Fetoprotein

Routine screening for the diabetic patient is essential for prenatal evaluation in view of the reported 20-fold increase in neural tube defects. It has been suggested that the maternal serum alpha-fetoprotein (MSAFP) values should be interpreted with caution in diabetic pregnancy, since they are lower per gestational age than in the nondiabetic pregnancy.

## Ultrasonic Evaluation

Routine screening of all diabetic pregnancies with ultrasonic evaluation should be made at approximately 20 weeks of gestation. This evaluation includes a general anatomical survey and fetal echocardiography. Sonographic examination of the fetal heart may be useful not only in the detection of malformations, but also to exclude diabetes-related cardiac hypertrophy.

## INSULIN ADMINISTRATION AND GLUCOSE EVALUATION

### Insulin Preparations

Advances in insulin delivery and monitoring of glucose have made the goal of stringent glycemic control feasible. Whenever insulin is used, dosages must be individualized and balanced with diet and exercise. A variety of insulin preparations exists, marketed by different manufacturers.

1. *Short-acting insulins*: regular and semi-Lente, with a peak activity of 2 to 4 hours
2. *Intermediate-acting insulins*: Lente and NPH with 5- to 12-hour span of peak activity
3. *Long-acting insulins*: protamine zinc insulin (PZI) and ultra-Lente with 12- to 24-hour-span of maximum activity

Insulin is injected into the subcutaneous tissue. In selecting a site, the variable absorption rates should be taken into consideration. The abdomen has the fastest rate of absorption, followed by the arms, thighs, and buttocks. Rotation of the injection site is recommended to prevent lipohypertrophy or lipoatrophy.

### Insulin Administration

In general, regimens that intend to achieve stringent metabolic control of diabetics must simulate the normal diurnal profile of endogenous insulin release.

### Self-Monitoring of Blood Glucose

The introduction of portable blood glucose meters has made it possible for diabetics to evaluate blood glucose several times per day in their homes. These devices have led to a decrease in hospital admissions, improved glucose control, and enhanced motivation among patients to achieve and maintain euglycemia.

Blood glucose determinations should be obtained six to eight times a day every day. Patients are instructed to test their blood for glucose whenever they feel symptoms of hypoglycemia. The patient and family members should be taught how to treat hypoglycemia, including the use of glucagon.

### Diet

Diet therapy is considered a standard treatment of diabetes mellitus. All patients are seen by the dietitian in the clinic, and individual meal plan adjustments are made. The American Diabetes Association (ADA) (1979) recommends 35 kcal/kg of ideal body weight, and a diet composed of 20% protein, 30% fat, and 50% carbohydrate. Restricted saturated fats and cholesterol and increased dietary fiber are suggested. Most patients are instructed on how to maintain a diet that consists of three meals and one to three snacks, the last snack usually being taken at bedtime. The bedtime snack should be composed of complex carbohydrates with proteins to maintain adequate blood glucose levels during the night, thereby avoiding nocturnal hypoglycemia.

Patient weight gains are assessed at each visit to the clinic, and caloric intake is adjusted accordingly. The aim is to prevent weight reduction and its associated ketogenic risk while ensuring optimal weight gain. It is desirable to increase weight by 2 to 4 lb (0.9 to 1.7 kg) in the first trimester and 0.5 to 1.0 lb (200 to 450 g) per week thereafter until term. A total weight gain of 22 to 30 lb (10 to 13 kg) during normal and diabetic pregnancy is recommended.

## MATERNAL COMPLICATIONS

Diabetic women have a markedly higher risk of a number of pregnancy complications. Because of a paucity of data regarding maternal complications during diabetic pregnancy, the exact relative risk for each complication is not known. Complications that have been reported to be more frequent in diabetic pregnancy include spontaneous abortion, preterm labor, pyelonephritis, hydramnios, and hypertensive disorders. Also directly related to metabolic control are hypoglycemia and diabetic ketoacidosis (DKA). These complications, together with the vascular alterations and the higher cesarean section rate, contribute to the higher maternal morbidity and mortality among diabetic pregnant patients.

### Maternal Mortality

The advent of insulin in 1922 brought about a dramatic fall in the maternal mortality from 45% to just over 2% shortly after the widespread introduction of insulin in 1935. Together with improved medical and obstetric care, maternal mortality has decreased to as low as 0.5%. More recently, a mortality rate of 0.11% was reported among 2614 pregnant diabetic patients.

### Diabetic Ketoacidosis

In recent years, the incidence of diabetic ketoacidosis (DKA) during pregnancy has decreased significantly. Ketoacidosis has been reported to occur in pregnant diabetic patients more rapidly and at lower blood glucose levels than in nonpregnant patients. It may be precipitated by stress, infection (e.g., urinary tract), or omission of insulin because of patient neglect. The use of B-sympathomimetic agents in pregnant diabetics may induce DKA.

Omission of insulin or insulin deficiency in IDDM pregnant patients results in hyperglycemia and glucosuria. Osmotic diuresis results in urinary potassium, sodium, and water losses. Hyperglycemia is aggravated, since, as a consequence of hypovolemia, there is an increase in the secretion of glucagon and cathecolamines. Lipolysis consequent to insulin deficiency leads to increased hepatic oxidation of fatty acids with the formation of ketone bodies (acetone, b-hydroxybutyrate, and acetoacetate), which leads, in turn, to the production of metabolic acidosis (Figure 37-2).

In recent years, treating DKA with a constant, low-dose insulin infusion regimen, and not with high-dose bolus therapy, has been recommended. The advan-

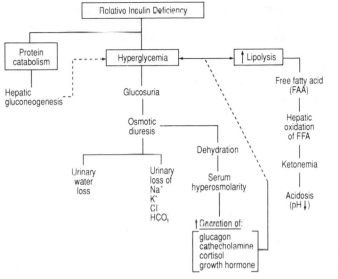

**FIGURE 37-2.** Metabolic alterations in diabetic ketoacidosis.

tage of a low-dose regimen is its simplicity, which reduces complications, such as hypoglycemia and hypokalemia, observed with the traditional high-dose bolus therapy. The following are some general guidelines for the treatment of diabetic ketoacidosis:

1. Insert two IV lines; obtain blood to assess levels of glucose, serum electrolytes and ketones, and arterial blood gases; administer oxygen by face mask. Frequently assess the clinical status and follow urinary output. Repeat blood and urinary test often.
2. Patients with DKA require simultaneous correction of fluid and electrolyte imbalance and treatment of hyperglycemia and acidosis.
   a. *Replacement of fluid.* The average fluid deficit is 3 to 5 L. It is therefore necessary to administer 1000 to 2000 mL of isotonic saline rapidly during the first hour. If hypernatremia is present, 0.45% sodium chloride is preferred. After the first hour, 300 to 500 mL/h is given, depending on hemodynamic status. Normal saline is given to hypotensive patients in larger amounts. In these cases, a central line may be necessary.
   b. *Insulin therapy.* Administer an initial bolus of 10 to 20 U of regular insulin intravenously. Follow this with a constant infusion of about 10 U/h. (Add 50 U of regular insulin per 500 mL of normal saline.) Larger doses of constant regular insulin infusion of 12 to 20 U/h may be required if acidosis does not begin to respond within 3 hours or if plasma glucose level does not fall by 30%.
   c. *Glucose administration.* To reduce the risk of hypoglycemia and cerebral edema, change the intravenous solution to 5% dextrose when the plasma glucose level reaches 200 to 250 mg/dL and simultaneously decrease the rate of the insulin infusion.

d. *Potassium administration.* On admission, hyperkalemia is usually present. At this point, potassium administration is not required, and, in fact, may be dangerous or even lethal, since hyperkalemia may rapidly reach cardiotoxic levels. Potassium administration is usually started after 3 to 4 hours of insulin therapy, when potassium begins to fall to normal or low levels. It is given by adding 40 mEq of potassium chloride per 1000 mL normal saline at a rate of 10 to 20 mEq/h, as needed. It should be stressed that when potassium is administered, it is given with extreme caution, and that potassium and urinary output are monitored carefully.

e. *Bicarbonate administration.* Add 44 mEq sodium bicarbonate to 1 L 0.45% saline and administer intravenously only if arterial pH is less than 7.1 or serum bicarbonate is less than 5 mEq. If the pH is less than 7, the sodium bicarbonate dose should be doubled (88 mEq). Bicarbonate administration should be terminated if arterial pH has been corrected to 7.2. Alkali administration in DKA is still controversial, because this therapy might aggravate tissue hypoxia.

## Hypoglycemia

The main symptoms of hypoglycemic reactions in patients with IDDM include sweating, tremors, blurred or double vision, weakness, hunger, confusion, paresthesia of lips and tongue, anxiety, palpitation, nausea, headache, and stupor. The increased risk of hypoglycemia in pregnant IDDM patients may be related to defective glucose counterregulatory hormone mechanisms.

In nonpregnant IDDM patients, the glucagon response to hypoglycemia is lost early in the disease and patients are dependent on epinephrine to promote recovery from hypoglycemia. Some nonpregnant IDDM patients with long-standing disease may develop deficient epinephrine secretory responses to hypoglycemia and may experience severe hypoglycemic episodes without the warning symptoms that allow the patient time to eat before hypoglycemia becomes severe.

The spectrum of potential adverse effects of maternal hypoglycemia on the human fetus has not been clearly established and awaits further investigation.

## Polyhydramnios

Polyhydramnios occurs commonly in diabetics, with a reported incidence that varies from 3% to 32%. Although this condition can be associated with central nervous system and gastrointestinal abnormalities, in almost 90% of diabetics with polyhydramnios, no etiology can be found.

The etiology of polyhydramnios in diabetics is not clear. Suggested mechanisms include increases in amniotic fluid osmolality caused by increases in glucose load, decreased fetal swallowing, high gastrointestinal tract obstruction, and fetal polyuria secondary to fetal hyperglycemia. Experimental work, however, has not provided strong evidence for any of these explanations. Although the most likely reason for the higher fluid volume is increased fetal urine production in diabetics, this was not demonstrated by sequential estimation of bladder volume over time.

Polyhydramnios complicating diabetes in pregnancy is associated with a higher perinatal mortality and morbidity rates than can be attributed to the higher rates of preterm delivery and congenital anomalies caused by this condition. In one report, the preterm delivery rate among diabetics with hydramnios was twice as high as that in diabetics without polyhydramnios (13% versus 6.1%, respectively).

## Preterm Labor

Magnesium sulfate therapy is considered the drug of choice in diabetic patients with premature labor, since this drug has no effect on diabetic control. In contrast, B-sympathomimetic tocolytic agents or glucocorticosteroids have been reported to induce hyperglycemia and ketoacidosis. Therefore, treatment with both medications in diabetics requires great caution, intensive monitoring of glucose levels, and treatment with intravenous insulin infusion as needed.

## Spontaneous Abortions

The rate of spontaneous abortion in pregestational pregnant diabetic patients varies considerably between reports, ranging from 6% to 29%.

## Diabetic Retinopathy

Diabetic retinopathy is usually classified as background simple diabetic retinopathy and proliferative diabetic retinopathy. The characteristic lesions of diabetic retinopathy are presented in Table 37-10.

**Pregnancy and Progression of Diabetic Retinopathy.** Investigators have reported controversial findings regarding the role of pregnancy in the development and progression of diabetic retinopathy. Most recent reports have shown that in some diabetic patients pregnancy is associated with progression of diabetic retinopathy, from minimal to marked deterioration of the retina. However, many changes during pregnancy have proved to be reversible, and many patients have experienced regression of their lesion after delivery.

**Principal Management of Diabetic Retinopathy in Pregnant Diabetics.** Diabetic retinopathy occurring during pregnancy should be treated in essentially the same manner as in the nonpregnant state. Laser treatment can be used safely during pregnancy when indicated. It is recommended that diabetic patients undergo careful retinal examination before conception and be treated with laser photocoagulation before pregnancy if necessary. It is our practice to perform ophthalmoscopy every trimester in pregnant IDDM patients and even more frequently in patients with documented retinopathy prior to pregnancy.

**TABLE 37-10.** Characteristic Lesions of Diabetic Retinopathy

Background Diabetic Retinopathy
    Microaneurysms
    Small vessel obstruction, soft exudate, intraretinal microvascular abnormalities
    Venous abnormalities
    Retinal hemorrhages
    Hard exudate
    Disk edema
    Maculopathy
Proliferative Diabetic Retinopathy
    Neovascularization
    Fibrous deposition
    Vitreous hemorrhage
    Retinal detachment

## Diabetic Nephropathy

The prevalence of diabetic nephropathy in IDDM pregnant patients is estimated at 6%. Five evolutionary stages of nephropathy in diabetics have been described for type I:

1. Early hypertrophy-hyperfunction
2. Glomerular lesions without clinical disease
3. Incipient nephropathy characterized by microproteinuria
4. Overt nephropathy characterized by macroproteinuria
5. End-stage diabetic renal disease

A diagnosis of diabetic nephropathy in pregnancy is made if there is persistent proteinuria of greater than 300 mg/day in the first half of pregnancy in the absence of urinary tract infection.

Acute worsening of hypertension is very common in patients with diabetic nephropathy and occurs in almost 60% of cases. The long-term maternal course was judged consistent with the expected course of diabetic nephropathy in nonpregnant women.

Perinatal mortality and morbidity in patients with diabetic nephropathy may be attributed to the higher incidence of early delivery (31%), a higher incidence of low-birth-weight infants (21%), an increased incidence of fetal distress, and preeclampsia. Pregnant patients with diabetic nephropathy require an intensive program of maternal and fetal evaluation; adequate bedrest during pregnancy; assessment of renal function and retinal status at regular intervals; blood pressure monitoring; and treatment of hypertension when required using methyldopa, arteriolar vasodilator, or beta blockers.

## ANTEPARTUM ASSESSMENT

### Maternal Assessment

Ophthalmologic and renal function tests, including creatinine clearance and total urinary protein excretion, are performed in each trimester, or more often if indicated. In patients with vasculopathy, an electrocardiogram is performed at the initial visit and repeated if clinically indicated. In patients in White's class H, the electrocardiogram is performed routinely in each trimester. The echocardiogram is performed at enrollment and repeated in the pregnancy, depending on the initial findings. It is extremely important to detect early signs of pregnancy-induced hypertension; therefore, assessment of blood pressure, signs of proteinuria, and edema formation is essential.

### Fetal Surveillance

All pregnancies complicated by diabetes require extra assessment. The use of ultrasonography provides essential information about the fetus. A first trimester scan is used to date the pregnancy, and to establish viability and fluid volume status. A second trimester scan is repeated at 18 to 20 weeks of gestation to rule out fetal anomalies. Subsequent ultrasound evaluations are then performed at 4- to 6-week intervals to assess fluid volume and fetal growth.

**Fetal Macrosomia.** Macrosomia, arbitrarily defined as fetal weight in excess of 4000 g, or as a birth weight above the 90th percentile for gestational age, occurs in about 10% of all pregnancies. Almost 30% of all diabetics will deliver infants weighing over 4000 g.

Fetal macrosomia is thought to be related to maternal hyperglycemia that induces fetal hyperglycemia and hyperinsulinemia. Fetal hyperinsulinemia results in enhanced glycogen synthesis, lipogenesis, increased protein synthesis, and, thus, fetal organomegaly and fat deposition. Macrosomia is much more frequent in IDDM patients without vasculopathy than in those with vasculopathy. Furthermore, infants delivered of patients with diabetic nephropathy are of significantly lower birth weight than those of controls.

Macrosomic fetuses have higher perinatal morbidity and mortality—a result caused mainly by the traumatic delivery. These fetuses are at increased risk of severe fetal asphyxia due to head and neck birth trauma. Shoulder dystocia is more common in macrosomic fetuses; therefore, infants of diabetics experience more shoulder dystocia than those of nondiabetics. Disproportional growth of the body compared with the head is believed to be the cause of shoulder dystocia.

**Antepartum Fetal Testing.** In pregnant diabetic patients, stillbirth occurs with increased frequency, particularly in the third trimester. Therefore, a program of fetal monitoring should be initiated, usually at 32 to 33 weeks. Currently, in most medical centers, outpatient protocols for antepartum fetal surveillance are used that include either once- or twice-weekly nonstress tests (NSTs) or a once-weekly oxytocin challenge test (OCT), or biophysical profiles.

Maternal assessment of fetal activity not only seems to be a practical approach toward evaluation of fetal condition but a simple, inexpensive, and valuable screening technique. Patients with diabetes are instructed to count fetal movements, beginning as early as 28 to 29 weeks of gestation, and to report any decrease in fetal movements so that further testing can be initiated if necessary.

Selecting the time of delivery is individualized in patients with diabetes and should take into account the following three factors:

1. Degree of glycemic control
2. Maternal complications
3. Fetal well-being

**Management During Labor and Delivery.** During labor and delivery, it is necessary to maintain maternal euglycemia to avoid neonatal hypoglycemia. Induced maternal hyperglycemia during labor in diabetics is associated with neonatal hypoglycemia.

Therefore, in patients undergoing induction of labor, the morning insulin doses should be withheld and glucose levels determined once every hour with a home glucometer. In well-controlled patients, 1 unit of insulin per hour and 3 to 6 g of glucose per hour are usually required to maintain a glucose level of 70 to 90 mg/dL. If the initial glucose level is between 80 and 120 mg/dL, 10 units of regular insulin can be added to 1000 mL of 5% dextrose in 0.5 normal saline or D5RL and administered at an infusion rate of 125 mL/h. However, if initial glucose levels are below 70 mg/dL, it is recommended that initially 5% dextrose in water without insulin at a rate of 100 to 120 mL/h be administered throughout labor.

If the patient presents in spontaneous labor and has already taken her morning intermediate-acting insulin, additional insulin may not be required throughout labor and delivery, but a continuous glucose infusion will be necessary (125 mL/h of 5% dextrose in water).

When an elective cesarean section is planned for a diabetic patient, the procedure should be scheduled early in the morning, when glucose levels are usually in the normal range because of the action of the intermediate-acting insulin dose given the night before. Infusion without glucose is preferred (i.e., normal saline), and glucose levels are monitored frequently. If the patient is under regional anesthesia, it is easier to detect signs of hypoglycemia.

After delivery, a dramatic decrease in the insulin requirement is almost the rule because of a significant decrease in the level of placental hormones that have anti-insulin action. At this time there is no need for stringent glucose control, and glucose levels below 200 mg/dL are satisfactory. In the first few days after delivery, it is preferable to give regular insulin subcutaneously before each meal on the basis of plasma glucose levels. After the patient is able to eat regular meals, she may receive one-half of the prepregnancy dosage of insulin, usually divided into two daily injections.

## MORBIDITY OF THE INFANT OF THE DIABETIC MOTHER

Neonatal morbidity is frequent in both gestational and pregestational diabetes mellitus but is much higher in the latter group. The exact etiology of many of these disorders remains unclear. However, there is evidence to show that neonatal morbidity is related to poor maternal metabolic control during pregnancy and that tight maternal glycemic control may prevent several major forms of morbidity.

### Hypoglycemia

The neonatal hypoglycemia in infants of diabetic mothers is probably related to the overproduction of insulin by the fetal pancreas that has been stimulated in utero by significant hyperglycemia.

Clinical signs of neonatal hypoglycemia include tremor, apathy, episodes of cyanosis, convulsions, weak or high-pitched cry, and episodes of sweating. Since prolonged and severe hypoglycemia may be associated with neurologic sequelae, initiation of treatment is advised in all neonates of diabetic mothers with plasma glucose levels of less than 40 mg/dL.

The most efficient means of therapy for hypoglycemia is continuous dextrose infusion at the rate of 4 to 6 mg/kg/min. The use of a bolus of a hypertonic glucose infusion should be avoided to prevent later rebound hypoglycemia.

### Hypocalcemia and Hypomagnesemia

There is a significant increase in the incidence of hypocalcemia and hypomagnesemia in infants of diabetic mothers. The incidence of neonatal hypocalcemia, defined as calcium levels at or below 7 mg/dL, has been reported to approach 20% in a group of infants with mean gestational age at delivery of 38 $\pm$ 0.2 weeks. Serum calcium levels in infants of diabetic mothers are lowest in the second to the third day of life. The etiology of hypocalcemia in neonates of diabetic mothers is not yet clear.

### Polycythemia

Polycythemia is diagnosed when venous hematocrit exceeds 65%. This condition has been reported to affect a third of neonates of diabetic mothers in the first few hours of life. The mechanism responsible for polycythemia in these babies may be related to chronic intrauterine hypoxia that leads to an increase in erythropoietin and a consequent increase in red cell production.

Usually, polycythemia is associated with hyperviscosity of the blood, which may impede the velocity of blood flow and increase the risk of microthrombus formation in multiple organs. Kidneys, adrenals, and lungs are the most commonly affected organs. Clinically, infants with polycythemia appear plethoric. Some of these infants have convulsions, respiratory distress, tachycardia, congestive heart failure, and hyperbilirubinemia. The treatment of polycythemia consists of partial exchange transfusion with a volume expander (i.e., plasma) to reduce the hematocrit to about 55%.

## Respiratory Distress Syndrome

Respiratory distress syndrome (RDS) is considered a common neonatal morbidity in the infants of diabetic mothers. Factors contributing to the development of RDS in these infants are preterm deliveries, delayed fetal lung maturation, and high rate of elective cesarean section.

Because a significant number of infants may develop RDS despite L/S ratio of ≥2, the use of an L/S ratio of more than 3.5 or at least 3.0 has been recommended as an indicator of fetal lung maturity in infants of diabetic mothers. Most authorities, however, prefer to analyze both L/S ratios and PG in the amniotic fluid before undertaking elective delivery.

## Hyperbilirubinemia

Prevention of hyperbilirubinemia in IDMs may be possible by reducing the incidence of prematurity, improvement of maternal metabolic control, and possibly reducing macrosomia by even more stringent glucose control. Finally, early treatment of polycythemia may further reduce the risk of hyperbilirubinemia.

## Birth Asphyxia

Birth asphyxia in neonates of diabetic mothers is much more common than that observed in the general obstetric population. Poorly controlled diabetics have an increased risk of macrosomia and chronic intrauterine hypoxia and therefore a greater risk of intrauterine or neonatal asphyxia.

Birth injuries in the macrosomic infants of diabetic mothers include Erb's palsy, fractured clavicle, facial paralysis, phrenic nerve injury, and intracranial hemorrhage. Severe birth injuries may result in permanent neonatal morbidity and sometimes in neonatal death.

## Cardiomyopathy

Infants of diabetic mothers have a higher risk of hypertrophic types of cardiomyopathy and congestive heart failure. The incidence of neonates of diabetic mothers with cardiomyopathy is not known. According to one study, 10% of infants of diabetic mothers may have evidence of myocardial and septal hypertrophy. The characteristic findings in echocardiography are generalized myocardial hypertrophy with disproportionate hypertrophy of the interventricular septum. Infants of diabetic mothers with severe cardiomyopathy may develop left ventricular outflow tract obstruction with reduced cardiac output and congestive heart failure. The natural history of cardiomyopathy in infants of diabetic mothers is different from other types of cardiomyopathy in that there is a complete regression of hypertrophic changes to normal after several months.

# 38. ENDOCRINE DISORDERS IN PREGNANCY

## HYPOTHALAMUS AND PITUITARY GLAND

Functional pituitary integrity is necessary for conception, and pregnancy is uncommon in women with pituitary abnormalities. Hypophysectomized women on full hormone replacement therapy are capable of normal conception, gestation, and parturition, indicating that an intact hypothalamic-pituitary arc is not required.

## ANATOMY AND HISTOLOGY

The pituitary gland is composed of three lobes—the anterior pituitary (adenohypophysis), the intermediate lobe (pars intermedia), and the posterior pituitary (neurohypophysis). The anterior pituitary comprises the bulk of the gland (75%) and enlarges up to three times during pregnancy. The intermediate lobe of the pituitary occupies a very small area in the adult and has an uncertain role in neuroendocrine function. The neurohypophysis (posterior pituitary) is a direct extension of cell bodies in the hypothalamic supraoptic and paraventricular nuclei responsible for the synthesis and secretion of the hormones oxytocin and vasopressin, and their carrier proteins neurophysin I and II.

## PATHOPHYSIOLOGY

Disorders resulting in either hyperfunction or hypofunction of the pituitary gland may occur during pregnancy—most commonly hyperprolactinemia secondary to a pituitary microadenoma, or panhypopituitarism from postpartum ischemic necrosis (Sheehan's syndrome). Pituitary tumors may involve any of the five cell types normally present in the pituitary. These may be microadenomas (<10 mm in size) or macroadenomas (>10 mm).

## DISORDERS OF HYPERSECRETION

Prolactin-secreting microadenomas are the most common pituitary tumors (40%) and are often associated with the syndrome of amenorrhea and galactorrhea. The infertility that occurs in about one-third of affected women is largely a result of impaired GnRH pulsatile secretion. The dopamine agonist bromocriptine will restore ovulatory cycles in over 80% of such women. Its use has been approved for ovulation induction in the presence of either a microadenoma (<1 cm size) or a macroadenoma (>1 cm size) confined to the sella turcica. Macroadenomas with suprasellar expansion should, however, probably be treated surgically prior to attempted pregnancy. Bromocriptine is the only dopamine agonist currently marketed in the United States. The usual adult oral dose of bromocriptine is

E. Albert Reece, John C. Hobbins, Maurice, J. Mahoney and Roy H. Petrie (Eds).
*Handbook of Medicine of the Fetus & Mother.* Copyright © 1995 by J.B. Lippincott Company

1.25 mg every 12 hours starting with an initial dose of 1.25 mg at bedtime. Bromocriptine crosses the placenta and should be discontinued as soon as possible after conception has occurred and reinstated only with evidence of tumor expansion. Large numbers of women have successfully undergone pregnancy with normal outcomes while receiving bromocriptine throughout gestation, but long-term studies have not yet been performed. Postpartum suckling does not further increase prolactin secretion in the presence of a prolactinoma and is not significantly associated with risks of tumor expansion. Therefore, patients who wish to breast-feed should not be discouraged from doing so. Eventually, postpartum nonlactating mothers should have the bromocriptine resumed, because chronic hyperprolactinemia is associated with hypoestrogenism and its attendant risks of bone loss. There is a risk of tumor expansion during pregnancy secondary to the rising estrogen and progesterone levels—1.6% for microadenomas and 15.5% for macroadenomas. Therefore, patients who become pregnant should be carefully followed by monthly visual field examinations by Goldman perimetry. Symptoms or signs of expansion, such as headaches, blurred vision, visual field or funduscopic changes, should be investigated with an imaging examination, preferably magnetic resonance imaging (MRI).

Growth hormone hypersecretion is usually secondary to a pituitary macroadenoma and results in the syndrome of acromegaly with its attendant bony overgrowth, visceromegaly, and hyperhidrosis. Hypertension and impaired glucose tolerance are often manifest, further complicating the success of pregnancy occurring simultaneously.

## DISORDERS OF HYPOSECRETION

Impaired pituitary hormone secretion may result from space-occupying lesions, head trauma, ischemic damage, or as a sequel to surgery or irradiation. Syndromes of hypopituitarism uniquely associated with pregnancy include lymphocytic hypophysitis and Sheehan's syndrome.

Lymphocytic hypophysitis is an autoimmune disorder associated with pituitary enlargement and functional insufficiency. In about half of the cases, the disease was detected in the postpartum period, and in two cases the onset was during gestation. This disorder occurs with increased frequency in association with multiple autoimmune glandular disease (diabetes mellitus, Hashimoto's thyroiditis, hypoparathyroidism), raising the possibility that it may be related to changes in autoimmunity during pregnancy and the postpartum period. The resultant inflammation may mimic a pituitary adenoma, and should be suspected with appearance of pituitary enlargement more than normal for pregnancy.

The most common cause of anterior pituitary insufficiency in the adult woman is Sheehan's syndrome. This syndrome of postpartum pituitary necrosis is associated with postpartum hemorrhage; however, cases with minimal known blood loss have been described.

An increased risk of pituitary necrosis also occurs in diabetics, heralded by a deep midline headache and falling insulin requirements in the third trimester.

## THYROID GLAND

Thyroid disorders are the most common endocrinopathies encountered during pregnancy—both hyperthyroidism and hypothyroidism are five to ten times more common in women than in men. The symptoms of hyperthyroidism may mimic the normal hypermetabolic state of pregnancy, and therefore a high index of suspicion is necessary to make the diagnosis. This is further complicated by the altered thyroid function tests that occur during normal pregnancy—most notably, a rise in thyroxine-binding globulin and total thyroxine levels. The free thyroid hormone levels remain normal, however, and therefore a state of euthyroidism state exists. Treatment of thyroid disorders is complicated by the presence of the fetus, because pharmacologic therapy beneficial to the mother may be harmful to the fetal thyroid.

## PHYSIOLOGIC ADAPTATIONS TO PREGNANCY

An increased glomerular filtration rate during pregnancy results in an early rise in renal iodine clearance and a subsequent decrease in the plasma inorganic iodine concentration. The thyroid responds by increasing its uptake of iodine and thus usually maintains euthyroid levels of thyroid hormone production. Dietary iodine may therefore be limiting in certain geographic locations, and result in formation of an iodine-deficient goiter. Supplemental iodine in order to achieve an intake of 250 μg/day is recommended during pregnancy and easily attained with prenatal vitamin supplements. Care must be taken to avoid excessive intake (>2000 μg/day), because this may also be harmful to the mother and fetus.

## LABORATORY INVESTIGATIONS

### Radioiodine Thyroid Uptake
The thyroid radioiodine uptake test is contraindicated during pregnancy, because radioisotopes cross the placenta and may be concentrated in the fetal thyroid (after 10 weeks gestation).

### Thyroid Hormones
The rise of TBG that occurs during pregnancy can be measured directly by radioimmunoassay. The T3 uptake test ($RT_3U$) measures uptake of exogenous [123]I-T3 by a binding resin, such that higher serum TBG levels result in a decreased [123]I-T3 resin uptake, and lower TBG levels have opposite effects. Thus, the $RT_3U$ is lower during pregnancy than during nonpregnancy and tends to be in the hypothyroid range. This test does not always accurately reflect absolute levels of TBG, because other serum proteins may affect the binding of [123]I-T3 to the resin, and thus result in misinterpretation of TBG levels. T4 and T3 concentrations measured by radioimmunoassay measure the total T4 and T3 (bound plus free fractions) and are therefore elevated during pregnancy. Despite this, levels of free thyroid hormones are usually within the normal range. An indirect estimate of free hormone concentrations may be made by determination of the free thyroxine index ($FT_4I$) = T4 × RT3U/100. However, due to failure of the $RT_3U$ test to accurately determine TBG concentrations, this estimate may not provide a true index of free T4 levels. In most cases, however, a normal $FT_4I$ and TSH level will exclude significant underlying thyroid pathology.

### Hypothalamic-Pituitary-Thyroid Axis
The TRH test is performed by injecting 200 to 400 μg TRH intravenously and monitoring the change in TSH 20 and 60 minutes after injection. TRH crosses the

placenta when administered in such pharmacologic doses, and may affect the fetal pituitary-thyroid axis. This test is therefore not recommended in pregnancy. The newer, more sensitive TSH assays are capable of differentiating normal from suppressed levels, and therefore should replace the TRH test as the best mode to diagnose hyperthyroidism in pregnancy. TSH levels are largely unchanged by normal pregnancy (minimal decrease in the first trimester), and the suppression that occurs with primary hyperthyroidism during pregnancy will be detectable by a sensitive TSH assay.

## Thyroid Autoantibodies

Thyroid-stimulating immunoglobulins may be detectable in the serum of women with either active or inactive Graves' disease (hyperthyroidism). These antibodies may cross the placenta and rarely (1%) induce a state of fetal or neonatal thyrotox-icosis. Thus, determination of the levels of these stimulating immunoglobulins (TSI) is recommended in women with evidence of past or present Graves' disease, especially in the presence of fetal tachycardia greater than 140 beats per minute. The levels of maternal thyroid autoantibodies tend to decline as pregnancy advances, and thus it is not uncommon to see amelioration of the thyroid hyperfunction with advancing gestation.

## PLACENTAL-FETAL THYROID PHYSIOLOGY

The placenta is relatively impermeable to the thyroid hormones T4 and T3 as well as TSH. The placenta contains deiodinase enzymes that degrade T4 and T3, and this may account in part for the difficulty of these hormones in crossing from the maternal to fetal circulation in an active form. Hyperthyroidism due to maternal Graves' disease may, however, result in fetal hyperthyroidism due to the placental transfer of thyroid-stimulating immunoglobulins. Furthermore, drugs used in treatment of such hyperfunction (thiouracils, propranolol, iodine) readily cross the placenta and may thus impair fetal thyroid function. When hCG levels are abnormally high, as in trophoblast disease, frank hyperthyroidism may rarely occur. Levels of 300,000 mIU/mL hCG are necessary to induce clinical hyper-thyroidism. hCG has an activity in the TSH bioassay of 0.2 $\mu$U TSH/$\mu$ hCG.

## Fetal Thyroid Function

The human fetal thyroid gland is capable of concentrating iodine by the 10th to 12th week of gestation, at which time TSH can be detected in the fetal pituitary and TRH in the hypothalamus. Serum TSH is first detectable in fetal serum at 10 weeks of age, and progressively rises from 20 to 30 weeks, reaching a peak of 15 $\mu$U/mL. At parturition, fetal thyroid function undergoes profound alterations, with a marked rise in TSH from 7.5 $\mu$U/mL to 30 $\mu$U/mL within 3 hours (Fig. 38-1). A surge in T3 > T4 then occurs in the neonatal serum, reaching a maximum by 24 hours and returning toward baseline by the end of the first week of life. Neonatal radioactive iodine uptake by the thyroid is elevated at 10 hours postpartum, reaching a peak by day 2 and returning toward adult normal limits by day 5 of life.

## Amniotic Fluid

During the first half of pregnancy, amniotic fluid thyroid hormone concentrations increase progressively, reaching peak concentrations at 25 to 30 weeks, although

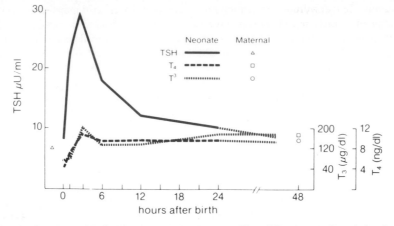

**FIGURE 38-1.** Serum (TSH), thyroid-stimulating hormone T4 and T3 concentrations during the first 48 hours in the neonate. (From Stubbe P, Gatz J, Heidemann P, Muhlen A, Hesch R. Thyroxine-binding globulin, triiodothyroxine, thyroxine and thyrotropin in newborn infants and children. Horm Metab Res 1978; 19: 58.)

levels of thyroxine are higher and rise more rapidly than triiodothyronine. During the latter half of pregnancy, the T4 levels decrease while T3 levels continue to increase. Reverse T3 concentrations are also elevated in the amniotic fluid, reaching peak levels at 17 to 20 weeks. Although the source of these thyroid hormones may be the fetus, the absolute level of amniotic fluid thyroid hormones does not necessarily correlate with fetal thyroid status.

## DISORDERS OF HYPOSECRETION

### Maternal Hypothyroidism
Although decreased thyroid function is not rare in women of reproductive age, its association with pregnancy is unusual. This most likely stems from the amenorrhea, menorrhagia, and anovulatory cycles, which frequently coexist and thus impair fertility. Hypothyroidism may be primary, with failure of the thyroid gland itself or secondary to loss of pituitary TSH stimulation. The latter usually occurs with either space-occupying lesions, such as macroadenomas and craniopharyngiomas, or ischemic necrosis. Cold intolerance, fatigability, constipation, dry skin, and weight gain accompany hypothyroidism in both the pregnant and nonpregnant state. Paresthesias are an early symptom in about 75% of patients. The thyroid gland is enlarged, firm, nontender, and bosselated (irregular) in Hashimoto's thyroiditis, whereas in idiopathic myxedema it is markedly atrophic and therefore impalpable. Physical examination may otherwise reveal a delayed relaxation phase of the deep tendon reflexes and, less commonly, frank myxedema with periorbital edema and vocal cord thickening may be observed.

**Diagnosis.** The laboratory diagnosis of primary hypothyroidism rests on the demonstration of an elevated serum TSH concentration, usually in association with a lower serum T4 concentration.

**Course.** Hypothyroid women who are inadequately treated during pregnancy have higher risks of spontaneous abortion, stillbirth, and abnormal offspring, with congenital defects and developmental retardation in some cases.

## TREATMENT

As soon as the diagnosis of primary hypothyroidism is established, L-thyroxine should be instituted in full replacement doses. Most patients require 100 to 125 μg per day of oral levothyroxine.

### Congenital and Neonatal Hypothyroidism

Most infants with congenital hypothyroidism appear clinically normal at birth, although thyroid hormone deficiency during the fetal and neonatal periods may be associated with developmental retardation. If hypothyroidism is diagnosed and treated before 3 months of age, four-fifths of affected children will have an intelligence quotient (IQ) above 90. Appearance of hypothyroidism after 2 years of age appears to have minimal effect on mental development.

**Etiology.** The most common cause of congenital primary sporadic hypothyroidism is thyroid dysgenesis, occurring approximately once in every 4000 births (Table 38-1).

**Diagnosis.** Cretinism is a syndrome of severe mental retardation, abnormal growth, deaf-mutism, spasticity, strabismus, and abnormal sexual maturation secondary to iodine deficiency occurring in utero. It occurs with higher frequency in regions of endemic goiter, such as the South American Andes, New Guinea, and Central Africa. Other causes of hypothyroidism are usually not apparent at birth, but may be associated with umbilical hernia, a large posterior fontanel, dry skin, hypothermia, constipation, and respiratory difficulties. Laboratory findings include a low serum T4 (<4 μg/100 mL) with a high TSH (>80 μU/mL), which should be determined after the peak TSH surge that normally occurs at 24 hours of life (See Fig. 38-1). Bone age determination may reveal the decreased maturation associated with deficiency of thyroid hormone. In particular, the lack of ossification of the distal femoral epiphysis suggests fetal hypothyroidism.

**Treatment.** Replacement therapy should begin as soon as the diagnosis of hypothyroidism is made in the neonatal period. The usual initial dose is 10 μg/kg per day of oral thyroxine as a single dose, which is then adjusted to maintain the serum free T4 concentration to the upper normal range and to suppress of serum TSH to 20 μU/ml. The requirements gradually decrease to approximately 5 μg/kg at the age of 24 months. At this time, cessation of thyroxine may be attempted with close follow-up of thyroid function tests.

**TABLE 38-1.** Etiology and Incidence of Congenital Hypothyroidism

| | |
|---|---|
| Primary hypothyroidism | |
| Thyroid dysgenesis | 1 in 4000 |
| Inborn errors of thyroid function | 1 in 30,000 |
| Drug-induced | 1 in 10,000 |
| Endemic hypothyroidism | 1 in 7 |
| Secondary and tertiary hypothyroidism | 1 in 60,000 |

## DISORDERS OF HYPERSECRETION

### Maternal Thyrotoxicosis

There is no proof that fertility is impaired in mild to moderate hyperthyroidism. The incidence of thyrotoxicosis during pregnancy is approximately 0.2%, with most women (95%) suffering from Graves' disease. Other causes of primary hyperthyroidism include toxic multinodular goiter (Plummer's disease), toxic uninodular goiter, subacute thyroiditis, and, very rarely, metastatic follicular cancer.

**Symptoms and Signs.** The clinical features of hyperthyroidism may closely mimic the normal pregnant state, because both conditions are associated with a hyperdynamic state. Heat intolerance, increased appetite, increased cardiac output with systolic flow murmurs and widened pulse pressure, skin warmth, and resting tachycardia occur in normal pregnancy. Thyrotoxicosis during pregnancy may also present with hyperemesis gravidarum, resulting in rapid weight loss early in pregnancy. This generally resolves following successful treatment of the hyperthyroidism.

**Diagnosis.** Hyperthyroidism during pregnancy may be confirmed by the finding of elevated free T4 hormone level. The newer, more sensitive TSH assays, if available, provide the best test for confirmation of hyperthyroidism where values are often below 0.05 $\mu$U/mL. Serum T4 levels above 15 $\mu$g/dL coincident with RT$_3$U values within the euthyroid or hypothyroid nonpregnant range are likely to occur in hyperthyroidism. The free T3 index = T4 × RT3U/100 is usually elevated in such cases. Unfortunately, because of elevated TBG in pregnancy, the free thyroxine index is not an accurate measure of the actual free thyroxine concentration. Occasionally the free T4 or free T4 index are normal when the T3 is elevated—so-called T3 toxicosis. This is more likely to occur with a toxic nodular goiter, and should be excluded if thyrotoxic symptoms are present with normal T4 values. Furthermore, determination of thyroid autoantibodies (especially thyroid-stimulating immunoglobulins) are important when Graves' disease is suspected, because high levels may warn of increased fetal risk.

**Course.** Untreated hyperthyroidism does not increase maternal mortality unless preeclampsia occurs, although there is an increase in neonatal morbidity (low birth weight, congenital malformations) and mortality in some reports. Down's syndrome has also been reported to occur more frequently in the offspring of thyrotoxic mothers, but these studies were not well controlled. There is no evidence that pregnancy makes hyperthyroidism more difficult to control; in fact, the severity of Graves' disease tends to decrease as pregnancy progresses. Furthermore, postpartum exacerbations can occur within weeks, presumably due to increasing thyroid-stimulating immunoglobulin (TSI) levels.

**Treatment.** Therapeutic intervention is recommended in all but the mildest forms of hyperthyroidism during pregnancy. Because radioactive iodine is contraindicated, treatment usually involves either antithyroid drugs (thionamides) or surgery.

The thionamide drugs propylthiouracil (PTU) and methimazole inhibit iodination of tyrosine and hence decrease thyroid hormone biosynthesis. PTU also decreases the peripheral conversion of T4 and T3, and this further enhances its efficacy in treatment. Because PTU inhibits formation of new thyroid hormone, but does not prevent release of previously formed hormone, its effect is slow in onset and requires 4 to 6 weeks to achieve a maximal effect. The dose of PTU should start at 100 to 150 mg three times daily, but may require 200 mg three times per day. Once clinical and biochemical improvement are evident, the dose should be decreased to 50 mg four times per day. If the patient remains euthyroid, the PTU could be decreased to 50 mg three times per day after 3 weeks. With monthly determination of the T4 level, the goal should be a serum level in the range of upper normal at a dose of less than 100 mg per day of PTU if possible. If thyrotoxicosis recurs, the PTU should again be increased to 300 mg per day. This should be especially noted in the postpartum period.

## COMPLICATIONS OF PTU

Approximately 2% of patients taking PTU will experience a mild, occasionally purpuric, skin rash, usually within the first 4 weeks of therapy. If this occurs, PTU should be stopped and may be replaced with methimazole. Pruritus, drug fever, and nausea may also occur in a small number of patients. More serious complications include the blood dyscrasias—leukopenia and agranulocytosis.

Antithyroid drugs cross the placenta and may block thyroid hormone biosynthesis in the fetal gland. The resultant rise in fetal TSH may result in goiter formation. When treatment is closely monitored to avoid excessive dosing, there does not appear to be any impairment of intellectual function in these children. Approximately 1% to 5% of children exposed to PTU develop transient hypothyroidism; usually sufficient maternal thyroid hormone crosses the placenta to prevent fetal goiter. Furthermore, because fetal loss is markedly reduced by treatment of maternal hyperthyroidism, and the long-term risks to offspring exposed in utero to propylthiouracil are minimal, these drugs should be the first line of treatment of thyrotoxicosis. In any case, if a mother desires to breast feed, it is recommended that close monitoring of neonatal thyroid function be performed.

## SEVERE HYPERTHYROIDISM

Although reports of intrauterine growth retardation, small placental size, and neonatal bradycardia, hypoglycemia, and respiratory depression have been associated with maternal beta-blocker ingestion, other investigators have reported successful outcomes. The recommended oral dose of propranolol is 40 mg every 6 hours.

Iodide treatment may also be instituted for not more than 1 week, because iodides readily cross the placenta and impair fetal thyroid function.

## THYROID STORM

This dramatic presentation of hyperthyroidism leads to a clinical picture of fever, dehydration, and cardiac decompensation, and has a mortality rate as high as 25%. An underlying cause should be sought and treated in order to gain control of the hyperthyroid state. Often, an infection or surgery may be the precipitating event, especially in a previously undiagnosed individual. Prompt treatment with intravenous fluids (losses may be as high as 5 L), oxygen, antipyretics, and antithyroid drugs are necessary. Propylthiouracil 400 mg orally every 8 hours or methimazole 30 to 40 mg via rectal suppository every 8 hours should be initiated. PTU is preferred because of its peripheral inhibition of T4 conversion to T3, an effect that is not mediated by methimazole. Sodium iodide 1 g intravenously in 500 mL of fluid may be administered once every 24 hours during the critical disease phase. This will sufficiently block thyroid hormone secretion. Lithium 300 mg orally every 8 hours will also block thyroid hormone secretion. Propranolol 40 mg orally every 6 hours should be administered, unless cardiac failure is present. Intravenous administration of small doses of 1 to 2 mg may be used if necessary, but should be done only with cardiac monitoring. Dexamethasone 2 mg orally or intramuscularly every 6 hours will block peripheral conversion of T4 to T3.

## SURGERY

When surgery is deemed necessary, it seems reasonable to continue thionamides until surgery is performed, if the patient is not experiencing side effects from their use. Further preoperative disease control may be attained by the use of propranolol 40 mg orally every 6 hours and Lugol's solution (iodide) 3 to 5 drops twice daily for a maximum of 1 week. Although the risk of spontaneous abortion is greatest during the first trimester, it is reasonable to perform surgery during the first trimester when absolutely necessary. However, the usual complications of thyroid surgery still exist during pregnancy. These include rarely a postoperative life-threatening hematoma, and an approximate 1% risk of recurrent laryngeal nerve damage or hypoparathyroidism.

## RADIOACTIVE IODINE

Although radioactive iodine ($^{131}$I) ablation of the thyroid is a therapeutic option in treatment of hyperthyroidism in the nonpregnant state, it is never considered justifiable to use radioactive isotopes of iodine for either diagnostic or therapeutic use during pregnancy.

### Fetal and Neonatal Thyrotoxicosis

**Etiology.** Transplacental passage of thyroid-stimulating immunoglobulins (TSI) in mothers with either active or apparently inactive Graves' disease may rarely result in fetal thyrotoxicosis. Neonatal thyrotoxicosis also results from maternal TSIs, but usually in the setting of maternal PTU ingestion. When the PTU is withdrawn at birth, the neonate remains under the influence of the abnormal circulating TSIs. Although the half-life of these abnormal stimulating antibodies is 4 to 10 days, disease activity may continue up to 2 to 3 months. The incidence of neonatal thyrotoxicosis is approximately 1% of all pregnant patients with Graves' disease.

**Symptoms and Signs.** Fetal tachycardia (>160 beats per minute) and IUGR are typical manifestations of intrauterine thyrotoxicosis. Neonatal thyrotoxicosis may be evident at birth with jaundice, tremulousness, diarrhea, tachycardia (>200 beats per minute), cardiac failure, hepatosplenomegaly, goiter, and eye signs of Graves' disease. However, when maternal PTU treatment has been used, the neonate may not demonstrate clinical signs of thyrotoxicosis until 2 to 14 days after birth. Both males and females are affected equally with this disorder, in contrast to the striking female predominance of adult Graves' disease.

**Diagnosis.** The diagnosis of fetal thyrotoxicosis must be made based on strong clinical suspicion in the presence of maternal Graves' disease.

**Course.** The mortality of this disease is high, approaching 15% to 25% in spite of treatment. For those infants who survive, the disease is usually transient, lasting up to 2 to 3 months. Neonatal thyrotoxicosis may result in long-term complications, such as craniosynostosis and minimal brain dysfunction.

**Treatment.** PTU in doses of 50 to 100 mg orally daily administered to the mother may ameliorate fetal thyrotoxicosis. The dose may be adjusted based on the fetal heart rate. Neonatal thyrotoxicosis should be treated with Lugol's iodide 1 drop orally every 8 hours (1 mg every 8 hours) and propranolol 2 mg/kg orally daily in divided doses if the disease severity is such that intervention is required. Additional measures include PTU 5 to 10 mg/kg per day in divided doses and digitalis if heart failure is present.

### Disordered Hyper- and Hyposecretion—Postpartum Thyroiditis

Postpartum autoimmune thyroiditis is a disorder known to occur in approximately 5.5% of women. It may present initially with symptoms of hyperthyroidism occurring 3 to 6 months after delivery and lasting typically 1 to 3 months. The subsequent hypothyroid phase is also transient, lasting usually up to 3 months as well. Patients may have a history of painless goiter prior to pregnancy, unassociated with the systemic symptoms typically accompanying subacute (de Quervain's) thyroiditis. The underlying disease is thought to be autoimmune in nature, with lymphocytic thyroid infiltration and high titers of thyroid autoantibodies. The diagnosis may be established by finding an elevated serum thyroxine level in the presence of a low thyroid radioiodine uptake (1% to 2% or less at 24 hours), which contrasts with the elevated uptake seen with Graves' disease (>30%). Spontaneous recovery occurs 90% of the time, although the disease tends to recur in future pregnancies.

### Thyroid Cancer

The occurrence of thyroid cancer in 15% to 20% of single thyroid nodules means that investigation and treatment of all such nodules is warranted during pregnancy. In any event, a fine needle aspiration biopsy of the nodule is necessary, and if cytologic diagnosis of malignancy is made, surgical resection is recommended. A benign lesion should be suppressed with L-thyroxine 0.15 mg orally daily for the remainder of pregnancy. Thyroid scanning should not be performed during pregnancy.

There is no evidence that pregnancy alters the natural course of thyroid carcinoma, and women previously treated for this disease may become pregnant without apparent sequelae.

## ADRENAL GLAND

Adrenal glucocorticoids are essential for survival, and disordered production has profound effects on the mother or her fetus. Maternal disease is most commonly found at the hypothalamic-pituitary level (ACTH), whereas fetal and neonatal disruption usually involves impaired adrenal steroidogenesis. Fortunately, adrenal diseases are not common during pregnancy, and when they do occur a high index of suspicion is necessary. Laboratory investigations are complicated by the normal rise of both ACTH and free cortisol known to occur in pregnancy.

## PHYSIOLOGIC ADAPTATIONS TO PREGNANCY

### Glucocorticoids
A rise of both total (bound) and free (unbound) cortisol occurs during normal pregnancy. The cortisol-binding globulin (CBG) level rises steadily to reach levels that stabilize at approximately twice the upper limit of normal by the end of the second trimester (Figs. 38-2 and 38-3).

### Mineralocorticoids
The renin-angiotensin-aldosterone axis is activated during pregnancy, and levels of all three hormones increase from early gestation. Renin levels peak at approximately the end of the first trimester, reaching levels twice that of the nonpregnant state.

### Sex Steroids
Pregnancy is associated with a rise in sex hormone-binding globulin, secondary to the elevated estrogen concentrations.

## LABORATORY INVESTIGATIONS

### Basal Hormone Determination (Glucocorticoids)
When glucocorticoid excess is suspected clinically, simple determination of plasma electrolytes and glucose should be performed. Although 24-hour urinary free

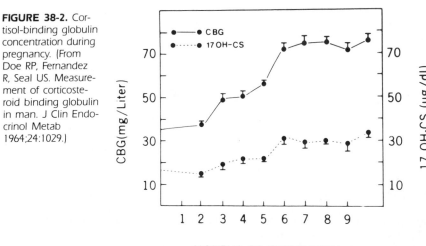

**FIGURE 38-2.** Cortisol-binding globulin concentration during pregnancy. (From Doe RP, Fernandez R, Seal US. Measurement of corticosteroid binding globulin in man. J Clin Endocrinol Metab 1964;24:1029.)

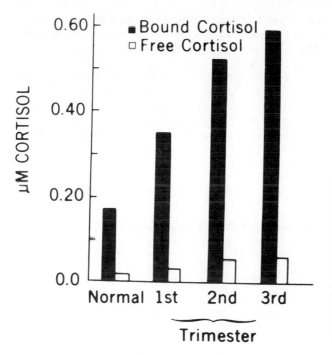

**FIGURE 38-3.** Free and bound cortisol concentrations during pregnancy. (From Rosenthal HE, Slaunwhite WR, Sandberg AA. Transcortin: a corticosteroid-binding protein of plasma. X: cortisol and progesterone interplay and unbound levels of these steroids in pregnancy. J Clin Endocrinol Metab 1969;29:352.)

cortisol is elevated in normal pregnancy, levels higher than 225 µg are more often associated with Cushing's syndrome.

## PLACENTAL-FETAL ADRENAL PHYSIOLOGY

The fetal adrenal plays an important role in maintenance of the necessary placental steroid hormone (estrogen) production.

In addition to its role in placental estrogen biosynthesis, the fetal adrenal independently functions under the influence of pituitary ACTH.

## DISORDERS OF HYPERSECRETION

### Maternal Cushing's Syndrome

The occurrence of glucocorticoid excess during pregnancy is rare and, when present, is associated with adverse fetal effects. The accompanying hyperglycemia and hypertension further increase the obstetrical risk of these patients. Two-thirds of cases are caused by pituitary ACTH secretion in excess of normal (Cushing's disease), which results in bilateral adrenal hyperplasia. Approximately one-third are due to either adrenal or ectopic causes.

**Symptoms and Signs.** Centripedal weight gain with a buffalo hump, moon facies and supraclavicular fat pads, thin fragile easy-bruising skin, purple striae, and hirsutism or acne may all manifest in the presence of glucocorticoid excess. The presence of virilizing signs such as male pattern hair loss, voice changes, and clitoromegaly should alert one to the possibility of an underlying adrenal tumor.

Complaints of muscle weakness and easy fatiguability may be inadvertently dismissed as features expected during normal pregnancy. Indeed, many of the clinical signs may be masked by the pregnant state.

**Diagnosis.** The diagnosis of Cushing's syndrome rests on demonstration of elevated plasma or urinary cortisol that fails to suppress after exogenous dexamethasone (see Table 38-2). Typically, pituitary sources of ACTH excess (Cushing's disease) fail to suppress after the overnight or low-dose dexamethasone suppression tests, but do suppress after high-dose dexamethasone administration.

**Course and Treatment.** If the results of dexamethasone testing indicate that a pituitary source of excess ACTH is likely, then transphenoidal resection is recommended, and results in successful treatment 85% to 95% of the time.

**TABLE 38-2.** Laboratory Investigations and Tests of Glucocorticoid Reserve to Diagnose Adrenal Cortical Failure

| Test | Comment |
|---|---|
| I. Basal Hormone Determination (Glucocorticoids) | |
|    A. Plasma electrolytes | Hyponatremia |
| | Hyperkalemia |
| | Acidosis associated with deficiency |
|    B. Glucose level | Hypoglycemia |
|    C. 24-hr urinary free cortisol | >225 mg associated with Cushing's Syndrome |
| II. Dynamic Tests (Glucocorticoids) | |
|    A. Dexamethasone Suppression Test | Levels associated with hormone excess |
|      Step 1. 1 mg at 11 p.m. | >5 μg/dL |
|      Step 2. Fail to suppress—0.5 mg dexamethasone orally every 6 hrs for 48 hrs | Urinary free cortisol >25 μg/day Urinary free cortisol (UFC) |
|      Step 3. Fail to suppress—2 mg orally every 6 hrs for 48 hrs | >50% suppression of UFC Adrenal or ectopic source of glucocorticoid excess is likely |
|      High-Dose Dexamethasone Suppression Test 8 mg oral dexamethasone at 11 p.m. | |
|      Plasma cortisol determination the following morning at 8 a.m. | 50% decline of plasma cortisol in adrenal or ectopic source |
|    B. ACTH Stimulation Test | |
|      1. Rapid test | Cortisol increases by 23 ± 3.3 mg/dl second trimester, 26 ± 5.5 third trimester |
|      2. Long test | No comparative testing available in pregnancy |
|    C. Basal Hormone Determination (mineralocorticoids) | Minimal value in pregnancy |
|    D. Dynamic Hormonal Evaluation (mineralocorticoids) | |
|      Volume expansion with oral or IV NaCl | Should inhibit renin production |
|    E. Basal Hormone Determination (catecholamines) | |
|      1. Plasma catecholamines | |
|      2. 24-hour urine VMA & metanephrines | |
|      3. Dynamic testing with clonidine suppression | Not recommended in pregnancy |

## Pheochromocytoma

This tumor usually occurs in the adrenal medulla (10% extraadrenal) and secretes the catecholamines norepinephrine and epinephrine. The resultant clinical picture of sporadic hypertension, palpitations, flushing, and sweating attacks may easily be dismissed as anxiety attacks. Diagnostic elevations of urinary catecholamines and their metabolites (see Table 38-2) occur, and subsequent treatment recommended is surgical if diagnosed before 24 weeks gestation. For women diagnosed after 24 weeks gestation, the treatment of choice is alpha-blockage alone until the fetus is sufficiently mature to be delivered by cesarean section. At this time, tumor removal should also be performed. Barbiturate anesthesia is preferred over other forms of general or local anesthesia. Both maternal (11%) and fetal (46%) mortality are high in this disorder, even when diagnosed during pregnancy. Indeed, maternal mortality reaches extraordinary rates of 55% when diagnosis is not made until the postpartum period.

## DISORDERS OF HYPOSECRETION

### Maternal Adrenal Insufficiency

Adrenal cortical insufficiency may be either primary, resulting from failure of the adrenal tissue itself, or secondary to loss of pituitary ACTH stimulation.

**Symptoms and Signs.** The rather vague and nonspecific complaints that accompany diminished adrenal glucocorticoid and mineralocorticoid secretion may easily go undetected. These include prominent anorexia, nausea, vomiting, and weight loss. Similar complaints occur during pregnancy and may be misdiagnosed as hyperemesis gravidarum. Other features include generalized weakness, postural hypotension, skin hyperpigmentation (especially in recent scars or pressure points), and areas of vitiligo.

**Diagnosis.** A definitive diagnosis rests on the demonstration of impaired glucocorticoid production in response to exogenous ACTH (see Table 38-2). The serum electrolytes show hyponatremia and hyperkalemic acidosis, with a tendency to hypoglycemia.

**Treatment.** Once diagnosed, immediate replacement with glucocorticoids (cortisone acetate 25 mg orally in the morning and 12.5 mg in the evening) and mineralocorticoids (0.05 to 0.10 mg 9-alpha-fluro-hydrocortisone daily) is necessary. If a patient with well-controlled Addison's disease is in labor or having a cesarean section, then an additional 100 mg cortisol may be infused over several hours.

**Course.** Patients with pregnancy and Addison's disease in whom treatment is begun before pregnancy have no apparent ill effects. If a pregnant patient with undiagnosed Addison's disease manages to complete a pregnancy successfully, then the neonate appears to suffer no serious effects either. However, a significant risk of maternal postpartum adrenal crisis exists in this setting. Furthermore, although maternal autoantibodies do cross the placenta, there does not appear to be any subsequent fetal or neonatal adrenal destruction. Finally, although a small proportion of maternal steroids do cross the placenta and could theoretically suppress fetal adrenal function, it is rarely necessary to administer glucocorticoids to the newborn.

## DISORDERED FETAL ADRENAL STEROIDOGENESIS

### Congenital Adrenal Hyperplasia

The congenital adrenal hyperplasias result from inherited defects in enzymes required in the biosynthetic pathways of steroid hormones of all three groups (gluco- and mineralocorticoids and sex steroids).

**Symptoms and Signs.** Over 90% of patients with congenital adrenal hyperplasia have defective 21-hydroxylase, which may present as severe salt-wasting, simple virilizing, attenuated, or cryptic disease. Severe salt-wasting disease is manifest at birth with ambiguous genitalia in the female and normal genitalia in the male. Finally, cryptic 21-hydroxylase deficiency refers to entirely asymptomatic individuals who are discovered to have abnormal 17-hydroxyprogesterone responses to ACTH stimulation (accentuated), usually in the course of family investigations. 21-hydroxylase deficiency is inherited as an autosomal recessive disorder, and the severity of the disease is based on allelic variation at the P450 c21 locus.

11-β-hydroxylase deficiency accounts for approximately 5% of cases of congenital adrenal hyperplasia. This defect results in diminished cortisol but elevated levels of deoxycorticosterone (DOC) and adrenal androgens. For this reason, hypertension may be a feature of this disorder, along with masculinization of the female fetus. This condition is also inherited as an autosomal recessive disorder.

**Diagnosis.** Because these disorders (21-hydroxylase and 11-β-hydroxylase deficiencies) may present later in life with menstrual irregularities, hirsutism, and acne, it is possible that a minority of individuals suffering from disturbances of fertility are actually undiagnosed patients.

Prenatal diagnosis of 21-hydroxylase deficiency is possible by HLA typing of amniotic cells in high-risk individuals. Both 17-hydroxyprogesterone and 11-deoxycortisol levels can be determined in amniotic fluid, and elevations suggest the presence of abnormal fetal adrenals.

**Treatment.** Replacement of glucocorticoids with 25 mg orally of cortisone acetate in the morning and 12.5 mg orally in the evening is adequate for maintenance both before and during pregnancy in the mother with CAH. This dose will suppress elevated ACTH levels and thereby diminish the excess adrenal androgen (21-hydroxylase and 11-β-hydroxylase) and DOC (11-β-hydroxylase) production.

**Course.** If maternal disease is adequately treated during pregnancy, then no untoward fetal or maternal effects are anticipated. However, the typically narrow android maternal pelvis often results in poor labor progression and thus cesarean section. Furthermore, hypertension appears commonly during these pregnancies and should be appropriately managed. Spontaneous abortion rates as high as 20% have been reported.

## CALCIUM AND PARATHYROID GLANDS

Calcium homeostasis is critical for normal development of the fetal skeleton, and maternal ingestion should be increased during pregnancy in order to accommodate these elevated demands.

## PHYSIOLOGY IN THE NONPREGNANT STATE

The serum calcium is normally regulated by both parathyroid hormone and vitamin D.

## PHYSIOLOGY IN THE PREGNANT STATE

Total serum calcium falls from the second or third month of gestation, along with declining levels of albumin (Fig. 38-4).

## LABORATORY INVESTIGATIONS

Evaluation of the serum calcium level must be done in conjunction with serum albumin, the major binding protein.

## FETAL PHYSIOLOGY

The fetus remains in positive calcium balance through gestation, and in doing so receives its calcium from the mother. At birth, a sudden withdrawal from maternal calcium sources occurs, and thus neonatal levels decline for the first 1 to 2 days of life. Thereafter, the neonatal parathyroids increase PTH production and calcium levels stabilize.

## DISORDERS OF HYPERSECRETION

### Maternal Hyperparathyroidism

Hyperparathyroidism may be quite insidious in its presentation, with such nonspecific complaints as fatigue, polyuria, and bone pain. It is usually caused by a

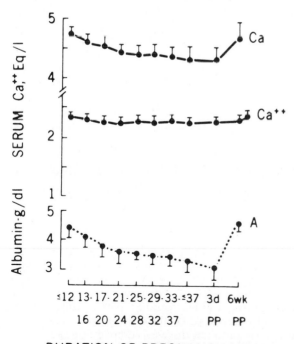

**FIGURE 38-4.** Serum calcium, ionized calcium, and albumin concentrations during pregnancy. (From Pitkin RM, Reynolds WA, Williams GA, Hargis GK. Calcium metabolism in normal pregnancy: a longitudinal study. Am J Obstet Gynecol 1979;133:781.)

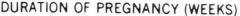

DURATION OF PREGNANCY (WEEKS)

single adenoma, but adenomatous hyperplasia of all four glands may also occur, especially in familial syndromes. Pregnancy may exacerbate preexisting hyperparathyroidism, and when this does occur, spontaneous abortion and late fetal deaths occur much more commonly than normal.

**Diagnosis.** The diagnosis is confirmed by finding elevated serum calcium levels (free), low serum phosphorous levels, and inappropriately normal (nonsuppressed) or high levels of parathyroid hormone.

**Treatment.** The preferred treatment is surgical removal of the adenomatous parathyroid tissue; successful results are often obtained.

**Fetal Effects.** A high percentage of neonates born to women with hyperparathyroidism experience subnormal calcium levels after birth. This is likely due to the prolonged exposure to elevated levels of maternal calcium in utero, and thus suppression of the fetal parathyroid gland. The effects are transient and often appear from 1 to 2 weeks of life.

## DISORDERS OF HYPOSECRETION

### Maternal Hypoparathyroidism

Hypoparathyroidism usually results from inadvertent removal at the time of thyroid surgery.

**Symptoms and Signs.** Most symptoms are related to the subnormal serum calcium that occurs in this condition, and include paresthesias, numbness and tingling, muscle cramps, and even tetany.

**Diagnosis and Treatment.** The diagnosis of hypoparathyroidism is made by demonstration of a subnormal serum calcium level with a low PTH serum determination.

Pregnancy is associated with increasing fetal calcium demands with advancing gestation, and therefore it is not surprising that dosages of calcium and vitamin D may need to be increased over time. If hypoparathyroidism is poorly controlled during pregnancy, then the fetus suffers from hypocalcemia and skeletal undermineralization.

---

# 39.  GASTROINTESTINAL DISEASES COMPLICATING PREGNANCY

---

Pregnancy can complicate almost any gastrointestinal disease. The pregnant woman may enter pregnancy with a gastrointestinal disorder, or it may develop during the pregnancy. The physiologic effects of pregnancy may cause gastrointestinal disturbances such as nausea, vomiting, hyperemesis gravidarum, and esophageal reflux. Conversely, gastrointestinal disorders such as ruptured appendix and inflammatory bowel disease may affect the course of pregnancy. This chapter discusses the various gastrointestinal diseases complicating pregnancy and their effect on the fetus and its mother.

# DISEASES WITHIN THE GASTROINTESTINAL TRACT

## NAUSEA, VOMITING, AND HYPEREMESIS GRAVIDARUM

Nausea with or without vomiting is an especially common symptom during early pregnancy. It usually occurs during the first trimester of pregnancy, and by midpregnancy most women no longer complain of these symptoms. The incidence has not been well studied, but it occurs in approximately 60% to 80% of pregnancies in the United States. In its mildest form, it is referred to as "morning sickness."

The cause of nausea and vomiting during pregnancy is unknown. The smooth muscle of the stomach does relax during pregnancy, and this physiologic change may play some role.

The management of nausea and vomiting during pregnancy is primarily supportive. Therapeutic regimens include reassurance, physical and psychological support, frequent small meals, the avoidance of foods that are unpleasant or that may initiate symptoms, adequate hydration and fluid intake, and selective, occasional use of antiemetics. There is no ideal antiemetic currently available for the treatment of morning sickness. When symptoms require treatment, both pyridoxine and doxylamine are still available over the counter as Unisom (25 mg). Antiemetic therapy should be used when supportive measures are not effective. Other antiemetics that have also been used successfully in the treatment of nausea and vomiting of pregnancy include the phenothiazines, trimethobenzamide, metoclopramide, and diphenhydramine.

Hyperemesis gravidarum is the abnormal condition of pregnancy associated with pernicious nausea and vomiting. Hyperemesis is both infrequent and uncommon. These patients experience persistent intractable nausea and vomiting associated with weight loss, fluid and electrolyte imbalance, ketonuria, and ketonemia. Electrolyte imbalance may include decreased sodium, potassium, and chloride, and metabolic alkalosis. The patient usually becomes clinically dehydrated and may even develop jaundice, hyperpyrexia, and peripheral neuritis. Recurrent hyperemesis gravidarum has caused recurrent first trimester jaundice. Outpatient therapy consisting of intravenous fluid hydration is usually sufficient, along with supportive therapy. Intravenous pyridoxine 100 mg/L of intravenous fluid has also been included as a part of the intravenous therapy. However, when the patient's condition does not improve, hospitalization with appropriate electrolyte, caloric, and fluid management is necessary.

## ORAL CAVITY COMPLICATIONS OF PREGNANCY

Pregnancy does not increase the amount of oral calculus present on the teeth. However, when oral hygiene is poor, calculus may lead to mild, moderate, or severe gingivitis and other periodontal disease.

Bleeding from the gingivae, a common complaint of pregnant women, due to pregnancy gingivitis, requires no treatment. Gingivitis that is due to poor dentition and hygiene is treated by a good cleaning of the teeth and by meticulous dental care. There is no basis for delaying dental care during pregnancy, and patients who require treatment should obtain it promptly. Pregnancy tumor is a granuloma that forms as a result of exaggerated gingival enlargement during pregnancy. It appears as a localized enlargement of the hyperplastic gingivae or pedunculated growth. Pregnancy tumors are pyogenic granulomas because they result from nonspecific inflammatory gingivitis secondary to poor oral hygiene, associated with deposits of plaque and calculus on the teeth. The tumors are typically pedunculated, lobulated, red due to their vascularity, and soft with a smooth surface. The lesion is painless and is first noticed by the patient as a mass, unless it is so large that it interferes with mastication. Consultation with a dentist is indicated. Biopsy is not usually necessary. Histology on the surgically removed tumor is always benign. The treatment for pregnancy tumor is complete surgical excision.

The treatment of dental problems associated with pregnancy is rarely contraindicated and, when several guidelines are used, may be performed safely. If the treatment is necessary but elective, it is best delayed until the second trimester, when there is the least risk for teratogenesis. Emergency treatment should be obtained whenever indicated. There is little or no harm to the fetus when dental radiographs are taken with the necessary precautions, good techniques, and modern equipment.

## REFLUX ESOPHAGITIS

Heartburn or pyrosis is really a symptom of reflux esophagitis. Reflux esophagitis is the pathophysiologic process in the esophagus that causes the symptom of heartburn. Heartburn is a very common, bothersome complaint during pregnancy and occurs in as many as 70% of pregnant patients. A quarter of pregnant patients experience some degree of heartburn daily. The symptoms of heartburn include burning and substernal discomfort radiating to the back of the neck. Heartburn usually is more severe after meals and is aggravated by recumbent positions. The pain is not limited to being substernal in nature, but may also be epigastric, between the shoulders, or, rarely, generalized chest pain. Usually, the symptoms of reflux esophagitis occur in the last trimester, but they can occur at any time during pregnancy. They subside after 36 weeks of gestation and improve, as expected, postpartum with the decrease in the size of the uterus.

Treatment of reflux esophagitis during pregnancy consists primarily of neutralizing the acid material that is being refluxed into the esophagus, thereby decreasing gastroesophageal reflux. Symptomatic strategies include dietary modification. Foods and drinks such as chocolate, caffeine, peppermint, and alcohol may actually decrease the lower esophageal sphincter pressure. Fatty or spicy foods aggravate the symptoms and are to be avoided. The avoidance of recumbency, particularly immediately after eating a meal, is likewise to be avoided. Elevation of the head of the bed while reclining may provide symptomatic relief. A variety of antacids have been prescribed for heartburn. All of these over-the-counter preparations neutralize gastric acid, which is responsible for the symptoms.

Prolonged esophageal reflux can result in complications such as peptic esophageal stricture, hemorrhagic esophagitis, gastrointestinal bleeding, and hemorrhage. Ulceration of the esophageal mucosa can also occur with significant bleeding. The symptoms of reflux esophagitis can be so severe or difficult to treat that esophagoscopy, parenteral hyperalimentation, and parenteral nutrition are necessary. These procedures may be performed safely during pregnancy.

## PEPTIC ULCER DISEASE

The development of peptic ulcer disease during pregnancy is uncommon and rare. Patients who have peptic ulcers before pregnancy frequently experience fewer symptoms during pregnancy and may even become totally asymptomatic. This is the primary reason why complications of ulcer disease, such as perforation, bleeding, and pyloric stenosis, are rare during pregnancy.

The symptoms of peptic ulcer disease are quite similar to those of reflux esophagitis. The diagnosis during pregnancy may therefore be delayed. The most common symptom of peptic ulcer disease is complaints of heartburn or dyspepsia. The patient may experience nausea and vomiting, which is a common complaint of pregnancy. She may also have anorexia, bloating, or epigastric pain and discomfort. Patients with duodenal ulcer disease more frequently have epigastric pain than those with gastric ulcers. There are no typical physical findings. Peptic ulcer disease is diagnosed by the visualization of the ulcer by radiography or endoscopy. Although the upper gastrointestinal series is frequently used to diagnose peptic ulcer disease in a nonpregnant patient, esophagoscopy when necessary should be used in the pregnant patient. This is usually not necessary except in the patient who has symptoms that do not respond to antacids.

The treatment of peptic ulcer disease consists primarily of the use of antacids, which are safe to use during pregnancy. A combination of magnesium trisilicate and aluminum hydroxide is found in most antacid preparations. Sodium bicarbonate should not be used as an antacid during pregnancy, because it can lead to the absorption of large amounts of sodium. Patients with peptic ulcer disease should avoid a diet of foods that cause their discomfort. Smoking, which should be avoided in both the pregnant and nonpregnant woman, and alcohol should certainly be eliminated from the diets of these patients. Aspirin and the nonsteroidal anti-inflammatory drugs such as indomethacin can produce gastric irritation and, with prolonged use, gastric ulcers.

Cimetidine is an $H_2$-receptor antagonist. There are several concerns about the use of cimetidine during pregnancy. It is an antiandrogen and has produced gynecomastia and impotence in a small number of male animals and male users. Cimetidine does cross the placenta.

Ranitidine is another $H_2$-receptor antagonist that has been used for ulcer therapy. It possesses no antiandrogen activity, but its use during pregnancy has been limited.

## ACUTE INTESTINAL OBSTRUCTION

Intestinal obstruction is a serious complication of pregnancy that is occurring with increasing frequency. The incidence is approximately 1 in 2500 to 1 in 3500 pregnancies. Acute intestinal obstruction is most common in the third trimester, less common in the second, and least likely in the first trimester.

The most common cause for intestinal obstruction in the pregnant and nonpregnant woman is adhesions. Intussusception and hernias are less common causes for intestinal obstruction during pregnancy. Adhesions may also form as the result of pelvic inflammatory disease or may rarely be congenital in origin.

The diagnosis of intestinal obstruction in pregnancy is not easy. As with appendicitis, delay in diagnosis is not uncommon. Pain, although usually present, may be constant, colicky, mild, severe, diffuse, or localized. Physical examination may or may not reveal guarding or rebound tenderness. Abdominal distention can easily be missed in late pregnancy because of the normally large uterus and abdomen. When present, it usually indicates large bowel rather than small bowel obstruction. Bowel sounds may be normal, absent, or high-pitched with rushes. Physical examination, however, can be completely nondiagnostic. The white count is usually not helpful because it is elevated normally in pregnancy. If there is considerable delay in diagnosis and the patient is not appropriately treated, then third spacing of fluids occurs. This results in dehydration, electrolyte imbalance, hypotension, oliguria, fever, tachycardia, and eventually shock and death.

Diagnosis, once expected clinically, can be made by radiographic studies showing bowel distention, intraluminal fluid levels, and decreased gas in the large bowel. The concern of obtaining radiographic studies during pregnancy should be tempered by the increased maternal and fetal mortality associated with delayed or misdiagnosis. X-ray or serial studies showing dilated, gas-filled loops of bowel with air-fluid levels is diagnostic.

Treatment of intestinal obstruction during pregnancy is the same as in the nonpregnant patient. Exploratory laparotomy is the treatment of choice. Prior to surgery, close attention must be paid to correction of fluid and electrolyte imbalance, maintenance of adequate urinary output, administration of blood and blood products, and fetal monitoring. Antibiotics may be indicated.

## INFLAMMATORY BOWEL DISEASE

The term *inflammatory bowel disease* refers to a group of idiopathic chronic inflammatory diseases of the intestinal tract. The two most commonly seen during pregnancy are ulcerative colitis and Crohn's disease, also called regional enteritis. Both of these disorders are not uncommon in women during their reproductive years and are frequently seen either before or during pregnancy.

The pathologic features of these two diseases distinguish and differentiate them. Ulcerative colitis is an inflammatory ulcerative pathologic process primarily of the mucosal lining of the left colon or rectum. It is characteristically not transmural. Crohn's disease is an inflammatory disease that may involve any area of the gastrointestinal tract, but the distal small intestine, colon, and anal rectal regions are most often affected. The pathologic process is transmural; that is, the granulomatous enteritis involves all layers of the bowel, mesentery, and lymph nodes.

These two disorders share a common cause, clinical findings, and management. Ulcerative colitis and Crohn's disease may be so similar clinically that a specific diagnosis of the type of inflammatory disease present cannot be made. They can be characterized as chronic disorders that go through periods of quiescence and exacerbation, making differentiation even more difficult. Ulcerative colitis primarily affects females, whereas both sexes are equally affected with Crohn's disease.

The best prognosis for pregnancy is in those patients who had inactive ulcerative colitis at the time of conception or whose active disease is limited to early pregnancy. Patients with inactive ulcerative colitis that becomes active during early pregnancy do not have an increased risk of spontaneous abortion; and patients who develop active disease later in pregnancy or postpartum are at increased risk for spontaneous abortion, stillbirth, and preterm labor. The effect of Crohn's disease on pregnancy is similar. Adverse pregnancy outcome, as reflected by prematurity, stillbirths, spontaneous abortion, or congenital anomalies, does not appear to be increased.

The route of delivery may be affected by inflammatory bowel disease. Cesarean section has been recommended if severe perineal fistulas or perineal scarring, which can occur as a complication of Crohn's disease, is present. Patients who have recently had a proctocolectomy performed to promote healing of perineal disease should also be delivered by cesarean section. Cesarean section is not indicated in patients who have had successful restorative surgery for inflammatory bowel disease.

Inflammatory bowel disease is treated by both medical and surgical measures during pregnancy. In general, the treatment is the same as in the nonpregnant patient.

Sulfasalazine is the most commonly used drug in the treatment of inflammatory bowel disease. It is a combination of sulfonamide, sulfapyridine, and 5-aminosalicylic acid. Several studies have shown that sulfasalazine can be safely used both during pregnancy and while the mother is breast-feeding. The drug should be started as soon as possible after delivery to prevent the possibility of a postpartum exacerbation. Although there is the theoretic possibility that sulfasalazine could bind to fetal albumin with the displacement of bilirubin and the development of hyperbilirubinemia, this does not appear to be a real clinical risk.

Corticosteroid therapy has been used in both of these diseases to suppress the inflammatory response present in the bowel. It is frequently used also in treating exacerbations of Crohn's disease. Doses of prednisone range from 40 to 60 mg daily for a period of several weeks to a month. Some pregnant patients who have been unable to be weaned from corticosteroids may enter pregnancy on a low dose. The continuation of their medication or even the institution of corticosteroid therapy during pregnancy is not contraindicated. The mother may experience the usual side effects of steroid therapy, but there are no proven adverse effects on the fetus from the use of steroids during pregnancy. Breast-feeding likewise is not contraindicated in the mother on corticosteroid therapy.

Medical management should include nutritional assessment and treatment, as in any patient with a chronic disease. Adequate calories should be provided to help in the prevention of weight loss. Parenteral nutrition, sometimes required in the management of some of the other gastrointestinal complications of pregnancy, is infrequently needed in these patients. If medically necessary to provide adequate caloric intake, total parenteral nutrition may be safely used during pregnancy. General therapeutic measures used include antidiarrheal drugs such as codeine, opium, paregoric, and diphenoxylate with atropine (Lomotil). As in the treatment of hyperemesis gravidarum, the patient should have the opportunity to discuss the psychological factors of pregnancy or other aspects of her life, which may be playing a part in the precipitation of inflammatory bowel disease.

Inflammatory bowel disease may require surgical treatment. The procedure most frequently used in the treatment of ulcerative colitis is total proctocolectomy with construction of an ileostomy. This procedure is curative. Indications for partial or total colectomy and ileostomy include perforation (with or without abscess formation), massive bleeding, and carcinoma of the colon. Patients who develop toxic megacolon and do not respond to other therapy may also be candidates for this surgical therapy. The procedure should not be done during pregnancy, because the surgery would not only be difficult to perform as the pregnant uterus enlarges, but could precipitate preterm labor. Surgical therapy for Crohn's disease or regional enteritis is the same as for ulcerative colitis. Intractability of symptoms is the most frequent indication for surgery. Perianal complications such as fistulas may also lead to total proctocolectomy with ileostomy or some other variance of this surgery.

A recent review of pregnancy and inflammatory bowel disease makes suggestions about the medical management of inflammatory bowel disease during pregnancy, with the following conclusions:

1. Judicious medical therapy is effective in controlling inflammatory bowel disease during pregnancy.
2. Sulfasalazine or steroid therapy should not be withdrawn in a patient who needs it to achieve or maintain a quiescent state of inflammatory bowel disease during the course of pregnancy.
3. Immunosuppressive therapy should be avoided.
4. Aggressive medical therapy with total parenteral nutrition and a team approach with a gastroenterologist, surgeon, and perinatologist usually will avoid the need for surgical intervention during pregnancy, with a good fetal outcome in a patient whose disease is active.
5. Contraception against pregnancy need only be considered in those patients whose disease is so severe that operative therapy is imminent.

## APPENDICITIS

Appendicitis remains the most common cause of an acute abdomen during pregnancy. The incidence during pregnancy has been reported to vary from 1 per 1000 to 1 per 2000 pregnancies, with an average incidence of 1 per 1500 deliveries. There appears to be no increased frequency during any particular trimester. Appendicitis occurring postpartum is particularly difficult to diagnose, because peritonitis is a less prominent finding.

The pregnant woman with appendicitis has symptoms and signs similar to those in the nonpregnant patient, but may not experience abdominal rigidity, rebound, or similar signs of peritonitis. Abdominal pain is present, but usually not at McBurney's point. This is due to the change in the position and direction of the appendix during pregnancy. As pregnancy advances, the cecum is displaced toward the iliac crest, thus moving the appendix laterally, superiorly, and posteriorly (Fig. 39-1). The abdominal pain of appendicitis typically is mild at its onset. During pregnancy it is even less severe. It may be intermittent or colicky, due to a fecalith within the appendix. The pain is followed within an hour or two by anorexia, nausea, and vomiting, symptoms frequently seen during a normal pregnancy. The temperature may be normal or there may be a low-grade fever. An increasing left shift may be helpful in making the diagnosis. The urinalysis is usually not helpful other than in excluding the diagnosis of urinary tract infection.

Appendectomy is the treatment of choice for appendicitis during pregnancy (Fig. 39-2). Surgeons suggest the use of a transverse muscle-splitting incision

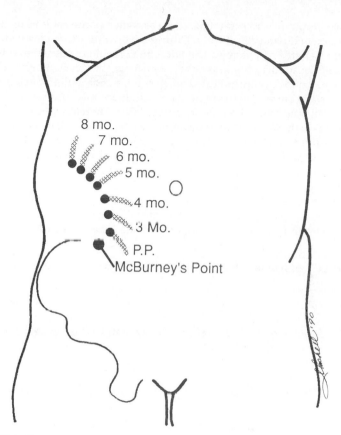

8 mo.
7 mo.
6 mo.
5 mo.
4 mo.
3 Mo.
P.P.
McBurney's Point

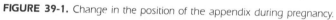

**FIGURE 39-1.** Change in the position of the appendix during pregnancy.

**FIGURE 39-2.**
Transverse ultrasound scan 12 days postappendectomy demonstrating embryo (E) at 6 weeks and showing echogenic fluid in the retrouterine cul-de-sac suspicious for abscess (A) in a patient with persistent postoperative fevers. The abscess resolved with intravenous antibiotic therapy. (Courtesy of Dr. Joseph C. Anderson.)

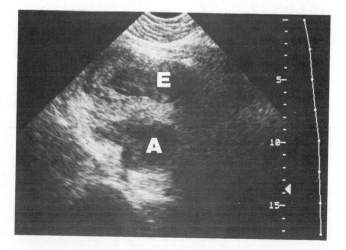

directly over the point of maximum tenderness. When necessary, this incision can be extended without much difficulty. During the operation, the uterus should be manipulated as little as possible. The left lateral position with uterine displacement should be used to minimize the chance for the development of supine hypotension. Antibiotics are indicated when the appendix is perforated or there is extensive inflammation. There are no data to indicate that tocolysis reduces the incidence of uterine contractions or premature labor. Therefore, the routine usage of such agents in these circumstances cannot be supported. When the diagnosis is made in the third trimester, there are few, if any, indications for a simultaneous cesarean delivery, except in the presence of obstetrical indications. Vaginal delivery is not precluded, with minilaparotomy and appendectomy immediately postpartum.

The complication rate with rupture of the appendix can be very high, including fetal loss and maternal morbidity. When the diagnosis is made promptly and procrastination in treatment does not occur, fetal loss is lowered.

## PREGNANCY FOLLOWING OPERATION FOR MORBID OBESITY

Most pregnant women with a jejunoileal bypass tolerate pregnancy quite well. It has been recommended that they receive supplemental iron, folic acid, vitamin $B_{12}$, and a prenatal vitamin-mineral preparation. An occasional patient appears to do poorly, developing intrauterine growth retardation and metabolic disorders. Pregnancy is not contraindicated after jejunoileal bypass, but a 2-year interval before pregnancy is undertaken has been suggested so the patient will not become pregnant during the highest phase of weight loss and so the weight loss will be allowed to plateau.

## CONSTIPATION

Constipation is a common symptom of pregnancy. Several authors have recently shown that the treatment of constipation during pregnancy should consist mainly of nutrition counseling, increased fluid intake, and dietary modification.

Constipation may result in the development of hemorrhoids. These can usually be treated by topical ointments or sprays, stool softeners, sitz baths, and over-the-counter preparations. When hemorrhoids develop during the puerperium after vigorous pushing, they may become thrombosed. Incision after local anesthesia may be necessary and beneficial.

## DISEASES ADJACENT TO THE GASTROINTESTINAL TRACT

### GALLBLADDER DISEASE

Classically, the female patient with gallbladder disease has been described as "fair, fat, forty, and fertile." Gallbladder disease is uncommon during pregnancy. It may occur as cholelithiasis or acute cholecystitis.

#### Cholelithiasis

Pregnancy predisposes to gallstones. Pregnancy increases the risk of cholesterol gallstones by causing incomplete emptying of the gallbladder, particularly in late pregnancy, leaving a large residual volume due to decreased gallbladder contractility.

Biliary colic, which is due to choledocholithiasis, is a form of chronic cholecystitis where the gallstones become impacted or pass through the biliary tract, and is the most common symptom that gallstones produce during pregnancy. It affects 15% of patients with cholecystolithiasis. The pain is due to the passage of the gallstones from the gallbladder into the cystic duct or the common bile duct. This produces a spasm of the gallbladder or the biliary duct involved. The pain is right upper quadrant and moderate to severe. It may be cramping or steady. The pain may come on abruptly, particularly after eating a fatty meal. It usually does not last more than a few hours. Although biliary colic is most frequently present in the right upper quadrant, it may also be epigastric, colicky, or steady in intensity. Unlike appendicitis, the pain of biliary colic is not altered in location or character. The patient may also experience nausea, vomiting, and, if cholangitis is present, fever. Jaundice may be present, although gallstones account for only 5% of the causes for jaundice during pregnancy. Depending on where the stone becomes impacted in the biliary tree, obstructive jaundice (common bile duct) or acute pancreatitis (ampulla of Vater) may occur. The symptoms of cholelithiasis may cease spontaneously once the stone is passed through the biliary tract or may persist, requiring surgical removal.

Laboratory diagnosis of gallstones in pregnancy is the same as during nonpregnancy. The leukocyte count and differential may be normal or slightly elevated, depending on the degree of cholangitis. Slight hyperbilirubinemia and slight elevation in the aspartate aminotransferase (AST, formerly SGOT) may be present. The serum alkaline phosphatase is elevated by biliary colic. This is not helpful during pregnancy because elevated serum alkaline phosphatase is normal in the pregnant patient as a result of placental production. The presence of acute pancreatitis as a result of common duct stones may cause pancreatitis and elevated serum amylase.

Real-time ultrasound has revolutionized the diagnosis of biliary tract disease during pregnancy. Several studies have shown ultrasound to be 95% to 98% sensitive in diagnosing both solitary and multiple gallstones in the gallbladder or biliary tract (Figs. 39-3, 39-4, and 39-5). Cholecystectomy is the second most frequent nonobstetrical abdominal surgical procedure performed in pregnancy. Nonoperative therapy consisting of hospitalization, antibiotics, analgesia, non per os, and nasogastric suction may be all that is necessary in patients who have mild illness. Patients with symptoms that do not improve with observation and medical therapy require prompt cholecystectomy. Many authors have demonstrated that a delay in surgery for biliary tract disease complications results in increased maternal and fetal morbidity and mortality. Cholecystectomy during pregnancy should be performed during the second trimester if possible. Several recommendations should be kept in mind when a patient requires cholecystectomy in the second half of pregnancy:

Tocolytic therapy may be necessary and should be instituted if preterm labor occurs.

There are no data to support or condemn the use of prophylactic tocolysis around the time of surgery.

**FIGURE 39-3.** Longitudinal ultrasound scan of solitary stone (GS) in the gallbladder (GB) in asymptomatic patient at 20 weeks gestation. The gallstone is stuck in the neck of the gallbladder and produces acoustic shadowing (S). False positives are uncommon. A small percentage of false negatives occur. (Courtesy of Jolene Snell, RDMS, BS, and Dr. John D. Terry.)

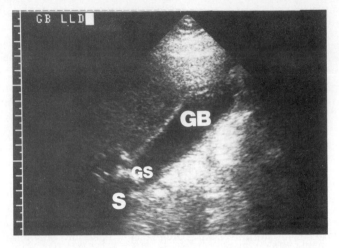

Surgery should be delayed until after delivery if possible if symptoms arise in the third trimester.

Agents to dissolve gallstones such as chenodeoxycholic acid (CDCA) are contraindicated during pregnancy.

## Acute Cholecystitis

The clinical manifestations of acute cholecystitis during pregnancy are the same as in the nonpregnant patient. Conservative medical management is the mainstay in the treatment of the pregnant patient with acute cholecystitis. This consists of nasogastric suction when necessary, analgesia, intravenous hydration, and antibiotics. Intravenous ampicillin or a cephalosporin are the drugs of choice. Most patients will respond to this medical management. Cholecystectomy should be

**FIGURE 39-4.** Longitudinal ultrasound scan of multiple gallstones, some floating in the gallbladder, at 30 weeks gestation in patient with recurrent episodes of biliary colic. A cholecystectomy was performed 7 days postpartum. (Courtesy of Jolene Snell, RDMS, BS.)

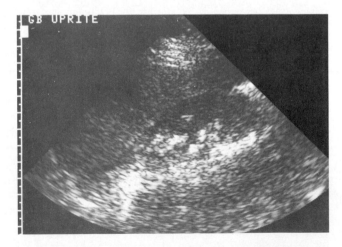

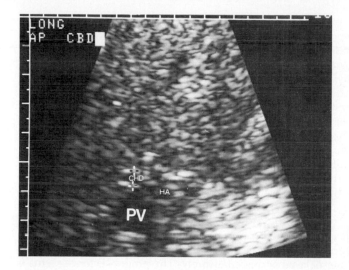

**FIGURE 39-5.**
Transverse ultra-sound scan showing the common hepatic duct (CHD) measuring 5.2 mm (less than 6 mm is normal) in patient with right upper quadrant pain at 20 weeks gestation. A normal portal vein (PV) and hepatic artery proper (HA) are also seen. No stones are visible in any of the biliary ducts. (Courtesy of Susan Crouch and Dr. John D. Terry.)

reserved for those patients who have gallstone pancreatitis, jaundice, repeated attacks, or who fail medical management.

## PANCREATITIS

The exact incidence of acute pancreatitis during pregnancy has been difficult to determine. It is not common and has been reported to occur in 1 per 1000 to 1 per 12,000 pregnancies. Pancreatitis can reoccur during the same or subsequent pregnancy or the puerperium. When pancreatitis develops in women less than age 30 years, half of them are pregnant.

The clinical picture of acute pancreatitis is characteristic. The symptoms and signs include a rapid onset of constant, central midepigastric pain that may radiate to the chest and back, and can be quite severe. In mild cases of pancreatitis, pain may be the only symptom that the patient experiences. Not infrequently, however, nausea and severe vomiting may occur alone or with pain. Low-grade fever and absent or decreased bowel sounds also aid in the diagnosis. The classic clinical presentation of a patient with pancreatitis is an individual rocking in the bed with her knees drawn up and trunk flexed in agony. The pain may also radiate to the flanks or shoulders due to the development of peritoneal irritation. Other symptoms include tachycardia in response to the pain, hypotension, ascites, pleural effusion, hypotonic bowel sounds or ileus, tenderness over the epigastrium, and generalized peritonitis. An adynamic ileus may be demonstrated on radiographic examination. The severity of the clinical features will depend on the severity of the pancreatitis and whether or not complications occur, such as pseudocyst or abscess formation.

Laboratory evaluation of the patient suspected to have pancreatitis may be helpful. Rarely is the white blood cell count above 30,000 cells/mm³. It may even be within the range for normal pregnancy, 10,000 to 20,000 cells/mm³. The serum amylase is the specific test used to diagnose pancreatitis and is usually elevated to at least 100 to 200 units/100 mL. A serum amylase above 1000 units/100 mL almost always is indicative of pancreatitis or an obstruction of the pancreatic duct. Serum amylase has been reported both increased and unchanged in the normal pregnancy.

The amylase/creatinine clearance ratio has been used in making the diagnosis of pancreatitis in pregnancy. As a result of an increased creatinine clearance during pregnancy, the amylase/creatinine clearance ratio is normally decreased.

Diagnostic ultrasound can be used to visualize the pancreas for the presence of infection, pseudocyst, or abscess. When inflamed, the pancreas can appear normal, swollen, or enlarged (Fig. 39-6). At the same time, the gallbladder and biliary ducts can be visualized to rule out the presence of gallstones. The pancreas can also be evaluated during pregnancy by a computed tomography (CT) scan.

Treatment for acute pancreatitis is primarily nonoperative. Management includes intravenous fluid hydration to correct hypovolemia and electrolyte imbalance, correction of hyperglycemia, enteric rest with nasogastric suction, broad-spectrum antibiotics, and adequate analgesia. Insulin may be necessary to reduce the blood sugar.

Maternal mortality is low when diagnosis is made promptly and appropriate management instituted. Pancreatitis is now a rare cause for maternal death unless the diagnosis is either delayed or missed entirely. The prognosis for the fetus is also good unless severe peritonitis occurs, which predisposes the patient to spontaneous abortion or preterm birth. Preterm labor occurs in 60% of patients when pancreatitis develops late in pregnancy. The mode of delivery is not affected by pancreatitis and, unless contraindicated for obstetric reasons, vaginal delivery is recommended.

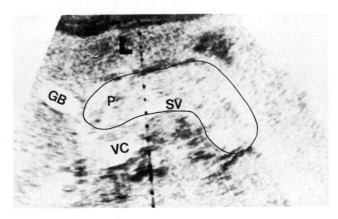

**FIGURE 39–6.** A 31-year-old G6 P4014 with history of alcohol and heroin abuse who at 35 weeks gestation developed severe vomiting, abdominal pain, and distention. Laboratory evaluation: serum amylase, 250; lipase, 290; LDH, 127; SGOT, 55; alkaline phosphatase, 66; WBC, 4400; and increased amylase/creatinine clearance ratio. Transverse ultrasound scan showing a 3.5-cm hypoechoic enlarged (normal is < 2.5 cm) body of the pancreas (P) due to acute pancreatitis. The liver (L) echogenicity is increased due to fatty infiltration of liver from alcoholism. The gallbladder (GB) was normal. The vena cava (VC) and splenic vein (SV) are also seen. A clinical, laboratory, and ultrasonographic diagnosis was made of acute pancreatitis. The patient improved with conservative medical therapy; however, the full-term infant weighed 4 lb, 3 oz and demonstrated the fetal alcohol syndrome. (Courtesy of Dr. Joseph C. Anderson.)

**TABLE 39-1.** Diseases Treated with Inpatient or Outpatient
Total Parenteral Nutrition During Pregnancy

Hyperemesis gravidarum
Reflux esophagitis
Peptic ulcer disease
Intestinal obstruction or failure
Inflammatory bowel disease
Pregnancy following operation for morbid obesity
Gallbladder disease
Pancreatitis
Malignancy
Diabetes mellitus with gastroenteropathy
Cystic fibrosis with marasmus
Anorexia nervosa
Maternal brain damage
End-stage renal disease

## TOTAL PARENTERAL NUTRITION IN PREGNANCY

Pregnant patients unable to consume sufficient nutrients orally require an effective method of feeding. Alternative forms of nutrition are being used more frequently in obstetrics. *Total parenteral nutrition (TPN), parenteral nutrition, hyperalimentation, intravenous hyperalimentation (IVH), and intravenous feedings* are used synonymously and interchangeably to describe the various methods of providing all required nutrients intravenously.

Recently, numerous authors have reported long-term parenteral nutrition being provided with good results to a variety of hospitalized or outpatient pregnant

**TABLE 39-2.** Patients at High Risk for Malnutrition During Pregnancy

1. Pregnancy weight 10% below ideal body weight
2. Adolescents: the younger the patient, the greater the nutritional risk
3. Neuropsychiatric problems
   a. Depression
   b. Dietary faddism
   c. Pica
   d. Eating disorder (anorexia nervosa, bulimia)
4. Prolonged dysfunction of the gastrointestinal tract
   a. Postoperative ileus
   b. Diabetic gastroenteropathy
   c. Inflammatory bowel disease
   d. Infectious gastrointestinal disease
   e. Hyperemesis gravidarum
   f. Cystic fibrosis with marasmus
5. Obstetrical conditions
   a. Rapid reproduction with short intervals between conceptions
   b. Repeated delivery of low-birth-weight infants
6. Low socioeconomic status

Adapted from Lee RV, Rodgers BD, Young C, Eddy E, Cardinal J. Total parenteral nutrition during pregnancy. Obstet Gynecol 1986;68:563, with permission.

**TABLE 39-3.** Pregnant Patients' Major Risk from Parenteral Nutrition

1. Complications of catheter placement
   a. Superficial thrombophlebitis (for PPN)
   b. Pneumothorax
   c. Mediastinal disturbances
   d. Catheter-related infection (for TPN)
   e. Hydrothorax
   f. Cardiac tamponade
2. Metabolic complications
   a. Hyperglycemia
   b. Hypoglycemia
   c. Hypophosphatemia
   d. Electrolyte derangements
3. Hepatocellular abnormalities
   a. Increased SGOT
   b. Increased SGPT
4. Vitamin and trace element deficiency syndromes

Adapted from data from Catanzarite VA, Argubright K, Mann BA, Brittain VL. Malnutrition during pregnancy? Consider parenteral feeding. Contemp Obstet Gynecol 1986;27:110, with permission.

patients at significant risk for malnutrition and poor fetal outcome (Table 39-1). Patients at high risk for malnutrition during pregnancy may also benefit from TPN (Table 39-2).

TPN, whether in the pregnant or nonpregnant patient, can be complicated by maternal death. Other complications include accidental pneumothorax or hemo-

**TABLE 39-4.** Criteria for Selection of Pregnant Patients for Total Parenteral Nutrition

I. Inaccessible or inadequate gastrointestinal nutrition route for any reason.
II. Maternal malnutrition
   A. Weight loss greater than 1 kg/wk for 4 wk consecutively
   B. Total weight loss of 6 kg or failure to gain weight
   C. Underlying chronic disease which increases basal nutritional requirements, including pre-conception malnutrition
   D. Biochemical markers of malnutrition
      1. Severe hypoalbuminemia less than 2.0 g/dL
      2. Persistent ketosis
      3. Hypocholesterolemia
      4. Lymphocytopenia
      5. Macrocytic anemia: diminished folic acid
      6. Microcytic anemia and decreased serum Fe
      7. Negative nitrogen balance
   E. Anthropometric markers of malnutrition
      1. Weight and height
      2. Growth rate
         a. Poor weight gain
         b. Delayed growth of adolescent
      3. Skin fold thickness
      4. Head, chest, waist, and arm circumference
   F. Intrauterine growth retardation of fetus

Adapted from Lee RV, Rodgers BD, Young C, Eddy E, Cardinal J. Total parenteral nutrition during pregnancy. Obstet Gynecol 1986;68:563, with permission.

thorax, catheter infection, various metabolic disorders, glycosuria, hypoglycemia and, rarely, clinical sepsis (Table 39-3).

It has been demonstrated that enteral or parenteral nutrition can be safely and effectively administered during pregnancy. An outline of selection criteria is given in Table 39-4. A team of qualified, knowledgeable individuals who are familiar with the technique being used should explain it to the patient, obtain a written consent, and manage the administration of the parenteral nutrition.

# 40. LIVER DISEASES IN PREGNANCY

## LIVER DISEASES UNIQUE TO PREGNANCY

Several liver diseases occur only in the pregnant woman and are considered to be associated etiologically with the pregnant state. As a rule, the obstetrician is more familiar with these disorders than is the consulting gastroenterologist. The major problem is that of differential diagnosis (Table 40-1).

## HYPEREMESIS GRAVIDARUM

Early-morning nausea is an extremely common symptom of pregnancy, indeed often the first. When the nausea is associated with intractable vomiting leading to dehydration and ketosis, hospitalization is required and the diagnosis of hyperemesis gravidarum is made. (See Chapter 39.) The pathogenesis of this disorder, and its attendant liver dysfunction, is unknown.

Liver dysfunction in patients with hyperemesis gravidarum has been reported. Abnormal liver tests (primarily elevated transaminases) are present in close to one-half of patients requiring hospitalization for hyperemesis gravidarum. Usually these are modest elevations, less than 250 units, but rarely they may approach 1000 units. The transaminase elevations parallel the vomiting. In the most severe cases, the bilirubin and prothrombin times may also be abnormal. Liver biopsy shows no inflammation, as would be characteristic of hepatitis, but rather central hepatocyte ballooning and vacuolization, as well as bile-stained Kupffer cells, suggestive of a cholestatic toxin.

Treatment of the liver dysfunction associated with hyperemesis gravidarum does not differ from that for the underlying disorder, namely, rehydration and antiemetic therapy. In severe cases, total parenteral nutrition is necessary. It is not unusual for severely affected patients to lose a significant percentage of their body weight. There are no known (or suspected) hepatic residua.

## CHOLESTASIS OF PREGNANCY

Cholestasis of pregnancy is the most common of the liver disorders unique to pregnant women. The clinical hallmark of this syndrome is pruritus. Any liver

**TABLE 40-1.** Differential Diagnosis of Liver Disease in Pregnancy

| Usual Trimester | Disorder | Symptoms | Lab | Liver Biopsy |
|---|---|---|---|---|
| First | Hyperemesis gravidarum | Vomiting | + Ketones, ↑ transaminases | Central vacuolization |
| Second | Cholestasis of pregnancy | Pruritus | ↑ GGTP, bile acids | Cholestasis |
| Third | HELLP | Abdominal pain | ↓ Plts, ↑ transaminase | Periportal hemorrhage |
| | Rupture | Abdominal pain, fever | ↑↑ Transaminases, + CT scan | |
| | Acute fatty liver of pregnancy | Nausea, vomiting | ↑ Protime | Microvesicular fat |
| Any | Viral hepatitis | Nausea, vomiting | ↑ Transaminase | Inflammation and necrosis |

+, positive findings; ↑, elevated; ↑↑, markedly elevated; ↓, decreased.

dysfunction in pregnancy associated with itching should be considered to be cholestasis of pregnancy until proved otherwise. In severe cases, the cholestasis progresses to jaundice.

The clinical characteristics of this syndrome, other than the associated pruritus, are variable. It may begin at almost any point in gestation, from early in the second trimester to late in the third. Itching is the first, and usually the only, symptom. Typical itching of cholestasis is generalized over all the body but worse on the palms and soles and worse at night. This symptom, when severe, is almost intolerable, and patients will beg to be delivered.

Laboratory tests show elevations in the serum bile acid levels, most conveniently measured as serum cholylglycine, a test that is widely available commercially. The "cholestatic" enzymes—alkaline phosphatase, γ-glutamyl transpeptidase, and 5'-nucleotidase—are elevated. The levels of transaminases vary but may rise above 1000 units in rare cases. Both the itching and the laboratory abnormalities may wax and wane during the pregnancy. All abnormalities resolve after delivery, but rarely this resolution may be delayed by several months.

Therapy for this condition is limited. Treatment with cholestyramine, a bile acid–binding resin, may help but will also exacerbate the steatorrhea associated with cholestasis. Phenobarbital therapy may help, presumably as a centrally acting sedative but perhaps also as a choleretic. Therapy with S-adenosylmethionine (SAM) has been suggested but has not been widely advocated. All affected patients should be assumed to be malabsorbing fat and should be supplemented with vitamin K via the parenteral route prior to delivery.

Generally, the outcome of this condition is benign. Some reports have documented an increase in both prematurity and stillbirths, and all affected pregnancies should be monitored with increased vigilance as term approaches. There is an increased incidence of gallstones in women previously affected with cholestasis of pregnancy. Patients affected in one pregnancy may have a recurrence of symptoms, either more or less severe, in subsequent pregnancies.

## LIVER INVOLVEMENT IN PREECLAMPSIA

Hepatic involvement in preeclampsia is increasingly recognized to be common and to have serious implications about the severity of this poorly understood systemic disorder. Given that preeclampsia exists as a broad spectrum, including normotensive preeclampsia, it is easy to comprehend that the spectrum of liver disease is also broad. It ranges from subclinical involvement, with the only manifestation of liver disease being deposition of fibrinogen along the hepatic sinusoids, to rupture of the liver, usually associated with maternal and fetal demise. Within these extremes fall the HELLP syndrome and hepatic infarction.

By far the most commonly encountered of these disorders is the syndrome dubbed the HELLP syndrome (for *hemolysis, elevated liver enzymes, and low platelets*) or some variant thereof. Affected patients can present with a variety of clinical pictures. The combination of thrombocytopenia with abnormal transaminases implies hepatic involvement, and this in turn implies serious disease, with a potentially fatal outcome. Indeed, elevated transaminases alone in the later half of pregnancy can presage the onset of preeclampsia. Thus, the combination of elevated transaminases and a platelet count that is known to be falling, even though still within the range of normal, has serious implications.

On physical examination, affected patients may have tenderness to palpation or to shock over their right upper quadrant or right lower chest. Jaundice is unusual. The transaminase elevations may be modest or may exceed 1000 to 2000 units. Usually, coagulation studies other than platelet count, including prothrombin time and fibrinogen, are normal. The liver biopsy may be normal or may show the periportal hemorrhage and fibrin deposition typical of preeclampsia (Fig. 40-1).

Definitive treatment is identical to that for the underlying disorder—namely, termination of the pregnancy. The timing and route are obstetrical judgments. Platelet transfusion is advisable if the count is severely depressed (<50,000). Recurrent HELLP syndrome has been reported, and any woman affected should be followed in subsequent pregnancies as a patient at increased risk. There are no hepatic sequelae.

Hepatic infarction is presumably a very severe, and fortunately very rare, extension of the HELLP syndrome. Affected patients complain of abdominal or chest pain and are febrile without an obvious source. There is often accompanying leukocytosis, and the transaminase values are extremely high, often above 5000 units. Severely affected women may have enough hepatic injury to experience true hepatic failure, with coagulopathy, encephalopathy, and jaundice. The infarcts are best visualized on CT scanning, since ultrasonography may fail to demonstrate the extensive areas of infarct. Despite the obviously extensive liver damage, most patients recover without sequelae, although there may be a fever of unknown etiology that lasts for several weeks.

Subcapsular hematoma and frank rupture of the liver are further extensions of this preeclamptic liver disease. When the rupture is contained within the capsule, the patient experiences severe pain but is hemodynamically stable. Again, the CT scan is the most reliable way to make this diagnosis. Patients who have hepatic rupture present in shock, with hemoperitoneum, and have a high mortality.

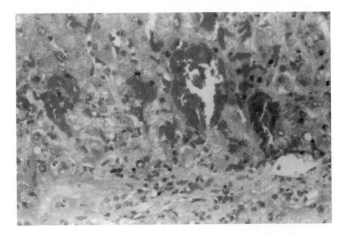

**FIGURE 40-1.** Liver biopsy in HELLP syndrome. The portal triad running along the bottom of the figure is surrounded by areas of hemorrhage and hepatocyte necrosis (hematoxylin and eosin stain, × 25).

## ACUTE FATTY LIVER OF PREGNANCY

Recent reports have expanded our knowledge of this once dreaded complication of late pregnancy. It is evident that this disorder is more common and less frequently fatal than previously thought. It also appears that acute fatty liver usually occurs in the setting of preeclampsia. This diagnosis is often difficult to make in affected patients, because acute fatty liver is a syndrome of fulminant hepatic failure, and hepatic failure is associated, almost invariably, with relative hypertension. Thus, affected patients have "normotensive preeclampsia." Interestingly, acute fatty liver of pregnancy is usually distinct clinically from the other liver conditions of preeclampsia discussed earlier. There may, however, be overlap between these syndromes, and fat in the liver has been reported in typical preeclamptic liver disease and in rupture of the liver. HELLP syndrome also has been reported in patients with typical acute fatty liver of pregnancy.

The clinical characteristics typical of acute fatty liver of pregnancy include presentation in the third trimester, near term, with signs and symptoms typical of both acute hepatitis and preeclampsia. Patients often have nausea, vomiting, and severe malaise and fatigue. Jaundice occurs frequently, but not invariably. Patients also complain of headache, thirst, and midepigastric or right upper quadrant pain. Rarely, a patient has no symptoms and is identified because of abnormal liver function tests. As the disease progresses, the patient can manifest typical hepatic failure, with agitation followed by stupor and coma, and severe coagulopathy with attendant bleeding.

Laboratory tests confirm the presence of hepatic failure, with elevations in prothrombin time, a decrease in serum fibrinogen below the usually elevated levels in pregnancy, hyperammonemia, and often hypoglycemia. The transaminase levels are elevated, but they are usually below 1000 units, and normal values at presentation have been reported. Typical severe cases show elevation in the serum bilirubin. In keeping with their preeclampsia, most patients have hyperuricemia. In severe cases, the patients may develop oliguric renal failure (the so-called hepatorenal syndrome) and may have complicating pancreatitis, both seen frequently in fulminant hepatic failure of any etiology.

Transient diabetes insipidus has been reported to be associated with preeclampsia and with acute fatty liver of pregnancy. Typical patients are hypernatremic and have an inappropriate diuresis and are often resistant to vasopressin.

The diagnosis of acute fatty liver of pregnancy should be suggested by the typical clinical picture and should be considered in the differential diagnosis of all patients with abnormal liver function tests in the third trimester. It can be a difficult diagnosis to confirm. The abdominal CT scan may be helpful if it shows a decrease in Houndsfield units in the liver, suggesting fatty infiltration. In cases of diagnostic uncertainty, liver biopsy is indicated. Using special stains, the typical microvesicular fatty infiltration can be seen (Fig. 40-2).

The course, in typical patients, is toward recovery, beginning with delivery. If the hepatic failure is severe, the patient may be in coma for several days prior to improvement.

Affected patients are left with no hepatic residua. There have been many reports of subsequent normal pregnancy in such patients. Patients with a history of acute fatty liver of pregnancy need not be dissuaded from becoming pregnant again but should be followed with care as high-risk pregnancies.

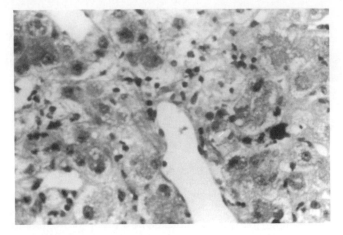

**FIGURE 40-2.** Liver biopsy in typical acute fatty liver of pregnancy. The hepatocytes surrounding this central vein are pleomorphic and vacuolated. There has been hepatocyte necrosis and there are scattered darkly stained pigment-laden macrophages (PAS with diastase stain, ×25).

## LIVER DISEASES EXACERBATED OR PRECIPITATED BY PREGNANCY

### BUDD-CHIARI SYNDROME

Veno-occlusive disease of the hepatic veins of the liver has been reported in patients taking oral contraceptives. This devastating disease is also reported to occur following pregnancy, primarily in India but rarely in the United States. The onset is usually in the weeks following delivery and is marked by abdominal pain and the abrupt onset of ascites and hepatomegaly. Liver function deteriorates, sometimes rapidly. Although this condition is usually fatal, successful pregnancy after Budd-Chiari syndrome has been reported.

Presumably, this condition results from the normal increase in coagulability that occurs in pregnancy as term approaches.

### CHOLELITHIASIS

Normal pregnancy is lithogenic. Gallbladder motility, like motility of other gut smooth muscle, is depressed during pregnancy. The usual enterohepatic cycling of bile acids, which solubilize cholesterol in bile, is decreased, and the bile becomes more lithogenic.

### HEPATITIS E

Recently, the virus associated with water-borne epidemics has been identified. It is known as hepatitis E and is an RNA virus that is found throughout the world in water contaminated with stool; so far it has not been seen in the United States. Why this virus should be so particularly lethal in pregnancy is unclear. Pregnant women should be discouraged from traveling to endemic areas, particularly India, Africa, Southeast Asia, and parts of Mexico and the Soviet Union, where outbreaks of this infection have been documented.

## HERPES SIMPLEX HEPATITIS

Like hepatitis E, infection with herpes simplex can cause fulminant hepatitis in pregnant women. There is usually an accompanying genital eruption. The diagnosis can be made by cultures of the lesions or by liver biopsy; in one case, suggestive "holes" were seen in the liver on CT scan. Therapy with acyclovir has been successful, but there is a high mortality rate among untreated women. Early diagnosis is crucial for both mother and infant.

## LIVER DISEASES OCCURRING CONCURRENT WITH PREGNANCY

### HEPATITIS A, B, AND C

Acute viral hepatitis due to one of the primary hepatotrophic viruses is not associated with increased morbidity or mortality in pregnant women, with the exception of hepatitis E. Diseases of pregnancy namely, preeclamptic liver disease and acute fatty liver of pregnancy—can mimic acute viral hepatitis and are often mistaken for it.

### DRUG-INDUCED HEPATOTOXICITY

Drug-induced hepatotoxicity should always be considered in the differential diagnosis of liver disease, and a careful history for drug ingestion should be obtained.

### METASTATIC MALIGNANCY

Rarely, malignant disease metastatic to the liver presents during pregnancy. Affected patients have palpable hepatomegaly, a very unusual finding during pregnancy and one that should prompt immediate evaluation.

### PREGNANCY IN PATIENTS WITH PREEXISTING LIVER DISEASE

Chronic liver disease is associated with decreased fertility, and such women rarely ovulate. Amenorrhea or premature menopause is a common symptom of chronic liver disease.

### CHRONIC HEPATITIS B

The hepatitis B virus may exist in a chronic carrier state, not associated with any clinical disease but still highly infectious. It is now the standard of care for all pregnant women to be screened for chronic hepatitis B early in gestation by testing them for hepatitis B surface antigen (HBsAg). If the mother is positive for this infection, then the infant is given hepatitis B hyperimmune globulin at birth and is begun on a three-dose regimen of vaccination with hepatitis B vaccine prior to discharge from the hospital. Cesarean section can lower the incidence of transmission but is not necessary if the infant is given correct immunoprophylaxis. Breastfeeding does not increase the risk of transmission and is not contraindicated.

## CHRONIC HEPATITIS C

The hepatitis C virus also exists in the population in a chronic carrier state, affecting approximately 1% of healthy blood donors. This virus appears to be less infectious than the hepatitis B virus and has less sexual and mother-infant transmission.

## STEROID-RESPONSIVE CHRONIC ACTIVE HEPATITIS

Steroid-responsive chronic active hepatitis, called autoimmune or lupoid chronic active hepatitis, occurs primarily in young women and is not rare. Affected patients respond (by definition) to immunosuppression with corticosteroids, often augmented with azathioprine. Pregnancy in such women can be successful, but is known to be associated with an increased incidence of stillbirths, prematurity, and obstetric complications such as preeclampsia. The immunosuppression must be continued, or the disease will recur. Despite its potential teratogenicity, azathioprine in the low doses used in these patients has not been associated with problems in their offspring.

## WILSON'S DISEASE

Wilson's disease, a disorder of copper metabolism, is associated with chronic liver disease, as well as chronic neurologic disease, and leads to death if untreated. Treatment with copper chelation, with either D-penicillamine or trientene, leads to a return to normal of hepatic function and to resumption of ovulation in affected young women. Such women may have successful pregnancies but must be maintained on their chelation therapy for the duration of the pregnancy. In this setting, there has been no associated teratogenicity of D-penicillamine.

## PORTAL HYPERTENSION

Patients with noncirrhotic portal hypertension have normal fertility. Such women may sustain variceal hemorrhage while pregnant but tolerate it well. Patients with cirrhosis fare less well. Fetal wastage and prematurity are more common in cirrhotic patients.

# 41. PREGNANCY COMPLICATED BY RENAL DISORDERS

## RENAL FUNCTION AND VOLUME HOMEOSTASIS DURING PREGNANCY

Normal pregnancy is characterized by a gradual cumulative retention of 500 to 900 mEq of sodium and 6 to 8 L of water, which are distributed between maternal extracellular fluid and the products of conception. Maternal plasma volume increases 30% to 45%; the incremental rise is most marked in the second trimester and is sustained until term. Renal plasma flow increases by 80% between conception and the second trimester, and subsequently falls to a level about 60% greater than the nonpregnant norm. The glomerular filtration rate (GFR) achieves an incremental increase of 30% to 50% by the 12th week, which is sustained until term, after which the rate rapidly falls to non-gravid levels (Fig. 41-1). The 24-hour creatinine clearance increases from $117 \pm 18$ to $136 \pm 11$ mL/min between early and midpregnancy.

In clinical practice, simple screening techniques for estimating the level of GFR usually rely on measurements of serum levels of urea nitrogen and creatinine. Because of the expansion of extracellular fluid and increased GFR, levels of these substances are substantially lower during gestation than in non-pregnant women. Compared to nonpregnant values of $13 \pm 3$ mg/dL (mean $\pm$ SD) of serum urea nitrogen and $0.67 \pm 0.14$ mg/dL of plasma creatinine, levels fall to $8.7 \pm 1.5$ mg/dL and $0.46 \pm 0.13$ mg/dL, respectively, in pregnancy. Concentrations that exceed 13 mg/dL of urea nitrogen and 0.8 mg/dL of creatinine suggest the possibility of renal insufficiency. In patients with known or suspected renal insufficiency, formal estimates of GFR are required. Two to three timed collections of urine of at least 30 minutes are obtained, along with a plasma sample, for the determination of creatinine clearance. Based on measurements obtained in normal gravidae, under this condition a $C_{cr} < 100$ mL/min is considered to be abnormal.

## EFFECT OF RENAL DISEASE ON PREGNANCY

Renal disease may be caused by many different types of tissue injury. Regardless of the type of injury, the functional consequences that result in morbidity usually take one or two non-exclusive forms—namely, the nephrotic syndrome and renal insufficiency.

## NEPHROTIC SYNDROME

The nephrotic syndrome is defined as heavy proteinuria of at least $3.0$ g/$1.73$ m$^2$/24 hours and a serum albumin level $< 3.0$ g/dL. Patients with this syndrome inevitably have a reduced capacity to excrete sodium and will retain salt and water as edema fluid if sodium intake exceeds their maximum excretory capacity. In

E. Albert Reece, John C. Hobbins, Maurice, J. Mahoney and Roy H. Petrie (Eds).
*Handbook of Medicine of the Fetus & Mother.* Copyright © 1995 by J.B. Lippincott Company

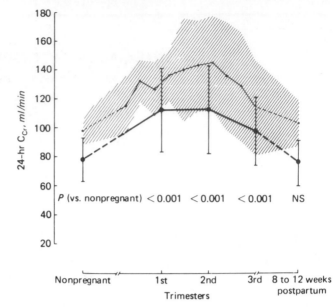

**FIGURE 41-1.** Alterations in 24-hour creatinine clearance determinations before conception, during each trimester, and 8 to 12 weeks postpartum, in 10 normal gravidas (mean ± 1 SD), shown in the shaded area and in 33 gravidas with primary renal disease and normal or near-normal renal functions, shown by solid line. (Katz AI, Davison JM, Hayslett JP, et al. Pregnancy in women with kidney disease. Kidney Int 1980;18:192.)

addition, and apparently as a consequence of hypoalbuminemia, these patients usually exhibit elevated cholesterol and triglyceride levels, due to increased lipid production. The GFR may be reduced, depending on the severity of the renal injury. Table 41-1 provides an overall classification of renal parenchymal diseases, but it should be emphasized that nephrotic syndrome always results from an injury reaction that affects the glomerulus, either in primary or in systemic diseases, which increases the rate of filtration of plasma proteins.

The clinical management of patients with nephrotic syndrome due to primary renal disease should aim to mitigate the severity of edema formation. Because proteinuria in patients with preexisting renal disease often increases during pregnancy to nephrotic levels, a low sodium intake can be introduced in early pregnancy (1.5 g Na) to reduce the rate of edema formation. In addition, frequent periods of bedrest with the subject lying on her side to promote a higher GFR, especially in late pregnancy, will enhance the rate of sodium excretion. In most patients, these conservative measures will suffice to prevent massive edema. In cases of primary renal disease where dietary salt restriction does not prevent massive symptomatic edema formation, diuretic agents, such as furosemide, can be employed on an intermittent basis to reduce edema to more tolerable levels. In the absence of significant hypertension or renal insufficiency, pregnancy is carried to term with the expectations of a vaginal delivery. In preeclamptic patients, the usual approach in the management of this condition is employed.

## RENAL DISEASE WITH NORMAL OR NEAR-NORMAL RENAL FUNCTION

Renal disease with normal or near-normal renal function is associated with a moderate incidence of reversible maternal complications and a moderate decrease

**TABLE 41-1.** Classification of Renal Parenchymal Disease

I. Glomerular
  A. Primary renal disease
    1. Epithelial disease
      a. Minimal-change disease
      b. Focal glomerulosclerosis
    2. Membranous nephropathy
    3. Proliferative glomerulonephritis
    4. Chronic glomerulonephritis
  B. Systemic disease
    1. Diabetic glomerulosclerosis
    2. Systemic lupus erythematosus
    3. Systemic vasculitis
    4. Amyloidosis
    5. Preeclampsia
II. Interstitial
  A. Acute interstitial nephritis
  B. Chronic interstitial nephritis
  C. Pyelonephritis
III. Vascular
  A. Arterionephrosclerosis
  B. Vasculitis
  C. Arterial emboli

From Hirch DJ, Hayslett JP. Renal disease during pregnancy. In: Berkowitz RL, ed. Critical care of the obstetric patient. New York: Churchill Livingstone, 1983:443.

in fetal survival. In general, pregnancy does not appear to affect the course of the underlying disease.

The management of this group of patients requires the skills of physicians trained in high-risk pregnancies and pediatric facilities designed to care for preterm and growth-retarded infants. Hypertension during pregnancy should be controlled to obviate further renal damage. Efforts to control edema formation in patients with nephrotic syndrome have been discussed. Anemia, sometimes of significant proportions, may also require direct intervention, and intermittent transfusions are advocated to maintain hematocrit levels above 25%. It should also be noted that patients with reduced renal function have a reduced capacity to excrete water and electrolytes. Therefore, they are at increased risk of developing dilutional hyponatremia when large amounts of solute-free water are administered, or hypernatremia, hyperkalemia, and metabolic acidosis after treatment with various types of electrolyte-containing intravenous solutions. Appropriate restrictions in the use of parenterally administered fluids are required during treatment of severe hypertension, prolonged labor, and other conditions requiring intensive therapy. As in other types of high-risk pregnancies, careful fetal monitoring is indicated in all cases.

## RENAL DISEASE WITH MODERATE RENAL INSUFFICIENCY

The effect of pregnancy on the course of renal disease in women with serum creatinine $\geq 1.5$ mg/dL but $<5.0$ mg/dL is less certain because of the paucity of data and lack of information on levels of renal function before conception in reported patients. Based on published reports, women with GFR levels between

15% and 40% of normal are likely to experience a hectic clinical course during pregnancy, due in large part to severe hypertension, and a successful pregnancy outcome of 50% to 75%. Table 41-2 illustrates the general correlations between functional renal status and maternal complications—fetal outcome derived from the recent literature; in this analysis, categories of renal insufficiency were based on serum creatinine levels in mg/dL: mild, <1.4; moderate, >1.4 and <2.5; and severe, >2.5.

## Acute Renal Failure

Acute renal failure is defined as a rapid decline in GFR toward a value that approaches zero. Hallmark clinical features include a near-linear increase in serum creatinine at a rate of 0.5 to 1.5 mg/dL/day, a progressive rapid rise in serum urea nitrogen, and usually a fall in urine flow rate to less than 400 to 500 mL/day. Sustained severe renal failure for more than a few days results in the manifestations of uremia and marked metabolic acidosis, hyperkalemia, and anemia. The general classification of acute renal failure is shown in Table 41-3.

**TABLE 41-2.** Pregnancy and Renal Disease: Functional Renal Status and Prospects

| | Category | | |
|---|---|---|---|
| Prospects | Mild | Moderate | Severe |
| Pregnancy complications | 22% | 41% | 84% |
| Successful obstetric outcome | 95% | 90% | 47% |
| Long-term sequelae | <5% | 25% | 53% |

Estimates are based on 804 women/1162 pregnancies (1973–1987) and do not include collagen diseases. From Davison JM, Lindheimer MD. Renal disorders. In: Creasy K, Risnik R, eds. Maternal-fetal medicine: principles and practice. 2nd ed. Philadelphia: WB Saunders, 1989;828.

**TABLE 41-3.** Classification of Causes of Acute Renal Failure

Prerenal
  Renal hypoperfusion due to
   1. Hypotension
   2. Decreased circulating plasma volume
   3. Decreased cardiac output
Renal Parenchymal
  Acute tubular necrosis—reversible
  Cortical necrosis—irreversible
  Caused by
   1. Renal hypoperfusion due to
    a. Hypotension
    b. Decreased circulating plasma volume
    c. Decreased cardiac output
    d. Disseminated intravascular coagulation (DIC)
   2. Nephrotoxins
Postrenal
  Obstruction of ureters or bladder outlet
  Extravasation of urine from urinary collecting system

The approach to a patient with the clinical findings of acute renal failure begins by determining the category of the most likely cause for the sudden decline in renal function. Postrenal causes are evaluated by simple straight catheterization of the urinary bladder and assessment of ureteral diameter by renal ultrasound. Evaluation of the urine for fractional sodium excretion and concentrating ability is helpful in distinguishing prerenal from acute tubular necrosis as a cause of acute renal failure. The presence of hypotension or clinically evident cardiac failure or dehydration demands prompt corrective measures to restore renal perfusion. Because effective plasma volume is often difficult to evaluate at the bedside, especially in edematous patients, Swan-Ganz catheterization to determine pulmonary wedge pressure is the most reliable means of evaluating volume status. In the presence of reduced filling pressures, isotonic fluids, or packed red blood cells (RBCs) when hemorrhage has occurred, should be administered until filling pressures are normalized.

If the diagnosis of acute tubular necrosis or cortical necrosis seems likely after exclusion of pre- and postrenal factors, therapy is begun to minimize the consequences of severe renal insufficiency. Fluid administration is restricted, after restoring volume status to normal, to match urine volume plus insensible losses of water (400 to 500 mL/day); calories are provided in the form of carbohydrates or lipids at a minimum of 2000 kcal/day; and the administration of sources of sodium, potassium, and metabolic acid are avoided. The hematocrit should be maintained at at least 25% with transfusion of packed RBCs, and hypertension should be controlled. After the patient is stabilized, a decision should be made regarding delivery. If delivery is performed, dialysis therapy should be instituted after the procedure. In the event that delivery is impractical because of fetal immaturity, dialysis therapy should be instituted within a few days to minimize the functional consequences of renal failure. Early dialysis also has the advantage of permitting the administration of protein and calories in the large amounts that are often required in severely catabolic patients.

## DIABETES MELLITUS AND RENAL DISEASE

Recent experience has shown that advances in perinatal and neonatal care have eliminated maternal mortality and reduced the perinatal death rate in diabetics in general to levels that approach the general population. The outlook, however, for patients with diabetes complicated by vascular disease has not improved in parallel with the general diabetic population. A 1977 report on the Joslin Clinic experience, for example, demonstrated a fetal survival of 84% in Class R, 72% in Class F, and 81% in Class FR, representing women with retinopathy (R), nephropathy (F), or a combination of both vascular complications (FR).* Recently, two studies with a total of 57 patients with diabetic nephropathy have described a more favorable outlook for this group of patients, managed with optimal perinatal technique and modern methods of fetal monitoring. Following delivery, changes in renal function, blood pressure, and protein excretion returned to values similar to that observed in the first trimester. The long-term maternal course was viewed

*Hare JW, White P. Pregnancy in diabetics complicated by vascular disease. Diabetes 1977;26:953.

as not differing from the expected course of diabetic nephropathy in subjects who had not become pregnant.

The fetal outcomes reported in these two studies are shown in Table 41-4, and are compared to results in a large series of patients with primary renal disease. Perinatal survival in the two groups of diabetic patients averaged 91%, a value that was not different from patients with primary renal disease and normal or near-normal renal function.

## SLE AND LUPUS NEPHROPATHY

In pregnant patients in whom clinical renal disease was present before pregnancy, the rate and severity of exacerbations correlate with disease activity during the 6 months prior to conception. Recent reports on patients with lupus nephropathy confirm a relationship between the level of disease activity at the onset of pregnancy and the subsequent course.

Regarding outcome for the product of conception, overall fetal survival was 76% in eight studies published since 1980. Inspection of these data, however, shows a relatively good outcome in some patients, especially in women who were in clinical remission at the time of conception, and fewer, mild flares during gestation. In patients who exhibited clinical remission prior to pregnancy, fetal survival varied between 88% and 100%. In contrast, when pregnancy occurred in women with active SLE, survivorship was reduced to 50% to 75% in the same series.

It should be noted that infants born to women with SLE have additional risks

**TABLE 41-4.** Perinatal Outcome of Patients with Nonsystemic Renal Disease and Patients with Diabetes-Associated Renal Disease**

|  | Pregnant Nondiabetic Patients with Renal Disease | Pregnant Diabetic Patients with Renal Disease (White Class F or FR) | |
| --- | --- | --- | --- |
| No. of patients | 121* | 26* | 31** |
| Fetal death | 7 (5.7%) | 2 (7.7%) | 2 (6.4%) |
| Preterm deliveries | 24 (20.0%) | 8 (30.8%) | 3 (37.5%) |
| Small for gestational age | 27 (24.3%) | 5 (20.8%) | 5 (16.0%) |
| Large for gestational age | 6 (5.4%) | 3 (12.5%) | 4 (12.9%) |
| Appropriate for gestational age | 78 (70.2%) | 18 (69.2%) | 22 (72.0%) |
| Major congenital anomalies | — | 3 (11.1%) | 3 (9.6%) |
| Neonatal | | | |
| Respiratory distress syndrome | — | 6 (23.0%) | 6 (19.3%) |
| Hypoglycemia | — | 11 (44.0%) | 2 (6.5%) |
| Hyperbilirubinemia phototherapy | — | 11 (44.0%) | 8 (25.8%) |
| Death | 6 (4.9%) | 1 (4.0%) | 0 (0.0%) |
| Perinatal survival | 90.0% | 88.9% | 93.6% |

* Data from Katz AI, Davison JM, Hayslett JP, et al. Kid Inter 1980;18:192 and Kitzmiller JL, Brown ER, Phillippe M, et al. Am J Obstet Gynecol 1981;141:741.
** Modified from Reece EA, Coustan DR, Hayslett JP, et al. Diabetic nephropathy: pregnancy performance and fetomaternal outcome. Am J Obstet Gynecol 1988;159:56.

besides impaired development in utero and preterm delivery. Transmission of autoantibodies to the fetus from maternal circulation is known to result in two types of disorders that are either transient or result in permanent tissue injury. Antinuclear antibodies and a positive lupus erythematosus (LE) cell test have been described in cord blood, but maternal antibodies disappear from neonatal blood within about 4 months. Although clinical involvement of the newborn with maternal SLE is uncommon, a few cases of discoid lupus, and of hemolytic anemia, neutropenia, and thrombocytopenia have been reported. These clinical episodes have been transient. A more important complication involves transmission of antibody to a soluble tissue ribonucleoprotein antigen called Ro (SS-A). Transmission of this antibody in utero has been associated with complete heart block in infants born to women with established SLE and to women with this circulating antibody in the absence of clinical features of connective tissue disease.

## DIALYSIS IN PREGNANCY

Because severe renal insufficiency is associated with infertility, the issue of renal dialysis usually arises in patients with acute renal failure or severe progressive renal failure who conceived before the appearance of renal failure. Pregnancy has occurred, however, in women on dialysis, and in most cases was diagnosed late in gestation because it was unexpected and menstrual irregularities are common under this condition. A comprehensive understanding of maternal and fetal complications incurred by this group of patients is not available, because information is based on case reports and small series, and probably tends to favor successful gestation.

Among patients who develop severe renal failure after the onset of pregnancy, the aim of dialysis is to prevent uremic complications in the mother and provide a more favorable environment for the fetus until the likelihood of extrauterine viability reaches a reasonable level. Because of limited experience with this procedure in pregnancy, guidelines for management have not been established. It is common practice, however, to initiate dialysis treatment earlier than is usually prescribed in nonpregnant individuals, when the blood urea nitrogen level reaches a value of about 100 mg/dL. When hemodialysis is selected as the mode of therapy, an arteriovenous fistula should be formed early in gestation of patients with a progressive decline in renal function to permit maturation. In acute renal failure, vascular access can be achieved rapidly at any time during pregnancy with a subclavian catheter. In cases where peritoneal dialysis is selected, the surgical placement of a permanent catheter can be performed when the decision to begin dialysis is made, even, as noted, in the later stages of gestation.

## RENAL TRANSPLANTATION AND PREGNANCY

Because a successful renal transplant restores fertility as well as renal function, it is not surprising that some women have become pregnant after transplantation or desire to do so after their sense of well-being returns. In a recent review, Davison (1987) reports a complication rate of 46% in pregnancies continuing beyond the first trimester, including uncontrolled hypertension, renal deterioration, and rejection.[†] Clinical differentiation between rejection of the graft and preeclampsia is difficult. The rate of successful obstetric outcome was 73% in women with complications before 28 weeks gestation and 92% in patients without early complications. The incidence of preterm delivery was 45% to 60%, and growth retardation was observed in 20%. Women desirous of pregnancy should be advised to avoid pregnancy for at least 18 months after surgery because of the higher incidence of rejection, infection, and permanent loss of graft function in this early postoperative interval.

# 42. NEUROLOGIC DISORDERS OF PREGNANCY

## CEREBROVASCULAR DISEASE

Cerebrovascular disease is a major cause of maternal mortality. Because cerebrovascular disease in young pregnant and puerperal women can be caused by a variety of unusual conditions, each case needs to be thoroughly investigated. Angiography is usually required to make a firm diagnosis and prognosis.

## SUBARACHNOID HEMORRHAGE

Spontaneous subarachnoid hemorrhage commonly results from rupture of an aneurysm and an arteriovenous malformation (AVM). Approximately one-third of instances are symptomatic of bleeding disorders, endocarditis, sickle cell disease, vasculitis, and, rarely, choriocarcinoma. Subarachnoid hemorrhage in gravidas under the age of 25 is more likely to be from an AVM, whereas in gravid women over age 25, often multiparas, the likely cause would be a ruptured congenital berry aneurysm. AVMs are more likely to initially bleed in the second trimester and during labor. The incidence of the initial rupture of aneurysms increases with each trimester of pregnancy. Intrapartum rebleeding is common for both conditions, and is probably related to the Valsalva maneuver.

If possible, the offending aneurysm should be surgically clipped or the AVM excised during pregnancy so that the woman may be delivered vaginally with no special risk. Surgery for unruptured aneurysms can be postponed, with the exception of aneurysms with diameters more than 10 mm.

If the lesion cannot be cured, vaginal delivery is a risk. Almost all women known to have an AVM and multiparas with aneurysms are delivered by elective cesarean section.

† Davison JM. Pregnancy in renal allograft recipients: prognosis and management. Baillieres Clin Obstet Gynecol 1987;1:1027.

## ARTERIAL ISCHEMIA

Pregnancy increases the risk of a cerebral ischemic event approximately tenfold. As many arterial occlusions occur during the first week postpartum as during the second and third trimesters combined. Almost all will be in the carotid territory. Approximately one-quarter of these strokes are caused by premature vascular disease accompanying diabetes mellitus, chronic hypertension, and familial hypercholesterolemia. For another quarter, no explanation will be found.

Management and prognosis depend on the underlying disease. Prophylactic anticoagulation is indicated for atrial fibrillation, cardiomyopathy, and the hypercoagulable state associated with antiphospholipid antibodies. The management of unexplained transient ischemic attacks (TIAs) during pregnancy is controversial. I recommend anticoagulation after the second TIA. The risk of having another unexplained cerebral ischemic episode during a subsequent pregnancy is undetermined, but probably is so rare that anticoagulation is not recommended. Heparin is the preferred anticoagulant during pregnancy.

## CEREBRAL VENOUS THROMBOSIS

Puerperal aseptic cerebral phlebothrombosis is now uncommon in Western industrialized nations, with an incidence of 1 to 4 per 10,000 deliveries. These cases occur from 4 days to 4 weeks postpartum. Some puerperal cases have been attributed to sickle cell crises, minor head trauma, paroxysmal nocturnal hemoglobinuria, and hyperviscosity due to leukemia, polycythemia, and cryofibrinoginemia. Deep vein thrombosis in the leg and pelvis coexists for approximately 10%.

The presentation depends on which veins are involved. A thrombosis of the superior sagittal sinus may present with headache and increased intracranial pressure. If a cortical vein is thrombosed, a focal seizure at the height of the headache's intensity is usually followed by weakness and aphasia. Intermittently progressive deficits, often punctuated by seizures, connote propagation of the clot. A quickly propagating clot prevents adequate drainage by collateral veins, increases the likelihood of hemorrhagic venous infarction, and predicts a poor prognosis. The presence of intracerebral bleeding, which can be detected by computed tomography (CT) scan, is a strong but not absolute contraindication to anticoagulation. Thus, rapid diagnosis by magnetic resonance imaging (MRI) and angiography can allow anticoagulation early enough to prevent clot propagation.

## EPILEPSY

Although the effect of pregnancy on epilepsy is unpredictable for any patient, the best indicator is the degree of control beforehand. Almost all women experiencing at least one convulsion per month can expect a worsening seizure state during pregnancy, whereas only 25% of those gravidas who were seizure-free for the 9 months before becoming pregnancy will have a seizure while pregnant. Those seizure-free for 2 years have only a 10% chance of convulsing during pregnancy.

The major factor responsible for an increased seizure frequency is an increased apparent plasma clearance (daily dose divided by blood level) of anticonvulsant.

This is especially true in the case of phenytoin. Other factors that can lower seizure thresholds include high estrogen levels and, in late pregnancy, insomnia.

The outcome of pregnancy depends more on socioeconomic status, regular prenatal care, and maternal factors such as age, parity, and other diseases, than on maternal epilepsy. There is usually no apparent harm caused by isolated seizures. Conversely, status epilepticus is a real threat: one-half of fetuses and one-third of mothers do not survive.

Infants of epileptic women do have a higher risk of major birth defects. The risk is present whether or not the fetus is exposed to an anticonvulsant, and increases with the severity of maternal epilepsy and the number of anticonvulsants used. The risk of orofacial cleft is increased fivefold. The incidence of congenital heart disease is not increased, except among infants exposed in utero to trimethadione, which is considered a human teratogen. The only malformation specifically related to an anticonvulsant is a defect in neural tube closure, which occurs in 1% to 2% of fetuses exposed to valproic acid in the first trimester.

Dysmorphic facial features have been described with various fetal anticonvulsant syndromes and are not specific to any one anticonvulsant. Usually these "minor" malformations become less recognizable as the child grows.

Epilepsy should be treated with the fewest drugs in the lowest dose needed to prevent convulsions. Single-drug therapy is recommended if possible.

The use of valproate during pregnancy is a special problem because it is associated with a 1% to 2% risk of a neural tube defect, which can usually be detected by ultrasonography and amniocentesis early enough to induce abortion, if desired. If a patient contemplating pregnancy understands this risk and accepts its consequences, I recommend valproate be continued for patients with a specific type of epilepsy for which valproate is the first choice, for those for whom valproate as monotherapy is more successful then any combination of polytherapy, and for those requiring valproate as a second drug.

Blood levels can be checked monthly and doses adjusted accordingly. Anticonvulsants should not be changed or added during pregnancy unless therapeutic doses of the previously proven regimen are no longer effective.

I recommend dietary supplementation with folic acid before and during pregnancy because it may decrease birth defects and third trimester bleeding. Inhibition of folate absorption by phenytoin and other anticonvulsants has been proposed as a teratogenic mechanism. An improved outcome of pregnancy in epileptic women has been associated with adequate progestational folate levels. Thus, starting a multivitamin tablet with folic acid, 0.5 or 1.0 mg, when a women stops using contraception seems reasonable.

Although mothers taking phenytoin, phenobarbital, and primidone have normal coagulation, about one-half of their newborns will have a deficiency of vitamin K–dependant clotting factors. This can be prevented by maternal administration of vitamin K near term. The lowest effective dose has not been determined, but vitamin K, 20 mg per day for 2 weeks before term, results in normal clotting of cord blood. A parenteral dose of 10 mg during early labor may be an adequate alternative.

## MULTIPLE SCLEROSIS

The course of multiple sclerosis is unpredictable. It is a consistent observation that the rate of exacerbations decreases with each successive trimester of pregnancy, only to rebound in the puerperium, when approximately 40% will have a relapse. For the entire pregnancy year, which includes the first 3 postpartum months, the exacerbation rate is at least as high as for a nonpregnancy year. An abortion during a relapse does not induce a remission.

For most women with mild multiple sclerosis, the management and outcome of pregnancy is unaffected. Spinal anesthesia is usually avoided. Epidural anesthesia, regional blocks, and general anesthesia can be administered as usual. The gravid uterus can complicate bladder control and increases the risk of cystitis. More seriously disabled women can have increased difficulty walking as weight increases. The incidence of congenital malformations among infants of women with multiple sclerosis is not increased.

## HEADACHE

Pregnancy can modify the frequency and severity of an established headache syndrome. A change in the quality of headache and the onset of headache during pregnancy may be symptomatic of an underlying condition, and should be evaluated accordingly just as for a nonpregnant woman. A thorough neurological examination including ophthalmoscopy is essential. Papilledema may be the only abnormality found in a patient with pseudotumor cerebri.

## CLASSIC MIGRAINE

Pregnancy usually improves classic migraine. The treatment of an acute migraine in a pregnant or lactating puerperal woman is complicated, because ergot alkaloids should not be used. Reliance is placed on analgesics (acetaminophen and, if needed, codeine or meperidine) and an antiemetic. If episodes are frequent and disabling, prophylactic therapy with a beta-adrenergic blocker is indicated. Both propranolol at 40 to 160 mg/day and atenolol at 50 or 100 mg/day are effective. An alternative is amitriptyline.

## TENSION HEADACHE

Chronic muscle contraction/tension headache is the most common headache during pregnancy and can be symptomatic of difficult psychological adjustments. Regular use of aspirin should be avoided because aspirin can increase intrapartum blood loss and impair neonatal hemostasis. Acetaminophen also crosses the placenta but has not been found to cause problems in 40 years of use. Recalcitrant tension headaches often respond to tricyclic antidepressants. Both amitriptyline and imipramine have an extensive record of reasonably safe use during pregnancy. The usual dose for either drug is 75 mg/day, with a range of 50 to 150 mg/day. Benzodiazepine tranquilizers should be avoided. Diazepam is poorly metabolized by the fetus and may cause neonatal depression.

## PSEUDOTUMOR CEREBRI

The typical patient with idiopathic pseudotumor cerebri is an overweight, fertile woman with headache and papilledema. Gestational pseudotumor cerebri begins in the third, fourth, or fifth months of pregnancy and usually lasts 1 to 3 months, although for a few it persists until the puerperium. The outcome of pregnancy is good; labor and delivery are normal. Epidural anesthesia may be used.

Treatment may be necessary to preserve vision. Visual acuity, visual fields, and optic discs should be evaluated regularly. A diet sufficient for maternal and fetal requirements but restrictive enough to curb excessive weight gain is recommended. If this is unsuccessful or if vision is already impaired, repeated lumbar punctures to drain cerebrospinal fluid and dexamethasone, 2 or 4 mg/day, are options. Shunting may be necessary for recalcitrant cases.

## BRAIN TUMOR

All types of primary brain tumors have occurred during pregnancy, usually presenting during the second half. A cerebral mass may be the signal lesion of metastatic choriocarcinoma. The treatment of the tumor and the management of pregnancy and delivery must be considered on a case-by-case basis. Surgery for meningiomas, some acoustic neuromas, and other slowly growing benign tumors can often be postponed until several weeks postpartum. Posterior fossa tumors are operated on during pregnancy to avoid the risk of tentorial herniation during delivery.

## PITUITARY ADENOMAS

If a woman with a prolactinoma becomes pregnant, the tumor will enlarge. Only 5% of microadenomas measuring less than 10 mm in diameter become symptomatic during pregnancy, whereas 15% to 35% of macroadenomas and extrasellar adenomas can be expected to do so. Women whose macroadenomas are excised before pregnancy revert to the low-risk group. Thus, patients with intrasellar macroadenomas commonly have transphenodial hypophysectomy before attempting pregnancy.

Headache routinely precedes visual deficits by 1 month. Visual acuity and visual fields can be done monthly by standard bedside techniques. CT or MRI is indicated if visual deficits develop and during the puerperium. Following prolactin levels is not helpful. If vision is impaired, bromocriptine therapy can be instituted. If corrected visual acuity becomes less than 20/50, or if the bitemporal hemianopia encroaches upon nasal sectors, more definitive treatment is indicated. One must recall that hypopituitarism may be developing. Surgery can be managed in any trimester; nevertheless, if the fetus has adequate pulmonary maturity, labor is often induced.

## NEUROPATHY

### BELL'S PALSY

Idiopathic unilateral facial paralysis is prone to occur in the third trimester and the first 2 weeks postpartum. The closer the onset to childbirth, the better the prognosis for complete spontaneous recovery. A brief course of high-dose corticosteroid therapy is indicated for patients with complete weakness, but may not improve cosmetic outcome for patients with partial weakness. In endemic areas, Lyme disease must be considered.

## CARPAL TUNNEL SYNDROME

Approximately 20% of pregnant women complain of nocturnal acroparesthesias. Most have a postural obstruction of blood flow. A few develop a carpal tunnel syndrome, commonly in the dominant hand, during the second half of pregnancy, which can be expected to remit within a few weeks postpartum. Most women respond to nocturnal splinting with the wrist in midposition or slightly flexed. Surgical division of transcarpal ligaments entrapping the median nerve is indicated during pregnancy if weakness exists and the diagnosis is confirmed by electromyography.

## MERALGIA PARESTHETICA

Meralgia paresthetica is a painful nuisance of the third trimester, which is presumably caused by an enlarged abdomen entrapping the purely sensory lateral femoral cutaneous nerve as it passes beneath the inguinal ligament. Symptoms typically resolve within 3 months after delivery.

## MATERNAL OBSTETRIC PALSY

The most common maternal obstetric palsy is foot drop caused by the fetal brow pressing against the lumbosacral trunk as it crosses the pelvic brim. Foot drop may also be caused by compression of the lateral peroneal nerve between the fibular head and a leg holder. Femoral neuropathy, sometimes coexisting with an obturator neuropathy, may be unilateral or bilateral and is associated with labor arrested in a transverse lie.

The prognosis of neuropractic lesions due to distortion of myelin sheaths is excellent, with full recovery within 6 weeks. If axons have been crushed, recovery is slower and may not be complete. During a subsequent pregnancy, women with previous neuropraxia may have a cautious trial of labor but should expect a cesarean section should dystocia develop. Women who had axonal degeneration from a previous delivery probably should be delivered by cesarean section in subsequent pregnancies.

## GUILLAIN-BARRÉ SYNDROME

Acute inflammatory demyelinating polyneuritis occurs randomly during pregnancy and runs its course seemingly independent of pregnancy. Early plasmapheresis decreases severity, and can be done during any trimester of pregnancy.

## MUSCLE DISEASE
## MYASTHENIA GRAVIS

Pregnancy has a profound but unpredictable effect on myasthenia gravis.

Previous thymectomy decreases the risk of pregnancy-associated exacerbations. In crisis, a series of plasmaphereses is certainly of less risk than prolonged immobilization with assisted ventilation. Postpartum presentations of my-asthenia gravis are not infrequent, and postpartum relapses occur in at least 40% of myasthenic women.

Myasthenia gravis does not affect the myometrium. Labor and delivery are normal. Magnesium sulfate will precipitate a myasthenic crisis. Regional anesthesia is preferred. Lidocaine is recommended for patients taking pyridostigmine and neostigmine, which would inhibit the hydrolysis of procaine by cholinesterase.

Maternal myasthenia gravis appears not to affect the fetus because intrauterine movements are forceful and polyhydramnios does not develop. At least 12% of infants of mothers with generalized myasthenia gravis develop neonatal my-asthenia due to maternal anti-acetylcholine receptor IgG that has crossed the placenta. Weakening during the first few days is typical. Thus, neonates at risk must be carefully watched for 4 days before leaving the hospital. Remission occurs spontaneously as the neonate's level of antibody declines, usually in 2 to 4 weeks.

## MYOTONIC DYSTROPHY

Women with myotonic muscular dystrophy usually weaken during the third trimester, and their myotonia can become more prominent. Breathing may be impaired.

Myotonic muscular dystrophy affects the myometrium in addition to skeletal and smooth muscle. Spontaneous abortion, premature labor, and uterine inertia during and after labor are common. Oxytocin stimulates uterine contractions. Regional anesthesia is preferred. Depolarizing muscle relaxants (e.g., succinyl-choline) can provoke rigor and hyperthermia.

The fetus can be affected, as manifested by polyhydramnios and arthrogryposis multiplex congenita. Affected neonates are floppy with facial diplegia and suck poorly.

---

# 43. THROMBOEMBOLIC DISORDERS OF PREGNANCY

---

## INCIDENCE OF VENOUS THROMBOEMBOLISM DURING PREGNANCY

A 1983 retrospective study by Kierkegaard estimated the risk of acute antepartum deep venous thrombosis at 0.13 per 1000, whereas the risk of puerperal DVT was estimated as 0.61 per 1000.* Women were at higher risk after a cesarean section.

---

*Kierkegaard A. Incidence and diagnosis of deep vein thrombosis associated with pregnancy. Acta Obstet Gynecol Scand 1983;62:239.

**TABLE 43-1.** Radiation Doses to Fetus with Procedures
Used to Diagnose Thromboembolic Disease

| Procedure | Estimated Fetal Radiation (mrad) |
|---|---|
| Bilateral venography without abdominal shield | 610 |
| Unilateral venography without abdominal shield | 305 |
| Limited venography | <50 |
| Pulmonary angiography via femoral route | 405 |
| Pulmonary angiography via brachial route | <50 |
| Perfusion lung scan | |
| $^{99m}$TcMAA | |
| 3 mCi | 18 |
| 1–2 mCi | 6–12 |
| Ventilation lung scan | |
| $^{133}$Xe | 3–20 |
| $^{99m}$TC-DTPA | 7–35 |
| $^{99m}$TC-SC | 1–5 |
| Radioisotope venography | 205 |
| $^{125}$I fibrinogen leg scanning | 2000 |

From Ginsberg JS, Hirsh J, Ranbow A, Coates G. Risks to the fetus of radiological procedures used in the diagnosis of maternal thromboembolic disease. Thromb Haemost 1989;61:189, with permission.

## DIAGNOSIS OF DEEP VEIN THROMBOSIS AND PULMONARY EMBOLISM

The diagnosis of DVT and PE during pregnancy presents special problems, because the clinical diagnosis is inaccurate and a number of key diagnostic tests expose the fetus to ionizing radiation.

The adverse effects of radiation on the fetus can be broadly classified into oncogenicity and teratogenicity. There is evidence that fetal exposure to radiation doses of even less than 5000 mrad is associated with a small increase in the risk of childhood cancer to the exposed individuals. However, most experts agree that fetal exposure to less than 5000 mrad of radiation is *not* associated with an increased risk of abortions, congenital malformations, or intrauterine growth retardation.

## RADIATION DOSES TO FETUS WITH PROCEDURES USED TO DIAGNOSE THROMBOEMBOLIC DISEASE

The doses of fetal radiation with venography and pulmonary angiography are calculations based on data obtained from McMaster University Medical Centre (Table 43-1). The dose for a given procedure can vary considerably between institutions.

### Contrast Venography
Contrast venography is the most definitive method available for diagnosing DVT in the nonpregnant patient. The total absorbed dose to the fetus for bilateral

venography *without* shielding of the abdomen is approximately 610 mrad. A limited venogram, which is performed by shielding the abdomen, is associated with fetal radiation exposure of well under 50 mrad.

## Lung Scanning

The perfusion lung scan is the pivotal test for the investigation of patients with suspected pulmonary embolism. A normal perfusion lung scan excludes PE, and a segmental or greater perfusion defect with normal ventilation (high probability scan) reliably diagnoses PE. Conversely, subsegmental perfusion defects or segmental perfusion defects with matching ventilation defects are inconclusive and require pulmonary angiography.

By using 1 mCi of $^{99m}$Tc-MAA for the perfusion scan and $^{99m}$Tc-SC for the ventilation scan, lung scanning can be done with fetal absorbed radiation of 11 mrad or less. Even performing full-dose perfusion lung scans and using a radiopharmaceutical other than $^{99m}$Tc-SC for the ventilation scan, it should be possible to do a full ventilation-perfusion lung scan with a fetal absorbed dose of less than 50 mrad.

## Pulmonary Angiography

Pulmonary angiography is the most definitive method for diagnosing pulmonary embolism. The examination is generally performed using fluoroscopy. Based on measurements performed on water phantoms at McMaster University, the total dose to the fetus is approximately 405 mrad. If performed by the brachial route and with appropriate abdominal shielding, the amount of radiation exposure should be well under 50 mrad.

## SUMMARY OF RADIATION HAZARDS OF DIAGNOSTIC PROCEDURES

Although every effort should be made to minimize radiation exposure, failure to make the correct diagnosis has important implications. Therefore, the best approach is the judicious selection of diagnostic procedures combined with efforts to minimize fetal radiation doses: lead shielding of the abdomen, reduction of doses of radioisotope for perfusion scanning, and pulmonary angiography by the brachial vein.

If bilateral venography is performed in a patient with suspected venous thrombosis, the fetal radiation exposure should not exceed 1000 mrad. If modified perfusion and ventilation lung scanning plus pulmonary angiography via the brachial route are performed, the fetal radiation exposure should again be well under 1000 mrad. The only likely adverse effect of in utero exposure to these doses of radiation is a small increase in the frequency of childhood cancers. Even assuming a doubling of childhood cancers, given a frequency of malignancy of approximately 1 per 1000 children, this level of exposure would give a frequency of childhood cancer of 0.2%.

## OTHER TECHNIQUES USED FOR THE DIAGNOSIS OF VENOUS THROMBOEMBOLISM

### Impedance Plethysmography

Impedance plethysmography (IPG) is a noninvasive method used for the diagnosis of proximal DVT. In the nonpregnant patient, this test is sensitive and specific for proximal vein thrombosis, but is insensitive to calf vein thrombosis. There is the potential for false-positive tests in the third trimester due to compression of the iliac veins by the uterus. This may be corrected by repeating the IPG with the patient lying on one side.

### Duplex Ultrasonography

Duplex ultrasonography is a new technique that is accurate for the detection of proximal DVT in nonpregnant patients. One potential disadvantage is the inability to consistently visualize the iliac veins, which can be the site of isolated thrombosis in pregnant patients.

## APPROACH TO THE DIAGNOSIS OF VENOUS THROMBOSIS DURING PREGNANCY

Our current approach to the diagnosis of suspected DVT during pregnancy favors the use of IPG as the initial test for this disorder. If the initial IPG is abnormal in patients during the first two trimesters of pregnancy, a diagnosis of proximal deep vein thrombosis is made, and the patient is treated with anticoagulants. If the IPG is abnormal during the third trimester, two options are available: (1) perform a venogram to differentiate between proximal deep vein thrombosis and compression of the iliac veins by the enlarged uterus, or (2) treat the patient with anticoagulants. If the initial IPG is normal, isolated calf DVT cannot be excluded, so the IPG is repeated the day following referral (day 1) and then at days 3, 5, 7, 10, and 14. Anticoagulant therapy is withheld if the test remains normal. If IPG is not available, a limited venogram should be performed; if the result is negative, the lead-lined apron should be removed and a complete venogram should be performed.

It is highly likely that duplex ultrasonography will complement the IPG for the diagnosis of DVT during pregnancy. If the duplex ultrasound is clearly abnormal and demonstrates noncompressibility of a venous segment, a diagnosis of venous thrombosis can be made.

It is our opinion that the risks of the tests used for the diagnosis of pulmonary embolism are less than the risks of not treating pulmonary embolism, or of treating patients with anticoagulants for symptoms which are not caused by pulmonary embolism. If the clinical features are compatible with pulmonary embolism, perfusion lung scanning is performed. If this test is normal, pulmonary embolism can be excluded. If the perfusion lung scan shows one or more segmental defects, a ventilation scan is performed and, if the perfusion defect(s) is mismatched, the patient is treated with anticoagulants. Patients with segmental matched defect(s), subsegmental perfusion defect(s), or indeterminate lung scans are candidates for pulmonary angiography because these scan patterns do not exclude pulmonary embolism.

## ANTICOAGULANTS

### SIDE EFFECTS OF ANTICOAGULANTS IN PREGNANCY

Heparin does not cross the placenta and therefore might not be expected to produce fetal complications, whereas oral anticoagulants cross the placenta, enter the fetal circulation, and have the potential to produce adverse effects in the fetus. Two recent studies suggest that heparin therapy is relatively safe to the fetus. The first study reviewed published studies through 1986 and demonstrated that, when pregnancies associated with comorbid maternal conditions that could independently cause adverse fetal outcomes were excluded, the rate of adverse fetal outcomes in heparin-treated patients was similar to that in a normal population. The second study demonstrated that the rate of adverse fetal/neonatal outcomes was comparable to that in a normal population. Thus, it is likely that heparin therapy is safe for the fetus, whereas oral anticoagulants may not be, particularly during the first trimester.

The reported fetopathic effects of warfarin include the warfarin embryopathy and central nervous system abnormalities. Warfarin embryopathy consists of nasal hypoplasia or stippled epiphyses after in utero exposure to oral anticoagulants in the first trimester of pregnancy. Central nervous system abnormalities include dorsal midline dysplasia, ventral midline dysplasia, and hemorrhage.

The report by Iturbe-Alessio and coworkers (1986), which documented warfarin use in 72 pregnancies, is the only prospective study that looked for congenital malformations following warfarin.[†] Warfarin embryopathy occurred in 10 of 35 (28.5%) infants after warfarin exposure during the 7th to the 12th week of gestation, and in none of the infants in whom warfarin was discontinued between 6 and 12 weeks of gestation. There were no central nervous system abnormalities reported.

## MATERNAL COMPLICATIONS

The most common maternal complication is hemorrhage. A recent study of 100 consecutive pregnancies associated with heparin therapy reported a bleeding rate of 2%.

## HEPARIN-INDUCED OSTEOPOROSIS

Two recent studies suggest that although symptomatic fractures are a rare complication of heparin therapy, a subclinical reduction in bone density occurs more commonly. The mechanism for heparin-associated osteoporosis is unknown. Although osteoporosis is an uncommon but real complication of heparin therapy, the true risk of developing heparin-induced osteoporosis is also unknown. There may be a dose effect. A subclinical reduction in bone density may be a relatively common sequel to long-term heparin therapy.

## TREATMENT OF VENOUS THROMBOEMBOLISM IN PREGNANCY

### ANTICOAGULANT THERAPY DURING PREGNANCY

Heparin is the anticoagulant of choice during pregnancy. Oral anticoagulants are probably contraindicated at all times during pregnancy unless heparin cannot be given.

---

[†] Iturbe-Allisio I, del Carmen Fonseca M, Mutchinik O, et al. Risks of anticoagulant therapy in pregnant women with artificial heart valves. N Engl J Med 1986;315:1390.

## USE OF ANTICOAGULANTS IN THE NURSING MOTHER

Heparin is not secreted into breast milk and can be safely administered to nursing mothers. There have been two convincing reports that warfarin does not induce an anticoagulant effect in the breast-fed infant when the drug is administered to a nursing mother.

## A SUGGESTED APPROACH TO THE TREATMENT OF VENOUS THROMBOEMBOLISM IN PREGNANCY

Patients who develop deep vein thrombosis or pulmonary embolism during pregnancy should be treated by continuous intravenous infusion of heparin for 5 to 14 days to maintain the activated partial thromboplastin time (aPTT) at 1.5 to 2 times control (equivalent to a heparin level of 0.2 to 0.5 U/mL). This should be followed by subcutaneous heparin given in therapeutic doses for the duration of the pregnancy. Subcutaneous heparin is administered every 12 hours in a dose that maintains the midinterval aPTT between 1.5 and 2 times control.

Patients with a past history of deep vein thrombosis or pulmonary embolism have a risk of recurrence that has been estimated at 5% to 12%. One option for these patients is to administer low-dose heparin in subsequent pregnancies during the first two trimesters and adjusted-dose subcutaneous heparin in therapeutic doses during the last trimester. The other option is to withhold anticoagulant prophylaxis and followup the patient with serial impedance plethysmography or duplex ultrasonography at weekly intervals.

## APPROACH TO THE PATIENT WHO IS BEING TREATED WITH LONG-TERM ANTICOAGULANTS AND PLANNING PREGNANCY

The correct approach to patients who are being treated with long-term oral anticoagulants and wish to become pregnant is problematic. Ideally, oral anticoagulant therapy should be replaced with heparin before conception. However, this may expose the patient to months of subcutaneous heparin therapy prior to conception. Results of a recently published cohort study suggest that there may be an alternative strategy that is more practical and reasonably safe. In this report, 12 patients with prosthetic heart valve replacements who were being treated with oral anticoagulants at the time of conception discontinued anticoagulant therapy at 6 weeks of pregnancy and none gave birth to children with warfarin embryopathy. It may therefore be reasonable to advise patients to have a diagnostic test for pregnancy performed frequently at appropriate times while they are attempting to conceive, and to replace oral anticoagulants with heparin when the test for pregnancy becomes positive, provided that pregnancy can be diagnosed within 6 weeks of conception.

# 44. COAGULATION DISORDERS IN PREGNANCY

Abnormal clotting may be identified when an unexpected aberration is noted on a routine laboratory bleeding profile or in association with a catastrophic event. Clotting abnormalities are commonly encountered in obstetrics, and hemorrhage remains a leading cause of maternal death.

## PHYSIOLOGY OF COAGULATION

The circulatory system depends on the interaction of platelets, the soluble coagulation components, and the vascular endothelium for both integrity and patency. An acquired or inherited abnormality affecting any subdivision can produce hypo- or hypercoagulability.

Hemostasis is commonly divided into two phases. First, a platelet plug forms at the site of endothelial disruption, effectively sealing the defect. Second, a fibrin cap forms over the platelet plug, strengthening and stabilizing it. Multiple regulatory systems exist to prevent extension of the clot past the site of endothelial damage.

## PREGNANCY-ASSOCIATED CHANGES IN COAGULATION

Pregnancy has a significant impact on the clotting system, presumably through enhanced hormonal synthesis (See Table 44-1). Interpretations of the various screening tests are listed in Table 44-2.

## SPECIALIZED TESTS

*Fibrin split products* (FSP) result from plasmin catabolism of fibrinogen and fibrin. Fragments X and Y are generated early in the degradation process; fragment Y is a particularly potent anticoagulant.

*Fibrinopeptide A* (FPA) is the first peptide cleaved from fibrinogen during thrombin-mediated fibrin generation. With a 3-minute half-life, the concentration of FPA directly reflects fibrin generation. A normal FPA during pregnancy is inconsistent with an acute thrombosis of any size.

*Antithrombin III* (AT III) inhibits most active soluble clotting components. AT III activity measurement has become one of the most useful laboratory parameters for monitoring the effect of therapy on DIC. Cessation of AT III consumption implies therapy has eliminated or blunted the causative process. The finding of a normal AT III value during pregnancy would be inconsistent with the diagnosis of DIC.

**460**

E. Albert Reece, John C. Hobbins, Maurice, J. Mahoney and Roy H. Petrie (Eds). *Handbook of Medicine of the Fetus & Mother.* Copyright © 1995 by J.B. Lippincott Company

**TABLE 44-1.** Changes in Coagulation During Pregnancy

| Increased | Unchanged | Decreased |
| --- | --- | --- |
| Fibrinogen (I) | II [ ↑ ] | XI |
| VII | V [ ↑ ] | XIII |
| VIII RC | IX [ ↑ ] | XIII platelets [→, ↑ ] |
| VIII RAg | Antithrombin III [ ↓ ] | |
| VIII RvWF | | |
| X | | |
| XII | | |
| Fibrinopeptide A | | |

[ ], controversial.
From Weiner CP. Evaluation of clotting disorders during pregnancy. In: Sciarra JJ, ed. Gynecology and obstetrics. Vol. 3. Philadelphia: JB Lippincott, 1988:5, with permission.

## DIAGNOSIS AND MANAGEMENT OF COAGULATION DISORDERS

### DISSEMINATED INTRAVASCULAR COAGULATION (DIC)

DIC is not a single clinical entity but an intermediate mechanism of a well-defined disease (Table 44-3). It exists whenever there is abnormal, intravascular activation of the clotting cascade, causing excess consumption of at least the soluble components. DIC is a continuum in which a variety of symptoms may appear. Its multiple presentations include hemorrhage, thrombosis, and laboratory abnormalities.

### Pathophysiology

The clinical disorders that trigger DIC produce excess systemic generation of thrombin and plasmin. Once abnormal coagulation has begun, the pathophysiology becomes intricate.

### Diagnosis

A patient who hemorrhages secondary to acute DIC has multiple hemostatic defects and bleeds from at least three sites at once (i.e., melena, hematuria, epistaxis, hemoptysis, oozing from puncture wounds, purpura, or petechiae). Shock associated with acute DIC is often out of proportion to the volume of blood loss. Renal failure is common. In contrast, patients with chronic DIC rarely have significant bleeding or other clinical findings. These patients are more likely to present with minor mucosal bleeding, hematuria, epistaxis, or easy bruisability. They are at greater risk to decompensate with an additional hemostatic stress. Settings for chronic DIC include malignancy, preeclampsia, and intrauterine fetal demise.

Laboratory confirmation of the clinical diagnosis should be obtained. Characteristic findings include prolongation of the PT, prolongation of the PTT, an abnormal platelet count (low and high), abnormal clotting factor concentrations, elevated FSP, abnormal clot retraction, reduced antithrombin III activity, a positive protamine sulfate test, leukocytosis, and schistocytosis on a smear of peripheral

**TABLE 44-2.** Laboratory Tests in Bleeding Disorders

| Bleed | PTT/PT | Bleeding Time | Platelet Count | Fibrinogen | Common Causes — Acquired | Common Causes — Hereditary |
|---|---|---|---|---|---|---|
| – | P/N | N | N | N | Lupus anticoagulant | High molecular weight kinogen, prekallikrein, factor XII deficiencies |
| + | P/N | N | N | N | Heparin, factor VIII inhibitors | Hemophilia A and B, factor XI deficiency |
| + | P/P | N | N | N | Heparin, coumarin, vitamin K deficiency, antibiotics | Deficiency in factors V, X, and II and dysfibrinogenemia |
| + | N/P | N | N | N |  | Factor VII deficiency |
| + | P/N | P | N | N | Lupus-like anticoagulant, factor VIII complex inhibitor | von Willebrand's syndrome |
| + | P/P | P | N |  |  | Afibrinogenemia |
| + | N/N | P |  | N | Thrombocytopenia secondary to immune thrombotic thrombocytopenia (ITP), drugs, etc. | Aldrich's syndrome, others |
| + | N/N | N | N | N |  | Factor XIII deficiency |
| + | P/P |  |  |  | DIC, liver disease |  |

–, absent; +, present; N, normal; P, prolonged.
Modified from Colman RW, Hirsh J, Marder VJ, Salzman EW. Approach to the bleeding patient. In: Colman RW, Hirsh J, Marder VJ, Salzman EW. Hemostasis and thrombosis. Philadelphia: JB Lippincott, 1982:700, with permission.

**TABLE 44-3.** Conditions Associated with DIC

Obstetrical Accidents
  Abruptio placentae
  Dead fetus syndrome
  Amniotic fluid embolus
  Saline abortion
  Preeclampsia eclampsia syndrome
Septicemia
  Gram-negative (endotoxin)
  Gram-positive (mucopolysaccharides?)
Viremia (varicella)
Intravascular Hemolysis
  Multiple transfusions (banked whole blood)
  Hemolytic transfusion reaction
Vascular Disorders
Acid-Base Imbalance
Hypoxic-ischemic Endothelial Damage

Modified from Wiener CP. Treatment of clotting disorders during pregnancy. In: Sciarra JJ, ed. Gynecology and obstetrics. Vol. 3. Philadelphia: JB Lippincott, 1988:2, with permission.

blood. In acute DIC, each parameter can be abnormal. In chronic DIC, only individual factor consumption rates may be elevated, while many of the previously noted tests remain normal.

Usually, the level of AT III declines as consumption exceeds production. However, in patients with malignancy and diabetes, AT III can behave as an acute phase reactant and may be normal or slightly increased despite rapid consumption. Thus, sensitivity of the test is reduced.

## Treatment

The primary therapeutic goal is to treat the underlying disorder and remove the triggering event (Table 44-4). When DIC is accompanied by hemorrhage, treatment must be accompanied by aggressive support of blood volume and pressure (i.e., volume replacement with crystalloids and colloids, antibiotic therapy, pressor medications). Underreplacement is a common error. Component replacement (platelets, cryoprecipitate, or fresh-frozen plasma) may occasionally be helpful to aid oozing from a wound associated with laboratory abnormalities.

Anticoagulation should be initiated only when the aforementioned measures fail to correct a clinically significant DIC. This situation is exceedingly rare in the obstetric patient. Observation for at least 4 hours after treatment of the underlying disease (if the hemorrhage is not severe) is recommended prior to starting anticoagulants. This allows adequate time for laboratory evaluation to identify the precise clotting defect. AT III activity should be determined during the observational period if heparin therapy is contemplated.

A reasonable approach consists of the subcutaneous administration of heparin (5000 U) every 8 to 12 hours. The PTT should normalize with treatment. AT III concentrate alone has been used successfully to treat acute DIC secondary to obstetric complications.

**TABLE 44-4.** Suggested Therapy for Acute DIC

---

Treatment or Removal of the Triggering Event
  Evacuation of the uterus
  Antibiotics
  Volume replacement and expansion (crystalloid, Plasmanate, albumin)
Component Therapy
  Packed red cells
  Platelets
  Fresh-frozen plasma
  Prothrombin complex
Anticoagulant Therapy
  Low-dose heparin
  Heparin
  Antiplatelet drugs (chronic DIC)
  Antithrombin III concentrates
Inhibition of Residual Fibrinolysis
  E-amino caproic acid
  Caution: ventricular arrhythmias, hypotension, hypokalemia

---

From Wiener CP. Treatment of clotting disorders during pregnancy. In: Sciarra JJ, ed. Gynecology and obstetrics. Vol 3. Philadelphia: JB Lippincott, 1988:4, with permission.

## Obstetric Causes

**Preeclampsia/Eclampsia Syndrome.** Overt DIC is uncommon in women with preeclampsia. Although thrombocytopenia is present in some 10% of women with severe preeclampsia/eclampsia, only a small percentage develop symptomatic bleeding.

There is now overwhelming evidence that a subclinical, consumptive coagulopathy is typical in women with the clinical diagnosis of preeclampsia. A decline in platelet number is one of the earliest laboratory signs of preeclampsia. A significant and pathologic decrease in AT III occurs in women with preeclampsia proportional to severity, which is secondary to increased consumption.

**Abruptio Placentae.** About 20% of women with abruptio placentae have a gross defect in clotting. Thus, placental abruption is probably the most common obstetric cause of acute DIC. One-fourth of patients with a gross clotting defect will hemorrhage postpartum.

The basic tenets of therapy for abruptio placentae follow the general guidelines for management of DIC. The uterus should be emptied and the blood volume vigorously supported with crystalloid, colloid, or blood products as necessary. Although coagulation components are rarely required antepartum for vaginal delivery, their use may be prudent if surgical intervention is contemplated. Oxytocin remains an effective stimulant of labor in most cases. Once emptied, even the Couvelaire uterus responds well to oxytocin. Patients with a suspected small abruption remote from term may be managed expectantly if their symptoms resolve, laboratory abnormalities do not exist, and fetal surveillance tests remain normal.

**Fetal Death Syndrome.** The onset of fetal death syndrome (FDS) is gradual. Most laboratory abnormalities are not detectable until 3 to 4 weeks after the demise, although the concentration of fibrinopeptide A rises within days. The laboratory picture is consistent with a true chronic DIC condition. Its cause is unknown.

Approximately 80% of women with an intrauterine fetal demise (IUFD) labor spontaneously within 2 to 3 weeks. The advent and availability of prostaglandin $E_2$ has simplified management considerably. The treatment of a medically stable patient with an intrauterine, singleton fetal demise is now delivery.

Heparin is the treatment of choice for the mother whose coagulopathy is associated with FDS. Most women require 5000 to 10,000 U subcutaneously twice a day rather than a larger dose of heparin.

**Septic Abortion.** Another well-documented obstetric cause of DIC is septic abortion.

*Pathophysiology.* There is a high correlation between the severity of the disease and the degree of coagulopathy. Bacterial endotoxin is likely the initiating mechanism. The main clinical findings of septic shock are attributable to DIC.

*Treatment.* The two goals of therapy are prevention and treatment of the underlying disease. The general protocol for the treatment of DIC applies with a few minor modifications. Aggressive antibiotic therapy and evacuation of the uterus in the absence of shock are the foundation of treatment.

When septic shock is present, crystalloid or colloid fluid replacement should be guided by a pulmonary artery catheter. The pulmonary capillary wedge pressure is nearly always low. Lactated Ringer's solution should also be avoided because it might potentiate the metabolic acidosis. High doses of corticosteroids (30 mg/kg) may be of use stabilizing biomembranes, exerting a positive inotropic effect upon the heart, dilating the vasculature, and preventing beta-endorphin release by the pituitary. In reference to the latter, pretreatment with naloxone may reduce the severity of septic shock.

In the absence of a definitive study, heparin therapy in septic shock becomes a matter of physician choice. Coagulation factor replacement is best done with fresh-frozen plasma, because cryoprecipitate has little AT III. However, in one situation, heparin administration does seem indicated. Prophylactic administration of heparin to women with septic abortions decreases the incidence of subsequent septic shock and reduces the level of soluble fibrin monomer to normal; 5000 U of subcutaneous heparin given two or three times daily is sufficient.

**Saline Abortion.** Increased consumption of intrinsic clotting cascade factors, increased FSP, and decreased platelet count occur during saline abortion. If one defines a significant hemorrhage as requiring a transfusion, 1% to 2% of women undergoing a saline abortion experience hemorrhage.

**Amniotic Fluid Embolus.** Amniotic fluid embolus (AFE) complicates between 1 per 7000 and 1 per 300,000 deliveries. Despite the small numbers of AFE cases, 5% to 10% of the maternal mortality in industrialized countries is attributed to AFE. The associated mortality rate approximates 80%.

*Diagnosis.* An AFE may occur at any time during the peripartal period, although the classic description involves an elderly multiparous woman with a large, term, meconium-stained infant, in the midst of or just having completed a vigorous labor with intact membranes when profound cardiovascular collapse occurs. This is considered Phase 1. Phase 2 begins 0.5 to 4 hours after the first phase, with the onset of uterine bleeding refractory to oxytocin, bleeding from old puncture sites, and easy bruisability. There are few adequately documented cases of hemorrhage associated with AFE without preceding cardiovascular symptoms.

The finding of fetal squames in a right-sided cardiac blood sample is consistent with but not diagnostic of AFE.

Only 45% of patients survive Phase 1. The survivors are at risk to develop severe coagulopathy and uterine atony during Phase 2.

**Treatment.** A well-documented, successful therapeutic protocol does not exist, due to the rarity of AFE. During Phase 1, therapy is directed toward cardiovascular and ventilatory support. A pulmonary artery catheter should be placed without delay. A clotting profile and heparinized sample for histologic study, as well as several extra tubes of citrated blood for later study, should next be drawn from the catheter. Liberal use of dopamine (or similar agent) and colloids as dictated by the information obtained from the pulmonary artery catheter is recommended for cardiovascular support. Fluid overload must be carefully avoided. Rapid digitalization may help. Intubation is the key to ventilatory support.

It is unclear whether the AFE-associated coagulopathy can be prevented. In one report, a patient survived a presumed AFE after administration of a small dose of heparin. Based on this one case report, a single intravenous heparin bolus of 3000 to 5000 U as soon as the diagnosis is made would appear to be an option.

Once fibrin-fibrinogenolysis is well established, component replacement alone may be adequate. Should the patient fail to respond to this plan, the administration of an antifibrinolytic agent (epsilon-amino caproic acid or aprotonin) should be considered. The dose of e-amino caproic acid is 4 g to 6 g every 4 to 6 hours.

**Other Obstetrically Related Causes.** Other purported causes of DIC include placenta previa, placenta accreta, degenerating leiomyomas, and hydatidiform mole.

### Nonobstetric Causes

**Antibiotics.** A continually growing number of broad-spectrum antibiotics are associated with hypoprothrombinemia and thrombocytopenia (Table 44-5).

**Acquired Inhibitors.** Specific inhibitors of individual clotting factors have been identified in previously healthy women during pregnancy. These frequently are antibodies. Inhibitors of factors V, VIII:C, VIII:RCoF, IX, XI, and XIII have all been reported. The two most common inhibitors are a lupus anticoagulant and an antifactor VIII antibody.

A factor deficit is most easily differentiated from an inhibitor by performing a 1:1 mix of the patient's plasma with normal plasma. If the clotting time remains prolonged, an inhibitor is present. However, a low-titer inhibitor may become apparent only after incubating the plasma mix. An antibody inhibitor usually shows progressive, time-dependent prolongation of the clotting time.

## HEREDITARY COAGULOPATHIES

The hereditary coagulopathies comprise the smallest group of patients suffering a clotting abnormality seen by the practicing obstetrician. A genetically determined defect has been identified at most points in the coagulation cascade. This discussion focuses on the more common of these defects.

**TABLE 44-5.** Antibiotics and Hemostasis

Hypoprothrombinemic
  Ampicillin
  Cephamandole
  Cefoperazone
  Moxalactam
  Penicillin G
  Tetracycline
  Chloramphenicol
Inhibit Platelet Function
  Carbenicillin
  Sulbenicillin
  Ticarcillin
  Piperacillin
  Mezlocillin
  Azlocillin
  Cephalothin (asymptomatic)
  Moxalactam
  Cefazolin (with uremia)
Coumadin Effect
  Nalidixic acid
  Sulfonamides
  Metronidazole
  Chloramphenicol
  Rifampin

From Weiner CP. Treatment of clotting disorders during pregnancy. In: Sciarra JJ, ed. Gynecology and obstetrics. Vol. 3. Philadelphia: JB Lippincott, 1988:12, with permission.

## Von Willebrand's Syndrome

Von Willebrand's syndrome (VWS) is a heterogeneous group of disorders usually inherited as an autosomal dominant trait. One especially severe form is inherited as an autosomal recessive trait.

The two most common forms of VWS are classic (Type I) and variant I (Type IIA). Each is associated with a prolonged bleeding time, decreased platelet adhesiveness, and decreased levels of VIII:C, VIII:RA, and VIII:RCoF. The variant is a qualitative VIII:RA disorder, whereas the classic is a deficiency state. Selective replacement of VIII:C does not correct the bleeding time. VIII:RCoF administration not only corrects the bleeding time, but also stimulates a transient increase in VIII:RA and VIII:C out of proportion to the amount of VIII:RCoF infused. The clinical risk of hemorrhage in patients with VWS correlates best with either the VIII:RCoF concentration or bleeding time.

VIII:C, VIII:RA, and VIII:RCoF usually increase to hemostatic levels during pregnancy. This gradual increase (when it occurs) starts after 11 to 12 weeks gestation. The increase is uniform in neither occurrence nor degree. Therefore, it should not be assumed that factor VIII complex is increasing. Further, the individual components decrease postpartum at a varying rate, which could account for the 20% incidence of postpartum hemorrhage. Patients who spontaneously or electively abort are at significant risk for hemorrhage. A baseline VIII:RCoF should be obtained early in pregnancy and again once or twice in the third trimester should the initial value be abnormal.

In the absence of a significant surgical challenge, a 50% level of VIII:RCoF is sufficient for most hemostatic stresses. But delivery constitutes a profound hemostatic challenge. An episiotomy should be avoided, as should the deep injection of a local anesthetic and conduction anesthesia. Cryoprecipitate should be available in case of emergency. Prophylactic transfusion of cryoprecipitate is indicated for vaginal delivery if the VIII:RCoF level fails to reach 80% by term. Postpartum, serial VIII:RCoF levels/bleeding times are obtained and cryoprecipitate therapy given for 7 days to prevent delayed hemorrhage. Cryoprecipitate should be given regardless of the laboratory parameters to all but the mildest cases of VWS if cesarean section is contemplated. Enough cryoprecipitate should be given to raise the VIII:RCoF level above 100%. Postoperatively, the VIII:RCoF level is maintained at 100% until the abdominal sutures are removed. The cryoprecipitate dose is empiric. Fifteen to 20 units are usually necessary twice daily in severe disease.

The fetus is assumed affected unless proven otherwise. The use of a scalp electrode is precluded. Fetal hemorrhage during labor due to VWS is rare. Prenatal diagnosis is possible from fetal blood. Type I is usually a mild condition, so that cordocentesis can usually be performed without significant risk of maternal hemorrhage. Type IIA, however, can be severe, and maternal transfusion of cryoprecipitate may be necessary prior to cordocentesis.

## Hemophilia A and B

Hemophilia A and B are characterized, respectively, by low levels of either factor VIII coagulant (VIII:C) or factor IX coagulant (IX:C) activity, and a normal to increased level of the factor-related antigen (RA). Both are X-linked and cannot be distinguished clinically from each other. Eighty-five percent of hemophilia is hemophilia A.

The task of the obstetrician in reference to hemophilia includes carrier identification, treatment of the symptomatic pregnant women, and prenatal diagnosis. Because one X chromosome is randomly inactivated in each cell (lyonization), the average ratio of the related antigen to coagulant activity is 2:1. Measurement of this ratio allows the diagnosis of 80% to 90% of nonpregnant carrier women. Although the ratio of antigen to coagulant activity increases with increasing gestational age to a variable degree, pregnant women should not be denied carrier analysis if prior to 20 weeks gestation.

Rarely, carriers of hemophilia are symptomatic. Those women whose VIII:C activity is less than 50% at delivery and who undergo cesarean section should be given cryoprecipitate adequate to elevate the VIII:C level above 80% prior to surgery and to keep it above 30% to 40% for 3 to 4 days postoperatively. If the VIII:C level is less than 30%, cryoprecipitate should be given prior to delivery regardless of the type. In contrast to hemophilia A, fresh-frozen plasma rather than cryoprecipitate is given to women with hemophilia B.

Hemophilia A and B may be diagnosed prenatally by either DNA analysis or direct study of fetal blood. By the midsecond trimester, definitive diagnosis of fetal hemophilia A is possible by measuring the ratio of VIII:RA to VIII:CA in a blood sample obtained by cordocentesis. Prenatal diagnosis of an affected fetus changes intrapartum and early postnatal management. Intrapartum use of scalp electrodes, the vacuum extractor, forceps, and prolonged labor should be avoided.

## Antithrombin III Deficiency

AT III is the major in vivo inhibitor of thrombin activity. The incidence of AT III deficiency in the general population is about 1 per 2000. This makes AT III deficiency the most common clotting disorder in women.

Pregnancy exponentially increases the risk of thrombosis in women with AT III deficiency. Approximately two-thirds of pregnant women with congenital AT III deficiency suffer thrombosis; 75% of these occur antepartum.

The ideal regimen for thrombosis prophylaxis during pregnancy of women with an AT III deficiency has been somewhat controversial. The most commonly recommended regimen employs subcutaneous heparin throughout the pregnancy. AT III concentrate can be given during labor or if a thrombosis develops.

Patients with AT III deficiency are resistant to heparin, so that a quantity of heparin required for a given effect is usually larger than in the nondeficient patient. Effective prophylaxis requires enough heparin administered subcutaneously to prolong the activated partial thromboplastin time 5 to 10 seconds above the patient's baseline throughout the pregnancy and puerperium. The PTT should be measured just prior to the next dose. Heparin therapy is continued at least 4 weeks after completion of the pregnancy, or the patient can be converted over to chronic warfarin anticoagulation postpartum. Danazol in a dose of 400 to 600 mg/day may increase the AT III activity so that anticoagulation is no longer necessary. The newborn delivered to a woman with AT III deficiency is at risk for inheriting the disease. Possible neonatal complications include fatal thrombosis. The newborn's plasma AT III activity should be measured.

## Protein C, Protein S, Other Inherited Coagulation Disorders

Protein C deficiency is an autosomal dominant trait with incomplete penetrance. The heterozygous disorder is associated with a propensity for venous thrombosis in early adulthood. Pregnant patients may exhibit manifestations of protein C deficiency, presenting with thromboembolism. Warfarin is the treatment of choice for this deficiency state, but during pregnancy full anticoagulation with heparin is advised. A deficiency of protein S, a protein C cofactor, is also associated with outcomes similar to protein C. Prenatal diagnosis is possible for each of these disorders, using cordocentesis.

Factor V deficiency is an autosomal recessive disorder. The major risk to the pregnant patient is postpartum hemorrhage. Fresh-frozen plasma is the treatment of choice.

Factor XI deficiency is an autosomal recessive disorder most common among Jewish families. Fresh-frozen plasma to maintain the activity level above 20% during the labor, delivery, and postpartum periods is recommended.

Factor XII deficiency is an autosomal dominant trait, and affected women tolerate pregnancy well.

Factor XIII deficiency is an autosomal recessive disorder. Factor XIII declines during normal pregnancy, although women with a factor XIII deficiency reportedly tolerate pregnancy well. The risk of postpartum hemorrhage seems increased.

## PLATELET DISORDERS

Quantitative or qualitative platelet disorders are common causes of abnormal coagulation in a pregnant woman. Platelet disorders often manifest as bleeding from mucous membranes or into the skin. Other findings include easy bruising, epistaxis, gastrointestinal or gingival bleeding, hematuria, menorrhagia, and petechiae. Maternal or fetal central nervous system hemorrhage is the most serious complication.

### Thrombocytopenia

Thrombocytopenia is defined as a platelet count less than 150,000 platelets/mm$^3$.

Thrombocytopenia may result from either decreased platelet production or increased platelet consumption/destruction. This distinction is based on measurement of the mean platelet volume and a bone marrow evaluation.

Environmental causes of thrombocytopenia include drugs, chemicals, and ionizing radiation (Table 44-6). Almost all medications have been implicated in one or more cases of thrombocytopenia. Because this is a very common cause of thrombocytopenia, a careful search for drug exposure should be made. Drug-induced thrombocytopenia usually resolves once the drug exposure ceases.

**Immune Thrombocytopenic Purpura.** The diagnosis of immune thrombocytopenic purpura (ITP) is made by demonstration of a platelet-associated antibody and the exclusion of all the other causes of thrombocytopenia. Abnormal skin and mucous membrane bleeding appear when the platelet count declines below 100,000 cells/mm$^3$. Counts below 20,000 cells/mm$^3$ are associated with spontaneous bleeding. Specific complications and bleeding severity vary greatly between patients.

**TABLE 44-6.** Drugs that May Produce Thrombocytopenia

Drugs That Suppress the Marrow
    Cytotoxic agents such as those used in cancer chemotherapy (nitrogen mustard, cyclophosphamide, 5-fluorouracil, methotrexate, and many others)

Drugs That by Immune Mechanisms Accelerate Platelet Destruction
    Chlorothiazides
    Chlorpropamide
    Diazepam
    Diphenylhydantoin
    Gold salts
    Quinidine
    Quinine
    Sulfisoxazole

Drugs Whose Mechanism of Antiplatelet Activity Is Unknown
    Acetaminophen
    Aminopyrine
    Chlorpromazine
    Cimetidine
    Furosemide
    Heparin
    Heroin
    Penicillamine
    Penicillin
    Phenylbutazone
    Various sulfonamides
    Tolbutamide

From Anderson HM. Maternal hematologic disorders. In: Creasy RK, Resnik R, eds. Maternal-fetal medicine: principles and practice. Philadelphia: WB Saunders, 1989:908, with permission.

Mild thrombocytopenia unassociated with other abnormalities needs no treatment. Epidural anesthesia is felt to be safe during the labor of a patient with an unexplained thrombocytopenia if the platelet count is at least 100,000 cells/mm$^3$.

**Treatment.** Corticosteroid therapy should be initiated when the platelet declines below 100,000/mm$^3$ secondary to an immune mechanism. Prednisone 80 to 100 mg/day in divided doses is given. Patient activity should be restricted if the count is below 50,000/mm$^3$ to avoid hemorrhage secondary to trauma. The platelet count should begin to improve within 3 to 10 days of initiating therapy. The steroid dose is tapered to the minimum value that permits a stable count once the platelet count exceeds 100,000/mm$^3$. Splenectomy during pregnancy may precipitate abortion and has been virtually replaced by steroid and other medical treatments. Platelet transfusion is only transiently effective in immune-mediated disorders.

Intravenous gamma globulin (400 mg/kg/day for 5 days) recently has been employed to treat immune thrombocytopenia during pregnancy. Most women respond to therapy with an increased platelet count within a few days of the initiation. The improvement may last from a few days to a few weeks. The neonatal response is more variable.

**Fetal Considerations.** The treatment of maternal ITP during pregnancy with steroids, splenectomy, or intravenous gamma globulin is successful. However, to date treatment has had no beneficial effect on the circulating antiplatelet IgG titers that cross the placenta to the fetus.

Cesarean section delivery was, in the past, recommended for all patients with thrombocytopenia. This was unnecessary for most pregnancies. Fetal scalp blood sampling permits a fetal platelet count early in labor (about 3 to 4 cm dilation). This technique is safe, with a low incidence of false-negative results. Vaginal delivery is considered safe if fetal platelet counts are >50,000.

The infant should be watched closely after birth. Infants not thrombocytopenic at birth may become so within the first few days of life.

**Alloimmune Thrombocytopenia in the Fetus.** Alloimmune thrombocytopenia is the platelet equivalent of Rh sensitization. The diagnosis is most often made following the birth of an affected sibling. The sensitized mother produces IgG antibodies to a foreign platelet antigen. The majority of cases of alloimmune thrombocytopenia are caused by PLA 1, PLGrLyC1, and PLGrLyB1, with greater than 50% of cases related to PLA 1. PLA 1 occurs in 98% of the population. By present laboratory methods, there is no correlation between the maternal antiplatelet antibody titers and the severity of the disease.

About 90% of children present with only mild bleeding, which resolves without residual deficits within 1 to 4 weeks after birth. However, there is still a high rate of perinatal morbidity and a 10% incidence of perinatal mortality, usually due to intracranial hemorrhage (ICH). About a third of ICHs occur in utero. The risk of early neonatal bleeding is 20%.

**Treatment.** Antepartum maternal therapy has met with varying success until recently. Corticosteroid therapy often has no effect on the fetal platelet count. Bussel and coworkers (1988) treated seven patients with intravenous gamma globulin 1.0 g/kg body weight, infused over 4 to 7 hours once a week.* Six patients

---

*Bussel JB, Berkowitz RL, McFarland JG, Lynch L, Chitkara V. Antenatal treatment of neonatal alloimmune thrombocytopenia. N Engl J Med 1988;319:1374. Also In utero platelet transfusion for alloimmune thrombocytopenia. Lancet 1988;2:1307.

had serial fetal blood samples performed prior to delivery (second sample 4 to 6 weeks after start of treatment), and all had improvement of the fetal platelet count. Other authors have been concerned that the incidence of fetal ICH increases markedly after 30 weeks gestation and have recommended intravenous fetal transfusion of maternal washed platelets (PLA 1 negative) to alleviate thrombocytopenia and prevent ICH.

We believe a combination of these approaches seems prudent. When an affected fetus is documented, intravenous gamma globulin therapy should be initiated. In the authors' hands, the addition of dexamethasone has benefited select fetuses. Only when the fetus was unresponsive to medical therapy would transfusion be necessary. This sequence would reduce the number of fetal platelet transfusions needed. Further investigation continues.

**Thrombotic Thrombocytopenic Purpura.** Classically, thrombotic thrombocytopenic purpura (TTP) is characterized by a diagnostic pentad of fever, microangiopathic hemolytic anemia, thrombocytopenia, central nervous system (CNS) symptoms, and renal impairment. An increase in the ratio of thromboxane to prostacyclin is thought to contribute to the development of widespread microvascular thrombi in TTP. The thrombi in TTP represent aggregated platelets without fibrin. DIC is uncommonly associated with TTP. The AT III level is normal in TTP. Unless treatment is successful, the usual course of this disease is progressive deterioration followed by death within 3 months.

Although TTP manifests as increased platelet destruction and decreased platelet survival similar to DIC, fibrinogen turnover is normal in TTP. Coagulation tests or factors are almost always normal in patients with TTP. TTP places both mother and fetus at extreme jeopardy. Only 25% (10/40) of maternal-infant pairs survived when antepartum TTP was present.

***Treatment.*** Based on literature review, the following treatment protocol for TTP in pregnancy is suggested. Plasma exchange with donor plasma should be initiated promptly, exchanging one plasma volume during the first 24 hours. The concentration of lactic dehydrogenase (LDH) levels is monitored as an indicator of ongoing hemolysis and ischemic tissue damage. If there is no or inadequate response, glucocorticoids (the equivalent of 1 to 2 mg/kg/day of prednisone) and antiplatelet agents are added. Splenectomy during pregnancy should be considered only as a last resort.

***Fetal Considerations.*** Maternal TTP does not improve with delivery. Successful treatment may allow the pregnancy to be lengthened by 4 weeks or more. Preterm delivery may be necessary because of fetal compromise.

**Other Disorders.** Other pregnancy-associated disorders may present similarly to TTP (Table 44-7).

***Preeclampsia.*** Preeclampsia can be confused with TTP, especially when its manifestations include thrombocytopenia, microangiopathic hemolysis, and renal failure. TTP may also be mistakenly diagnosed as severe preeclampsia. The differences in maternal serum AT III activity may aid in the diagnosis. AT III activity is decreased in women with severe preeclampsia, but remains stable in TTP and hemolytic uremic syndrome.

The following management protocol is suggested when the differential diagnosis is TTP versus severe atypical preeclampsia. If the AT III activity level is normal, the fetus is not compromised, and the amniotic fluid studies are incom-

**TABLE 44-7.** Differentiating Causes of Thrombocytopenia in Pregnancy

|  | TTP | HUS | Preeclampsia | ITP |
|---|---|---|---|---|
| Clinics |  |  |  |  |
| CNS | + | − | + | − |
| Fever | + | − | − | − |
| Hypertension | − | − | + | − |
| Petechiae | + | − | + | + |
| Laboratory |  |  |  |  |
| Hemolytic anemia | + | + | + | − |
| Lactate dehydrogenase | ↑ | ↑ | ↑ | N |
| SGOT/SGPT | N | N | ↑ | N |
| Antithrombin III activity | N | N | ↓ | N |
| Autoantibodies | − | − | − | I |
| Proteinuria | + | + | + | − |
| Serum creatinine | ↑ | ↑ | ↑ | N |
| Blood urea nitrogen | ↑ | ↑ | ↑ | N |

CNS, central nervous system symptoms; HUS, hemolytic uremic syndrome; ITP, idiopathic thrombocytopenic purpura; N, normal; SGOT, serum glutamic-oxalacetic transaminase; SGPT, serum glutamic-pyruvic transaminase; TTP, thrombotic thrombocytopenia purpura; +, present; -, absent; ↑, increased; ↓, decreased.

patible with fetal lung maturity, a trial of plasma therapy should be instituted and continued until the postpartum period, when a remission has been achieved. It should not be discontinued during the pregnancy. The likelihood of relapse is increased during pregnancy. If the patient does not respond, she should be delivered.

**Postpartum Hemolytic Uremic Syndrome.** Hemolytic uremic syndrome (HUS) is often confused with TTP. It too can present with microangiopathic anemia, thrombocytopenia, and renal failure. HUS may be associated with seizures due to renal failure or hypertension, but is rarely associated with neurologic changes. Other distinguishing features of HUS include the following:

- History of a prodromal gastrointestinal disorder with diarrhea
- Early, severe renal failure with anuria and hypertension
- Milder bleeding and thrombocytopenia than in TTP
- Onset 48hours after a normal delivery.

The primary coagulation defect in HUS involves the platelet. Thrombocytopenia is often but not always present. AT III activity is usually normal. In contrast to TTP, FSP are frequently increased, possibly due to fibrinogen rather than fibrin degradation. Urinary free hemoglobin is common secondary to hemolysis. Treatment recommendations for HUS are similar to those for TTP, with the addition of dialysis.

## Functional Platelet Defects
Acquired disorders of platelet function can occur in conjunction with medical illnesses such as uremia, myeloproliferative disorders, and congestive heart failure. Drug-induced platelet dysfunction is much more common in pregnancy.

# 45. HEMATOLOGIC DISORDERS OF PREGNANCY

## DEFINITION

Anemia is usually defined as a hemoglobin (Hgb) value below the lower limits of normal not explained by the state of hydration. The normal hemoglobin level for the adult female is $14.0 \pm 2.0 \, g/dL$. The above definition has physiologic validity in that it is the amount of Hgb per unit volume of blood that determines the $O_2$ carrying capacity of blood. On the basis of the above normal value, 20% to 60% of prenatal patients will be found to be anemic at some time during their pregnancy. Some centers choose to use slightly lower Hgb values (11.0 or 10.5 g/dL) to define anemia during pregnancy. Symptoms due to anemia are those of tissue hypoxia, those of the cardiovascular system's attempts to compensate for the anemia, and/or symptoms due to an underlying disease. Tissue hypoxia produces fatigue, lightheadedness, weakness, and exertional dyspnea. Cardiovascular compensation leads to symptoms of a hyperdynamic circulation such as palpitations and tachycardia. However, in obstetric patients anemia is most commonly discovered because a complete blood count (CBC) is obtained as part of routine laboratory evaluation either at the initial prenatal or at 28 to 32 weeks gestation.

## USE OF THE COMPLETE BLOOD COUNT (CBC)

Anemia is not a diagnosis but rather a sign such as fever or edema. The key issue in the evaluation of anemia is to define the mechanism or disease process. To properly evaluate and cure anemia, one must resolve the following:

1. What is the morphology of the anemia?
2. What is the reticulocyte count?
3. What is the mechanism of the anemia?
4. Is there an underlying disease?
5. What is appropriate treatment?

The CBC and the reticulocyte count provide the answers to the first three questions and are really the hematologist's "critical biopsy." These data allow a morphological classification of the anemia and define whether the marrow is hyper- or hypoproliferative. Table 45-1 presents normal values for women. The peripheral blood smear also allows evaluation of the white cells (WBCs). In most cases of leukemia, abnormal granulocytes or lymphocytes appear. The presence of nucleated RBCs in association with marked poikilocytosis suggests erythroleukemia, myeloid metaplasia, or marrow infiltration with solid tumor or granulomatous infection. Although use of the CBC allows an excellent first approximate at the diagnosis of anemia, additional studies are usually necessary to confirm the diagnosis. Table 45-2 details laboratory studies frequently used in the evaluation of an anemic patient.

E. Albert Reece, John C. Hobbins, Maurice, J. Mahoney and Roy H. Petrie (Eds). *Handbook of Medicine of the Fetus & Mother.* Copyright © 1995 by J.B. Lippincott Company

**TABLE 45-1.** Normal Values for Red Blood Cells

| | |
|---|---|
| Erythroid values | |
| Hemoglobin (HgB) | 12–16 g/dL |
| Hematocrit (Hct) | 36–46% |
| Red cell count (RBC) | 4.0–5.2 × $10^{12}$/L |
| Erythroid indices | |
| Mean corpuscular volume (MCV) | 80–100 fL |
| Mean corpuscular hemoglobin concentration (MCHC) | 31–36 g/dL |
| Red cell morphology | |
| Anisocytosis | Variation in cell size |
| Poikilocytosis | Variation in cell shape |
| Polychromatophilia | Amount of "blueness" |
| Hypochromia | Amount of central pallor |
| Platelet estimate | 5–10 platelets per oil immersion field |
| Reticulocyte count | 48–152 × $10^9$/L |
| White blood cell count | 5–14 × $10^9$/L |

**TABLE 45-2.** Laboratory Studies Useful in Evaluation of Anemia

| Study | Normal Value |
|---|---|
| Serum hemoglobin | <1.0 mg/dL |
| Serum haptoglobin | 30–200 mg/dL |
| Total bilirubin | 0.1–1.2 mg/dL |
| Direct Coombs' text | Negative |
| G-6-PD | |
| Electrophoresis | B+ (A+, A−, B− 150 others are abnormal) |
| Quantitative study | 4–8 U/g of Hgb |
| Hemoglobin electrophoresis | >98% A <br> <3.5% A2 <br> <2% F |
| RBC enzymes | Multiple types; pyruvate kinase most common |
| Osmotic fragility | Preincubation: 0.40–0.46% NaCl <br> Postincubation: 0.48–0.60% NaCl |
| Serum ferritin | >10 µg/L |
| Free erythrocyte protoporphyrin (FEP) | <3.0 µg/g |
| Plasma iron | 40–175 µg/dL |
| Plasma total iron-binding capacity | 216–400 µg/dL |
| Transferrin saturation | 16–60% |
| Stool guaiac | Negative |
| Serum folate | 6–12 µg/L |
| RBC folate | 165–760 µg/L |
| Serum $B_{12}$ | 190–950 ng/L |
| Anti-intrinsic factor antibody (AIF) | Negative |
| Bone marrow | Normal distribution of erythroid and myeloid precursors |

## NORMAL HEMATOLOGIC EVENTS ASSOCIATED WITH PREGNANCY

### BLOOD VOLUME CHANGES

Figure 45-1 depicts the changes in blood volume and RBC mass during pregnancy. Relative hemodilution is evident from early pregnancy and is maximum at 28 to 34 weeks. Although this dilutional effect will lower the Hgb, Hct, and RBC count, it causes no change in the mean corpuscular volume (MCV) or in the mean corpuscular hemoglobin concentration (MCHC). Thus, serial evaluation of these two indices is useful in differentiating dilutional anemia from progressive iron deficiency anemia during pregnancy. In the former, the indices do not change, whereas in the latter they decrease progressively.

### IRON KINETICS

Most healthy women have marginal iron stores and thus easily become iron deficient when subjected to the increased demands for iron imposed by pregnancy. Table 45-3 lists the iron requirements for pregnancy. If there is insufficient iron available to meet the demands of pregnancy, iron-deficient erythropoiesis will result, and finally anemia develops.

### FOLATE

During pregnancy there is a significant increase over the nonpregnant state requirement of folate from 50 μg/day to 800 to 1000 μg/day. When folate depletion occurs the usual sequence of events is a decreased serum folate, hypersegmentation of polymorphonuclear leukocytes, a decrease in RBC folate, the appearance of ovalocytes in the blood, development of an abnormal marrow, and finally anemia.

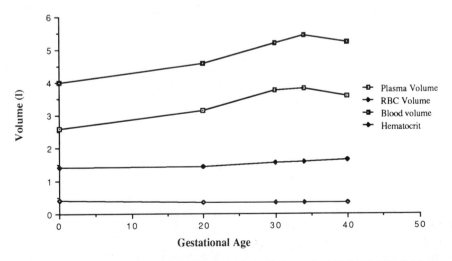

**FIGURE 45-1.** Hematologic changes during pregnancy. (Redrawn from Peck TM, Arias F. Hematologic changes associated with pregnancy. Clin Obstet Gynecol 1979; 22:785.)

**TABLE 45-3.** Iron Requirements for Pregnancy

| Required For | Average (mg) | Range (mg) |
|---|---|---|
| External iron loss | 170 | 150–200 |
| Expansion of RBC mass | 450 | 200–600 |
| Fetal iron | 270 | 200–370 |
| Iron in placenta and cord | 90 | 30–170 |
| Blood loss at delivery | 150 | 90–310 |
| Total requirement | 980 | 580–1340 |
| Requirement less RBC expansion | 840 | 440–1050 |

## VITAMIN B₁₂

Vitamin $B_{12}$ is also abundantly available in the diet bound to animal protein. Absorption requires hydrochloric acid and pepsin to free the cobalamine molecule from protein. Intrinsic factor is also essential for absorption. Once absorbed, transport occurs by binding to transcobalamine II. The majority of storage is in the liver, and most humans have a 2- to 3-year store available.

## MORPHOLOGIC CLASSIFICATION OF ANEMIA

### MICROCYTIC

This group of anemias is characterized by abnormal Hgb synthesis with normal RBC production. Figure 45-2 presents a logical progression of diagnostic steps for evaluation of a microcytic anemia. The first step is to rule in or out iron deficiency. If present, it is also essential to consider whether or not chronic blood loss from the gastrointestinal or genitourinary tract is a factor in the etiology.

When a microcytic anemia is not due to an iron deficiency, one must then differentiate cases due to hemoglobinopathy, chronic infection, or various sideroblastic anemias. Differentiation is based on plasma iron and iron-binding capacity, FEP, hemoglobin electrophoresis, DNA probing for alpha-genes and bone marrow examination.

### NORMOCYTIC

The difficulty in evaluating a normocytic anemia is due to the diverse nature of this group. Figure 45-3 presents a diagnostic algorithm for normocytic anemias and macrocytic anemias with normoblastic erythropoiesis. The reticulocyte count differentiates between cases with increased versus normal or decreased RBC production. If erythropoiesis is increased, one must then differentiate between hemorrhage and an increased rate of destruction. The blood smear may reveal a type of RBC that is virtually diagnostic. Fragmented cells are seen in microangiopathic hemolysis (the HELLP syndrome of preeclampsia/eclampsia and thrombotic thrombocytopenic purpura) and in association with prosthetic heart valves. Other types of named poikilocytes include sickle cells, target cells, stomatocytes, ovalocytes, spherocytes, elliptocytes, and acanthrocytes.

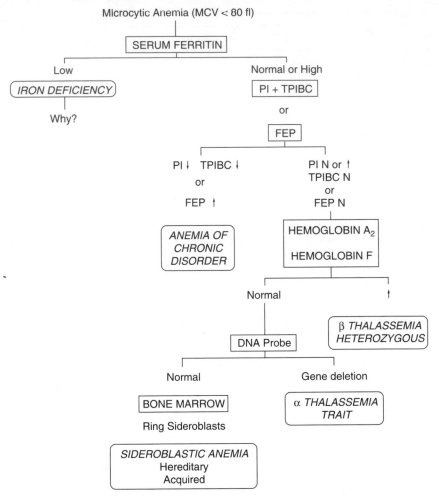

**FIGURE 45-2.** Diagnostic algorithm for microcystosis (PI-plasma iron, TPIBC, total plasma iron-binding capacity; FEP, free erythrocyte protoporphyrin.)

The Coombs' test will differentiate immune from nonimmune causes of hemolysis. Immune hemolysis is related to alloantibodies, drug-induced antibodies, and autoantibodies. Nonimmune causes of hemolysis include various hemoglobinopathies, hereditary disorders of the RBC membrane (spherocytosis and elliptocytosis), hereditary deficiency of an RBC enzyme, and the porphyrias. Acquired, nonimmune hemolysis is due either to paroxysmal nocturnal hemoglobinuria or lead poisoning.

Bone marrow examination is essential for evaluation of patients with hypoproliferative anemias with normal iron studies. If erythropoiesis is megaloblastic, folate or $B_{12}$ deficiency are likely causes. If sideroblastic, both acquired and hereditary forms of sideroblastic anemia must be considered. Finally, if erythropoiesis is

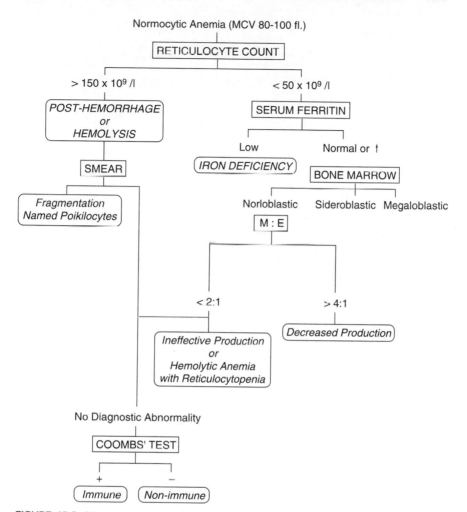

**FIGURE 45-3.** Diagnostic algorithm for normocytic anemia. (M:E, myeloid:erythroid ratio.)

normoblastic, etiologies fall into two major categories. The first show myeloid: erythroid (M:E) ratios of >4:1 and include aplasia, infiltration, the effects of chronic diseases, and endocrine disorders such as hypothyroidism and hypopituitarism. Ineffective erythropoiesis, usually associated with M:E ratio of <2:1 is the second group.

## MACROCYTIC

Macrocytic anemia is associated either with an increased rate of RBC production with release of less than fully mature RBCs or with disorders of impaired DNA synthesis. Figure 45-4 outlines an algorithm for evaluation of macrocytosis. One

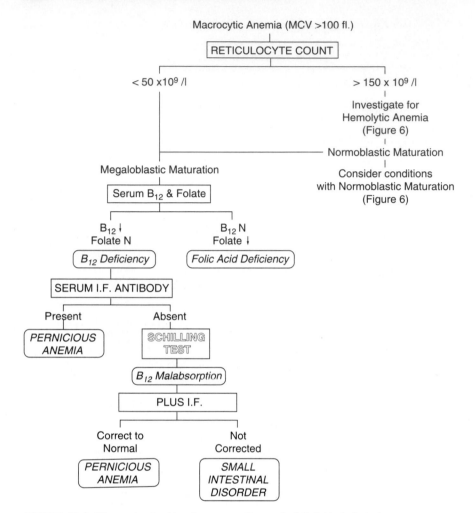

**FIGURE 45-4.** Diagnostic algorithm for macrocytic anemia (I.F., intrinsic factor.)

quickly notes that there are substantial areas of overlap between the evaluation of a normocytic and a macrocytic anemia. Early use of a bone marrow examination is very helpful in pointing the investigation in the correct direction.

When maturation is megaloblastic, serum $B_{12}$ and RBC folate levels will allow a diagnosis of $B_{12}$ or folate deficiency. When folate deficiency is diagnosed, the various causes of decreased deconjugation of the polyglutamate and malabsorption must be considered. If anti-intrinsic factor antibodies are present a diagnosis of pernicious anemia (PA) is assured. If absent, a Schilling test is required to differentiate between PA and a small bowel malabsorption syndrome.

## ANEMIA AND PERINATAL MORBIDITY AND MORTALITY

### THE EFFECTS OF ANEMIA

Although traditional instruction suggests that significant maternal anemia is associated with suboptimal fetal outcome, the data supporting this concept are scarce. Several studies in developing countries have compared fetal outcome in groups of women with hemoglobins above or below 6 to 7 g/dL. Although improved reproductive function was observed in women with higher hemoglobin levels, the studies lacked controls for protein malnutrition and chronic parasitic infestation. Studies in sheep show that fetal $O_2$ consumption is maintained until the maternal Hct is reduced by 50%.

### GENETIC IMPLICATIONS

Many of the hemolytic anemias are inherited as either autosomal dominant or autosomal recessive traits. Thus, once the correct diagnosis has been made, the genetic implications should be thoroughly discussed with the patient and her partner. Where appropriate, the discussion should include antenatal diagnosis.

### SPECIFIC ANEMIAS

### IRON DEFICIENCY ANEMIA

Iron deficiency is one of the most common causes of anemia during pregnancy, with symptoms of easy fatigue, lethargy, and headache. Pica involving clay, dirt, ice, or starch is a classic manifestation of iron deficiency. Clinical findings include pallor, glossitis, and cheilitis. Koilonychia has been associated with iron deficiency anemia but is a rare finding. The laboratory characteristics of iron deficiency anemia are a microcytic, hypochromic anemia with evidence of depleted iron stores. The plasma iron is low, and the total iron binding capacity high, the serum ferritin is low and/or the free erythrocyte protoporphyrin is elevated.

The specific treatment is oral ferrous sulfate, usually in a dose of 320 mg three times daily. Reticulocytosis should be observed after 7 to 10 days of therapy, and the Hgb can rise by as much as 1 gram per week in severely anemic individuals. Absorption from the gastrointestinal tract can be enhanced by administration of 500 mg of ascorbic acid with each dose of iron. Once the anemia has resolved, the patient should continue receiving iron therapy for an additional 6 months in order to replace iron stores.

### MEGALOBLASTIC ANEMIA

Megaloblastic anemia is the second most common nutritional anemia seen during pregnancy. Its etiology is most commonly folate deficiency, but vitamin $B_{12}$ deficiency also must be considered.

Patients with folate deficiency present with the typical symptoms of anemia plus roughness of the skin and glossitis. The CBC reveals a macrocytic, normochromic (or normocytic, normochromic) anemia with hypersegmentation of the polymorphonuclear leukocytes. The reticulocyte count is normal or low and the WBC and platelet count are frequently decreased. Bone marrow examination is usually not necessary to make the diagnosis but if done shows megaloblastic erythropoiesis. The RBC folate is decreased to >165 µg/dl and the vitamin $B_{12}$ level is normal.

Treatment consists of oral folic acid in a dose of 1 mg three times daily. Parenteral folic acid may be indicated in individuals with malabsorption. A reticulocyte response should be seen in 48 to 72 hours and the platelet count will normalize within a few days. The neutrophils will normalize after 1 to 2 weeks.

In addition to anemia, individuals with $B_{12}$ deficiency may also show neurologic defects related to damage of the posterior columns of the spinal cord. It is critical that individuals with $B_{12}$ deficiency are not treated with folic acid alone. Such treatment may well improve the anemia but will have absolutely no salutary effect on the neuropathy and in fact may make it worse. Appropriate treatment for pernicious anemia consists of 1000 µg of vitamin $B_{12}$ administered parenterally weekly for 6 weeks followed by monthly administration for life in cases of pernicious anemia. Again a prompt reticulocyte response is anticipated after 3 to 5 days of therapy.

## HEREDITARY SPHEROCYTOSIS AND ELLIPTOCYTOSIS

Spherocytosis is the most common form of inherited hemolytic anemia. The inheritance is as an autosomal dominant with variable penetrance. A hemolytic crisis can be precipitated by many conditions, including infection, trauma, or pregnancy itself.

The diagnosis is suspected on the basis of family history and by findings in the CBC and reticulocyte count that suggest the hyperproliferative branches of the diagnostic algorithms in Figures 45-3 and 45-4. Confirmation is obtained with the osmotic fragility test.

Prenatal care of women with hereditary spherocytosis who have not had a splenectomy requires vigilance for hemolytic crisis and folate supplementation to ensure adequate marrow function. A hemolytic crisis can be treated conservatively with replacement transfusions or with splenectomy. Splenectomy is mechanically difficult to accomplish during the third trimester of pregnancy unless preceded by cesarean section. In the absence of severe, untreated anemia, spherocytosis does not contribute to perinatal morbidity or mortality.

## AUTOIMMUNE HEMOLYTIC ANEMIA (AIHA)

There are two major types of antibodies responsible for AIHA, warm-reactive and cold-reactive. Most warm-reactive antibodies are of IgG class and are directed against some component of the Rh system on the surface of the red cell. In contrast, most cold-reactive antibodies are IgM and usually are specific for anti-I or anti-i. AIHA with warm-reactive antibodies is frequently seen in association with various hematologic malignancies (chronic lymphocytic leukemia, lymphoma), lupus erythematosus, viral infections, and drug ingestion. Penicillin, stibophen and alpha-methyldopa all have been reported to cause AIHA. Cold-reacting antibodies can be seen in association with mycoplasma infections, infectious mononucleosis, and lymphoreticular neoplasms. Unfortunately, in a large number of cases no specific inciting event can be identified.

Diagnosis is suspected by identifying a hyperproliferative, macrocytic anemia. The stained smear of the peripheral blood often reveals microcytes, polychromatophilia, poikilocytosis, and the presence of normoblasts. Leukocytosis is frequently seen and is a result of marrow hyperactivity. The critical study to confirm the diagnosis is a positive direct Coombs' test.

Treatment of AIHA is directed toward both the hemolytic process and the underlying disease. Blood transfusion, corticosteroid therapy, immunosuppression and splenectomy are the most frequently used measures. In cases with warm-reactive antibodies, corticosteroids should be tried initially because approximately 80% of patients will respond dramatically. Splenectomy is an effective form of treatment in approximately 60% of patients with warm-reactive antibodies. If the patient is refractory to both corticosteroid therapy and splenectomy, a trial of immunosuppression is warranted.

The treatment of cold-reactive antibodies depends on the severity of the hemolytic process. In patients with mild anemia, avoidance of cold temperatures is all that is required. Corticosteroid therapy and splenectomy are usually not effective if the majority of CBC breakdown occurs intravascularly. In patients with severe anemia, a trial of immunosuppressive or plasmapheresis should be considered.

## APLASTIC AND HYPOPLASTIC ANEMIA

Aplastic anemia is characterized by a reduction in the number of circulating RBCs, neutrophils, and platelets, and by the presence of a hypocellular bone marrow. Although a number of drugs, chemical agents, and irradiation are known marrow depressants, in about half of all cases careful search does not reveal any causative agents.

Some 80 cases of hypoplastic anemia of pregnancy have been reported and are characterized by hypoplasia during pregnancy with spontaneous remission after delivery. The bone marrow was described as hypocellular with an increase in megakaryocytes. Cases reported to date present a spectrum of clinical and bone marrow findings that make it difficult to substantiate the existence of hypoplastic anemia specifically related to pregnancy.

Patients with aplastic anemia seek medical attention because of symptoms relating to profound anemia, bleeding, or infection. The CBC reveals pancytopenia with a hypoproliferative reticulocyte count. Examination of the bone marrow reveals hypoplasia with normoblastic erythropoiesis.

Severe aplastic anemia is fatal for more than 50% of affected patients. Bone marrow transplantation is now the treatment of choice, and long-term survival of 50 to 70% can be expected. During pregnancy, supportive therapy remains the major objective. In recent years, with modern supportive therapy, the maternal mortality rate has been only 15%, and more than 90% of patients survive in remission. Supportive treatment consists of maintenance of hemoglobin levels by periodic transfusion, prevention and treatment of infection, stimulation of hematopoiesis with androgens, splenectomy, therapeutic abortion and premature delivery, intravenous gamma globulin, and marrow transplantation.

Androgen therapy can be effective at stimulating erythropoiesis. However, androgens are contraindicated during pregnancy unless the fetus is demonstrated to be male. Agents commonly used include fluoxymesterone (0.25 mg/kg per day), oxymetholone (3 to 5 mg/kg per day), nandrolone decanate (3 to 4 mg/kg weekly), or testosterone ethanate (1 to 3 mg/kg per week). Adrenocorticosteroids have also been widely used with some benefit. Unfortunately, the remission rate with steroids is only 12%.

## PAROXYSMAL NOCTURNAL HEMOGLOBINURIA (PNH)

Hemolysis occurs in PNH due to an unexplained structural defect in the RBC. There are distinct cohorts of long-lived and short-lived cells. The inherent defect makes the RBCs unusually susceptible to lysis by complement. PNH usually begins insidiously, and there is no familial tendency. There is considerable variability in severity of the disease, and the classic presentation of hemoglobinuria is seen in only 25% of patients. Exacerbations of the hemolytic process are precipitated by infection, menstruation, transfusion, surgery, and ingestion of iron.

The most serious complications associated with PNH are marrow aplasia, thrombosis, and infection. Thrombosis accounts for 50% of deaths and is of particular concern during pregnancy. Although anemia is the most prominent hematologic feature of PNH, leukopenia and thrombocytopenia also occur frequently. The diagnosis of PNH is based on a series of special tests that demonstrate the sensitivity of the patient's RBCs to complement.

The ideal treatment for PNH is replacement of the abnormal stem cell with cells capable of producing the normal cellular components. This has been accomplished by bone marrow transplantation. The major therapeutic modalities during pregnancy are iron therapy, androgen treatment, corticosteroids and transfusions. Iron can be administered orally to replace the considerable amount lost in the urine. Unfortunately, in significantly iron-deficient patients, such treatment may lead to a burst of erythropoiesis with delivery of a cohort of cells susceptible to the lytic action of complement. If a hemolytic episode follows iron therapy, it should be treated with either suppression of erythropoiesis by transfusion or suppression of hemolysis with corticosteroids. Prednisone in a dose of 1 mg/kg per day is an effective regimen.

When acute hemolytic episodes occur, treatment is aimed at diminishing hemolysis and preventing complications. Because patients with PNH have frequent episodes of venous thrombosis, this must be watched for carefully. In cases of acute deep venous thromboses, anticoagulation should be begun. Care must be taken in the use of heparin because hemolytic episodes clearly can be related to its use. During pregnancy heparin is the anticoagulant of choice; however, during the puerperium or nonpregnant state, warfarin is preferred. Only a few pregnancies have been reported in women with PNH, and both spontaneous abortion and thrombotic events appear to be increased in frequency.

# 46. MATERNAL ALLOIMMUNIZATION AND FETAL HEMOLYTIC DISEASE

Fetal hemolytic disease was first described in twins in 1609, one dying a hydropic death shortly after birth, the other dying of kernicterus at a few days of age. The postulate that fetal hemolysis was due to the development of a blood group antibody in the mother directed against a blood group antigen present on the red cells of her fetus was proved in 1941 following the discovery of the Rh blood group system in 1940.

## THE RH BLOOD GROUP SYSTEM

Although other blood group systems are assuming greater importance as the prevalence of maternal Rh immunization diminishes, the Rh blood group system is still the most common system causing serious alloimmunization and fetal hemolytic disease.

There are three pairs of antigens—commonly Dd, Cc, Ee—which are inherited in two sets of three, one from each parent. The presence or absence of the antigen D determines whether an individual is Rh-positive or Rh-negative. About 45% of D-positive individuals are homozygous for D, having inherited a D-containing set from both parents; the remaining 55% are heterozygous, having inherited a D-containing set from only one parent. If the Rh-positive husband of an Rh-negative woman is homozygous, all his children will be D-positive; if he is heterozygous, in each pregnancy there is an equal chance that the fetus will be D-negative or D-positive. Only D-positive fetuses provoke Rh immunization, and only D-positive fetuses will be affected by the Rh antibody provoked (Table 46-1).

Rh-negativity is primarily a Caucasian trait. In most Caucasian populations, the incidence of Rh-negativity is 15% to 16%. In Chinese and Japanese populations it is less than 1%. About 1% to 2% of North American Indians and Inuit are Rh-negative, as are about 2% of Indo-Eurasians. In blacks the incidence ranges from 4% to 8%, being higher in North American than in African blacks.

## PATHOGENESIS OF MATERNAL ALLOIMMUNIZATION

Following the discovery of the Rh blood group system and the interdiction of transfusion of Rh(D)-compatible blood, the prevalence of Rh immunization diminished only very slightly. That fetal transplacental hemorrhage (TPH) into the mother caused Rh immunization, was proved in 1954.

The Kleihauer acid elution test is an accurate and very sensitive method of determining the incidence and size of TPH. Seventy-five percent of women have evidence of fetal TPH at some time during pregnancy or at the time of delivery. The size of the hemorrhage is usually small, but about 1% of women will have as

E. Albert Reece, John C. Hobbins, Maurice, J. Mahoney and Roy H. Petrie (Eds).
*Handbook of Medicine of the Fetus & Mother.* Copyright © 1995 by J.B. Lippincott Company

**TABLE 46-1.** Zygosity for Rh(D) of D-Positive Husband (D-Negative Wife)

| Antigens Present In Husband | A (Most Likely Rh Genotype) | B (Less Likely Rh Genotype) | C (Least Likely Rh Genotype) |
|---|---|---|---|
| 1. CDe | $CDe/CDe(R^1R^1)$* <br> Homozygous | $CDe/Cde(R^1r')$ <br> Heterozygous | |
| 2. CDce | $CDe/cde(R^1r)$ <br> Heterozygous | $CDe/cDe(R^1R^0)$ <br> Homozygous | $cDe/Cde(R^0r')$ <br> Heterozygous |
| 3. CDEce | $CDe/cDE(R^1R^2)$ <br> Homozygous | $cDE/Cde(R^2r')$ <br> $CDe/cdE(R^1r'')$ <br> Heterozygous | $CDE/cDe(R^2R^0)$ <br> Homozygous |
| 4. DEc | $cDE/cDE(R^2R^2)$* <br> Homozygous | $cDE/cdE(R^2r'')$ <br> Heterozygous | |
| 5. DEce | $cDE/cde(R^2r)$ <br> Heterozygous | $cDE/cDe(R^2R^0)$ <br> Homozygous | $cDe/cdE(R^0r'')$ <br> Heterozygous |
| 6. Dce | $cDe/cde(R^0r)$ <br> Heterozygous | $cDe/cDe(R^0R^0)$ <br> Homozygous | |

* Genotypes 1A and 4A can very infrequently be proved because the infant will usually be of only one paternal genotype (CDe in 1A and cDE in 4A). The remainder of the husband's possible genotypes can be proved only if he produces children of two different genotypes. (From Bowman JM, Friesen RF. Rh-isoimmunization. In: Goodwin JW, Godden JO, Chance G, eds. Perinatal medicine. Baltimore: Williams & Wilkins, 1976:92-107.)

much as 5 mL, and 0.25% will have 30 mL or more of fetal blood in their circulation. Abortion carries a risk of TPH, usually of less than 0.1 mL. After a therapeutic abortion, the risk may be as high as 20% to 25%.

## ANTIBODY DETECTION AND MEASUREMENT METHODS

The following are some of the methods used to measure and detect antibodies:

1. *Saline*. Rh-positive erythrocytes suspended in isotonic saline are agglutinated only by IgM anti-D.
2. *Colloid*. Rh-positive red cells suspended in more viscous colloid media such as albumin are agglutinated by IgG anti-D. Bovine serum albumin is the most frequently used colloid medium.
3. *Indirect antiglobulin (IDAT)*. Antihuman globulin antibody (Coombs' serum, AHG) is produced by injection of human serum (or specific human IgG) into other animal species. Following incubation of Rh-positive red cells with serum being screened for Rh antibody, anti-D, if present, adheres to the red cells. The red cells are then suspended in the AHG serum. If the red cells are coated with antibody, they agglutinate, a positive indirect antiglobulin test (IDAT, or indirect Coombs, test). IDAT screening is more sensitive than albumin screening. IDAT titers are usually one to three dilutions higher than albumin titers.
4. *Enzyme*. Red cells incubated with enzymes and then suspended in saline lie closer together and are agglutinated by IgG anti-D. Enzyme techniques are the most sensitive manual methods for detecting Rh immunization.

# THE PREVALENCE OF RH IMMUNIZATION

The risk of Rh immunization appearing within 6 months after delivery of the first Rh-positive ABO-compatible baby is 8% to 9%. However, an equal number of women will demonstrate that they also were immunized by the first pregnancy, but at an undetectable antibody level, until they mount a secondary immune response in the next Rh-positive pregnancy. Therefore, the overall risk of Rh immunization occurring as a result of the first Rh-positive ABO-compatible pregnancy is about 16%. After a woman has undergone five Rh-positive ABO-compatible pregnancies, there is a 50% likelihood that she will be Rh-immunized. About 30% of Rh-negative women are nonresponders and will not become Rh-immunized despite exposure to repeated doses of Rh-positive red cells.

ABO incompatibility between the Rh-positive fetus and the Rh-negative mother reduces her risk of becoming Rh-immunized to 1.5% to 2%. However, once Rh immunization has developed, ABO incompatibility of the Rh-positive fetus confers no protection at all against the development of severe fetal hemolytic disease.

A significant incidence of Rh immunization occurs during pregnancy. In one study, 1.8% of Rh-negative women carrying Rh-positive fetuses were Rh-immunized by the time of delivery. About 13% of all instances of Rh immunization occur during pregnancy.

The woman who has an abortion is at risk of becoming Rh-immunized. The risk is about 2% after spontaneous abortion and 4% to 5% after therapeutic abortion.

# PATHOGENESIS OF FETAL HEMOLYTIC DISEASE

Blood production starts in the third week of gestation. Rh antigen is present in the red cell membrane by the sixth week. Erythropoiesis begins in the liver and spleen, shifting to the bone marrow by the sixth month. Maternal IgG anti-D traverses the placenta and coats the D-positive fetal red cells (the reason for the direct positive antiglobulin or Coombs' test). Anti-D does not fix complement. The fetal red cells are destroyed extravascularly, primarily in the spleen. The resulting anemia stimulates erythropoietin production and increased erythropoiesis. When marrow red cell production cannot compensate for the increased hemolysis, extramedullary erythropoiesis recurs, primarily in liver and spleen.

Control of erythrocyte maturation in this situation is poor. Nucleated red cell precursors from normoblasts to very primitive erythroblasts are released into the circulation (Fig. 46-1).

Severity of hemolytic disease is determined by the amount of maternal IgG anti-D (the titer), its affinity or avidity for the fetal red cell membrane D antigen (the binding constant), and the ability of the fetus to keep up with the red cell destruction without becoming hydropic.

# MILD DISEASE—NO TREATMENT

About one-half of all affected fetuses do not require treatment after birth (Table 46-2). They are only mildly anemic and are not severely hyperbilirubinemic. The hemoglobin levels do not drop below 11.0 g/L, nor do the serum indirect bilirubin levels exceed 340 μmol/L (20 mg/dL) in the neonatal period, and 260 to 300 μmol/L

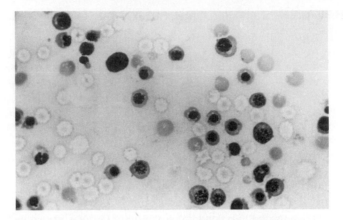

**FIGURE 46-1.** Cord blood of baby with severe Rh erythroblastosis fetalis who required multiple fetal transfusions and exchange transfusions. Smear treated by Kleihauer technique and Wright's stain. Note adult donor ghost red cells, dark fetal red cells, and early fetal erythroid series from erythroblasts through to normoblasts. (From Bowman JM. The management of Rh-isoimmunization. Obstet Gynecol 1978;52:3.)

(15 to 17.5 mg/dL) in premature infants. These babies are normal and survive without treatment now.

## INTERMEDIATE DISEASE—KERNICTERUS

About 25% to 30% of affected fetuses are born at term or near term in good condition, without severe anemia (cord blood hemoglobin levels greater than 9.0 g/L). Prior to birth, products of blood destruction are metabolized and excreted by the mother. After delivery, the baby must use his own resources.

In fetal hemolytic disease, there is increased production of indirect bilirubin. The newborn liver is deficient in glucuronyl transferase and Y transport protein. Thus, in the presence of increased indirect bilirubin production and the inability of the newborn infant to conjugate and excrete it as water-soluble bilirubin diglucuronide serum, indirect bilirubin increases.

**TABLE 46-2.** Classification of Severity of Rh Hemolytic Disease

| Degree of Severity | Description | Incidence (%) |
| --- | --- | --- |
| Mild | Indirect bilirubin does not exceed 16–20 mg/100 mL. No anemia. No treatment needed. | 45–50 |
| Moderate | Fetal hydrops does not develop. Moderate anemia. Severe jaundice with risk of kernicterus unless treated after birth. | 25–30 |
| Severe | Fetal hydrops develops in utero | 20–25 |
| | Before 34 weeks gestation | 10–12 |
| | After 34 weeks gestation | 10–12 |

From Bowman JM. Maternal blood group immunization. In: Creasy R, Resnik R. eds. Maternal-fetal medicine: principles and practice. Philadelphia: WB Saunders, 1984:561-602.

Indirect bilirubin is water insoluble and can remain in the plasma only when bound to albumin. When the albumin-binding capacity of the neonate's plasma is exceeded, "free" indirect bilirubin appears. Being water-insoluble and lipid-soluble, it cannot remain in the plasma but diffuses across the lipid neuron membrane. Within the neuron it interferes with vital cellular metabolism. The dead neurons with accumulated bilirubin appear yellow at autopsy (kernicterus).

Babies who develop bilirubin encephalopathy (kernicterus) become deeply jaundiced. On the third to the fifth day they become lethargic and then hypertonic. They lie in a position of opisthotonos with neck hyperextended, back arched. Death occurs in about 90% of babies with kernicterus.

The 10% who survive show evidence of severe central nervous system dysfunction. Most have profound neurosensory deafness and choreoathetoid spastic cerebral palsy.

## SEVERE DISEASE—HYDROPS FETALIS

The 20% to 25% of most severely affected fetuses, despite maximal red cell production, become progressively more anemic. Ascites with anasarca occurs. Although heart failure may develop in hydropic infants after birth, it is not commonly the underlying cause of hydrops fetalis caused by fetal hemolytic disease. Hepatic circulatory obstruction and hepatocellular damage are the probable causes of alloimmune hydrops fetalis.

Expanding islets of erythropoiesis distort hepatic cords and obstruct portal venous blood flow, causing portal hypertension. Ascites develops; albumin production diminishes; hypoalbuminemia occurs; anasarca appears. The fetus usually dies.

## MONITORING THE MOTHER AND HER FETUS AT RISK

### PRENATAL BLOOD TESTING

A blood sample must be obtained from every woman at her first prenatal visit for blood grouping and antibody screening. There must be no deviation from this policy no matter what the woman's parity or what screening tests showed in her previous pregnancies. Mistyping of an Rh-negative woman may have occurred in a prior pregnancy. An Rh-positive woman, particularly if she has been transfused, may have developed a dangerous atypical blood group antibody.

### THE UNIMMUNIZED PREGNANT WOMAN

The Rh-positive woman without demonstrable blood group antibodies at her first prenatal visit is not likely to develop dangerous atypical blood group antibodies later in her pregnancy. Since, on occasion, significant atypical antibodies may develop, we do recommend repeat screening at 34 to 38 weeks gestation.

The Rh-negative woman without Rh antibodies should be ABO grouped and the Rh status of her husband should be determined. The risk of Rh immunization can be estimated (Table 46-3).

**TABLE 46-3.** Approximate Risk of Rh Immunization

| Husband | Baby | Risk (%) |
|---|---|---|
| D-negative | D-negative | 0 |
| D-positive<br>Homozygous<br>ABO-compatible | D-positive<br>ABO-compatible | 16 |
| D-positive<br>Homozygous<br>ABO-incompatible | D-positive<br>ABO-unknown | 7 |
| | D-positive<br>ABO-incompatible | 2 |
| D-positive<br>Heterozygous<br>ABO-compatible | D status unknown<br>ABO-compatible | 8 |
| D-positive<br>Heterozygous<br>ABO-incompatible | D status unknown<br>ABO unknown | 3.5 |

The Rh-negative pregnant woman whose husband is Rh-positive should be rescreened at 18 weeks gestation and every 4 weeks thereafter. Cesarean section and manual removal of the placenta increase the frequency and size of fetal-maternal TPH. Amniocentesis carried out for genetic purposes or for determination of pulmonary maturity carries a risk of TPH. If carried out under ultrasound guidance, the risk is about 2%. At delivery, cord and maternal blood must be tested—cord blood for the ABO and Rh type of the infant and the direct antiglobulin (Coombs') status of the infant's red cells, and maternal blood for the presence of Rh antibody and fetal red cells (TPH).

## PREDICTING SEVERITY OF RH HEMOLYTIC DISEASE

### HISTORY

Disease may remain of about the same degree of severity from baby to baby (mild, moderate, or severe), but it is just as likely to become progressively more severe from pregnancy to pregnancy. Infrequently, disease may become less severe. If a woman has had a hydropic baby, there is a 90% chance that the next affected fetus will also become hydropic. In a first sensitized pregnancy the risk of hydrops is 8% to 10%. When hydrops has developed in a prior pregnancy and the father is heterozygous, the fetus may be Rh-negative and unaffected or Rh-positive and severely affected.

### RH ANTIBODY TITERS

If Rh antibody titers are measured in the same laboratory by the same experienced personnel using the same methods and test red cells, the results are reproducible and of some value in predicting the risk of severe hemolytic disease. The maternal antibody titer that puts the fetus at risk must be determined for each laboratory. Generally speaking, an albumin titer of 16 or an indirect antiglobulin titer of 32 to

64 puts the fetus at about a 10% risk of becoming hydropic. Because it is the Rh antibody titer that selects the immunized woman who has a fetus at risk, titers should be repeated at 16 to 18 weeks gestation, at 22 weeks gestation, and at 2-week periods thereafter.

## AMNIOTIC FLUID SPECTROPHOTOMETRY

Amniotic fluid surrounding severely affected fetuses is stained yellow. The pigment, which absorbs visual light at 450 nm, is bilirubin. Amniotic fluid is predominantly fetal in origin.

Amniotic fluid after centrifugation and filtration has optical density readings made over the visual wavelength spectrum 700 to 350 nm. The readings are plotted on semilogarithmic graph paper (wavelength the horizontal linear coordinate, optical density the vertical logarithmic coordinate). The readings are joined. The deviation from linearity at 450 nm (the $\Delta$OD 450 reading) is directly related to severity of disease.

The $\Delta$OD 450 reading must be plotted according to gestation, since early in gestation unaffected fetuses produce bilirubin. Readings in zone 3 indicate severe disease, usually hydrops within 7 to 10 days. Readings falling into zone 1 indicate mild or no disease. Readings in zone 2 indicate intermediate disease, increasing in severity as the zone 3 boundary is approached.

The zone boundaries slope downward because of the diminishing amount of bilirubin normally produced as pregnancy progresses. This is not true before 24 weeks gestation, since the zone boundaries are parabolic, reaching their highest levels at 24 weeks gestation.

Although single $\Delta$OD 450 measurements before 26 weeks gestation may be misleading unless they are very high ($\geq$0.400), serial measurements, often as frequent as every 5 to 7 days, do give a reasonable prediction of severity of hemolytic disease in the second trimester. Nevertheless, since 1986, in the face of rising $\Delta$OD 450 readings, direct fetal blood sampling is strongly recommended prior to undertaking fetal treatment measures.

Amniocentesis must be preceded by ultrasound placental localization. If the placenta is anterior, amniocentesis should be carried out under direct ultrasound guidance. Every effort must be made to avoid traversing the placenta with the amniocentesis needle. Without ultrasound placental localization, amniocentesis carries with it a 10% likelihood of causing placental trauma, TPH, and a rising antibody titer. A clotted maternal blood sample is obtained before and 5 minutes after the procedure. A 20- or 22-gauge spinal puncture needle is introduced into the amniotic cavity to the depth at which ultrasonography has determined fluid to be present, and 10 to 15 mL of fluid are aspirated gently. The fluid will have a varying degree of yellow pigmentation and will be slightly to moderately turbid later in gestation. The fluid, protected from light, is sent for a $\Delta$OD 450 measurement and for fetal pulmonary maturity measurements if the pregnancy is past 32 weeks gestation. The maternal blood samples are sent for antibody measurement and fetal red cell screening.

Maternal or fetal blood produces sharp 580-, 540-, and 415-nm oxyhemoglobin peaks, which obscure the $\Delta$OD 450 readings, making the fluid valueless. Heme produces a 405-nm peak, which may obscure the 450-nm peak but is in itself indicative of severe hemolytic disease. Meconium in amniotic fluid distorts and increases the 450-nm peak. Exposure of the sample to light (particularly fluorescent light) decolorizes bilirubin, reducing the ΔOD 450 peak. Congenital anomalies such as anencephaly, open meningomyelocele, and upper gastrointestinal obstruction produce hydramnios and markedly elevated ΔOD 450 readings, which may be misleading if the mother is immunized.

Amniocentesis should be carried out only when the history or titer is such that the fetus is at risk of hydrops and death. Amniocentesis is required in only about 1 half of Rh-immunized pregnancies. If a previously affected perinate has died or required fetal transfusion or exchange transfusion after birth, fetal assessment and amniocentesis are required at 18 to 19 weeks gestation. If the placenta is anterior and cannot be avoided, fetal blood sampling is a better alternative than amniocentesis. Failing such a history, amniocentesis is carried out only if the antibody titer (≥16 in albumin, ≥32 to 64 by indirect antiglobulin) indicates a risk of fetal hydrops. Amniocenteses are repeated at 5- to 28-day intervals, the interval depending on the ΔOD 450 measurement of the immediately preceding fluid sample.

## FETAL ULTRASONOGRAPHY

Because ultrasound is noninvasive, it can be used serially (often daily) to determine severity of hemolytic disease and to monitor fetal condition over time and in relation to specific treatment measures. Ultrasound allows a determination of placental and hepatic size and the presence or absence of edema and effusions. Unfortunately, it may not give as accurate a prediction of impending hydrops as do serial amniotic fluid ΔOD 450 readings.

Ultrasonography has improved the accuracy and reduced the trauma from needle insertion at intraperitoneal fetal transfusion and is essential when direct intravascular fetal transfusions are being carried out. Following intraperitoneal transfusions, serial ultrasound examinations confirm the presence of blood in the peritoneal cavity and its rate of absorption. Following both intraperitoneal and intravascular transfusions, ultrasound biophysical profile scoring provides an accurate assessment of fetal well-being and whether improvement or deterioration in fetal condition is occurring.

## FETAL BLOOD SAMPLING

Percutaneous umbilical blood sampling (PUBS) allows a measurement of all blood parameters that can be measured after birth (hemoglobin, hematocrit, serum bilirubin, direct and indirect platelet count, leukocyte count, serum proteins, and blood gases). Fetal blood sampling is by far the most accurate means of determining the degree of severity of hemolytic disease in the absence of hydrops fetalis.

This is a surprisingly benign procedure, carrying with it a fetal mortality rate of a fraction of 1%. Since it carries with it a very high risk of fetal transplacental hemorrhage, its use is recommended in two situations: (1) where serial amniotic fluid ΔOD 450 readings are rising into the upper 65% level of zone 2; (2) where an anterior placenta cannot be avoided at amniocentesis and maternal history and antibody titer put the fetus at risk. Direct fetal blood sampling may be possible as early as 16 to 18 weeks gestation; it is usually feasible by 20 to 21 weeks gestation.

## MANAGEMENT OF THE RH-IMMUNIZED WOMAN AND HER FETUS

In the 50% of pregnancies not requiring amniocentesis (or fetal blood sampling) and in those where the Δ450 reading has been consistently below the middle of zone 2, spontaneous delivery at term may be allowed to occur. If there is a bad history or a high titer, a heterozygous husband and serial readings in zone 1 or low zone 2, the fetus is Rh-negative. Again, delivery should be allowed to take place spontaneously. If the readings rise into the 50% to 75% level of zone 2 by 35 to 37 weeks gestation, delivery should be carried out at 36 to 38 weeks gestation, provided that there is evidence of pulmonary maturity. If pulmonary maturity is not demonstrated and if the fluid reading is in the 70% to 75% level of zone 2, a fetal blood-sampling procedure may be considered. These fetuses should not be left undelivered after 38 weeks gestation.

If the ΔOD 450 reading falls in the 80% to 85% level of zone 2 at 34 weeks gestation or later, prompt delivery should be undertaken, provided again that there is evidence of pulmonary maturity. Failing this evidence, a blood-sampling procedure should be carried out, followed by a direct intravascular transfusion, if fetal blood parameters indicate the need for it. If fetal blood sampling in this situation is not feasible and if the fetus appears appropriate for gestational age (≥34 weeks gestation), administration of corticosteroids for 48 hours followed by delivery is recommended.

## INTRAPERITONEAL FETAL TRANSFUSIONS (IPT)

In the absence of fetal hydrops, 10% to 12% of transfused red cells are absorbed each 24 hours following IPT. In the presence of hydrops, absorption is very capricious but may be very reasonable. When the fetus is moribund (not breathing), little or no absorption will occur. The volume of blood injected is limited by the size of the peritoneal cavity. If the volume transfused is such that intraperitoneal pressure exceeds umbilical venous pressure, blood flow from the placenta to the fetus will stop and the fetus will die. Fetuses usually tolerate IPT volumes calculated by the following formula:

$$\text{IPT volume} = (\text{weeks gestation} - 20) \times 10 \text{ mL},$$

(i.e., 50 mL at 25 weeks, 90 mL at 29 weeks). A second IPT is carried out as soon as the red cells from the first IPT have been absorbed (9 to 12 days). Subsequent IPT intervals are about 4 weeks, the last one rarely after 32 weeks gestation. The aim is delivery 3.5 to 4 weeks after the last IPT at greater than 33.5 to 34 weeks gestation.

## DIRECT INTRAVASCULAR FETAL TRANSFUSION (IVT)

Fetal blood sampling and direct intravascular transfusion are now carried out in most, if not all, tertiary-level centers by the insertion of the tip of a 20- or 22-gauge spinal needle, under careful ultrasound guidance, into an umbilical blood vessel (preferably the umbilical vein, preferably at its insertion into the placenta).

## SELECTION OF PATIENTS FOR IUT

Only fetuses at risk of hydrops or hydropic before 33 to 34 weeks gestation are candidates for IUT. Patients are selected based on history or titer (or both) for either amniocentesis or direct blood sampling, the procedure chosen being dependent on placental site and ultrasound findings. If a pregnant woman meets the history or titer criteria for further investigation, she is assessed by ultrasound at 16 to 18 weeks gestation or as soon (later in gestation) as she meets the criteria.

If the fetus looks well and if the placenta is not anterior and can be avoided at amniocentesis, an initial amniocentesis is carried out. The interval between further amniocenteses will be determined by the prior $\Delta$OD 450 reading. If the placenta is anterior and the amniotic cavity cannot be reached without traversing it, amniocentesis is not carried out. Depending on the gestation of the assessment and the size and accessibility of the umbilical vein placental insertion, a direct blood-sampling procedure may be carried out. If there is ultrasound evidence of prehydrops or hydrops, immediate fetal blood sampling and IVT are carried out no matter what the gestation or placental site. If the fetus continues to look well but serial amniotic fluid $\Delta$OD 450 measurements rise into the 75th percentile of zone 2, prompt fetal blood sampling is carried out followed by IVT, if there is significant fetal anemia (a fetal circulating hemoglobin concentration of less than 110 g/L at any gestation).

Because of the availability of fetal blood sampling, we no longer recommend IUT based on serial amniotic fluid $\Delta$OD 450 readings or a very high single zone 3 reading, but use these criteria to have blood available for immediate transfusion if fetal blood sampling indicates its need. Only if fetal blood sampling is not possible due to fetal vessel inaccessibility would we now carry out IUT (an IPT in this circumstance), based on amniotic fluid findings alone (a single high zone 3 fluid or $\Delta$OD 450 readings rising into the 80th to 85th percentile of zone 2).

## SUITABLE BLOOD FOR IUT

Blood for IUT (either IPT or IVT) should be drawn from the donor no more than 5 days before the transfusion is planned. It should be group O and missing the antigen (or antigens) to which the mother is sensitized (D-negative if the mother is Rh-negative with anti-D). Careful cross-match of the donor red cells with the mother's serum is imperative immediately prior to each transfusion. A second antibody may become manifest after one or two IUT, jeopardizing the lifespan of the donor red cells infused at the previous IUT.

The blood unit should be centrifuged, the red cells tightly packed, and the supernatant plasma with buffy coat expressed and discarded. X-ray irradiation of the donor red cells is recommended. Immediately prior to the IUT, sterile isotonic saline should be added to the packed red cells (10 to 12 mL in the case of IVT, 12 to 18 mL in the case of IPT).

## TECHNIQUE OF IUT

IVT has almost completely replaced IPT. Nevertheless, on occasion, particularly after 30 to 32 weeks gestation, in the situation where a growing fetus completely obscures the cord vessel insertion into a posteriorly implanted placenta, IPT may be a preferable alternative to the placement of a needle tip into a cord blood vessel inserted into the fetal abdomen.

## Technique of IPT

The mother is premedicated with an analgesic and muscle relaxant but is not anesthetized. The perinatal ultrasonographer, using real-time scan, localizes the target area, the fetal abdomen. Meticulous asepsis is observed. Under ultrasound guidance, the perinatal obstetrician directs a 16-gauge, 18-cm Tuohy needle into the fetal abdomen. If the fetal abdomen is in an anterior position (Fig. 46-2), care should be taken to insert the needle well below the midabdomen, to avoid the umbilical area through which the cord vessels travel. If the fetal back is anterior, IPT should not be undertaken until the fetus has assumed a more favorable position. If the placenta is anterior and the fetal abdomen cannot be approached without traversing it, the cord vessel insertion into the placenta is readily accessible. Fetal blood sampling and IVT are the procedures of choice.

As the IPT needle reaches the depth of the fetal abdomen, the needle tip can be seen (by ultrasonography) indenting the abdomen and then penetrating the fetal peritoneal cavity. A size 16 epidural catheter, with the blind tip and side holes removed, is threaded down the needle. As the catheter is threaded through the needle, its tip often may be seen ultrasonographically moving around the peritoneal cavity. After about 30 cm of catheter have been threaded down the needle, the needle is withdrawn over the catheter to lie on the maternal abdomen. Under careful ultrasonographic observation, 0.5 to 1 mL of well-shaken saline is then

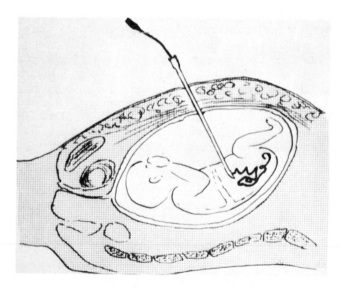

**FIGURE 46-2.** IPT diagram. The Tuohy needle has been inserted across the maternal abdominal wall and uterine wall into the fetal peritoneal cavity, and the epidural catheter has been threaded into the peritoneal cavity of the fetus. The safest position for the fetus at IPT is not with the abdomen anterior (as shown in this diagram), because the umbilical fetal vessels then lie in the center of the target area. (From Bowman JM. Blood-group incompatibilities. In: Iffy L, Kaminetzky HA, eds. Principles and practice of obstetrics and perinatology. New York: John Wiley, 1981:1213.)

injected down the catheter. If the saline and air bubbles produce a sonographic opacity rising promptly and freely to lie under the most upper part of the fetal abdominal cavity, indicating beyond doubt that the tip of the catheter is indeed free in the peritoneal cavity, the transfusion is carried out. If the tip cannot be demonstrated with certainty to be lying free in the peritoneal cavity, the woman is transferred to the radiology department. Two milliliters of radio contrast (76% meglumine diatrizoate) are injected through the catheter, and an anteroposterior x-ray is taken. If the catheter tip is free in the peritoneal cavity, in the absence of ascites, semilunes of contrast outline fetal bowel and contrast can be seen around the liver. If ascites is present, contrast can be seen diffusing into the ascitic fluid.

The red cells are infused in 10-mL aliquots to a total volume calculated according to the IPT transfusion formula already outlined. The fetal heart rate is monitored by Doppler ultrasound. If the fetus is in good condition, the heart rate increases to 160 to 190 beats per minute. Early bradycardia is rare but very ominous. Late bradycardia is an indication for prompt termination of the IPT, since intraperitoneal pressure may be approaching umbilical venous pressure. As intraperitoneal red cells increase in volume, real-time ultrasound will reveal an enlarging crescent of sonar lucency between the diaphragm and liver, further confirming the successful placement of the catheter tip. The mother is discharged about 24 hours after the IPT and is examined every 3 to 7 days by real-time ultrasound to assess both fetal condition and the adequacy of absorption of the intraperitoneal red cells.

### Technique of IVT

Neither fetoscopic nor intracardiac IVT will be discussed in this chapter. Only IVT under ultrasound direction will be considered. Most teams prefer to insert the needle tip into an umbilical vessel at its insertion into the placenta (usually a vein but occasionally an artery). In the same manner as for IPT, the mother is given full analgesic and muscle-relaxant premedication.

Prior to preparation of the maternal abdomen, the perinatal ultrasonographer takes considerable time and great care in identifying the cord vessel insertion, the target for the IVT needle (Figure 46-3). After aseptic preparation of the maternal abdomen, the obstetrician-venipuncturist, under real-time ultrasound guidance (the transducer being enclosed in sterile plastic), directs a spinal puncture needle (22 gauge if the fetus is between 20 and 30 weeks gestation; 20 gauge if between 30 and 34 weeks gestation), toward the target vessel. The transducer is positioned in such a plane that there can be simultaneous identification of the target vessel and the needle tip.

When the needle appears to be in the vessel, the stylet is withdrawn and aspiration of fetal blood (0.8 mL) into a lightly heparinized 1-mL tuberculin syringe is attempted. If free-flow blood is obtained, confirmation that the needle is correctly placed is determined in two ways:

1. A small aliquot of the blood is tested immediately for fetal hemoglobin by alkaline denaturation. If the hemoglobin solution resists alkaline denaturation (remains pink), the blood is fetal and the needle is correctly placed. An immediate hemoglobin examination of the fetal blood sample also is carried out. Subsequently, the fetal red cells are blood-grouped and direct anti-

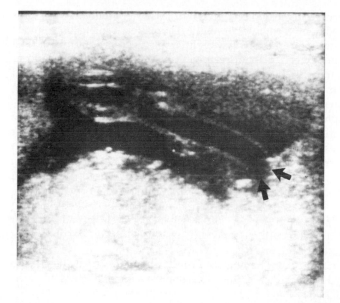

**FIGURE 46-3.** Real-time scan ultrasound view of insertion of the umbilical vein into the placenta (*arrows*). The lumen of the umbilical vein is sonar lucent. (From Bowman JM. Maternal blood group immunization. In: Creasy R, Resnik R, eds. Maternal-fetal medicine: principles and practice. 2nd ed. Philadelphia: WB Saunders, 1989:637.)

globulin tested. The hemoglobin is repeated and hematocrit, serum bilirubin, serum protein, platelet, and blood gas measurements are carried out in the laboratory.

2. Further confirmation of the proper placement of the needle is obtained by injecting 0.5 to 1.0 mL of sterile isotonic saline down the needle and observing characteristic ultrasound turbulence as the saline courses down the vein. If fetal movements are likely to disturb the needle insertion, pancuronium is injected into the fetal vessel to stop fetal movement temporarily. If the circulating red cell hemoglobin criterion ($\leq$110 g/L) is met, the donor red cells are injected in aliquots of 10 mL, the injection of each aliquot taking 1 to 2 minutes. The transfusion is monitored continuously by the perinatal ultrasonographer. Streaming turbulence is seen as the donor red cells pass down the vein. Conversely, if the needle tip is in an umbilical artery, turbulence is seen coursing in the opposite direction onto the fetal surface of the placenta. If characteristic turbulence is not seen, no blood should be transfused. If turbulence, once present, disappears, the transfusion must be stopped at once. Since only 2 to 3 mm of needle are in the fetal vessel, there is a significant risk of dislodgment, either into the amniotic cavity (easily recognized and not hazardous—the needle needs to be promptly reinserted into the vessel) or into the cord substance. The latter is potentially very dangerous, since further infusion of blood will produce a cord hematoma with great risk of umbilical venous compression, interference with venous blood flow, and serious fetal compromise.

The fetus, connected to its expansile placental vascular bed, can tolerate large volumes of blood. The actual volume infused varies from 40 mL/kg to 60 mL/kg, depending on the pretransfusion hemoglobin concentration and fetal condition. If the pretransfusion hemoglobin concentration is greater than 90 g/L or if the fetus is severely hydropic with a hemoglobin of 40 g/L or less, the initial IVT volume is 40 mL/kg of estimated nonhydropic fetal weight. Thereafter, transfusion volumes are usually of the order of 50 mL/kg body weight, rarely as great as 60 mL/kg. The aim is to reach, but not exceed, a donor-recipient circulating hemoglobin concentration of 200 g/L. A transfusion of 50 mL per estimated kg body weight of packed red cells, with a hemoglobin concentration of 280 g/L, will raise the circulating donor-recipient hemoglobin concentration 112 g/L.

The ultrasonographer monitors the fetal heart rate and size of the right ventricle during the IVT. On the very rare occasions when the fetal heart rate slows (under 110 beats per minute) or there is evidence of significant right ventricular dilation before the planned transfusion volume is reached, the IVT is discontinued.

When the desired packed red cell volume has been transfused, two 0.8-mL posttransfusion blood samples are withdrawn. The first is sent for blood gas measurements. The second sample is tested for hemoglobin, hematocrit, platelet count, serum bilirubin, serum protein, and Kleihauer acid elution adult donor fetal red cell ratio estimations. All the preceding tests are done on all subsequent pre- and post-IVT blood samples.

By raising the donor-recipient hemoglobin concentration to about 200 g/L, we aim to stop fetal erythropoiesis altogether. This donor-recipient hemoglobin level can be attained with two IVT spaced 2 to 7 days apart (the actual interval depending on the condition of the fetus and the initial pretransfusion circulating fetal hemoglobin level). Thereafter, transfusion intervals are determined by the donor-recipient red cell hemoglobin attrition rate (4 g/L/day), the posttransfusion donor-recipient hemoglobin concentration, and our desire not to let the circulating hemoglobin concentration in the fetus fall below 90 g/L.

## IUT IN THE PRESENCE OF HYDROPS FETALIS

If gross ascites is present, IVT is the procedure of choice; indeed, it is the only hope for the fetus so severely affected that no breathing movements are present. Without diaphragmatic movement, no absorption of intraperitoneal blood occurs. Only if venous access is impossible (a very rare occurrence) and the fetus is not moribund should IPT be carried out in the hydropic fetus. If the fetus is moribund and venous access is not possible, an intracardiac tranfusion should be undertaken.

If feasible, subsequent procedures should be IVTs. If further IPTs must be carried out, a second IPT should be given in 4 to 12 days, with the interval depending on ultrasound assessment of fetal condition and whether the hydrops is becoming more severe (increasing ascites, the appearance of pleural and pericardial effusions, increasing edema).

If IVTs are feasible in the hydropic fetus, and they nearly always are, we restrict the volume of the first IVT to 40 mL/kg, increasing to 50 mL/kg thereafter. The very anemic hydropic fetus may be very thrombocytopenic (platelet counts below 20,000/mm³) and at risk of exsanguinating hemorrhage. On several occasions, faced with this situation, transfusions of platelet concentrate have been required.

Since again our aim is to raise the total donor-recipient circulating hemoglobin to 200 g/L as quickly as possible, the second IVT is carried out within 1 to 7 days, at a time when the calculated donor-recipient hemoglobin level will be in the range of

90 to 100 g/L. Subsequent transfusion intervals do not differ from those in nonhydropic fetuses and are calculated in the same manner. Provided that the mother does not deliver, IVT invariably reverses fetal hydrops.

## SURVIVAL AFTER FETAL TRANSFUSION

Winnipeg IPT experience in the ultrasound era is shown in Table 46-4, column 1. The overall IPT survival rate was 76.0% (86.7% when the fetus was not hydropic, 60% when the fetus was hydropic). Of the 8 moribund nonbreathing hydropic fetuses, none survived.

Survival rates with IVT are set out in Table 46-4, column 2. Overall IVT survival rates were 93.2% (41 of 44 fetuses transfused and delivered). Of the 28 non-hydropic fetuses transfused, 27 (96.4%) survived. Fourteen of 16 hydropic fetuses (87.5%) survived; 6 of the 16 were moribund and 5 survived.

## RISKS OF IUT

Maternal risks with either IPT or IVT are very low. Both carry some risk to the fetus (see Table 46-5).

The risk of fetal-maternal transplacental hemorrhage with increasing maternal antibody titer is great with IVT because of needle insertion into the fetal vessel at its placental end, fetal TPH occurring in at least 50% of cases. TPH at IPT will occur only if the placenta is inadvertently transfixed.

There is a risk of overtransfusion with specific different hazards, such as intraperitoneal pressures exceeding umbilical venous pressures at IPT, compromising umbilical venous blood flow; and hypervolemia at IVT, precipitating fetal

**TABLE 46-4.** Intrauterine Transfusions Winnipeg Ultrasound Era

| | 204 IPT (July 1980–October 1986) | 163 IVT* (May 1986–February 1989) |
|---|---|---|
| Total Fetuses | 75 | 44 |
| Survivors | 57 (76.0%) | 41 (93.2%) |
| Nonhydrops | 45 | 28 |
| Survivors | 39 (86.7%) | 27 (96.4%) |
| Hydrops | 30 | 16 |
| Incidence of hydrops | 40.0% | 35.6% |
| Survival of hydrops | 18 (60.0%) | 14 (87.5%) |
| Moribund hydrops | 8 | 6 |
| Survival | 0 (0.0%) | 5 (83.3%) |
| Nonmoribund hydrops | 22 | 10 |
| Survival | 18 (81.8%) | 9 (90.0%) |
| IUT per fetus | 2.7 | 4 |
| Traumatic deaths | 7 (10.0%) | 1 (2.3%) |
| Risk of death per IUT | 3.5% | 0.62% |

*Fourteen IPT were carried out on the 44 IVT fetuses whose management was primarily IVT.

**TABLE 46-5.** Hazards of IUT

IPT-IVT
  Maternal or fetal infection
  Maternal or fetal tissue trauma
  Exsanguination
  Precipitation of labor
  Fetal–maternal transplacental hemorrhage
  Graft versus host disease
  Transient susceptibility to infection
IPT
  Overtransfusion, increased intraperitoneal pressure, obstruction to umbilical venous
    circulation
IVT
  Overtransfusion with fetal heart failure
  Umbilical cord hematoma, obstruction to umbilical venous circulation

heart failure. The IPT problem can be circumvented by not exceeding the IPT volume formula already outlined and by discontinuing the transfusion at the first sign of fetal bradycardia. Hypervolemia at IVT, precipitating fetal heart failure, will undoubtedly occur if excessive volumes are transfused. We have been pleasantly surprised by the large volumes that the fetus will tolerate without going into heart failure. We never exceed 60 mL/kg estimated nonhydropic fetal weight and usually restrict the volume to 50 mL/kg. We discontinue the transfusion at smaller volumes if fetal bradycardia or marked cardiac dilation occurs, but the situation rarely arises.

A potentially serious and never-to-be-forgotten hazard at IVT is the risk of producing a cord hematoma if the needle tip inadvertently is in the cord substance. Such a hematoma may cause interference with venous blood flow and compromise the fetus. A skilled, experienced perinatal ultrasonographer will forestall such an accident by quickly having the transfusion stopped at the first sign of a cord hematoma forming.

## THE ADVANTAGES AND DISADVANTAGES OF IVT VERSUS IPT

The ability to sample fetal blood directly and infuse blood into the fetal circulation is a major advance in the management of the fetus with severe erythroblastosis. Because diagnosis of severity of disease is rendered much more accurate and because the response to direct transfusion occurs immediately, not over an 8- to 10-day period as it is with IPT, IVT is unquestionably the superior procedure and is the transfusion method of choice wherever possible.

There are certain situations in which IPT may be the only feasible procedure. On rare occasions in early pregnancy (before 20 to 22 weeks gestation), the fetal vessels may be too small to access. In such a situation, if there is an ominous amniotic fluid reading and ultrasound evidence of early but not severe hydrops, an initial IPT is indicated. More frequently, after serial IVT early in gestation— when the placenta and cord insertion are posterior and venous access is obstructed by the fetus (32 to 33 weeks)—we will elect a final IPT to carry the fetus to 36 to 37 weeks gestation.

## DELIVERY OF THE FETUS FOLLOWING IUT

The availability of fetal blood sampling and IVT with low risk (0.62% in our hands) has altered the gestation at which delivery is recommended. Where IVT is feasible, the fetus should not be delivered before 36 weeks gestation. An IVT at 34 weeks gestation will allow delivery at 37.5 to 38 weeks gestation. If IVT is not possible and IPT must be used, we would not carry out IPT after 31 to 31.5 weeks gestation, preferring delivery at 34.5 to 35 weeks gestation. These delivery times may be modified by the presence in amniotic fluid of evidence of pulmonary maturity. Nevertheless, even with such evidence, we would not recommend delivery before 32 to 33 weeks gestation, and if IVT were feasible, we would not deliver the infant before 36 weeks gestation.

## SUPPRESSION OF RH IMMUNIZATION

### PLASMA EXCHANGE

Intensive plasma exchange—whereby large amounts of maternal antibody-containing plasma (3 L/day, 5 days/week) are removed and replaced with saline, 5% albumin, and small amounts of fresh-frozen plasma—will reduce circulating maternal blood group antibody levels by 75% to 80%. Such reductions are transient and may delay the need for IUT by 2 or 3 weeks. The procedure is very costly, in both professional time and resources. With the advent of fetal blood sampling and IVT as early as 18 to 20 weeks gestation, intensive plasmapheresis, which carries minor risks to the mother, including the need for transfusion of small amounts of plasma, is rarely indicated. We would recommend its use only for the woman with an extremely high antibody level ($\geq256$), with a documented history of prior hydropic fetal death before 22 to 24 weeks gestation, and with a husband homozygous for the antigen to which she is sensitized.

### INTRAVENOUS IMMUNE SERUM GLOBULIN

Intravenous immune serum globulin (IVIG) administration has been reported to reduce severity of hemolytic disease. Doses required are 400 mg/kg maternal body weight administered for 5 days and repeated every 3 to 4 weeks. High-dose IVIG is expensive and is of modest benefit. Again, with the advent of very early fetal blood sampling and IVT, administration of high-dose IVIG is rarely indicated. It may be used as an alternative treatment measure to intensive plasma exchange.

### PREVENTION OF RH IMMUNIZATION

The ability to prevent Rh immunization is a major advance in the management of the Rh-negative pregnant woman. Experiments, carried out on Rh-negative male volunteers, in which the volunteers were given Rh-positive red cells and Rh antibody in the form of Rh-immune globulin (RhIG, anti-D IgG), showed that the anti-D prevented Rh immunization from developing.

Clinical trials followed, in which Rh-negative unimmunized women after delivery of Rh-positive infants and therefore at risk of Rh immunization were give

RhIG. All such trials were uniformly successful. One such trial is set out in Table 46-6.

## STANDARD RH PROPHYLAXIS RECOMMENDATIONS

Standard Rh prophylaxis recommendations are that one prophylactic dose of RhIG should be given to the Rh-negative unimmunized mother as soon as her baby has been determined to be Rh-positive, and in no event later than 72 hours after delivery. If the Rh status of the baby is not known within 72 hours, the mother should be given RhIG regardless of the fact that in one-third of such instances the baby will be Rh-negative and she will not be at risk. It is obviously better to treat unnecessarily than to fail to treat a mother who is at risk. Rh-negative mothers of all Rh-positive babies should be protected irrespective of the ABO status of the mother and baby. If there is inadvertent failure to administer RhIG within the 72-hour deadline, Rh prophylaxis should still be administered up to 28 days after delivery.

## RH PROPHYLAXIS PROBLEMS

In the past 21 years, standard postdelivery Rh prophylaxis problems have greatly reduced but have not entirely eliminated Rh immunization. Residual problems are outlined in Table 46-7.

Occasional failures to provide protection to the Rh-negative woman after delivery of an Rh-positive infant arise. There are three reasons:

1. The mother may not have attended for prenatal care.
2. The physician may not have had prenatal blood samples tested.
3. The hospital obstetric unit may not have sent cord and maternal samples for testing.

**TABLE 46-6.** Western Canadian Rh Immunization Prevention Trial (March 1, 1967, to January 31, 1968)

| Treatment and Parity | Number of Patients in Trial* | Patients Rh-Immunized 6–9 Months Later | |
|---|---|---|---|
| | | Number | % |
| RhIG, 145–435 μg, given within 72 hours postpartum | | | |
| Primiparas | 481 | 0 | 0 |
| Multiparas | 735 | 0 | 0 |
| TOTAL | 1216 | 0 | 0 |
| No treatment | | | |
| Primiparas | 203 | 18 | 8.9 |
| Multiparas | 297 | 18 | 6.1 |
| TOTAL | 500 | 36 | 7.2 |

* Only Rh-negative women who had just produced ABO-compatible, Rh-positive babies were entered in the trial. (Adapted from Chown B, Duff AM, James J, et al. Prevention of primary Rh immunization: first report of the Western Canadian Trial. Can Med Assoc J 1969;100:1021.)

**TABLE 46-7.** Residual Problems in Rh Prophylaxis

1. Failure of compliance after delivery
2. Failure to give prophylaxis after abortion
3. Failure to give prophylaxis after amniocentesis
4. Failure of protection after massive fetal TPH
5. Failure to protect against Rh immunization during pregnancy
6. The question of augmentation of the risk of Rh immunization
7. The question of Rh immunization during infancy
8. The question of the $D^u$ mother
9. The question of suppression of weak Rh immunization

Therapeutic abortion carries with it a 4% to 5% risk of Rh immunization; spontaneous abortion carries a 2% risk. It is mandatory that the Rh-negative woman who aborts or is aborted be given Rh prophylaxis. If minidoses of RhIG (50 µg) are available, they will provide protection for first trimester spontaneous abortions. The woman who has antepartum bleeding (threatened abortion) should be given 300 µg of RhIG. If the pregnancy continues, this dose should be repeated every 12 weeks until delivery.

If the placenta is situated on the anterior uterine wall, there is a risk that it will be traversed by the amniocentesis needle. Although this risk has been very much reduced by prior ultrasonographic placental localization, it still occurs in about 2% of amniocenteses. The unimmunized Rh-negative woman undergoing genetic amniocentesis or later amniocentesis for determination of pulmonary maturity should be given RhIG. The dose should be 300 µg, repeated in 12 weeks if she remains undelivered. Chorionic villus sampling carries a similar risk. Prophylaxis after chorionic villus sampling should be carried out in exactly the same manner as after amniocentesis. RhIG given to the pregnant woman, for any reason at any gestation, will not harm her Rh-positive conceptus.

Protection against Rh immunization is dose dependent. It has been shown experimentally that 300 µg of RhIG administered IM will prevent Rh immunization up to an exposure to 30 mL of Rh-positive blood (12 to 15 mL of red cells). Since only about one woman in 400 will be exposed to greater than 30 mL of blood, Rh immunization due to failure to diagnose massive fetal TPH and therefore failure to give more than 300 µg of RhIG will occur very rarely. Nevertheless, screening the Rh-negative woman for massive fetal TPH after delivery is recommended.

If massive TPH is diagnosed after delivery of an Rh-positive baby, 300 µg of RhIG should be given IM if the TPH is 25 mL or less, 600 µg (two vials) if the TPH is greater than 25 mL but less than 50 mL, 900 µg (three vials) if the TPH is greater than 50 mL but less than 75 mL, and so on. Up to 1200 µg (four vials) IM should be given every 12 hours until the total dose has been administered.

Rh immunization during pregnancy constitutes about 13% of all instances of Rh immunization if no prophylaxis is carried out. In the Manitoba experience, 1.8% (62) of 3533 mothers carrying Rh-positive fetuses, without evidence of Rh immunization at the beginning of their pregnancies, were Rh-immunized during pregnancy or within 3 days after delivery.

A clinical trial of antenatal Rh prophylaxis, whereby 300 μg of RhIG was given IM at 28 and again at 34 weeks gestation, was successful and reduced the incidence of Rh immunization from 1.8% to 0.1%. Antenatal prophylaxis consists of one injection of 300 μg of RhIG at as close to 28 weeks gestation as possible. The single dose at 28 weeks gestation has been highly successful. Universal antenatal prophylaxis combined with universal postpartum, postabortion, and postamniocentesis prophylaxis will reduce the prevalence of Rh immunization from the preprophylaxis incidence of about 13% to 0.27% (i.e., by about 97%).

Because of the likelihood of augmentation of the risk of Rh immunization if passive anti-D levels become very low, it is strongly recommended that a further 300-μg dose of RhIG be given if a woman given RhIG antepartum, for any reason, has not delivered within 12 weeks after her first 300-μg injection. If she then delivers within 3 weeks after administration of a second (or a third) dose, postdelivery RhIG need not be given if she has no evidence of a fetal TPH greater than 0.1 mL of fetal red cells.

It has been hypothesized that reverse maternal TPH of Rh-positive red cells into an Rh-negative fetus at the time of delivery will cause Rh immunization (60% of the mothers of Rh-negative babies are Rh-positive). The true incidence of maternal reverse TPH is 2% and the volumes are usually minute, equivalent to 0.005 mL fetal TPH. Rh immunization during infancy is exceedingly rare. Administration of RhIG to Rh-negative infants born of Rh-positive mothers is not indicated.

The great majority of "D$^u$" mothers are genetically Rh(D)-positive, the weakened expression of D being "environmental," because of the presence of C on the other chromosome [i.e., C(d)ecDe]. They are not at risk of Rh immunization and do not require RhIG. The less common D variant (genetic D$^u$) mother is missing part of the D antigen and is at risk of Rh immunization, but very much less so than the true Rh(D)-negative woman. If the genetic D$^u$ mother can be differentiated from the "environmental" D$^u$ mother, we recommend that she be given postpartum RhIG, although the risk of Rh immunization is very small.

Not infrequently, an Rh-negative woman will be determined to have a very weak Rh antibody. If the Rh antibody is demonstrable, even if only very weakly, by the most sensitive manual technique (enzyme), she is truly Rh-immunized, and RhIG administration will not prevent progression of her Rh immunization. Nevertheless, if there is any question about the specificity of such an antibody, it should be given, because RhIG will do no harm.

## CURRENT RECOMMENDATIONS FOR RH PROPHYLAXIS

The following are the current recommendations for Rh prophylaxis:

1. Every Rh-negative unimmunized woman who delivers an Rh-positive baby must be given one prophylactic dose of RhIG as soon as possible after delivery.
2. Every Rh-negative unimmunized woman, unless her husband is known to be Rh-negative, who aborts or threatens to abort must be given RhIG.
3. Every Rh-negative unimmunized woman who undergoes amniocentesis or chorionic villus sampling, unless her husband is known to be Rh-negative, must be given 300 μg of RhIG at the time of the procedure, with subsequent doses at 12-week intervals until delivery.

4. Every Rh-negative unimmunized woman whose husband is either Rh-positive or Rh-unknown should be given 300 μg of RhIG at 28 weeks gestation. A second dose should be given in 12.5 weeks if delivery has not taken place and need not be repeated postpartum if delivery occurs within 3 weeks.
5. If massive TPH is diagnosed, 300 μg of RhIG should be given IM for every 25 mL of blood or fraction thereof in the maternal circulation.

## NON-RH(D) BLOOD GROUP IMMUNIZATION

## ABO HEMOLYTIC DISEASE

Although ABO-incompatible hemolytic transfusion reactions are intravascular and much more serious than extravascular Rh-incompatible hemolytic transfusion reactions, ABO hemolytic disease is much milder than Rh hemolytic disease. Kernicterus due to hyperbilirubinemia in ABO hemolytic disease may occur, but the author has never seen hydrops caused by ABO hemolytic disease. ABO hemolytic disease is mild because A and B antigens are not well developed on the fetal red cell membrane, most anti-A and anti-B is IgM and does not cross the placenta, and most of the small amounts of IgG anti-A and anti-B that do cross the placenta become attached to the numerous other tissue and fluid A or B antigens. The cord blood direct antiglobulin test is only weakly positive and may be negative unless a sensitive test is used. Serologically, ABO hemolytic disease is by far the most common hemolytic disease. Management of ABO erythroblastosis is entirely pediatric. Amniocentesis and other fetal investigative measures are not required in the ABO-incompatible pregnancy.

## HEMOLYTIC DISEASE CAUSED BY ATYPICAL BLOOD GROUP ANTIBODIES

With the reduction in incidence of Rh(D) immunization, the increased prevalence of blood transfusion, and the greater screening of Rh-positive pregnant women,

**TABLE 46-8.** Association of Hemolytic Disease with Atypical Maternal Blood Group Antibodies

---

Common
  c(cE): incidence high, disease common, may be severe
  Kell: incidence high, disease uncommon but if present may be severe
  E: incidence high, disease common, usually mild, rarely may be severe
  C(Ce): incidence moderate, disease common, usually mild, rarely may be severe
Uncommon
  k: rarely present but when present may be very severe
  $Kp^a(Kp^b)$: rare, disease may require treatment, very rarely severe
  $Jk^a$: uncommon, may require treatment, rarely may be severe
  $Fy^a$: uncommon, usually mild, may require treatment, rarely severe
  S: uncommon, usually mild, may require treatment, rarely severe
Rarely, if Ever, Cause Hemolytic Disease
  s, U, M, $Fy^b$, N, $Do^a$, $Di^a$, $Di^b$, $Lu^a$, $Yt^a$, $Jk^b$, $C^w$
Never Cause Hemolytic Disease
  $Le^a$, $Le^b$, P

---

hemolytic disease due to other blood group antibodies is becoming relatively and absolutely more common. Many atypical blood group antibodies are without consequence. Others are potentially as hazardous as anti-D. Atypical blood group antibodies which have produced very severe disease (hydrops) in Manitoba were anti-Kell, anti-c or anti-cE, anti-Fy$^a$, anti-Jk$^a$, anti-CC, anti-k, and anti-E.

Anti-c and anti-Kell are potentially as lethal as anti-D. However, whereas the woman with anti-c has a 65% likelihood of having an affected baby and a 9% likelihood that the affected baby will become hydropic or will require IUT to prevent hydrops, the woman with anti-Kell has only a 4.5% likelihood of having an affected fetus. Anti-E is usually very benign. However, one of our referred patients had a prior hydrops due to anti-E and lost her fetus at IUT.

Table 46-8 lists four categories of atypical blood group antibodies and their potential for hemolytic disease. Pregnant women with atypical antibodies listed in the common and uncommon group should be managed in exactly the same manner as if they were Rh-negative and Rh(D)-immunized. Antibodies that never cause hemolytic disease may be disregarded, as those rarely, if ever, cause hemolytic disease. However, if the antibody is in the latter group and appears very potent and of high titer, amniocentesis and/or fetal blood sampling is indicated. As with Rh hemolytic disease, interpretation of atypical hemolytic disease is based on history, titer, amniotic fluid measurements, and ultrasound assessment. If these parameters indicate severe disease, fetal blood sampling, if possible, and IUT (IVT if possible) should be carried out.

# 47. MATERNAL INFECTIONS DURING PREGNANCY

The altered immune state of pregnancy increases the risk of infection for the adult host. Both the frequency and severity of infection can be increased.

There are conflicting laboratory data about a reduced immunologic response during pregnancy. For purposes of discussion, any evaluation of immunity is divided into two categories: humoral and cellular. Most of the studies of humoral immune response in pregnancy show reactions similar to those found in nonpregnant women. In contrast, the cellular immune response has generally been diminished. Although the mechanism remains in question, pregnancy generally has been associated with a depressed cell-mediated immunity.

Pregnant women have an increase in both the incidence and complications of malaria, and in endemic regions coccidioidomycosis is a leading cause of maternal death. All of these different disease entities, caused by bacteria, viruses, protozoa, and fungi, share two similar traits—they are normally held in check by cell-mediated immune mechanisms, and all are more serious in pregnancy.

Poverty is an important factor in maternal infection during pregnancy. Poor women have more frequent and severe infections than middle class or upper class women, for many reasons. The first is that poor women in America do not have the same access to antepartum medical care as women of higher economic levels. In addition, there is good experimental evidence that malnutrition can diminish the immune response. The morbidity associated with all infections is greater in the pregnant poor than in women of higher economic levels in the United States.

## URINARY TRACT INFECTIONS

Increased stasis of urine during pregnancy makes the urinary tract the most common site of infection. This altered state is caused by the convergence of a number of normal pregnancy changes. The capacity of the urinary tract is usually increased. Although there are few radiologic observations of the urinary tract in normal pregnant women, the available data indicate that dilation is mild in the first half of pregnancy, although this dilation is not a uniform phenomenon. After midpregnancy, the right side is dilated in three-quarters of cases, and the left side is dilated in a third. In addition, there is expansion of the renal pelves and calyces; there is also an increase in bladder capacity. At the same time, the collecting capacity is increased, and more urine is delivered to this dilated urinary excretion system in pregnancy as renal blood flow and glomerular filtration rate increase. Increased progesterone production effects urinary tract function. Ureteral peristalsis slows, and transit time from kidneys to bladder is prolonged. The impact on the bladder is hypotonia with an increase in the residual volume of urine. All of these changes increase the risk of urinary tract infection. Urine is an excellent growth medium for bacteria, and the stagnant urine provides an environment that encourages overgrowth of bacteria and subsequent clinical infection. The bacterial nidus for infection is present in the 2% to 10% of pregnant women with asymptomatic bacteriuria. It is small wonder that urinary tract infections are seen so frequently in pregnant women.

## PREVENTION OF PYELONEPHRITIS

It is estimated that 25% to 30% of women with asymptomatic bacteriuria at the time of their first antepartum visit will develop pyelonephritis later in pregnancy. Probably 80% of all cases of pyelonephritis in pregnancy could be eliminated if this population were identified and treated.

These results support the use of a standardized approach for pregnant women who are seeing the obstetrician for the first time. All should have a culture of voided urine to test for significant bacteriuria.

When urine culture tests are used to detect asymptomatic bacteriuria, a significant colony count is >100,000 colonies of one bacterial species. Women in high-risk categories for pyelonephritis should be rescreened during pregnancy. These include patients with a past history of pyelonephritis, those with sickle cell trait or disease, and those with diabetes.

For treatment, one choice is the use of a nitrofurantoin for 10 days after the 12th week of pregnancy. This family of drugs is chosen because there is minimal alteration in the fecal flora of the women taking them, which minimizes the risk of subsequent infections with some resistant organisms. There are many safe and effective alternative antibiotics that can be prescribed. Cure rates similar to those of the nitrofurantoins have been demonstrated with ampicillin, the cephalosporins, or sulfas. If a high percentage of the bacterial isolates in any individual practice are *Klebsiella*, ampicillin could be a bad choice, because so many of these strains are resistant. Similarly, if enterococcus is a frequent isolate, a cephalosporin often is inappropriate. Following treatment, the patient should have another urine culture to determine if the bacteriuria has been eliminated. If the repeat urine culture is positive for the same bacterial species and it is not resistant, treatment should be done with an antibiotic effective against the isolate. In those women who are culture negative after treatment, clean voided urine cultures should be repeated in each subsequent trimester of pregnancy, because many patients will have a recurrence of bacteriuria later in pregnancy.

## CYSTITIS AND PYELONEPHRITIS

Cystitis during pregnancy is a confusing disease. Despite universal screening and treatment of women with asymptomatic bacteriuria, the incidence of cystitis has remained the same, even though the frequency of pyelonephritis has diminished fivefold.

The diagnosis of cystitis should be suspected in any pregnant woman with frequency and dysuria, with or without a fever. Patients with these symptoms can have other problems, such as a vaginitis or urethritis. Because of this, they should have a hanging drop examination of vaginal secretions to determine whether or not the patient has candida vaginitis, trichomonas vaginitis, or bacterial vaginosis. An endocervical culture for *Neisseria gonorrhoeae* and *Chlamydia trachomatis* should also be obtained in these patients to rule out those infections. If the clinician notes on the request slip that the clinical diagnosis is cystitis, the laboratory must agree to continue to work up any *E. coli* isolates, even when more than one species is recovered, and do antibiotic susceptibility studies. Colony counts of less than 100,000 have meaning in these women. A 10-day regimen with a nitrofurantoin is my choice; alternatively, ampicillin, cephalosporins, or sulfas can be used. Although there is a theoretical concern about the use of sulfas in a woman about to deliver a premature baby, this class of drugs can be prescribed and then discontinued if there is any evidence of labor. All of these patients require a posttreatment culture. If positive, long-term suppression with the nitrofurantoins is often used.

The treatment of patients with pyelonephritis during pregnancy is much more intense. These patients are sicker and will usually benefit from in-patient therapy so that problems of fever, hydration, and electrolyte imbalance, as well as the infection, can be treated. In addition, premature labor can occur in these women. Occasionally, some of these women become critically ill. In a series with a large number of pregnant women with pyelonephritis, 3 of 99 (3%) had evidence of septic shock. In addition, adult respiratory distress syndrome has been reported in pregnant women with pyelonephritis.

All of these potential problems require a broad therapeutic approach to the pregnant patient with pyelonephritis. The uterus should be assessed immediately to be sure there is not a pattern of uterine contractions, and there should be immediate fetal heart rate monitoring to ascertain the health of the fetus. A vaginal examination should be done to be sure there is no cervical dilatation, and cultures obtained to rule out maternal colonization with Group B β-hemolytic streptococcus, *C. trachomatis* and *N. gonorrhoeae*. As soon as a voided urine sample can be obtained from the patient, a portion should be examined microscopically for the presence of bacteria. Uncentrifuged urine samples have been used by the author, but a recent survey of laboratory studies in patients with bacteriuria recommended oil immersion microscopy of a gram-stained centrifuged urine. A portion of the urine should be sent for culture. Fluid replacement should be an important part of therapy. Many of these women are dehydrated, a condition which is further aggravated because they are febrile with an increased insensible fluid loss. They need sufficient intravenous fluid replacement with a balanced electrolyte solution to ensure a urine output of at least 50 mL/hour. Because septic shock and respiratory distress have been reported in these women, they should be frequently observed with regular monitoring of vital signs. In addition, these patients must be monitored for premature labor. If it occurs, tocolytic agents can be employed. Because respiratory distress can occur when these agents are used, an electrocardiogram (ECG) should be obtained before treatment begins. If the patient has unrelenting flank pain, an ultrasound evaluation for the presence of urinary tract calculi should be done. If electrolyte abnormalities are noted in the initial screening blood chemistries, these can be corrected and repeat electrolyte determinations done until they are normal. Intravenous antibiotics should be given for treatment. Either ampicillin or one of the cephalosporins is acceptable. Both are usually well tolerated during pregnancy. Both of these antibiotics achieve high levels in urine. Because of this, a laboratory report of bacterial resistance can still be associated with a clinical cure. If such a report is obtained in a patient who has shown a good clinical response, the culture should be repeated. Only if the culture is positive with an organism resistant to the antibiotic should the regimen be changed. If the patient is allergic to penicillin, an aminoglycoside can be given. All patients should have a repeat culture done at 48 hours after the initiation of treatment. If bacteria are still recovered, consideration should be given to switching antibiotics to an agent more effective against the organism to avoid later recurrence of infection. When patients have been afebrile for 24 to 48 hours, they can be switched to an oral penicillin or cephalosporin to complete 10 days of therapy. (In the case of aminoglycosides, there is no alternative oral antibiotic.) All of these women should have a posttreatment culture obtained, and if it is positive, they should be treated with a different agent that is effective against the isolates. In those women who remain culture positive after a full course of treatment, it would be appropriate to get an ultrasound examination to check for the presence of urinary tract calculi. If the follow-up culture is negative, there is controversy about the subsequent care of these women for the rest of the pregnancy. One authority has championed antibiotic suppression of these women for the remainder of the pregnancy.

## RESPIRATORY TRACT INFECTION

### UPPER RESPIRATORY TRACT

Upper respiratory infections occur frequently in the wintertime. Most are viral in origin and antibiotics will not be beneficial. If the throat is inflamed or if tonsillitis is present, a culture for the group A β-hemolytic streptococcus should be obtained. If there is clinical suspicion of a group A β-hemolytic streptococcus infection, penicillin should be prescribed. If the patient is allergic to penicillin, erythromycin can be started. If the clinician suspects a viral cause for a sore throat, it is appropriate to wait for the culture report before starting therapy.

## LOWER RESPIRATORY TRACT

Although uncommon, pneumonia is a serious disease for a pregnant woman.

However, the prognosis for pregnant women with pneumonia has markedly improved in the last 20 years. The key to the care of these women is early diagnosis. The evaluation begins with careful percussion and auscultation. A sputum sample should be obtained for Gram's stain and culture. A chest radiograph should be obtained, as well as an arterial $po_2$. Blood studies, including a complete blood count and electrolytes, can be helpful. In most cases, the diagnosis is established by the roentgen findings.

The most frequent organism causing pneumonia in pregnant women is *Streptococcus pneumoniae*. This pathogen should be suspected in the febrile patient with lobar consolidation on chest radiograph and with white cells with gram-positive diplococci present on microscopic examination of a smear of the expectorate. Penicillin remains the drug of choice in the treatment of these women. Premature labor can be a problem. Adequate hydration and close monitoring of uterine activity is important. Because cardiopulmonary problems can occur with ritodrine, the use of magnesium sulfate is the best choice if tocolytic therapy is indicated in such patients.

A wide variety of other organisms can be implicated in the pneumonia in pregnancy in which the patient is febrile with an elevated white count. There are three pathogens other than *S. pneumoniae* that cause pneumonia: *Haemophilus influenzae*, group A β-hemolytic *streptococcus*, and the coagulase-positive Staphylococcus.

Another category of patients with pneumonia includes those with an atypical clinical presentation. These are the patients with roentgen evidence of pneumonia who may not be febrile. The most important diagnostic clue to these atypical pneumonias is the microscopic examination of the expectorate. If few or no bacteria are found, *Legionella pneumophila* and *Mycoplasma* are prime concerns. The antibiotic of choice for both of these organisms is erythromycin.

There are other uncommon pneumonias. Varicella pneumonia can be life-threatening. This diagnosis can be confirmed by roentgen examination of the lungs of a very ill patient with cutaneous manifestations of chickenpox. Fortunately, acyclovir, a potent antiviral agent, is available for the treatment of these women. In addition, assisted ventilation can be necessary in some women with extensive pulmonary involvement. First trimester varicella can result in the fetal varicella syndrome, and can be the rationale for termination of the pregnancy. There are other pneumonias that have serious implications. The first is tuberculosis. This should be part of the differential diagnosis in the patient with apical changes on radiograph who has no resolution of lung findings on treatment, particularly in the patient from an urban poor population or part of a population of recent immigrants to the United States. Another atypical pneumonia is caused by *P. carinii*. These patients usually have high fever, have a lowered $po_2$, and may have no changes initially on chest radiograph, but subsequently have diffuse bilateral alveolar disease. If this diagnosis is made, appropriate testing for anti-bodies to HIV should be done. In endemic areas, pulmonary infection due to yeast can occur. The most common pathogens in these patients are *Coccidioides immitis* and *Histoplasma capsulatum*.

## MENINGITIS

Primary meningitis in pregnancy is very uncommon, but when it occurs, it is life-threatening. The possibility of meningitis should be considered in any patient who has had generalized malaise for a period of time, followed by headache, nausea, vomiting, and hyperthermia. If this patient also has convulsions, the concern about meningitis should be high.

In adults, *Neisseria meningitidis* and *S. pneumoniae* are the most common causes, whereas *H. influenzae* is rarely seen. A presumptive diagnosis can be made of *N. meningitidis* by the presence of gram-negative cocci on Gram's stains and for *S. pneumoniae* by the presence of gram-positive diplococci.

There are some cases in which the spinal fluid examination is not diagnostic, because bacteria are not present and the glucose level is not reduced. In these situations, the major diagnostic concern is a viral meningitis such as coxsackie-virus B2. Viral cultures should be done on the cerebrospinal fluid (CSF) and antibiotics discontinued if studies of the spinal fluid are positive for a virus. Listeria meningitis can be confused with a viral meningitis. Many such patients will have no bacteria seen on Gram's stain and normal or borderline CSF glucose levels are found. A positive culture for *Listeria monocytogenes* will confirm the diagnosis.

## BACTERIAL ENDOCARDITIS

Bacterial endocarditis is another rare but serious infection for a pregnant woman. Although bacterial endocarditis occurs infrequently, it can be life-threatening. This is a difficult diagnosis for the obstetrician. It is an uncommon disease, and the clinical and laboratory findings can be subtle. The most diagnostic clinical sign is a changing heart murmur. At least three blood cultures should be drawn 30 to 60 minutes apart. An ECG should be obtained and an echocardiograph done to determine if there is vegetation on any of the valves.

Patients should be treated with intravenous bactericidal antibiotics for at least 28 days. Women with bacterial endocarditis are at risk for preterm labor with the delivery of premature infants. Careful monitoring of uterine activity and meticu-lous attention to fluid balance is important in this population.

## GASTROINTESTINAL INFECTIONS

Gastrointestinal infections have a broad range of presentation in a pregnant population.

## APPENDICITIS

Acute appendicitis illustrates how pregnancy can modify many of the clinical manifestations of intra-abdominal disease. Appendicitis in pregnancy usually presents with no fever, no leukocytosis, and right midquadrant pain. If the obstetrician makes the diagnosis of appendicitis in pregnancy, a surgical exploration of the abdomen should be carried out.

## CHOLECYSTITIS

Acute cholecystitis is another gastrointestinal problem seen in pregnant women. It should be suspected in the patient with nausea, vomiting, and right upper quadrant pain. New sophisticated imaging techniques that do not use radiation can be used to detect the presence of stones in the gall bladder or the collecting ducts. An important differential diagnosis in urban poor patients is the presence of an amoebic liver abscess. This abscess will respond to medical treatment with metronidazole, which should be given to avoid intra-abdominal rupture of the abscess.

## PERITONITIS

Primary bacterial peritonitis is a rare but life-threatening condition in pregnant women. In pregnant women, it has been associated with underlying disease or acute salpingitis. The diagnosis should be considered in any pregnant woman with fever and abdominal tenderness. Paracentesis and microscopic examination of peritoneal fluid should confirm this diagnosis, and the treatment should be with systemic antibiotics. Some of these women are critically ill, and they should be monitored closely for evidence of premature labor.

## DIARRHEA

Diarrhea is seen with some frequency in any large obstetrical practice. Fortunately, it is usually self-limited and without complication. If it is explosive in nature or persists beyond 24 hours, the associated dehydration can be accompanied by premature labor.

The patient is advised to take adequate oral fluids and to limit the use of medications in the first 24 hours to Kaopectate, a nonabsorbed local medicine that does not alter intestinal motility. Acute diarrhea in these women can be caused by rotaviruses or by Norwalk-like viruses. These infections are usually self-limited, and the diarrhea represents the response of the host's gastrointestinal tract to eliminate pathogens and toxins. If the diarrhea persists beyond 24 hours, the patient should be seen, evaluated for dehydration and uterine activity, and a stool specimen obtained. A portion of stool should be examined in the laboratory for ova, parasites, and fecal leukocytes. Another portion will be sent for culture to see if such organisms as *E. coli, Campylobacter, Yersinia enterocolitis, Salmonella*, or *Shigella* are recovered. The treatment of these isolates will be guided by antibiotic susceptibility studies. In the United States, it is rare for the diarrhea to be so severe that the patient requires admission and treatment with intravenous fluids for the dehydration.

## CHRONIC DIARRHEA

There is another category of women who require evaluation of the gastrointestinal tract. These are women with chronic diarrhea. They need to be evaluated for ova

**TABLE 47-1.** Treatment of Parasitic Infections During Pregnancy

| | Treat During Pregnancy? | Therapy |
|---|---|---|
| Malaria | | |
| *Plasmodium vivax* | Yes | Chloroquine phosphate, 1 g initially, 500 mg at 6, 24 and 48 hr, continued 500 mg weekly until end of pregnancy. Postpone primaquine until after pregnancy for radical cure |
| *P. malariae* | Yes | If sensitive to chloroquine, treat with same regimen as for *P. vivax* |
| *P. falciparum* | | |
| *P. falciparum* resistant to chloroquine or if severe infection | Yes | Quinine. If necessary, pyrimethamine and sulfadoxine (Fansidar). If Fansidar-resistant, then tetracycline |
| *Entamoeba histoylica* | | |
| Asymptomatic | No | Treat as asymptomatic cyst carrier postpartum with diloxanide furoate (Furamide) |
| Symptomatic* | Yes | Paromomycin (Humatin) if no intestinal ulcerations |
| | | Metronidazole for severe cases or if paromomycin unsuccessful |
| *Chlonochis sinensis* (liver fluke)* | No | Treat with praziquantel if complicated by cholecystitis, preferably postpartum |
| *Enterobious vermicularis* (pinworm) | No | Pyrantel pamoate (Antiminth) |
| *Giardia lamblia* | | |
| Asymptomatic or mild | No | |
| Symptomatic (poor weight gain) | Yes | Paromomycin; if fails, then metronidazole |
| Hookworm (*Necator americanus, Ancyclostoma duodenale*) | Yes Yes | Iron therapy; if fails, or heavy worm burden then, pyrantel pamoate |
| *Taenia solium* | No | Quinacrine, postpone until after delivery |
| *T. saginata* | No | Niclosamide |
| *Strongyloides stercoralis* | | |
| Asymptomatic | No | |
| Symptomatic* | Yes | After first trimester, thiabendazole (known teratogen) |
| *Tricuris trichuria* (whipworm)* | No | Severe disease rare, mebendazole (known teratogen) |
| *Hymenolepsis nana* (tapeworm)* | No | Niclosamide |
| *Ascaris lumbricoides* | Yes | Pyrantel pamoate in the late third trimester |

*Breast-feeding not allowed.
From Roberts NS, Copel JA, Bhutani V, et al. Intestinal parasites and other infections during pregnancy in Southeast Asian refugees. J Reprod Med 1985;30:720, with permission.

and parasites, particularly *Giardia lamblia* and *Entamoeba histolytica*. Therapeutic guidelines for parasitic infections in pregnancy are given in Table 47-1.

## LYME DISEASE

Lyme disease is a new infection for obstetricians. It is caused by a tick-borne spirochete, *Borrelia burgdorferi*, and is spread by the bite of infected ticks, *Ixodes dammini*, or related ixodid ticks. It is a multisystem disorder that usually begins in the summer with a spreading skin eruption, to be followed weeks to months later with cardiac, neurologic, or arthritic abnormalities. This is a transplacental infection that can result in intrauterine fetal death or impairment of cerebral function because of in utero acquired central nervous system infection. This pathogen is susceptible to antibiotics.

The diagnosis of Lyme disease will depend on the clinical awareness of the obstetrician, backed by appropriate laboratory testing. In the United States, most of the cases to date have been clustered in three areas: the Northeast from Massachusetts to Maryland, the Midwest in Wisconsin and Minnesota, and the West in California and Oregon. Clinically, the disease begins as a red macule or papule at the site of the tick bite, and this lesion spreads. Concomitant with this, the patient complains of malaise, fatigue, headache, chills, and fever. Blood should be drawn for IgM antibodies. In pregnancy, phenoxymethyl penicillin would seem to be the drug of choice for early disease. For patients who are first diagnosed with late disease, including arthritis, ceftriaxone seems to be the drug of choice, because of its long half-life.

# 48. HIV AND OTHER SEXUALLY TRANSMITTED DISEASES IN PREGNANCY

As might be expected, all of the STDs regularly occur in pregnancy, with varying effects on mother, fetus, and neonate (Table 48-1). This chapter will focus on issues related to HIV, gonorrhea, syphilis, chlamydia, HPV, and HSV infections in pregnant women and their fetuses.

## HUMAN IMMUNODEFICIENCY VIRUS

Infection with HIV results in a systemic, degenerative, and ultimately fatal disease that assaults the immune and central nervous systems. Its pathognomonic finding is a selective depletion of CD4$^+$ helper T lymphocytes. The final stage of infection, called the acquired immunodeficiency syndrome (AIDS), is characterized by complete derangement of the immune system, with occurrence of opportunistic infections (OIs) or neoplasms.

**TABLE 48-1.** Sexually Transmitted Pathogens

| Bacterial Agents | Viral Agents |
|---|---|
| *Neisseria gonorrhoeae* | Human papilloma virus |
| *Chlamydia trachomatis* | Herpes simplex virus |
| *Gardnerella vaginalis* | Hepatitis B virus |
| *Haemophilus ducreyi* | Cytomegalovirus |
| *Shigella* sp. | *Molluscum contagiosum* virus |
| Group B Streptococcus | Human immunodeficiency virus |
| *Treponema pallidum* | Protozoan Agents |
| Mycoplasma Agents | *Trichomonas vaginalis* |
| *Mycoplasma hominis* | *Entamoeba histolytica* |
| *Ureaplasma* | *Giardia lambia* |
| *urealyticum* | Fungal Agents |
| Ectoparasites | *Candida albicans* |
| *Phthirius pubis* | |
| *Sarcoptes scabiei* | |

## EPIDEMIOLOGY

From early in the epidemic, the transmission of HIV was well understood. Modes of acquisition include contact with blood or blood products, intimate sexual contact, and vertical transmission from mother to fetus or neonate.

### Intravenous Drug Use

Although as of May 1990 IVDU transmission was reported in 21% of AIDS cases, a disproportionate share of female AIDS patients were either inravenous drug users (IVDUs) (52%) or heterosexual partners of IVDUs (20%). The predominant source of spread in IVDUs is the sharing of needles contaminated with HIV-infected blood.

### Heterosexual Sexual Activity

Although the vast majority (60%) of AIDS cases in the United States have occurred in homosexual or bisexual men, heterosexual transmission is more common worldwide and is increasing in the United States. Although this mode of acquisition accounts for only 5% of AIDS cases overall, it ranks second after IVDU as a risk behavior for American women, currently accounting for 32% of female AIDS cases.

HIV appears to be much less contagious than most other STDs. The chance of acquiring HIV infection per sexual contact in the general population ranges from 1:1,000,000 to 1:100,000,000. This risk rises to 1:10,000 for a single heterosexual contact with an HIV-infected person using a condom, and to 1:1000 for a single instance of unprotected intercourse with an infected partner.

### Transfusion

Transfusion-associated HIV infection occurred as the result of the parenteral administration of infected whole blood, blood cellular components, plasma, or clotting factors between 1978 and 1985, at which time routine screening practices for HIV antibody were instituted. The current risk of infection after receiving a unit of blood ranges from 1:100,000 to 1:1,000,000.

## PATHOGENESIS

HIV-1 is one of the more complex members of the retrovirus family. It is composed of core (p 18, p 24, and p 27) and surface (gp 120 and gp 41) proteins, genomic RNA, and the reverse transcriptase enzyme, surrounded by a lipid bilayer envelope. The virion contains three structural genes (*gag*, *pol*, and *env*), and an intricate set of regulatory genes that control, among other things, each other and the rate of HIV production. Two of these genes (*tat* and *vif*) speed viral replication, while two more (*nef* and *vpu*) restrain growth. One last gene (*rev*) appears to operate as a switch, promoting protein expression and viral replication. It may direct the progression from latent to active infection.

HIV gains access to host cells via the binding of its surface protein gp 120 to CD4 receptors on helper T lymphocytes, B lymphocytes, macrophages, lymph nodes, Langerhans' cells of the skin, and some brain cells. The virion then fuses directly with the host cell membrane, an action apparently mediated by the gp 41 surface protein. Once inside, its reverse transcriptase converts its RNA genome to DNA, which is incorporated into the host genome.

A latent period of variable length ensues, during which HIV replication is restricted. The triggers for activation are poorly understood, and may include mitogenic, antigenic, or allogenic stimulation. An interesting finding is that in vitro HIV infection of resting helper T cells results in latent viral behavior, whereas infection of activated helper T cells, usually a very small percentage of the total T-cell population, leads to prolific HIV replication. Multiple infections (e.g., cytomegalovirus [CMV], HBV, HSV) and inflammatory processes (e.g., contact with semen, blood, allografts) induce T cell activation and may play a role in activating the virus.

Once activated, the infected host genome transcribes mRNA and virion RNA, the latter of which is packaged and transported to the cell surface for exocytosis. The host cell is killed during HIV replication. It is this latter phenomenon that results in the depletion of helper T lymphocytes and the subsequent immunodeficiency associated with clinical disease.

## CLINICAL MANIFESTATIONS

The CDC classification scheme for HIV infection is given in Table 48-2. The average incubation time from HIV exposure to primary infection is 2 to 4 weeks, with a range from 3 days to 3 months. When patients are symptomatic, most report the sudden onset of a flu-like syndrome with fever, malaise, lassitude, headache, myalgias, arthralgias, diarrhea, sore throat, lymphadenopathy, and a maculopapular rash on the trunk. Less frequent findings are elevated liver function tests and neurologic abnormalities. Symptoms can persist for 2 weeks. Patients suffering from primary infection will not have circulating antibodies to HIV, although viral cultures and tests identifying antigen or viral DNA should be positive.

Following this, the infection enters a latent phase of variable duration. Most HIV-infected persons fall into this category. Dormant HIV infection has been

**TABLE 48-2.** Centers for Disease Control HIV Infection Classification Scheme

Group I: Acute HIV Infection
Group II: Asymptomatic HIV seropositivity
Group III: Persistent generalized lymphadenopathy (PGL)
Group IV: Severe AIDS-related diseases
    A: Constitutional symptoms (formerly called AIDS-related complex or ARC)
    B: Neurologic disease
    C-1: Opportunistic infections listed in CDC surveillance definition
    C-2: Other recurrent infections
    D: Opportunistic malignancies listed in CDC surveillance definition
    E: Other serious conditions

reported to last longer than 10 years in some individuals, although progression to symptomatic disease and death appear inevitable.

Evidence of more substantial immunocompromise can take many forms. Constitutional symptoms such as weight loss, fevers, night sweats, and diarrhea are worrisome. Neurologic involvement either from direct HIV infection or opportunistic infection or neoplasm is common. Histologic central nervous system involvement has been documented in 40% to 80% of those dying of AIDS. Opportunistic infections included in the CDC surveillance definition of AIDS are listed in Table 48-3, and other recurrent infections associated with HIV disease progression are listed in Table 48-4. Finally, a number of opportunistic malignancies characteristic of HIV infection have been included in Table 48-5.

## MATERNAL AND FETAL RISKS

### Effects of HIV Infection on Pregnancy Outcomes

Preliminary data suggested a number of adverse perinatal outcomes in pregnancies complicated by HIV infection. They indicated an increase in the rates of preterm delivery and intrauterine growth retardation. Subsequent studies that controlled for IVDU failed to support this contention.

**TABLE 48-3.** Opportunistic Infections Included in the CDC Definition of AIDS (Group IV-C$_1$)

*Pneumocystis carinii* pneumonia
Chronic cryptosporidiosis
Extraintestinal strongyloidiasis
Cytomegalovirus infection (other than liver, spleen, or lymph nodes)
*Mycobacterium avium* complex or *M. kansasi* disease, disseminated
Candidiasis of esophagus, trachea, bronchi or lungs
Herpes simplex virus infection, disseminated or chronic mucocutaneous
Toxoplasmosis of the brain
Cryptococcosis, extrapulmonary
Histoplasmosis, extrapulmonary
Isosporiasis
Progressive multifocal leukoencephalopathy

**TABLE 48-4.** Recurrent Infections Commonly Complicating HIV Infection (CDC Group IV-C₂)

Recurrent Salmonella bacteremia
Multidermatomal *Herpes zoster*
Nocardiosis
Tuberculosis
Oral candidiasis
Oral hairy leukoplakia

## Perinatal HIV Transmission

Although it is accepted that perinatal transmission occurs, little is understood about the rate, timing, mode of spread, or cofactors involved in the process. First trimester transplacental infection has been hypothesized, based on the description of an AIDS embryopathy syndrome and viral antigen identification from electively aborted fetuses. Intrapartum transmission resulting from exposure to infected bodily secretions seems plausible, but has not been proved. HIV infection has developed in infants born by cesarean section with intact membranes. Transmission of HIV through breast-feeding has been documented in a limited number of cases. This has prompted authorities to recommend breast-feeding only for HIV-infected mothers in undeveloped countries; bottle-feeding is advocated for women living in industrialized countries.

Vertical transmission rates were initially thought to be 36% to 65%, but current estimates are much lower, ranging from 17% to 41%. The major difficulty in assessing vertical transmission is that infants will carry passively acquired HIV IgG antibody for up to 15 months. Because our mainstay tests involve antibody recognition, the diagnosis must be delayed in many children.

## PHYSICAL DIAGNOSIS

Close attention and thoroughness are necessary in the antepartum assessment of HIV-infected women. Periodic review of systems should uncover constitutional symptoms such as weight loss, malaise, fatigue, persistent fevers, chills, and night sweats; respiratory symptoms; and neurologic abnormalities. Physical examination should be meticulous. Ocular hallmarks include cotton-wool spots in *Pneumocystic carinii* pneumonia (PCP) and diffuse hemorrhages in cytomegalovirus (CMV). Mucous membranes may harbor candidal infection or Kaposi's sarcoma (KS) lesions. Skin lesions in the form of seborrheic dermatitis, herpes zoster, tinea, molluscum, or KS are typical, and generalized lymphadenopathy is common. A dry cough with rales is the rule with PCP; hepatosplenomegaly is often encountered in hepatitis, ideopathic thrombocytopenic purpura, and persistent generalized lymphadenopathy (PGL). Neurologic abnormalities can be remarkably subtle. Gynecologic manifestations include candidal vaginitis, rapidly growing condylomata acuminata, secondary syphilis, HPV, and KS lesions.

**TABLE 48-5.** Opportunistic Malignancies Commonly Complicating HIV Infection (CDC Group IV-D)

Kaposi's sarcoma
B-cell non-Hodgkin's lymphoma

## LABORATORY DIAGNOSIS

Common laboratory abnormalities during HIV infection include the following:

- Decreased CD4 levels
- Decreased helper/suppressor T cell ratio
- Absolute leukopenia, lymphopenia, anemia, or thrombocytopenia
- Elevated serum globulins
- Abnormal delayed cutaneous hypersensitivity

Numerous researchers have attempted to identify markers foreshadowing progression to AIDS. The most suggestive are:

- Elevated levels of β2 microglobulin
- HIV p 24 antigenemia
- Anemia
- Low helper T cell count
- High proportion of suppressor T cells
- Absolute lymphocytopenia
- Reduced level of HIV antibody
- Elevated level of CMV antibody
- Sexual contact with someone in whom AIDS has developed

The most common tests for HIV infection include detection of antibody or antigen and direct culture. Antibody tests include enzyme-linked immunoabsorbent assay (ELISA), immunofluorescent antibody (IFA), or Western blot. ELISA testing is highly sensitive and specific. False-negative ELISA results have been obtained in the brief window of time during early infection before antibody production has occurred. Finally, there is great enthusiasm for polymerase chain reaction (PCR), the new rapid technique for the detection of viral DNA.

## TREATMENT

### Zidovudine

Zidovudine (AZT) functions as an inhibitor of the reverse transcriptase enzyme of HIV, thus preventing viral DNA incorporation into the host genome. It has been shown to reduce opportunistic infections and prolong survival in AIDS patients.

The current recommendation is a dosage of 500 to 600 mg/day (much lower than the original dose of 1500 mg). This lower dose has significantly reduced the toxicity associated with AZT use.

### Sulfamethoxazole-Trimethoprim

This is the first-line drug of choice for PCP. Although many patients are treated orally, reduced gastric absorption during pregnancy favors parenteral administration. Both elements of this therapy cross the placenta, and although sulfa use is usually not recommended in the third trimester, the morbidity associated with PCP outweighs the minimal risk to the fetus.

### Pentamidine

There are two main uses for pentamidine in HIV disease. The first is in patients who have failed first-line treatment for PCP. Although its use in pregnancy has not been well studied, the hazards of untreated PCP override concern for the fetus. Aerosolized pentamidine is also being used for its prophylactic ability against the development of PCP, although its effects in pregnancy are unknown.

## PREVENTION

Early diagnosis in the asymptomatic phase of infection may allow for prophylactic therapy that could slow the disease progression.

## GONORRHEA

*Neisseria gonorrhoeae* infects both columnar and transitional epithelian, including the endocervix, urethra, anal canal, pharynx, and conjunctivae. Local spread in women results in endometritis, salpingitis, and bartholinitis, and systemic manifestations include arthritis, dermatitis, endocarditis, meningitis, myocarditis, and hepatitis. It is estimated that 2 to 3 million cases occur annually in the United States, with an incidence in pregnancy reported at 0.6% to 7.5%.

A number of risk markers for gonorrhea have been identified. These include age less than 30 years, nonwhite race, early onset of sexual activity, low socioeconomic status, unmarried status, urban dwelling, illicit drug use, and prostitution. The use of condoms, diaphragms, and spermicidal foams all have been shown to decrease the rate of sexual transmission of gonorrhea.

Women appear to be at higher risk than men for contracting gonorrhea. The chance of becoming infected as the result of a single sexual encounter with an infected heterosexual partner is estimated to be 20% to 25% for men and 80% to 90% for women.

## CLINICAL MANIFESTATIONS

The clinical presentation depends on the site of inoculation, duration of infection, and whether the infection has remained local or has spread systemically. The percentage of women with asymptomatic infection ranges between 25% and 80%. Gonococcal infections in pregnant patients are commonly asymptomatic.

### Anogenital Gonorrhea

Acute symptomatic anogenital infections in women are characterized by dysuria, increased urinary frequency, increased vaginal discharge secondary to an exudative endocervicitis, abnormal menstrual bleeding, or anorectal discomfort. Most women who become symptomatic do so within 3 to 5 days of inoculation, or during menstruation. Inflammation of the Skene's or Bartholin's glands is usually unilateral and acute in nature. Only 15% of all women with gonorrhea will have extension of infection to the upper genital tract, although this is rarely seen during pregnancy.

### MATERNAL AND FETAL RISKS

The association between maternal gonorrheal infection and ophthalmia neonatorum has been appreciated for over a century. Before routine administration of silver nitrate, this disease occurred in 10% of newborns. The institution of routine neonatal prophylaxis reduced this rate dramatically, although recently there has been a resurgence. Gonococcal infection is transmitted to 30% to 35% of babies who pass through an infected cervix. After an incubation period of between 4 and 21 days, bilateral purulent conjunctivitis is the usual manifestation, with rapid progression to corneal ulceration, scarring, and blindness in the absence of treatment. More recently, gonococcal infection during gestation has been linked with a wide variety of perinatal complications.

The most reliable method of gonorrhea detection in women is culture of the cervix and any other symptomatic site. Given the high percentage of asymptomatic gonococcal infection in sexually active women under the age of 30 years, routine annual endocervical screening is advocated. During pregnancy, cultures should be obtained from all patients at the first antenatal visit and again in the third trimester in those at high risk for infection. Factors identifying those at high risk include sex with a symptomatic partner, bleeding induced by cervical swab, Medicaid as a method of payment, age at first intercourse ≤16 years, and low abdominal or pelvic pain.

## TREATMENT

### Anogenital and Pharyngeal Infection
The factors to consider in the treatment of uncomplicated anogenital gonococcal infection are (1) the incidence in many urban areas of resistant strains of *N. gonorrhoeae*, (2) the availability of effective single-dose agents against *N. gonorrhoeae*, (3) the coexistence of chlamydial infection in up to 50% of patients, and (4) the absence of a rapid, reliable, inexpensive means of making the diagnosis of *C. trachomatis*. With these in mind, patients with gonococcal infections should be treated with regimens effective against both pathogens. The CDC has recently updated their recommendations. For pregnant women, ceftriaxone plus erythromycin is suggested (Table 48-6).

### Extragenital Disseminated Infection
Inpatient treatment is advisable for patients with disseminated gonococcal infection (DGI), particularly those with endocarditis, meningitis, synovial effusions, or

**TABLE 48-6.** Centers for Disease Control 1989 Recommended Treatment Guidelines for Uncomplicated Anogenital Gonorrhea During Pregnancy

---

Recommended Regimen
  Ceftriaxone 250 mg intramuscularly once
                    *plus*
  Erythromycin 500 mg orally 4 times daily for 7 days
                    *or*
  Erythromycin ethylsuccinate 800 mg orally 4 times a day for 7 days
Alternatives to Ceftriaxone
  Spectinomycin 2 g intramuscularly once
  Cefuroxime axetil 1 g orally once with probenecid 1 g orally
  Cefotaxime 1 g intramuscularly once
  Ceftizoxime 500 mg intramuscularly once

---

compliance problems. CDC recommendations for treatment include ceftriaxone, ceftizoxime, cefotaxime, or spectinomycin (Table 48-7).

## PREVENTION

Efforts to reduce the incidence of gonococcal infections rest with screening programs to identify asymptomatic cases; careful tracing of the sexual contacts of infected persons; rapid, adequate treatment strategies; education in safe sexual practices; and the neonatal use of prophylactic silver nitrate ointment or eyedrops containing either erythromycin or tetracycline.

## SYPHILIS

Syphilis is a chronic, debilitating systemic infection, characterized by infrequent but severe and varied exacerbations, caused by the spirochete *Treponema pallidum*.

## PATHOGENESIS

Syphilis is efficiently transmitted during sexual contact, with 60% of partners acquiring the infection after a single sexual encounter. Spirochetes require a break in the integument in order to gain access to the host. Microscopic tears in genital mucosa occur almost universally during sexual intercourse. There follows a mean incubation period of 21 days, with a range of 10 to 90 days. The organism sets up a local infection and eventually disseminates widely via lymphatic drainage. Wherever it lodges, it stimulates an immune response.

## CLINICAL MANIFESTATIONS

### Primary
The first sign of primary infection is the development of a single, nontender lesion at the site of entry. The most customary sites of infection in the female include the

**TABLE 48-7.** Centers for Disease Control 1989 Recommended Treatment Guidelines for Disseminated Gonococcal Infection During Pregnancy

---

Recommended Inpatient Regimens
    Ceftriaxone 1 g IM or IV every 24 hrs
        *or*
    Ceftizoxime 1 g IV every 8 hrs
        *or*
    Cefotaxime 1 g IV every 8 hrs
        *or*
    Spectinomycin 2 g IM every 12 hrs
        *or*
    Ampicillin 1 gm IV every 6 hrs, for strains known to be penicillin-sensitive
Recommended Ambulatory Follow-up Regimens
    Cefuroxime axetil 500 mg orally 2 times daily
        *or*
    Amoxicillin 500 mg plus clavulanic acid orally 3 times daily

---

vulva, introitus, or cervix. Extragenital sites include the lips, tongue, tonsils, breasts, and fingers. The lesion is a painless, dull red macule, which becomes a papule and then ulcerates. Ulcers are rounded with a well-defined margin and a rubbery, indurated, weeping base. The ulcer persists for 3 to 6 weeks without treatment and then heals spontaneously.

Painless unilateral or bilateral inguinal lymphadenopathy often develops a week after the appearance of the lesion. Nodes are small, rubbery, and nonsuppurative. Worth noting is that both ulcers and lymph nodes may become tender in the face of secondary infection.

## Secondary

The symptoms of secondary syphilis typically emerge 3 to 6 weeks later. By this time, the infection is widely disseminated and most symptoms are due to immune completion. Nonspecific complaints include fever, malaise, sore throat, headache, musculoskeletal pains, and weight loss.

A classic faint macular rash develops over the trunk and flexor surfaces in the vast majority of infected individuals. Its lesions are pink, rounded, and ordinarily less than 1 cm in diameter. The rash spreads over the whole body, including the palms and soles, and becomes first dull red and papular, then squamous. Superficial ulcerations called mucous patches appear in the mucous membranes in 30% of patients. Also, generalized lymphadenopathy is present in the majority.

Fewer than 10% of patients have other manifestations. They include arthritis, bursitis, osteitis, hepatitis, glomerulonephritis, gastritis, hypersplenism, and iritis.

## Tertiary

In the absence of appropriate treatment, one-third of patients develop tertiary syphilis. This is characterized by involvement of the cardiovascular, central nervous, or musculoskeletal systems. The presence of gummas in various tissues designates late benign tertiary syphilis. Aortic aneurysms and aortic insufficiency are characteristic cardiovascular lesions, and generalized paresis, tabes dorsalis, and optic atrophy with the Argyll Robertson pupil that accommodates but does not react to light are all features of neurosyphilis.

## LABORATORY DIAGNOSIS

The gold standard for diagnosis of early syphilis is the detection of treponemes on dark-field examination of ulcer scrapings or tissue samples. It is inexpensive and easy, and provides immediate results.

Indirect diagnosis of syphilis can be made with the use of two types of serologic tests. Nontreponemal tests such as the Venereal Disease Research Laboratory (VDRL) and rapid plasma reagin (RPR) become reactive approximately 2 weeks following development of the initial lesion. If more than one specimen has been drawn, a rising titer is also evidence of primary infection. In secondary syphilis, the VDRL titer is usually ≥1:16. Following successful treatment, the VDRL should decrease fourfold in 3 months and eightfold in 6 months. It should be nonreactive 1 year after therapy for primary infection, and 2 years for secondary disease.

The diagnosis of latent syphilis is made on the basis of two elevated nontreponemal serologic tests taken at least 1 year apart. A further diagnostic workup includes evaluation of the cerebrospinal fluid (CSF) and a chest radiograph to screen for calcification of the ascending aorta.

The diagnosis of neurosyphilis is challenging, because no one test is reliable. The CSF should be tested for cell count, protein, and VDRL. An elevated count of >5 white blood cells (WBC) per mm$^3$ is a relatively sensitive indicator of active infection. A positive CSF VDRL is diagnostic for neurosyphilis. Alternatively, a negative result cannot be used to rule out syphilis. In such cases, an FTA-ABS may be ordered; although less specific, it is highly sensitive, meaning that a negative result rules out the diagnosis of syphilis.

## TREATMENT

Treatment regimens in pregnancy are listed in Table 48-8.

## MATERNAL AND FETAL RISKS

Pregnancy does not appear to alter the course of syphilis; however, *T. pallidum* adversely affects pregnancy. It crosses the placenta and has been associated with preterm delivery, stillbirth, congenital infection, and neonatal death, depending on the timing of infection. The majority of infants with congenital syphilis are born to mothers with early syphilis, particularly recent or current secondary infection. Fetal infection during the first and second trimesters carries significant morbidity, and third trimester exposure results in asymptomatic infection.

Infants with early congenital syphilis are usually asymptomatic at birth, but develop symptoms at 10 to 14 days of life. A maculopapular rash arises and often desquamates or becomes vesicular. Many develop a flu-like syndrome with a copious nasal discharge, commonly referred to as "snuffles." Other symptoms include oropharyngeal mucous patches, lymphadenopathy, hepatosplenomegaly, jaundice, osteochondritis, iritis, and chorioretinitis. Untreated early congenital syphilis progresses to the late phase, marked by Hutchinson teeth, mulberry molars, deafness, saddle nose, saber shins, mental retardation, hydrocephalus, general paresis, and optic nerve atrophy.

**TABLE 48-8.** Centers for Disease Control 1989 Recommended Treatment Guidelines for Syphilis in Pregnancy

Early Syphilis Recommended Regimen
  Benzathine penicillin G 2.4 million units IM once (1.2 million units in each buttock)
Late Latent, Gummas, and Cardiovascular Syphilis Recommended Regimen
  Benzathine penicillin G 7.2 million units total administered as three doses of 2.4 million units IM given 1 week apart for 3 consecutive weeks
Neurosyphilis Recommended Regimen
  Aqueous crystalline penicillin G 12–24 million units administered 2–4 million units IV every 4 hours for 10–14 days
Neurosyphilis Alternative Regimens
  Procaine penicillin 2–4 million units IM daily
              with
  Probenecid 500 mg orally 4 times daily, both for 10–14 days

## CHLAMYDIAL INFECTIONS

*Chlamydia trachomatis* is probably the most frequently diagnosed sexually transmitted disease in the United States today, with an estimated prevalence of over 4 million cases, and an annual cost of over $1 billion. Lower genital tract infection predisposes in nonpregnant women to pelvic inflammatory disease (PID) and in pregnant women to a variety of maternal and neonatal infections.

## CLINICAL MANIFESTATIONS

The incubation period for genital chlamydial infections ranges from 6 to 14 days. A variety of clinical manifestations, from bartholinitis to PID with peritonitis and perihepatitis, have been described. The most common perinatal syndromes are briefly described below.

### Endocervicitis

The most commonly infected site in the female genital tract is the endocervix. As mentioned above, the majority of infected women are asymptomatic. Findings on physical examination extend from normal to cervical erosion and mucopurulent cervicitis (MPC). Requisite components of the diagnosis of MPC include endocervical friability; erythema or edema; the presence of yellow or green endocervical mucopus; and >10 polymorphonuclear leukocytes (PMNs) per high-power field of a cervical Gram's stain.

### Acute Urethral Syndrome

Chlamydial infection has also been implicated in the etiology of 25% of patients with acute urethral syndrome. Such women present with dysuria and increased urinary frequency in the face of sterile urine or low-level bacteriuria.

### Endometritis

It has been well established that the incidence of postabortion endometritis is higher among women with chlamydial cervicitis. Because up to 35% of women with chlamydial cervical infection who undergo elective termination develop endometritis, antibiotic prophylaxis is recommended for high-risk women.

### Acute Pelvic Inflammatory Disease

The association between maternal lower genital tract *C. trachomatis* infection, neonatal inclusion conjunctivitis, and the subsequent development of postpartum pelvic inflammatory disease (PID) has been recognized for over half a century.

## MATERNAL AND FETAL RISKS

Vertical transmission rates secondary to passage through an infected cervix are as high as 60% to 70%. Inclusion conjunctivitis develops during the first 2 weeks of life in 25% to 50% of these neonates, and another 10% to 20% will develop chlamydial pneumonia within 4 months of birth. Although the use of erythromycin eye prophylaxis has markedly decreased the incidence of conjunctivitis, this topical preparation has no protection against pneumonia.

Culture remains the optimal means of making the diagnosis of chlamydial infection. Isolation of *C. trachomatis* remains challenging, because the organism requires a susceptible tissue culture cell line. The McCoy cell is most commonly employed, using a technically arduous procedure whereby these cells are inoculated with specimen and then examined 24 to 72 hours later for the development of inclusions. Recent improvements that have increased the sensitivity of culture include the performance of a second passage for specimens initially negative, and the use of a cytobrush for sample collection.

Two chlamydial antigen detection products have become available recently. One uses fluorescent monoclonal antibody staining of chlamydial EBs (Microtrac-Syva Company, Palo Alto, CA), and the other is an enzyme-linked immunosorbent assay (ELISA) (Chlamydiazyme, Abbott Laboratories, Chicago, IL). The sensitivities and specificities of both products are comparable at over 90%. Their most appropriate use is in populations with a high prevalence of chlamydial infection, because their positive predictive value decreases markedly in low-prevalence populations.

## TREATMENT

The optimal treatment for uncomplicated chlamydial infection during pregnancy remains debatable. The CDC recommends erythromycin base or ethylsuccinate, given its good performance in multiple treatment trials, and reserves amoxicillin, which has been shown in limited trials to reduce vertical transmission, for an alternative regimen (Table 48-9). Erythromycin estolate can cause hepatotoxicity and is thus contraindicated during pregnancy.

## HUMAN PAPILLOMA VIRUS

Among women in the United States today, genital warts caused by human papilloma virus (HPV) is the most common viral STD. The association of HPV with genital intraepithelial neoplasias and squamous cell carcinomas has been publicized widely, resulting in an increased public awareness of the problem.

## PATHOGENESIS

HPV is a member of the papovavirus family, and is composed of double-stranded DNA. Over 50 types have been identified.

**TABLE 48-9.** Centers for Disease Control 1989 Recommended Treatment Guidelines for Chlamydial Infections in Pregnancy

---

Recommended Regimen
  Erythromycin base 500 mg orally 4 times a day for 7 days
Alternative Regimens
  Erythromycin base 250 mg orally 4 times a day for 14 days
*or*
  Erythromycin ethylsuccinate 800 mg orally 4 times a day for 7 days
*or*
  Erythromycin ethylsuccinate 400 mg orally 4 times a day for 14 days
    *or, if erythromycin cannot be tolerated,*
  Amoxicillin 500 mg orally 3 times a day for 7 days (limited data)

---

## CLINICAL MANIFESTATIONS

The majority of HPV lesions are subclinical, identified only with the use of colposcopy, cytology, tissue examination, or in situ hybridization techniques. They can be found on the vulva, vagina, cervix, and anorectal region. Exophytic warts, also called condyloma acuminata, are typically caused by HPV types 6 and 11. They appear as friable, pink, fleshy skin appendages that vary greatly in size and are either broad-based or pedunculated. Many lesions, however, are not visible to the naked eye. These flat endophytic condylomata are found with the use of colposcopy on the cervix, vagina, and vulva.

## LABORATORY DIAGNOSIS

The diagnosis of condyloma acuminata is usually made on clinical grounds. Given the high prevalence of subclinical disease, cytology, tissue biopsy, and in situ hybridization techniques are often necessary to make the diagnosis.

## TREATMENT

The most critical concept in HPV treatment is that none of our currently used regimens eradicates the virus. Remedies that are expensive, toxic, or scarring are of no known benefit to patients. Thus, therapy must be aimed at the removal of visible or dysplastic warts and symptomatic improvement.

### External Genital and Perianal Warts

Cryotherapy using liquid nitrogen or a cryoprobe is preferred in the treatment of external genital and perianal warts (Table 48-10). Topical application of trichloroacetic acid (TCA) and electrodessication or electrocautery are recommended as alternatives. These remedies are inexpensive, nontoxic, and, when used correctly, do not harm normal surrounding tissue.

**TABLE 48-10.** Centers for Disease Control 1989 Recommended Treatment Guidelines for HPV in Pregnancy

---

External Genital or Perianal Warts
  Recommended Regimen
    Cryotherapy with liquid nitrogen or cryoprobe
  Alternative Regimens
    Trichloroacetic acid (TCA) (80%–90%): Applied to warts weekly.
                            *or*
    Electrodessication/electrocautery
Cervical Warts
  Dysplasia must be ruled out prior to the institution of any therapy. Treatment should be performed with the aid of one trained in the treatment of dysplasia.
Vaginal or Anal Warts
  Recommended Regimen
    Cryotherapy with liquid nitrogen
  Alternative Regimen
    TCA as above

---

## Cervical Warts

For women with cervical warts, dysplasia must be ruled out. Cryotherapy, laser, and surgical approaches must be carried out in consultation with someone trained in the treatment of dysplasia.

## Vaginal and Anal Warts

Warty lesions in the vagina and anus can be treated using liquid nitrogen cryotherapy. The use of a cryoprobe for vaginal lesions is not recommended. The only alternative during pregnancy is TCA, using the same technique as for external lesions. Extensive or persistent lesions should be treated by an expert.

## MATERNAL AND FETAL RISKS

Warty lesions have a tendency to grow and become more vascularized during pregnancy. The only contraindications to a vaginal delivery are extensive lesions that might result in dystocia and lesions that might bleed heavily with birth trauma. Although some suggest removal of large warts during pregnancy, this practice is of uncertain benefit. Vertical transmission of HPV is rare, but can result in respiratory papillomatosis in the exposed infant. The exact mode of spread is unknown.

## HERPES SIMPLEX VIRUS

Genital herpes is an infection caused by sexual transmission of herpes simplex virus types 1 and 2 (HSV-1 and HSV-2).

## PATHOGENESIS

The majority of genital herpetic infections are caused by HSV-2, although up to 15% may be due to HSV-1. HSV is a double-stranded DNA virus that infects susceptible mucosal surfaces. It has an incubation period of 2 to 10 days, which is followed by a primary infection characterized by focal vesicle formation and a pronounced cellular immune response. The infection enters a latent phase, with the virus ascending peripheral sensory nerves and coming to rest in nerve root ganglia. Recurrent exacerbations occur intermittently, stimulated by poorly understood mechanisms.

## CLINICAL MANIFESTATIONS

There are three types of herpetic episodes. Primary infections occur in previously unexposed hosts, and are characterized by multiple painful vesicular lesions that ulcerate, with inguinal lymphadenopathy, and flu-like symptoms including fever, malaise, nausea, headaches, and myalgias. Symptoms usually persist for about 2 weeks, with viral shedding for about 12 days. Nearly 4% will progress to viral meningitis.

First episode nonprimary (secondary) genital herpes occurs in an individual with previous nongenital exposure to HSV-1 or HSV-2. Its presentation is generally much milder than primary infections.

Recurrent HSV is more frequent following HSV-2 infection. Approximately one-half of infected individuals will experience a recurrence within 6 months. Most of these episodes are prefaced by a 1- or 2-day prodrome consisting of localized pruritus, pain, and paresthesias. Systemic manifestations are absent. The episode usually lasts about half as long as the primary outbreak, with only 4 to 5 days of viral shedding.

## LABORATORY DIAGNOSIS

The diagnosis can be made using a number of laboratory techniques. Culture remains the gold standard. Results are typically available within 72 hours. Its sensitivity ranges from 70% to 95%, and is highest early in the course of primary infection.

## MATERNAL AND FETAL RISKS

Maternal HSV infection does not seem to confer any deleterious effect on pregnancy itself. The infection may be vertically transmitted, however, either transplacentally or perinatally. Fortunately, transplacental transmission is rare. Neonatal symptoms typically arise during the first 7 days of life. The infection is characterized by vesicular skin lesions and CNS abnormalities such as microcephaly, hydranencephaly, and microphthalmia. Death occurs in approximately one-third of infants, and neurologic sequelae are noted in most survivors. Perinatal acquisition occurs either with passage through an infected birth canal or from contact with orolabial lesions in the parents or hospital workers.

Infectivity appears to be enhanced during maternal primary infection. Also, the severity of perinatal morbidity is worsened in primary maternal infection; spontaneous abortion secondary to herpetic chorioamnionitis, preterm delivery, intrauterine growth retardation, neonatal infection, and death have all been described.

The Infectious Disease Society for Obstetrics and Gynecology developed a position paper on the peripartum management of women with a history of HSV. They made the following suggestions:

Weekly antenatal cultures should be abandoned.

In the absence of genital lesions, cesarean sections should be performed for obstetric considerations only.

A culture should be obtained from mother or neonate at delivery in order to identify exposed infants.

Women with genital lesions should undergo cesarean section, preferably within 6 hours of membrane rupture, to prevent HSV exposure in the neonate.

The mother should not be isolated from her infant.

## TREATMENT

Because there is no known cure for this virus, HSV becomes a chronic and usually recurrent infection. Acyclovir (Zovirax) is an antiviral agent that inhibits viral DNA synthesis. It has been shown to ameliorate the symptoms of primary infections, and when given prophylactically, may reduce the frequency and intensity of recurrences.

The safety of acyclovir in pregnancy has not been fully established. However, experience to date has not identified adverse fetal effects. In nonpregnant patients oral acyclovir has safely been used to suppress severe recurrent HSV for up to 3 years.

# 49. ARTHRITIS AND PREGNANCY

## APPROACH TO THE PREGNANT PATIENT WITH ARTHRITIS

Musculoskeletal complaints are common among pregnant patients. Certain *structural* changes are secondary to hormonal changes (sacroiliac relaxation), due to an alteration in weight (postural back pain), or related to redistribution of body fluid (entrapment neuropathy), and common overuse syndromes and minor trauma unrelated to pregnancy may be responsible for tendinitis or bursitis.

## RHEUMATOID ARTHRITIS AND PREGNANCY

Rheumatoid arthritis (RA), a systemic inflammatory disorder, causes pain and swelling of synovial joints in a symmetrical distribution. The smaller, peripheral joints are typically affected, and the arthritis is associated with morning stiffness and fatigue. The disease may be complicated by extra-articular manifestations.

In addition to chronic peripheral joint swelling, the diagnosis of RA is supported by the presence of serum rheumatoid factor (an autoantibody which binds the Fc portion of IgG), normochromic normocytic anemia, and elevated sedimentation rate. The 1987 American Rheumatism Association Criteria for RA (Table 49-1) allow proper diagnosis with greater than 90% sensitivity and specificity.

## EFFECT OF PREGNANCY ON RHEUMATOID ARTHRITIS

Since the earliest description of RA, physicians and pregnant women have observed gestational remission of symptoms. Improvement usually begins early in pregnancy, with a gradual reduction of pain, swelling, and stiffness, a decrease in the requirement for analgesics, and a sense of well-being that peaks near term. Of these patients, 75% improve during the first trimester, 20% during the second trimester, and 5% during the third trimester. In women with a history of juvenile rheumatoid arthritis, a flare is common 3 to 6 months postpartum. However, the outcome of pregnancy is good in JRA and the arthritis does not appear to be permanently reactivated.

It is difficult to determine which women will improve, because gestational remission of RA is independent of rheumatoid factor, the type of joint involvement, disease duration, number of children, or sex of the fetus. The cause of

**TABLE 49-1.** The 1987 Revised Criteria for the Classification of Rheumatoid Arthritis (Traditional Format)*

| Criterion | Definition |
| --- | --- |
| 1. Morning stiffness | Morning stiffness in and around the joints, lasting at least 1 hour before maximal improvement |
| 2. Arthritis of 3 or more joint areas | At least 3 joint areas simultaneously have had soft tissue swelling or fluid (not bony overgrowth alone) observed; bilateral involvement of PIP, MCP, wrist, elbow, knee, ankle, and MTP joints |
| 3. Arthritis of hand joints | At least 1 area swollen (as defined above) in a wrist, MCP, or PIP joint |
| 4. Symmetric arthritis | Simultaneous involvement of the same joint areas (as defined in **2**); bilateral involvement of PIPs, MCPs or MTPs is acceptable |
| 5. Rheumatoid nodules | Subcutaneous nodules, over bony prominences, or extensor surfaces, or in juxta-articular regions |
| 6. Serum rheumatoid factor | Abnormal serum rheumatoid factor positive in <5% of normal control subjects |
| 7. Radiographic changes | Posteroanterior hand and wrist radiographs, must include erosions or unequivocal bony decalcification |

* Diagnosis satisfied by at least 4 of these 7 criteria. Criteria 1 through 4 must have been present for at least 6 weeks. Patients with 2 clinical diagnoses are not excluded.
PIP, proximal interphalangeal; MCP, metacarpophalangeal; MTP, metatarsophalangeal.
Modified from Arnett FC, Edworthy SM, Bloch DA, et al The American Rheumatism Association 1987 revised criteria for the classification of rheumatoid arthritis. Arthritis Rheum 1988;31:315, with permission.

gestational remission in RA appears multifactorial, including hormonal changes (increased serum cortisol and estrogen), depressed cellular immunity, and protective humoral factors such as blocking antibodies or alteration of IgG carbohydrate composition.

## POSTPARTUM

At least 90% of women will have an exacerbation of RA, generally between 2 and 10 weeks after delivery. The rest (10%) may enjoy a prolonged postpartum remission, which rarely exceeds 8 months. Breast-feeding provides no protection against this postpartum flare. Likewise, abortion, either spontaneous or therapeutic, is often followed by exacerbation of RA.

## EFFECT OF RA ON PREGNANCY

RA patients usually deliver healthy newborns of normal birth weight. When compared to healthy pregnant women, those with RA have no increased frequency of spontaneous abortion, premature labor, or complications at delivery. Complications in both the mother and fetus are more likely to arise with antirheumatic drugs, which are not withdrawn in 25% of cases due to activity of disease.

Recent surveys have shown no decrease of fertility among women with RA.

## ANTIRHEUMATIC DRUG THERAPY

The symptoms of RA usually improve during pregnancy, and the need for drug treatment is often reduced. However, the patient whose disease does not improve presents an interesting and difficult problem for the clinician. To minimize any harmful effects on the fetus, only well-known drugs with short elimination half-lives should be used, in the lowest possible dose for limited periods. In this section, the approach to drug therapy is primarily directed at the 25% of women whose RA remains active, the 2% of women who experience the *onset* of RA during pregnancy, and the 90% of women whose disease flares postpartum during lactation.

### Acetaminophen

Acetaminophen, although not necessarily effective for symptoms of acute inflammation in rheumatoid arthritis, is nevertheless commonly prescribed for pain relief in patients with rheumatic diseases. It freely crosses the placenta, although there is no clear evidence that it causes congenital anomalies.

### Salicylates

Aspirin is inexpensive and efficacious, and remains the initial drug of choice for RA. Its role, and that of other nonsteroidal anti-inflammatory agents (see below) in the inhibition of prostaglandin synthesis, has an obvious effect on fetal development. Most notably, it inhibits the synthesis of prostaglandin $E_2$, which maintains pulmonary and systemic vessel relaxation, as well as patency of the ductus arteriosus. Toxicity of aspirin is often dose-related, including tinnitus, respiratory alkalosis, gastrointestinal erosion, and elevation of transaminases.

### Nonsteroidal Anti-Inflammatory Drugs

Even though there have been no reports of NSAID-related teratogenicity in humans, the reluctance to use them routinely during pregnancy has stemmed largely from the lack of controlled trials and a suitable alternative in aspirin.

### Gold

Intramuscular gold salts have been the standard of RA therapy for over 50 years, inducing remission in roughly 70% of patients by an unclear mechanism. Potential side effects of these agents include dermatitis, membranous nephropathy, bone marrow suppression, hepatotoxicity, and interstitial pneumonitis.

**Oral Gold.** In humans, 13 women with RA who continued oral gold therapy during pregnancy reportedly developed healthy infants. This report is encouraging, but further investigation is needed before oral gold can be considered safe during pregnancy and lactation.

### Corticosteroids

Corticosteroids are commonly used during a flare of rheumatoid synovitis and during serious extra-articular manifestations of RA. Prednisone is a popular choice because it is inexpensive and well absorbed when given orally. Adrenal suppression may occur in doses greater than 5 mg to 7.5 mg per day (prednisone or equivalent), especially when administered in divided doses. Therefore, corticosteroids should be tapered slowly when adrenal-suppressive doses are given for longer than 14 days.

Corticosteroids are generally safe in pregnancy. The placenta provides an effective barrier to prednisone and prednisolone due to placental 11-β dehydrogenase, which partially inactivates cortisone. Dexamethasone, conversely, is not reliably deactivated in the placenta, and is not recommended during pregnancy.

During lactation, low-dose corticosteroids are acceptable. Less than 1% of an oral dose of 5 mg prednisolone accumulates in mother's milk, but the effect of higher doses in the nursing infant has not been fully studied. When high doses (>30 mg) of cortisone or equivalent are required in the setting of a postpartum flare, consideration may be given to discontinuation of breast-feeding.

### Penicillamine
The more current and conservative posture recommends withdrawal of penicillamine when a pregnancy is being planned.

### Sulfasalazine
Sulfasalazine, widely used for inflammatory bowel disease, was originally formulated for treating RA, and is now enjoying increased use as a disease-modifying agent. Both the 5-amino salicylic acid and sulfapyridine components of sulfasalazine cross the placenta, without a known increase in congenital abnormalities. Reversible azoospermia and infertility have been reported in men receiving sulfasalazine, although infertility is not known to be a side effect among women. Until further reports of the risks and benefits of sulfasalazine in pregnant women with RA become clear, this useful agent should probably be withheld during pregnancy and lactation.

### Hydroxychloroquine
If a woman on hydroxychloroquine becomes pregnant, the drug should be withdrawn.

## IMMUNOSUPPRESSIVE THERAPY

Methotrexate and azathioprine are useful in RA, but should be avoided during pregnancy. Neither has been proven to impair fertility.

## SURGERY

Surgery, including synovectomy, arthrodesis, and prosthetic joint replacement, has greatly contributed to the preservation of ambulation and performance of activities of daily living for patients with severe RA. When possible, surgery should be deferred until the postpartum state.

## ADDITIONAL CONCERNS

Flexion films of the cervical spine are important for women with RA, even in the absence of neck pain, to search for atlantoaxial (C1–C2) subluxation. Greater than

3 mm of subluxation should alert the anesthesiologist to avoid excessive neck manipulation. These women should arrive in the delivery room wearing a soft cervical collar. If there is no subluxation, the anesthesiologist should still be aware of the presence of RA due to the potential exacerbation of temporomandibular joint arthritis, or the possibility of a narrowed trachea if cricoarytenoid arthritis is present.

If remission is achieved, this is an ideal time for muscle strengthening, toning, and joint mobility exercises, preferably through the physiotherapy department. A balance between rest and exercise is preferred, with at least two daily rest periods of 1 hour each. Exercise in a heated swimming pool is ideal, allowing muscle toning without undue stress on joints. In preparation for the post–delivery period, mothers should be informed about the likelihood of arthritis exacerbation, fatigue, and postpartum depression. Baby clothes should have Velcro ties or zippers instead of buttons, and occupational therapy should be specifically geared toward bathing and holding the infant. Reassurance with regard to self-esteem, body image, sexuality, and independence requires particular sensitivity in dealing with the woman with RA and other disabilities.

## ANKYLOSING SPONDYLITIS AND OTHER SPONDYLOARTHROPATHIES

Ankylosing spondylitis is characterized by progressive stiffness and discomfort of the spine, which may be seen radiographically as squaring of the vertebral bodies, progressing to calcification of the outer fibers of the annulus fibrosus, giving a "bamboo spine" appearance. The resulting loss of spinal mobility is characterized by flattening of the normal lordosis, poor chest expansion, and increased susceptibility to spinal fractures. Sacroiliitis, when present, is initially painful, and may lead to fusion of the sacroiliac joints. Several other conditions, including Reiter's syndrome, psoriatic arthritis, and ulcerative colitis-associated arthritis, belong to the spondyloarthropathy family, and can present like ankylosing spondylitis. Sclerosis of the lateral aspect of the sacroiliac joint, or *osteitis condensans ilii*, is an occasional postpartum phenomenon that is not necessarily associated with spondylitis.

Pregnancy does not usually induce remission in women with ankylosing spondylitis, most of whom experience aggravated disease during the second and third trimester, including spinal tenderness, morning stiffness, nocturnal pain, and increased need for NSAID therapy. Among spondylitis patients whose disease is active during gestation, relief of symptoms is typically not felt until a few days after delivery, lasting 4 to 8 weeks, after which an exacerbation of spinal disease may be accompanied by peripheral arthritis in up to 50% of patients, and anterior uveitis in up to 20%.

Women with psoriatic arthritis are similar to those with RA in that they enjoy improvement during the first trimester, and typically throughout the pregnancy. As in RA, the postpartum period may be difficult for those women with psoriatic arthritis.

Despite maternal difficulties during gestation, it should be noted that in a 1988 survey of pregnancy in 50 women with spondylitis, all 50 had uneventful pregnancies and gave birth to 120 healthy children (Eleventh European Congress of Rheumatology).

## RUBELLA-ASSOCIATED ARTHRITIS

Transient arthralgias lasting up to 1 month develop in 30% of women during rubella infection or after rubella vaccination. Less commonly, women may develop an acute symmetric polyarthritis involving the fingers, wrists, and knees, typically several days after the onset of the morbilliform rash, sometimes with notable tenosynovitis and painful stiff hands. Although arthritis may result when the rubella vaccine is inadvertently given during pregnancy, there have been no reports of vaccine-induced congenital malformation. Rubella-associated arthritis is treated with analgesics, and generally lasts several weeks, rarely if ever progressing to chronic arthritis.

## PARVOVIRUS-ASSOCIATED ARTHRITIS

Human parvovirus B19, the etiologic agent in erythema infectiosum or fifth disease, causes transient, symmetric polyarthritis in adults. The illness typically occurs during the winter, 4 to 14 days after exposure, and is characterized by a mild upper respiratory infection accompanied by a bright red rash on the face and followed by a lace-like eruption over the arms and legs. During this time, moderate synovitis of the small joints of the hands, wrists, and knees lasting several weeks to months may occur. Positive serology for human parvovirus-specific IgM antibody helps confirm the diagnosis.

There is increased risk of fetal death and aplastic anemia, particularly if exposure is during the first 18 weeks of pregnancy. These complications are monitored by ultrasound (hydrops fetalis and ascites), and maternal serum alphafetoprotein levels. During the course of monitoring, women should be reassured that the vast majority of pregnancy outcomes will be normal.

## REGIONAL PAIN

### FIBROMYALGIA

On occasion, women with musculoskeletal pain who have no objective abnormalities will describe sleep disturbance, tiredness, and typical trigger points indicative of fibromyalgia syndrome. This remains a diagnosis of exclusion, and is best treated with reassurance and gentle conditioning during pregnancy.

## TRANSIENT OSTEOPOROSIS

Transient osteoporosis in pregnant women in their third trimester with painful demineralization of one or both hips, the knee, or ankle may be involved, sometimes in a migratory fashion, with severe pain upon motion or weight bearing lasting several months before gradually resolving completely. Erythema and swelling may be present with no organisms. Radiographs may be initially normal, but within 4 to 8 weeks severe osteopenia of subchondral cortical bone is seen, with normal overlying cartilage.

Treatment is conservative, with rest and protected weight bearing for pain relief and prevention of fracture. Ibuprofen or naproxen can be used until 4 weeks prior to term. Low-dose prednisone is commonly used, although it does not always hasten recovery.

## SCOLIOSIS AND PREGNANCY

In pregnancy, scoliosis may be associated with increased breathlessness and back pain, neither of which are correlated with the severity of the spinal curve. In a study of 118 pregnancies in 64 women with scoliosis (two-thirds in excess of 60 degrees), there were no serious cardiorespiratory complications attributed to the spinal deformity, and the majority had normal vaginal deliveries.

## LOW BACK PAIN AND PELVIC ARTHROPATHY

Back pain is a frequent complaint among pregnant women, usually due to an exaggerated lumbosacral lordosis with decreased abdominal tone, causing undue stress of the ligaments and muscles of the lower spine. This condition is more common among those with underlying back disease such as spondylitis or scoliosis, prior trauma of disc disease, poor posture, and perhaps among older pregnant women. Conservative treatment with rest on a firm mattress, acetaminophen, and periodic moist heat are usually adequate. When pain is localized and fever is present, MRI is useful to rule out pyogenic infection of the sacroiliac joint, particularly if the pregnant patient is an intravenous drug abuser.

Pelvic relaxation, or pelvic arthropathy, occurs during the second or third trimester due to excess hormone-induced relaxation of the sacroiliac joints and pubic symphysis. The patient experiences pain and instability of these joints. Rest and analgesia usually suffice, and delivery can proceed vaginally. Severe instability may require a sturdy fitted girdle, securing the sacrum and symphysis for several months until joint stability returns to normal.

Several weeks after delivery, laxity of the pubic symphysis, coupled with the trauma of childbirth, may lead to osteitis pubis. These patients develop pain over the symphysis pubis, radiating down the inner aspect of the thigh, often aggravated by coughing or straining. Radiographs may be normal initially, but osteolysis and irregular joint margins develop within 2 to 4 weeks. Treatment is similar to that for pelvic relaxation, and remission occurs in several months.

Coccydynia, seen after a difficult delivery, is associated with pain and soreness of the coccyx radiating to the low back, aggravated by climbing stairs or during a bowel movement. A careful bimanual examination and radiographs should be performed to rule out abscess or bony lesion. A ring-cushion may relieve pressure while sitting, and stool softeners may prove invaluable. Some patients find relief from a local injection of anesthetic with steroids. Spontaneous recovery over weeks to months can be expected.

## REGIONAL PAIN DUE TO ENTRAPMENT NEUROPATHY

Carpal tunnel syndrome due to compression of the median nerve may cause episodic numbness, wrist or forearm pain, and weakness of grasp. Splinting of the wrist in a neutral position usually provides adequate relief until delivery, and low-dose salicylates, if given, should be stopped several weeks prior to expected delivery. If pain is severe, a carefully placed steroid injection into the carpal tunnel may help, particularly when there is underlying inflammatory arthritis. Surgical release and evaluation for underlying endocrine or inflammatory conditions should be considered if symptoms persist beyond delivery.

Compression of the lateral femoral cutaneous nerve as it emerges from the inguinal ligament may cause a burning dysesthesia or hypesthesia over the anterior and lateral thigh. This phenomenon, known as a meralgia paresthetica, is exacerbated by direct palpation of the superficial perineural tissue in the antero-lateral thigh. Acetaminophen, salicylates, and moist heat offer relief of symptoms. When necessary, a local steroid injection, targeting the region of greatest discomfort, is useful. Compression and symptoms abate on delivery.

# 50. SELECTED IMMUNOLOGIC AND CONNECTIVE TISSUE DISORDERS IN PREGNANCY

For a more thorough discussion of this topic, please see Chapter 74 in Reece EA, Hobbins JC, Mahoney MJ, and Petrie RH, eds. Medicine of the fetus & mother J.B. Lippincott, 1992.

## SYSTEMIC LUPUS ERYTHEMATOSUS

Systemic lupus erythematosus (SLE) is a multisystem disease that most frequently presents in young women. The apparent prevalence has increased as more mild forms of the disease are recognized. In 1974 Fessel found a prevalence of 1 in 700 women aged 15 to 64 years. In black women the prevalence was 1 in 245.*

In pregnancy, proteinuria and thrombocytopenia can lead to confusion with preeclampsia. The clinical features of preeclampsia, which usually run a much more acute course, remit after delivery, and are not associated with other features summarized in Table 50-1, normally distinguish the two conditions.

## EFFECT OF PREGNANCY ON SLE

As with most illnesses that run a fluctuating course, such as asthma or disseminated sclerosis, it is difficult to document any special effect of pregnancy on SLE. Certainly a simple comparison of the prevalence of autoantibodies in a normal population has shown no difference between pregnancy and the nonpregnant state. The general consensus is that pregnancy does not affect the long-term prognosis of SLE but that pregnancy itself may be associated with more "flare-ups," particularly in the puerperium. In a comparison with the prepregnancy period, Garsenstein and coworkers (1962) found that the exacerbation rate was

---

*Fessel WJ. Systemic lupus erythematosus in the community. Incidence, prevalence, outcome and first symptoms; the high prevalence in black women. Arch Intern Med 1974;134:1027

**TABLE 50-1.** Criteria for the Diagnosis of SLE as Suggested by the American Rheumatism Association

1. Facial butterfly rash
2. Discoid lupus
3. Photosensitivity—skin rash as a result of unusual reaction to sunlight
4. Oral or nasopharyngeal ulceration
5. Nonerosive arthritis involving two or more peripheral joints
6. Pleurisy or pericarditis
7. Proteinuria > 0.5 g/day or cellular casts
8. Psychosis or convulsions
9. One of the following:
   a. Hemolytic anemia
   b. Leukopenia, WBC < 4000 μL on two or more occasions
   c. Lymphopenia < 1500/μL on two or more occasions
   d. Thrombocytopenia < 100,000 μL
10. Immunologic disorder:
    a. Positive LE preparation
    b. Antibody to native DNA in abnormal titer
    c. Antibody to SM nuclear antigen
    d. Chronic false-positive syphilis serology for 6 months
11. Antinuclear antibody in abnormal titer

From Tan EM, Cohan AS, Aries JF, Masi AT, McShane DJ, Rothfield N, et al. The 1982 revised criteria for the classification of systemic lupus erythematosus. Arthritis Rheum 1982;25:1271.

three times greater in the first half of pregnancy, one and one half times greater in the second half, and at least six times greater in the puerperium.[†] Chorea gravidarum is a rare complication of SLE in pregnancy.

## EFFECT OF SLE ON PREGNANCY

SLE affects pregnancy and its outcome in three main ways. First, it increases the risks of late pregnancy losses due to hypertension and renal failure. Second, it is an important cause of heart block and other cardiac defects in the newborn. This effect may be part of a more general neonatal lupus syndrome. Third, it increases the risk of abortion. Although technically most of the latter cases, being pregnancy losses before 28 weeks, should be classified as abortions, it is clear that they are quite different from most abortions, which occur at about 12 weeks. The losses in association with SLE may occur at gestations up to and even after 28 weeks with a bias toward the later part of pregnancy.

### Hypertension and Renal Failure

Houser and colleagues (1980) studied 18 pregnancies in patients with SLE.[‡] Ten occurred in patients with no evidence of renal disease and were uncomplicated. The remaining eight occurred in patients with renal disease. There were four

---

[†] Sarsenstein M, Pollak VE, Karils RM. Systemic lupus erythematosus and pregnancy. N Engl J Med 1962;267:165.

[‡] Houser MT, Fish AJ, Tagatz GE, Wilhaims PP, Michael AF. Pregnancy and systemic lupus erythematosus. Am J Obstet Gynecol 1980;138:409.

abortions (one elective), three premature deliveries, and only one normal-term delivery. A creatinine clearance of less than 65 mL/min/m$^3$ or proteinuria greater than 2.4 g in 24 hours would be ominous. Hayslett and Lynn noted a 50% fetal loss rate in mothers with a serum creatinine in excess of 132 mol/L (1.5 mg/dL).§

## The Neonatal Lupus Syndrome

The neonatal lupus syndrome includes hematologic complications, cardiac abnormalities, babies in whom skin lesions are present or are the only abnormalities, and neonates who develop SLE in the absence of any involvement in the mother. Maternal IgG antibodies have been shown to cross the placenta.

The hematologic abnormalities are hemolytic anemia, leukopenia, and thrombocytopenia. They are usually transient and not a major problem.

By far the most common cardiac abnormality is complete heart block, which may be present and detected antenatally. Although the majority of infants born to mothers with SLE are normal, about one in three mothers (38%) who deliver babies with isolated congenital heart block have, or will have, a connective tissue disease. Most frequently, the disease is SLE.

About 60% of mothers who deliver a child with congenital heart block have antibodies to soluble tissue ribonucleoprotein antigen (anti-Ro and anti-La antibodies). Antibody has been found in the site of the conducting tissue in the heart of a fetus that died with complete heart block. More recently, it has been shown that the mothers and their offspring may also have an IgG antibody that reacts with fetal cardiac tissue. This antibody may also be involved in the pathogenesis of congenital heart block, and the presence of this and other autoantibodies may explain why the fetal prognosis is not invariably good even in the absence of well-established markers for fetal death such as anticardiolipin antibodies (see Abortion and the Cardiolipin Syndrome). In addition, fatal cases may be associated with endomyocardial fibrosis or pericarditis. Of course, fetuses may have congenital heart block because of a primary cardiac abnormality, frequently an atrioventricular canal defect.

## Abortion and the Cardiolipin Syndrome

The incidence of abortion in patients with SLE may be as high as 40%. On reviewing previous pregnancies, even those occurring before the onset of SLE, some researchers found that the incidence of abortion was 23%—about twice as high as that in a group of control patients. In another study of the outcome of 630 pregnancies in mothers with SLE, there was a 36% failure rate. The risk of abortion is not related to the severity of the condition.

In the last 5 years it has been realized that the presence of lupus anticoagulant and cardiolipin antibodies may be closely related to the risk of abortion and later fetal loss. It is probable that those women with clinical lupus who do not have significant cardiolipin antibodies or lupus anticoagulant do not have excess fetal risk.

Anticardiolipin antibodies are active against certain phospholipid components of cell walls. They are responsible for the "false-positive" Wasserman reaction, which has been known to occur in SLE. The higher the titer of anticardiolipin

§ Hayslett JP, Lynn RI. Effect of pregnancy in patients with lupus nephropathy. Kidney Int 1980;18:207.

antibodies, the greater the risk to the fetus. Other clinical features of the "anti-cardiolipin syndrome" are summarized in Table 50-2.

## MANAGEMENT OF SLE IN PREGNANCY

### Maternal Considerations

The drugs most frequently used for the treatment of SLE are simple analgesics, such as acetaminophen, and nonsteroidal anti-inflammatory drugs, including aspirin. In more severe cases antimalarial drugs, corticosteroids, and cytotoxic agents are used.

Acetaminophen (paracetamol) has been used widely in pregnancy with no adverse effects in normal therapeutic doses. Aspirin has been extensively studied. Three large prospective studies, including the Perinatal Collaborative Project of over 14,000 women exposed to aspirin in the United States, have shown no teratogenic risk. However, salicylate and other nonsteroidal anti-inflammatory agents have been associated with neonatal hemorrhage because of their action in inhibiting platelet function. In addition, there is the risk that prostaglandin synthetase inhibitors will cause premature closure of the ductus arteriosus and pulmonary hypertension. This appears to be more a theoretical than a practical risk. Chloroquine causes choroidoretinitis and should be avoided. Prednisone, at least in doses up to 30 mg/day, and hydrocortisone should be considered safe in pregnancy. Although an association between steroid therapy and facial clefts in the fetus has been claimed, the only data to support this are in rabbits. There is always concern that steroid hormones may cross the placenta, suppressing the fetal hypothalamus-pituitary-adrenal axis, and predisposing the fetus to Addisonian collapse after delivery. In practice, this occurs very rarely, if at all, probably because these steroids, in contrast to dexamethasone and betamethasone, are metabolized by the placenta and therefore do not enter the fetal circulation in significant quantities. If a woman has taken regular glucocorticoid therapy for more than 1 month in the year before delivery, parenteral steroids such as hydrocortisone (100 mg every 6 hours) should be given to prevent Addisonian collapse at this time. Azathioprine is the cytotoxic agent most commonly used in rheumatic conditions and the only cytotoxic agent that can be considered for use in pregnancy. Azathioprine has been used rather widely in pregnancy, chiefly in patients with renal transplants. There have not been any specific ill effects reported in the fetus. The worry concerning azathioprine is that it induces chro-

---

**TABLE 50-2.** Clinical Features of the Anticardiolipin Syndrome

1. Abortion: Recurrent IUD, placental thrombosis, and infarction
2. Thrombosis
   a. Venous: Recurrent DVT (also axillary, IVC, and retinal vein thrombosis)
   b. Arterial: Cerebrovascular accidents, peripheral arterial gangrene, coronary thrombosis, retinal artery thrombosis
   c. Other: Pulmonary hypertension, ? avascular necrosis
3. Thrombocytopenia: intermittent, often acute
4. Other occasional features: Coombs' positivity, livedo reticularis, migraine, chorea, epilepsy, ?endocardial disease, ? progressive dementia due to repeated cerebrovascular thromboses

From Hughes GRV, Harris EN, Gharavi AE. The anticardiolipin syndrome. J Rheumatol 1986;13:486.

mosome breaks. These have been observed in peripheral blood leukocytes in neonates exposed to maternal azathioprine therapy. They disappear as the infants grow older and the cells are replaced by others that have not been in contact with azathioprine. But the female fetus contains all the ova that the woman will ever shed during ovulation. It is therefore possible that these ova may be affected and that azathioprine will have impaired the future reproductive capacity of the female fetus.

In summary, acetaminophen is the best agent to use as an analgesic and an antirheumatic in pregnancy. Nonsteroidal anti-inflammatory agents are best avoided in normal therapeutic doses in the last trimester; if a patient requires extra therapy for this relatively short time, corticosteroids should be used. Since the ESR is elevated in normal pregnancy, it cannot be taken as an index of disease activity, and reduction of $C_3$ complement may be used instead. In patients taking long-term corticosteroids, parenteral steroid cover should be given in labor (see previous paragraph). Because of the risk of dangerous exacerbation of SLE in the puerperium, steroid dosage should only be reduced with great care after delivery. The use of azathioprine should be reserved for cases where steroid therapy has failed or is contraindicated.

In breast-feeding women the nonsteroidal anti-inflammatory drugs with short half-lives and rapidly eliminated or inactive metabolites are best (i.e., ibuprofen, flurbiprofen, and diclofenac). Salicylates and antimalarial drugs should be avoided for the reasons given earlier. Minute quantities of prednisolone are secreted in breast milk, and this drug should therefore be considered safe.

## Fetal Considerations

It was originally hoped that the use of corticosteroids would decrease the high abortion rate associated with SLE. In general, this has not been the case. However, more recently it has been reported that aggressive treatment with aspirin 75 to 300 mg/day and prednisone in doses increasing to 60 mg/day can suppress lupus anticoagulant and anticardiolipin antibodies and consequently improve fetal outcome. However, the dose of prednisone often makes the patients Cushingoid and induces diabetes that requires further treatment. Even with such treatment the pregnancies are usually complicated by hypertension or growth retardation and require very careful monitoring of both mother and fetus. Removal of anticardiolipin antibodies and lupus anticoagulant is not a guarantee of success, nor is failure to remove the antibodies a guarantee of fetal death. Furthermore, we still do not know the significance in fetal terms of these antibodies in an unselected population (see section on Abortion and the Cardiolipin Syndrome). Therefore, controlled clinical trials of this aggressive form of therapy are urgently required.

Monitoring of the fetus of the mother with cardiolipin syndrome requires all the resources that can be mustered in each department, since delivery may be necessary from 26 weeks gestation onward. Such monitoring should include clinical judgment, ultrasound measurement of growth, and cardiotocography. Even nonspecific bradycardia at the end of the second trimester may be an indication for elective delivery. In addition, many departments will use Doppler estimation of maternal uterine and fetal umbilical blood flows.

Patients who also have a history of thromboembolism, arterial or venous, should be treated with subcutaneous heparin throughout pregnancy in addition to any aspirin and prednisone therapy that might be considered necessary. The heparin is given as described for patients with thromboembolism in pregnancy (see Chaps. 43 and 44). Although this treatment will exacerbate any bone loss associated with steroid therapy, I believe it to be necessary in view of the dire consequences, particularly of cerebral arterial thrombosis.

The timing of delivery in patients with SLE without the cardiolipin syndrome depends on the severity of the condition and whether the patients have renal involvement or hypertension. If there are none of these complications, the patient should be delivered at term. Increasing degrees of renal failure or hypertension will necessitate early delivery, either for these reasons alone or because of evidence of fetal compromise, as judged earlier.

Congenital heart block should be diagnosed before delivery from routine auscultation of the fetal heart and subsequent cardiotocography when bradycardia is discovered. If possible, a detailed ultrasound examination of the fetal heart should then be performed. This will show atrioventricular dissociation confirming complete heart block and also demonstrates any structural heart disease that is present in 15% to 20% of cases and that may occur in the absence of maternal connective tissue disease. If the fetus has complete heart block, it is difficult to assess its general condition in utero, since accurate assessment usually depends on measurement of fetal heart rate and its variability. Measurement of umbilical blood flow by Doppler ultrasound can be of value, and antenatal fetal blood sampling to measure fetal blood gases could be of real value. In this situation the fetus can be monitored by repeated fetal blood gas estimation during labor, but many such fetuses are understandably delivered by elective cesarean section.

## SCLERODERMA

Scleroderma is a connective tissue disease affecting skin, gastrointestinal tract (esophagus), kidneys, and lungs. Scleroderma has been divided into localized cutaneous and diffuse cutaneous forms. In the localized cutaneous form, the scleroderma process is localized usually to the hands; it is associated with Raynaud's phenomenon and without organ involvement. The prognosis is good in general and particularly good in pregnancy. Diffuse cutaneous scleroderma has more widespread cutaneous manifestations and is a much more aggressive illness. The prognosis in general, and in pregnancy in particular, is far worse than that for localized scleroderma. Fetal outcome is poor. In a review of 17 pregnancies reported in the literature, Karlen and Cook (1974) documented 5 perinatal deaths and 5 instances of premature delivery.[*] These patients often have sclerotic skin and blood vessels, making venipuncture, venous access, and blood pressure measurement difficult. Both regional and general anesthesia are associated with technical problems, particularly the difficulty of endotracheal intubation. Such patients should see an anesthetist early in their pregnancy so that anesthetic management can be planned rather than guessed at in an emergency. Captopril has been advocated as treatment for crises in patients with scleroderma. It is usually used as an antihypertensive drug but should be avoided in pregnancy because of concern about the fetus.

[*] Karlen JG, Cook WA. Renal scleroderma and pregnancy. Obstet Gynecol 1974;44:349.

# 51. DERMATOLOGIC DISORDERS OF PREGNANCY

Skin changes in pregnancy include alterations common to most gestations (Table 51-1) as well as unique cutaneous eruptions specific to pregnancy (Table 51-2). (For a more thorough discussion of this topic, please see Chapter 75 in Reece EA, Hobbins JC, Mahoney MJ, and Petrie RH, eds. Medicine of the fetus & mother. J.B. Lippincott, 1992.)

## CUTANEOUS CHANGES IN PREGNANCY

### PIGMENTARY CHANGES

#### Hyperpigmentation

Darkening of skin during pregnancy is common. Areas usually affected are the arcolae of the breasts (so-called secondary areolae), the abdominal midline (darkening of the linea alba to form the linea nigra), and the axillae, perineum, perianal area, and genitalia. Freckles, nevi, and scars may also darken during gestation. Hyperpigmentation usually appears during the first trimester of pregnancy, progresses until delivery, and regresses postpartum; it may persist in the areolae and the linea nigra. Although the exact physiologic basis of this hyperpigmentation is unknown, estrogen and progesterone are believed to be mainly responsible for these alterations.

#### Melasma (Chloasma Gravidarum, the Mask of Pregnancy)

Melasma affects 50% to 75% of pregnant women and up to one-third of nonpregnant women exposed to oral contraceptives. Its onset is usually in the second half of gestation. Melasma is characterized by blotchy, brownish macules or patches on the cheeks, forehead, chin, upper lip, or mandible. Melasma in pregnancy is probably caused by a combination of hormonal changes, a genetic predisposition, and sun exposure.

### VASCULAR CHANGES

#### Spider Angiomas (Spider Nevi, Nevus Araneus)

Spider angiomas are small vascular lesions characterized by a pulsatile central red punctum and radiating branches. Spider angiomas usually begin to appear during the second to the fifth month of pregnancy and may increase in size and number until delivery. Pregnancy-associated spider angiomas usually occur in areas drained by the superior vena cava, such as the neck, throat, face (especially the periorbital area), and arms.

#### Palmar Erythema

Palmar erythema is a frequent finding in pregnancy. Its onset usually begins in the first trimester. Clinically, there are two forms of this disorder—erythematous

**TABLE 51-1.** Cutaneous Changes in Pregnancy

**Pigmentary Changes**
 Hyperpigmentation
 Melasma (chloasma gravidarum, mask of pregnancy)
**Vascular Changes**
 Spider angiomas (spider nevi, nevus araneus)
 Palmar erythema
 Varicosities
 Hemangioma
 Purpura
 Granuloma gravidarum
 Edema
 Vasomotor instability
**Hair Changes**
 Postpartum telogen effluvium
 Increased hair growth
**Connective Tissue Changes**
 Striae gravidarum (striae distensae, stretch marks)
 Molluscum fibrosum gravidarum
**Miscellaneous Changes**
 Changes in nails
 Changes in eccrine sweat glands
 Changes in apocrine sweat glands
 Changes in sebaceous glands

areas that are sharply separated from adjacent normal skin, or (more commonly) a diffuse erythematous mottling of the entire palm. This finding usually resolves postpartum and requires no specific therapy.

### Varicosities

Varicosities are common during pregnancy and frequently involve the saphenous and hemorrhoidal veins as well as vessels in the vulvar region. Varicosities may develop as early as the first trimester in response to a combination of factors (e.g., increased intrapelvic pressure due to the gravid uterus, hormonally induced

**TABLE 51-2.** Cutaneous Eruptions Associated with Pregnancy

**Dermatoses of Pregnancy**
 Herpes gestationis
 Pruritic urticarial papules and plaques of pregnancy (PUPPP)
 Impetigo herpetiformis
 Prurigo gravidarum/recurrent cholestasis of pregnancy
**Less Well Defined Eruptions Reported in Association with Pregnancy**
 Prurigo gestations of Besnier
 Spangler's papular dermatitis of pregnancy
 Autoimmune progesterone dermatitis of pregnancy
 Pruritic folliculitis of pregnancy
 Prurigo of pregnancy
 Toxemic rash of pregnancy
 Linear IgM dermatosis of pregnancy

vascular relaxation, fluid retention, or predisposing genetic factors). Treatment consists of frequent elevation of the legs sleeping in Trendelenburg's position, avoidance of clothing that interferes with venous return, and elastic support for the legs. Varicosities tend to improve after delivery.

## Hemangioma

Small superficial or subcutaneous hemangiomas may develop during pregnancy. These lesions usually appear at the end of the first trimester and enlarge slowly until delivery. They usually regress postpartum and require no specific treatment.

## Purpura

Purpura on the legs is common during the final trimester due (perhaps) to increased capillary permeability and/or fragility.

## Hyperemia, Gingival Hypertrophy, and Granuloma Gravidarum

Hyperemia and hypertrophy of the gingiva occur in a large percentage of pregnant women. Proliferation of capillaries within hypertrophic gingiva can result in the formation of granuloma gravidarum (also known as pregnancy tumor). These lesions clinically and histologically resemble pyogenic granulomas—dull red, vascular nodules that grow rapidly in size. They are usually located in the gingival papillae between adjacent teeth or on the buccal or lingual surface of the marginal gingival mucosa. Like pyogenic granulomas, these lesions bleed and ulcerate easily when traumatized. They usually regress after delivery. Proper dental hygiene and avoidance of trauma are appropriate therapy for most patients. Selected cases may require surgical treatment.

## Edema

Nonpitting edema of the eyelids, face, and extremities is a common feature of pregnancy. Fluid and sodium retention in these patients is thought to be related in part to increased levels of circulating adrenocortical, ovarian, and placental hormones. Moreover, the gravid uterus increases hydrostatic pressure within lower-extremity vessels and contributes to increased capillary permeability in dependent regions. It is important that cardiac and renal abnormalities as well as preeclampsia-eclampsia can be excluded as causes of this problem. Treatment includes dietary restrictions as well as physical measures (see section regarding varicosities).

## Vasomotor Instability

Vasomotor instability accounts for such symptoms as pallor, facial flushing, hot and cold sensations, and cutis marmorata (a transitory bluish-red mottling of the skin occurring on exposure to cold) that occur during pregnancy. These changes resolve upon delivery and usually require no specific therapy.

## HAIR CHANGES

### Postpartum Telogen Effluvium

Postpartum telogen effluvium is a rapid hair loss that begins roughly 4 to 20 weeks after delivery and often continues for several months. This condition requires no specific treatment. Hair regrowth within 6 to 15 months is the rule.

### Increased Hair Growth

The growth of coarse, terminal, male-patterned hair is sometimes seen during pregnancy. A common site of this problem is the face, especially the upper lip, chin, and cheeks; the arms, legs, back, suprapubic region, and abdominal midline may also be affected. Excessive body hair usually regresses within 6 months of delivery, but coarse terminal hair may persist. Patients who develop a substantial number of coarse terminal hairs may need to be evaluated for virilizing tumors or syndromes.

## CONNECTIVE TISSUE CHANGES

### Striae Gravidarum (Stretch Marks, Striae Distensae)

Striae gravidarum develop in a large percentage of pregnant women during the latter part of gestation. Striae gravidarum appear as irregular, linear, pink-to-violet lesions that are initially edematous and pruritic. Lesions eventually become atrophic and hypopigmented. Although their exact etiology is unknown, stretching of the skin, adrenocortical hormones, and genetic predisposition have been suggested to play roles in their pathogenesis. No specific treatment other than symptomatic or supportive measures are available.

### Molluscum Fibrosum Gravidarum

Molluscum fibrosum gravidarum, which clinically and histologically resembles a skin tag, often develops during the second or the third trimester of pregnancy. These lesions are commonly found on the sides of the face, neck, upper portion of the chest, or beneath the breasts. Their diameter ranges from 1 to 5 mm; lesions are pedunculated, skin-colored or slightly pigmented, and soft. These lesions may or may not regress after delivery. Persistent lesions may be treated with shave excision or light electrodesiccation.

## MISCELLANEOUS CHANGES

### Nail Changes

Nail changes during pregnancy develop in selected patients and may consist of transverse grooving, brittleness, and onycholysis (i.e., distal separation of the nail plate from the nail bed). Supportive treatment is advised, as is ruling out other causes of these abnormalities.

### Changes in Eccrine Sweat Glands

Eccrine sweat gland activity increases in pregnancy and may lead to an increased incidence of miliaria (heat rash), hyperhidrosis (increased sweating), and dyshidrotic eczema. Treatment is largely supportive.

### Changes in Apocrine Sweat Glands

Apocrine sweating, which occurs mainly in the axillae and groin, tends to decrease during pregnancy and may contribute to an improvement in preexisting Fox-Fordyce disease (an occlusive disorder involving apocrine pilosebaceous units) or hidradenitis suppurative (a chronic, recurrent, deep-seated pyoderma of apocrine pilosebaceous units).

## Changes In Sebaceous Glands

Sebaceous glands on the areolae of the breasts tend to enlarge during pregnancy and appear as small brown papules called Montgomery's tubercles. These papules may appear as early as 6 weeks of gestation. They tend to regress postpartum.

# DERMATOSES OF PREGNANCY

## HERPES GESTATIONS

Herpes gestations is (HG) is a rare, pruritic, blistering eruption of pregnancy and the immediate postpartum period. It may also occur in association with hydatidiform mole or choriocarcinoma. This disorder is not related to an active or prior herpes virus infection. HG is rare. The most recent estimate of its incidence is 1 in 50,000 Caucasian births. HG is less common among blacks. It usually begins in the second or third trimester but may develop as early as the ninth week of gestation or as late as 1 week postpartum. HG tends to recur in subsequent pregnancies; in recurrent cases, the onset tends to be at an earlier phase of the gestation.

HG is a polymorphous (i.e., many forms of lesions) eruption characterized by intense pruritus. The morphology of lesions in these patients may include urticarial papules and plaques, vesicles, bullae, and excoriations. Vesicles or bullae rimming inflammatory urticarial plaques is a classic (but not specific) morphologic feature of HG. In many cases, lesions initially appear within the umbilicus and then spread over the abdomen. The chest, back, buttocks, and extremities are also frequently involved in a generalized, symmetric pattern. Lesions may also develop on the palms and soles. Facial or mucosal lesions are unusual and occur in less than 10% of cases. Because HG is quite pruritic, numerous crusts and excoriations are commonly seen in these patients. Healing usually proceeds without scar formation unless bacterial infection or severe excoriation have occurred. Postinflammatory hyperpigmentation at lesional sites is common and typically resolves with time.

HG often improves late during pregnancy only to flare at the time of delivery. In fact, postpartum flares (or onset of disease) are seen in a large percentage of patients with HG. Clearing of lesions generally occurs within 3 months of delivery or soon thereafter. Temporary exacerbations or recurrences may also be noted at menses during the first few months postpartum. Flares can also occur if patients with a prior history of HG are exposed to oral contraceptives (both estrogens and progestins). Although there is no increased risk of maternal mortality in HG, maternal morbidity may be substantial because of severe pruritus, generalized malaise, fever, cutaneous erosions, or secondary bacterial infections. The incidence of fetal morbidity and mortality in patients with HG is controversial. At present, evidence suggests that there is an increased risk of prematurity in these patients. Cutaneous lesions in newborns are occasionally seen and may consist of urticarial, vesicular, or bullous eruptions. In general, these lesions are mild, transient, resolve within several weeks, and require no specific therapy.

Treatment of mild cases of HG may require only frequent applications of potent topical glucocorticosteroids. For more extensive and symptomatic disease, systemic glucocorticosteroids are required. Moderate doses of daily prednisone (i.e., 20 to 40 mg) usually control the eruption and relieve pruritus. Some patients respond faster to divided daily doses of glucocorticosteroids. All patients should be continually monitored to ensure that they are receiving the lowest possible dose of glucocorticosteroids for control of their disease. In fact, some degree of disease activity (i.e., a few new lesions every few days) in these patients is acceptable. Infants of mothers exposed to systemic glucocorticosteroids should be evaluated at birth for evidence of adrenal insufficiency.

## PRURITIC URTICARIAL PAPULES AND PLAQUES OF PREGNANCY (PUPPP)

PUPPP is a distinct dermatosis of pregnancy that has characteristic clinical features that separate it from other dermatoses of pregnancy. These clinical findings are important because no specific laboratory abnormality has been demonstrated in these patients. Although the exact incidence of PUPPP is unknown, it is reasonable to believe that it is a relatively common disorder because several large series have been reported.

PUPPP usually resolves within 1 week of delivery and may abate prior to parturition. PUPPP is not associated with an increased risk of maternal mortality, fetal morbidity, or fetal mortality. In general, PUPPP does not recur in subsequent pregnancies, though anecdotal reports of recurrent disease have been made.

Most patients with PUPPP respond to frequent applications of potent topical glucocorticosteroids. With this approach, lesions usually stop appearing within 2 to 3 days and patients can begin to taper their frequency of treatment.

## IMPETIGO HERPETIFORMIS

Impetigo herpetiformis is the nosologic designation for a rare form of pustular psoriasis that develops during pregnancy. This disorder is accompanied by significant constitutional symptoms, including fever, chills, nausea, vomiting, diarrhea, and in severe cases, tetany secondary to hypocalcemia. This disease is considered a life-threatening dermatosis.

Clinically, impetigo herpetiformis is characterized by erythematous plaques surmounted at their margins by tiny superficial sterile pustules. The plaques expand peripherally with new pustules forming at their leading edges. Lesions commonly begin in flexural areas but may extend to involve a substantial portion of the body surface area. In advanced cases, involvement of mucous membranes and nails (i.e., subungual pustules and onycholysis) occurs.

Biopsies of early lesional skin from patients with this disorder reveal changes identical to those seen in pustular psoriasis. Additional laboratory abnormalities in these patients may include elevated peripheral blood leukocyte counts, elevated erythrocyte sedimentation rates, hypoalbuminemia, and/or hypocalcemia. Patients requires careful monitoring, supportive treatment, and specific therapy for their skin disease. Some reports have suggested an increased risk of fetal morbidity and mortality in these patients. Impetigo herpetiformis tends to remit promptly after delivery but may recur in subsequent gestations.

## PRURIGO GRAVIDARUM/RECURRENT CHOLESTASIS OF PREGNANCY

Prurigo gravidarum (also called intrahepatic cholestasis of pregnancy or benign recurrent intrahepatic cholestasis) is a hepatic disorder characterized by severe pruritus that may be followed by jaundice in selected patients. It usually first presents in the third trimester but may begin earlier. Pruritus is often localized initially and later becomes generalized. Although no specific skin lesions are associated with this pruritus, excoriations may be seen. In general, pruritus precedes the onset of jaundice by 2 to 4 weeks; selected patients may develop malaise, fatigue, anorexia, nausea, or vomiting. Liver function tests in these patients often demonstrate elevated levels of alkaline phosphatase, leucine aminopeptidase, and bilirubin.

Recurrent cholestasis of pregnancy tends to remit soon after delivery, but as its name suggests it usually recurs in subsequent gestations. Although the exact etiology of this disorder is not known, it is believed to be hormonally induced in susceptible patients. Some patients with a history of this disorder have developed cholestatic jaundice when exposed to oral contraceptives. Current data suggest that there is an increased incidence of prematurity and postpartum hemorrhage in these patients. Although controversial, several studies have suggested that there is an increased incidence of fetal loss.

Dermatologic therapy in these patients is entirely symptomatic. Emollients, topical antipruritics, and in selected cases systemic antihistamines with or without cholestyramine may be beneficial.

## OTHER ERUPTIONS REPORTED IN ASSOCIATION WITH PREGNANCY

A number of cutaneous eruptions have been reported in association with pregnancy. However, most of these eruptions have been incompletely characterized clinically, histologically, and immunopathologically. In some instances, the existence of these disorders is controversial. A listing of these disorders is presented in Table 51-2.

---

# 52. CANCER IN PREGNANCY

---

Cancer during pregnancy is unusual. Recent observation suggests that, as a result of physiologic changes that normally occur in pregnancy, cancer during pregnancy may become more advanced because the diagnosis is not recognized as early as it otherwise might have been. Stage for stage, cancer during pregnancy is no more virulent than cancer occurring in the nonpregnant state. The routine interruption of pregnancy to influence cancer progression has not been established.

Chemotherapy experiences have been reported in a sufficient number of patients to state that congenital malformations will not routinely occur in patients treated in the second or third trimesters of pregnancy, and selective use of chemotherapy in the first trimester of pregnancy may obviate congenital malformations previously reported when patients had been exposed to alkylating and antifolate agents. However, prematurity and low birth weight remain problems in a substantial number of infants exposed in utero to chemotherapeutic agents during any trimester of pregnancy. (For a more thorough discussion of this topic, please see Chapter 76 in Reece EA, Hobbins JC, Mahoney MJ, and Petrie RH, eds. *Medicine of the fetus & mother*, J.B. Lippincott, 1992.)

## INCIDENCE

Estimates of cancer during pregnancy vary considerably (Table 52-1). The uterine cervix remains the most common site for neoplasia to develop in pregnancy. It is estimated that 1 in 770 pregnancies will be associated with cervical intraepithelial neoplasia and that invasive cervical cancer will occur in 1 of every 2200 pregnancies. The breast is the second most common site. The incidence of cancer during pregnancy as compared to that in control nonpregnant women suggests that there may be a significantly reduced incidence of cancer in pregnancy. Transplacental metastasis is extremely unusual, and metastases to the fetus are so rare as to preclude this as an indication for termination of a pregnancy complicated by cancer. The most common malignancy to be associated with fetal metastases is malignant melanoma.

## SURGERY IN PREGNANCY

Patients may undergo successful surgical procedures when they are pregnant without interfering with the fetus. In general, surgery should be delayed until the second trimester, which seems to be the safest time in terms of avoiding patients going into labor. Spontaneous abortion frequently occurs when surgery is performed in the first trimester, and premature labor has been associated with surgery in the third trimester. Corpus luteum function is replaced by the placenta after the 12th week of gestation. Pathologic ovaries may be safely removed once the patient has entered into the second trimester.

In preparing the patient for a surgical procedure, simple technical considerations may have an important impact on the success of the operation. For example,

**TABLE 52-1.** Estimates of Cancer Occurring in Pregnancy

| Site | Estimated Incidence |
| --- | --- |
| Cervix | |
|   Carcinoma in situ | 1/767 |
|   Invasive | 1/2205 |
| Breast | 1/3000 |
| | 10–39/100,000 |
| | 1/1008 |
| Vulva | 1/8000 |
| Ovary | 1/9000 |
| | 1/25,000 |
| Leukemia | <1/75,000 |
| | 1/100,000 |
| Hodgkin's disease | 1/1000 |
| | 1/6000 |
| Colorectal | 1/100,000 |
| Skin–melanoma | 2.8/1000 |

placing the patient in a lateral position to avoid vena cava and aortic compression is an important factor in considering anesthetic consequences of surgery. This will help avoid fetal complications of hypoxemia or hypertension. The gastroesophageal junction in pregnancy tends to be relaxed, and its ability to control regurgitation is diminished. The patient should be operated on only after one is certain that her stomach is emptied. Anesthesiologists must always act as if a pregnant woman has a full stomach, since progesterone relaxes the gastroesophageal sphincter and pyloric displacement by the gravid uterus impedes gastric emptying.

## RADIATION IN PREGNANCY

Radiation is commonly employed in the routine management of cancers that may occur in pregnancy. Deleterious effects that the fetus may experience from being exposed to radiation therapy have been recognized for many years. Three phases of pregnancy must be considered with regard to radiation damage. The preimplantation phase lasts for approximately 7 to 10 days and represents the time from fertilization to the implantation of the blastocyst into the uterine wall. Spontaneous abortion is the most likely consequence of an embryo being exposed to radiation in the preimplantation phase. For many patients the pregnancy may not be clinically recognized.

Organogenesis, the period from the first to 10th week of gestation, represents the most sensitive time for the fetus with regard to radiation injury. This is the time of major organ formation and the time the fetus is most susceptible to teratogenic agents. However, the central nervous system, the eyes, and the hematopoietic system remain highly sensitive to the effect of radiation throughout the entire pregnancy. Radiation has been associated with microcephaly—the most common malformation observed in humans exposed to high-dose radiation during pregnancy—and mental retardation. In general, such effects are seen in fetuses exposed to amounts greater than 50 rads (0.5 cGy) of low-energy-transfer (LET) radiation. Embryonic exposure to 5 rads (0.05 cGy) or less is rarely associated with anomalies.

Radiation exposure between the 11th and 20th weeks has been associated with a significant decline in anomalies. Exposure after the 20th week of gestation is usually limited to anemia, skin pigmentation changes, and dermal erythema. The risks of growth retardation and abnormalities of the eye and central nervous system increase throughout the later period of fetal radiation exposure. It has been suggested that fetuses exposed to radiation doses higher than 10 rads should be considered for therapeutic abortion.

## CHEMOTHERAPY AND PREGNANCY

Although certain drugs must be avoided during early pregnancy, others might be life-saving and might not cause congenital anomalies in the fetus. Prematurity and low birth weight are frequent complications of chemotherapy exposure in any trimester of pregnancy. The fear of exposure in the second and third trimesters of pregnancy resulting in congenital anomalies no longer appears to be a major concern, provided that the selection of drugs is appropriate. Children who have been born after in utero exposure to chemotherapeutic agents during the second and third trimesters have not been noted to have significant congenital abnormalities. See Table 52-2.

Physiologic effects of pregnancy may have an impact on the efficacy and toxicity of chemotherapeutic agents. For example, renal blood flow, glomerular filtration rate, and creatinine clearance increases may lead to increased clearance of drugs from the body. It has been suggested that amniotic fluid may act as a pharmacologic third space for such drugs as methotrexate, in a fashion somewhat analogous to ascites or pleural effusions that may then increase methotrexate toxicity. Gastrointestinal absorption of drugs may be decreased due to delayed gastric motility. The distribution and kinetics of antineoplastic agents may be substantially affected by the physiologic increase of body water in a pregnant woman in association with a 15% increase in plasma volume and changes in plasma protein concentrations. Drugs that cross the placenta have low molecular weight, have high lipid solubility, are nonionized, and are loosely bound to plasma proteins. However, knowledge regarding transplacental passage of chemotherapeutic agents is extremely limited.

In assessing the teratogenic effects of chemotherapeutic agents administered in pregnancy it must be kept in mind that up to 3% of children have associated major congenital anomalies and 9% have minor anomalies in pregnancies not complicated by cancer treatments or exposure to a chemotherapeutic agent.

## ASSESSING FETAL MATURITY

The early delivery of a child has been incorporated into the management strategy in treating pregnant cancer patients. This strategy requires that highly sophisticated newborn special care units be available for maintaining such infants. Infants born after 30 weeks of gestation have a definite survival advantage.

The use of the lecithin-to-sphingomyelin (L/S) ratio in amniotic fluid is extremely important. Corticosteroid therapy may hasten fetal lung maturation and avoid respiratory distress syndrome, provided the fetus is at least 30 weeks gestation. Dexamethasone therapy administered to the mother between 24 hours and 7 days prior to delivery appears to be most beneficial to infants.

## GYNECOLOGICAL MALIGNANCIES

### CERVICAL CANCER

The cervix remains the most common site for precancerous and cancerous changes in pregnancy. Epidemiologic studies suggest that women who develop cervical intraepithelial neoplasia and invasive cancer in pregnancy tend to be married at an earlier age, have an earlier age of diagnosis of cervical intraepithelial neoplasia and invasive cancer, and have a higher parity than a control population. The most common histologic types of cancer occurring in the cervix are squamous cell (93.1%), adenocarcinoma (3%), anaplastic carcinoma (2.6%), adenosquamous carcinoma (1.1%), adenoacanthoma (0.1%), and sarcoma (0.1%).

### CERVICAL INTRAEPITHELIAL NEOPLASIA

The presence of cervical intraepithelial neoplasia (CIN) in pregnancy is usually identified by Pap smear and confirmed by colposcopically directed biopsies. In

**TABLE 52-2.** Chemotherapeutic Agents and Reported Associated Anomalies by Trimester

| Chemotherapeutic Agents | Mechanism of Action | Reported Significant Anomalies by Trimester* | | |
|---|---|---|---|---|
| | | 1st | 2nd | 3rd |
| **Alkylating Agents** | | | | |
| Melphalan, chlorambucil, cyclophosphamide, triethylene thiophosphoramide, CIS-diammine-dichloroplatinum, streptozotacin, BCNU, CCNU, methyl-CCNU, busulfan | Cell cycle nonspecific; forms cross-linkages with DNA | Yes[†] | No | No |
| **Antimetabolites** | | | | |
| Amethopterin (methotrexate),[‡] aminopterin, 5-fluorouracil,[‡] cytosine arabinoside, 6-thioguanine, 5-azacytidine, hydroxyurea, hexamethylmelamine, L-asparaginase | Cell cycle specific; structural analogue of precursor purine and pyrimidine bases; lead to nonfunctional DNA and cell death | Yes[§] | No | No |
| **Antibiotics** | | | | |
| Actinomycin D, doxorubicin, daunorubicin, bleomycin, mitomycin C, mithramycin | Cell cycle nonspecific; interferes with DNA-dependent RNA synthesis; cell death from lack of RNA and an inability to produce cell proteins | No | No | No |
| **Vinca alkyloids** | | | | |
| Vincristine, Vinblastine, VP16, VM26 | Cell phase specific | Yes | No | No |
| **Glucocorticoids** | | | | |
| Cortisone, presnisolone, prednisone, methylprednisone, dexamethasone | Inhibition of DNA, RNA and protein synthesis | Yes[*] | No | No |

\* Reports of anomalies are limited and should be viewed with caution.
† Chlorambucil syndrome—renal aplasia, cleft palate, skeletal abnormalities.
‡ Abortifacients in first trimester.
§ Aminopterin syndrome—cranial dysostosis, hypertelorism, anomalies of the external ears, micrognathia, cleft palate.
# Cleft lip, cleft palate.

553

general, colposcopy will show the entire transformation zone, since the squamocolumnar junction tends to be present well out on the exocervix during pregnancy. If the entire transformation zone is not seen in early pregnancy, it is usually safe to wait a few weeks and repeat the colposcopy before making any definitive decisions regarding additional patient management, provided the Pap smear is consistent with cervical intraepithelial neoplasia and not invasive cancer. The latter diagnosis requires immediate evaluation. Cone biopsies of the cervix are avoided, since they are associated with hemorrhage, abortion, and premature labor.

It has been a successful policy to biopsy the worst colposcopically identified site, and if the cervical biopsy and Pap smear are consistent, simply to follow the patient throughout the pregnancy with Pap smears every 3 months. Patients are reevaluated at approximately 36 weeks gestation with repeat colposcopy and Pap smears to be as certain as possible that the lesion has not progressed.

If the assessment at 36 weeks remains consistent with cervical intraepithelial neoplasia, the patient and her physician are advised that the patient may deliver vaginally, if obstetrical indications are appropriate. No attempt is routinely made to perform cesarean hysterectomies in the management of cervical intraepithelial neoplasia. Assessment of precancerous changes can be readily done 8 to 12 weeks following delivery. In general, regression rather than progression is observed when one assesses patients postpartum for cervical intraepithelial neoplasia.

## MICROINVASIVE CANCER OF THE CERVIX

Microinvasive cancer of the cervix is defined as a lesion that has only microscopically penetrated through the basement membrane. The current International Federation of Gynecologsits and Obstetricians (FIGO) staging system is given in Table 52-3. In general, patients with microinvasive cancer are found to have abnormal Pap smears and undergo routine colposcopic assessment. The confirmation of extent of disease is extremely important in pregnancy. It may require a more extensive biopsy in the form of a hemicone biopsy or a cone biopsy of the cervix. If surgical margins are histologically free of disease on the cervical biopsy, patients may safely continue with the pregnancy as long as they are willing to be assessed with frequent Pap smears and colposcopy. Stage Ia2 patients have more extensive microinvasive cancer. Patients with microinvasive cancer who wish to undergo prompt therapy are usually successfully managed with a simple hysterectomy and leaving the ovaries in place. Patients who wish to have definitive surgery performed following completion of pregnancy may be delivered vaginally and have a subsequent hysterectomy or may be delivered by cesarean section followed by an extrafascial hysterectomy.

## INVASIVE CANCER OF THE CERVIX

The identification of invasive cancer of the cervix requires prompt treatment, except for patients in the third trimester, when one may briefly delay therapy until fetal viability is established. Patients with stage IB and stage IIA cervical cancer recognized in the first trimester of pregnancy are routinely recommended to be

**TABLE 52-3.** International Federation of Gynecologists and Obstetricians (FIGO) Cervical Cancer Staging Classification

| | |
|---|---|
| 0 | Carcinoma in situ, intraepithelial carcinoma; cases of stage 0 should not be included in any therapeutic statistics for invasive carcinoma |
| I | The carcinoma is strictly confined to the cervix (extension to the corpus should be disregarded) |
| Ia | Preclinical carcinoma of the cervix; that is, those diagnosed only by microscopy |
| Ia1 | Minimal microscopically evident stromal invasion |
| Ia2 | Lesions detected microscopically that can be measured; the upper limit of the measurement should not show a depth of invasion of >5 mm taken from the base of the epithelium, either surface or glandular, from which it originates; a second dimension, the horizontal spread, must not exceed 7 mm; larger should be staged as Ib |
| Ib | Lesions of greater dimension than stage Ia2, whether seen clinically or not; performed space involvement should not alter the staging but should be specifically recorded so as to determine whether it should affect treatment decisions in the future |
| II | The carcinoma extends beyond the cervix but has not extended onto the pelvic wall; the carcinoma involves the vagina, but not as far as the lower third |
| IIa | No obvious parametrial involvement |
| IIb | Obvious parametrial involvement |
| III | The carcinoma has extended onto the pelvic wall; on rectal examination there is no cancer-free space between the tumor and the pelvic wall; the tumor involves the lower third of the vagina; all cases with a hydronephrosis or nonfunctioning kidney should be included, unless they are known to be due to other cause |
| IIIa | No extension onto the pelvic wall, but involvement to the lower third of the vagina |
| IIIb | Extension onto the pelvic wall or hydronephrosis or nonfunctioning kidney |
| IV | The carcinoma has extended beyond the true pelvis or has clinically involved the mucosa of the bladder or rectum |
| IVa | Spread of the growth to adjacent organs |
| IVb | Spread to distant organs |

From Gynecol Oncol 1986;25:383.

treated with a type III radical hysterectomy and bilateral deep pelvic lymphadenectomies.

The surgical approach to the management of invasive cancer of the cervix in pregnancy has had mixed reviews in the literature. Some physicians believe that there is an increase in complications secondary to major blood loss and that postoperative complications, such as fistulae, are more likely. Other investigators have not found this to be as significant a problem. My personal experience suggests that for most patients radical hysterectomy in pregnancy is not particularly difficult, since there is substantial tissue edema and tissue planes are easy to establish.

Patients with more advanced cervical cancer are treated with radiation therapy. External beam radiation therapy has generally been employed first and will induce spontaneous abortion. Some physicians have recommended that a hysterotomy and termination of pregnancy be performed prior to initiating radiation therapy in second trimester cervical cancer patients, rather than waiting until the onset of labor secondary to the radiation.

Advanced-stage cervical cancer has a particularly poor response to standard radiation therapy. A major effort in the past few years has resulted in the development of neoadjuvant chemotherapy protocols for the management of such disease. The role for neoadjuvant chemotherapy in the control and treatment of patients with cervical cancer in pregnancy has yet to be assessed.

## BREAST CANCER

The breast is the second most common site for invasive cancers in pregnant women. It is estimated that approximately 1 in 3000 pregnancies will be associated with breast cancer. The average age for patients to develop breast cancer in pregnancy is between 32 and 38 years. Breast self-examination as well as physician examinations should be a routine part of prenatal care. The diagnosis of cancer in pregnancy is complicated by the physiologic enlargement of the breast and associated hyperemia. Breast cancer diagnosed in pregnancy tends to be more advanced because of the misinterpretation of the significance of the mass and the ascription of that lesion to being part of normal pregnancy changes. Mammography may be employed safely in pregnancy, provided the abdomen is shielded. Suspicious breast masses in pregnancy must be biopsied.

The upper outer quadrants of the breasts are the most likely sites to identify breast cancer, as 50% of breast cancer will arise in these quadrants. Fine-needle-aspiration biopsy techniques have now been perfected and should be liberally used to separate benign masses from malignancy. Most malignant breast masses occurring in pregnancy are first discovered by the patient.

Excisional biopsy is the best way to confirm the nature of a breast mass. The biopsy can be done either under local anesthesia or under general anesthesia. The frequencies of the histologic types of breast cancer occurring in pregnancy are similar to those in the nonpregnant state. However, an occasional lactational mastitis can be confused with an inflammatory breast carcinoma. The differential diagnosis of neoplastic diseases occurring in breast masses in pregnancy includes Hodgkin's disease, Burkitt's lymphoma, acute myelogenous leukemia, and sarcomas.

It is routine to send a piece of the excised breast mass for estrogen and progestin receptor protein analysis. However, 23 of 32 patients with diagnosed breast cancer in pregnancy had cancer specimens that were negative for estrogen receptor, and the three cancers assayed for progestin receptors also were lacking that receptor. These findings were also compatible with an earlier report suggesting that breast cancer arising in pregnancy is not hormonally sensitive. The best success in treating pregnant patients with breast cancer is achieved in early-stage cancers. However, stage for stage, the prognosis for breast cancer patients in pregnancy is similar to that in the nonpregnant state. Breast cancer occurring in pregnancy should be treated in a manner similar to that occurring in the nonpregnant state.

The survival for patients with breast cancer is influenced by the presence of metastases to the axillary lymph nodes. Patients with metastatic disease to these lymph nodes benefit from adjuvant cytotoxic chemotherapy in the nonpregnant state. Because chemotherapy has teratogenic effects, pregnant women in the first trimester should be counseled regarding the possibility of a pregnancy termination. Patients in the third trimester may wish to delay chemotherapy until fetal maturity is achieved and the baby is delivered. Terminating a pregnancy in the presence of breast cancer has no effect on patient survival. Prophylactic castration of the pregnant woman with breast cancer does not influence her survival.

Previously, it was recommended that patients who developed cancer in pregnancy not become pregnant again. It now seems that delaying 3 to 5 years before conceiving might be wise, since most patients with breast cancer in whom the cancer recurs have those recurrences within the first few years of the diagnosis. Such patients may be placed on birth control pills without incurring a risk of reactivating the cancer.

## OVARIAN CANCER

Most ovarian cancers in the United States are epithelial in origin and occur in women over age 35. Most ovarian cancers complicating pregnancy are either borderline malignant potential epithelial cancers or germ cell malignancies. Invasive epithelial cancers are rare in pregnancy, and sex cord stromal tumors occur extremely infrequently.

Ovarian malignancies occurring in pregnancy are estimated to complicate 1 in 9000 to 1 in 25,000 pregnancies. Ovarian neoplasms are usually observed in the first trimester and are operated upon in the second trimester. These lesions tend to be asymptomatic when recognized. However, torsion is a relatively frequent presentation for a germ cell malignancy of the ovary and requires prompt surgical intervention. Simple cysts of the ovary may be followed with serial ultrasound examinations until the cysts resolve. Lesions greater than 6 cm in diameter, complex cysts (i.e., cysts containing both solid and cystic elements), and solid tumors are the usual indications for operative intervention in pregnancy.

In general, surgical management of ovarian neoplasms occurring in pregnancy is delayed until the second trimester, provided the patient is asymptomatic and the tumor is not suspicious for malignancy by diagnostic imaging techniques. Symptomatic patients and patients with tumors suspicious for malignancy should promptly undergo surgery to diagnose and initiate the treatment of the cancer. The final decision regarding management must be based on the histologic assessment of the operative specimens.

## SURGICAL STAGING

Surgical staging for ovarian cancer in pregnancy should be the same as that recommended for surgical staging in the nonpregnant state. A vertical incision should be used. On entering the abdomen, any free fluid should be aspirated and sent for cytology. If no free fluid is present, washings of the paracolic spaces, the pelvis, and subdiaphragmatic spaces should be obtained. The ovarian lesion should then be removed and sent for frozen section histologic analysis. Every effort should be made to remove the tumor intact. The remaining ovary should be carefully inspected and biopsied. Any peritoneal abnormalities should be sampled. Any retroperitoneal nodularities should also be sampled. Sampling of periaortic lymph nodes should be attempted. It is inappropriate to remove both ovaries when a germ cell ovarian malignancy is diagnosed by frozen section techniques. The most common neoplasm in the contralateral ovary of a woman with a germ cell malignancy is a benign cystic teratoma. Germ cell ovarian malignancies are almost invariably unilateral. Removing the contralateral ovary does not affect prognosis for the patient. The current FIGO staging system for ovarian cancer is presented in Table 52-4.

## EPITHELIAL OVARIAN CANCER

Borderline malignant potential tumors are the most common epithelial ovarian cancers in pregnancy. Stage IA and IB borderline malignant potential tumor patients appeared to be adequately treated with surgery alone. More advanced-stage ovarian borderline malignant potential tumors are also treated surgically, chemotherapy being reserved only for the unusual group of patients with invasive metastases in association with borderline malignant potential tumors of the ovary.

## GERM CELL OVARIAN MALIGNANCIES

Germ cell ovarian malignancies are infrequently occurring tumors that present in women in their second and third decades of life. The dysgerminoma is the most common malignancy in pregnancy. Management of dysgerminoma requires re-

**TABLE 52-4.** FIGO Ovarian Cancer Staging Classification

| | |
|---|---|
| I | Growth limited to the ovaries |
| Ia | Growth limited to one ovary; no ascites; no tumor on the external surface; capsule intact |
| Ib | Growth limited to both ovaries; no ascites; no tumor on the external surfaces; capsule intact |
| Ic | Tumor either stage Ia or Ib, but with tumor on surface of one or both ovaries; or with capsule ruptured; or with ascites present containing malignant cells; or with positive peritoneal washings |
| II | Growth involving one or both ovaries with pelvic extension |
| IIa | Extension and/or metastases to the uterus and/or tubes |
| IIb | Extension to other pelvic tissues |
| IIc | Tumor either stage IIa or IIb but with tumor on surface of one or both ovaries; or with capsule ruptured; or with ascites present containing malignant cells; or with positive peritoneal washings |
| III | Tumor involving one or both ovaries with peritoneal implants outside the pelvis and/or positive retroperitoneal or inguinal nodes; superficial liver metastases equals stage III; tumor is limited to the true pelvis but with histologically proven malignant extension to small bowel or omentum |
| IIIa. | Tumor grossly limited to the true pelvis with negative nodes but with histologically confirmed microscopic seeding of abdominal peritoneal surfaces |
| IIIb. | Tumor involving one or both ovaries with histologically confirmed implants of abdominal peritoneal surfaces none exceeding 2 cm in diameter; nodes are negative |
| IIIc | Abdominal implants greater than 2 cm in diameter and/or positive retroperitoneal or inguinal nodes |
| IV | Growth involving one or both ovaries with distant metastases. If pleural effusion present, there must be positive cytology to allot a case to stage IV; parenchymal liver metastasis equals stage IV |

Gynecol Oncol 1986;25:383.

moval of the primary tumor and careful surgical staging, as described earlier. Dysgerminomas are the only germ cell malignancies of the ovary to frequently (5% to 15%) involve both ovaries. Biopsying the contralateral ovary is appropriate even if it grossly appears to be normal. Dysgerminomas also have a tendency to spread to the para-aortic nodes. Every effort should be made to sample the para-aortic lymph nodes surgically at the time of the extirpation for the dysgerminoma.

Dysgerminomas are exquisitely sensitive to radiation therapy. Recent data suggest that they are also exquisitely sensitive to combination chemotherapy. Stage Ia dysgerminoma may be very effectively treated with surgery. Advanced-stage dysgerminoma should be treated with chemotherapy. Pregnant women should be given the chance to maintain the pregnancy if a dysgerminoma is present. They may be given chemotherapy in the second or third trimesters to control and possibly cure them of the cancer. The bleomycin, etoposide, and platinum (BEP) regime and the vincristine, actinomycin D, and cyclophosphamide (VAC) regimen require only short-term administration. They are usually administered every 3 to 4 weeks. A cesarean section is used to deliver the fetus at the time of fetal viability.

## SEX CORD STROMAL TUMORS

Sex cord stromal tumors are rare tumors that may complicate pregnancy. The granulosa theca cell tumor is the most common member of this category and is associated with estrogen production. The Sertoli-Leydig cell tumor is rare and is associated with androgen production. In a report of 36 sex cord stromal tumors diagnosed in pregnancy, all were stage I. Thirteen of the 36 patients presented with pain due to rupture of the tumor; two of the latter patients were in hemorrhagic shock. Treatment was limited to removing the tumor. Only one of these tumors has subsequently recurred. Advanced-stage sex cord stromal tumors require more aggressive chemotherapy. Our current recommendation in the nonpregnant state is bleomycin, etoposide, and platinum.

## UTERINE CARCINOMA

Adenocarcinoma of the endometrium is an extremely unusual disease in pregnant women, and only 8% of endometrial cancers have reported to recur in women under age 40. Infertility has been a factor associated with women who develop adenocarcinoma of the endometrium.

## VULVA CANCER

Vulvar carcinoma in situ has been increasing, according to data from the Connecticut Tumor Registry. Forty percent of patients with vulvar carcinoma in situ are under age 40. Thus, it can be anticipated that more women will be diagnosed in pregnancy to have vulvar carcinoma in situ. The management of a vulvar lesion in pregnancy is a local excision. Vulvar carcinoma in situ does not progress rapidly to invasive cancer unless associated with an immune deficiency. Definitive therapy in terms of a wide local excision or vulvectomy can be delayed in most cases until after completion of the pregnancy.

## VAGINAL CANCER

Carcinoma of the vagina occurs infrequently and usually is a squamous carcinoma presenting in a peri- or postmenopausal woman. Its management is similar to that of cervical cancer.

## NONSPECIFIC MESENCHYME MALIGNANCIES

Nonspecific mesenchyme malignancies are rare in the pregnant state. The most frequent histologic type is the mixed mesodermal tumor that occurs in older women.

## HODGKIN'S DISEASE

Hodgkin's disease generally occurs during the reproductive years, the peak incidence being between ages 18 and 30. It is estimated that one-third of women with Hodgkin's disease are pregnant or have delivered within 1 year of the diagnosis. As with almost all malignancies associated with pregnancy, Hodgkin's disease has not been reported to be affected by the pregnancy. It is a disease that is extremely sensitive to therapy. The cure rate for localized disease treated with radiation therapy is 80%, and patients with advanced disease treated with chemotherapy can anticipate a long-term disease-free survival of 65%. Peripheral lymphadenopathy is the most common presenting symptom for patients with Hodgkin's disease. Between 60% and 80% of Hodgkin's disease patients have enlarged cervical lymph nodes. In addition, patients may be asymptomatic or may have a history of fever, night sweats, weight loss, malaise, and pruritus.

The diagnosis of Hodgkin's disease is based on the histologic demonstration of the Reed-Sternberg cell, a dedifferentiated histiocyte. The most important prognostic factors for Hodgkin's disease are the histologic appearance and the pattern of spread. The lymphocyte-predominant histologic type has the best prognosis, followed by mixed-cellularity, lymphocyte-depleted, and nodular sclerosis Hodgkin's disease. Nodular sclerosis Hodgkin's disease is the most common type in women and usually involves the neck, supraclavicular, anterior, and superior mediastinal regions.

Selection of local radiation or systemic chemotherapy is based on the staging system (Table 52-5). Staging studies recommended for a patient with Hodgkin's disease are done in an attempt to identify extranodal disease. If such a finding is made, no further detailed studies are necessary prior to commencing treatment. The minimal studies necessary, in addition to the routine history and physical examination, are a chest x-ray, complete blood count, an erythrocyte sedimentation rate, renal and liver function tests, and a bone marrow aspirate and biopsy. Pregnant women may undergo ultrasound or magnetic resonance imaging studies of the liver, spleen, and retroperitoneal lymph nodes to avoid the hazard of diagnostic imaging radiation exposure to the fetus.

Strategies for treating patients with stage I and stage II Hodgkin's disease usually are radiotherapeutic, with reported 5-year survivals of 89% and 67%, respectively. Radiation is the only modality necessary for patients with stage IIIA lymphocyte-predominant or nodular-sclerosing Hodgkin's disease. Stage IIIA

**TABLE 52-5.** Ann Arbor Staging Classifications for Hodgkin's Disease

| | |
|---|---|
| Stage I | Involvement of a single lymph node region (I) or a single extralymphatic organ or site ($I_E$) |
| Stage II | Involvement of two or more lymph node regions on the same side of the diaphragm (II) or localized involvement of an extralymphatic organ or site ($II_E$) |
| Stage III | Involvement of lymph node regions on both sides of the diaphragm (III) or localized involvement of an extralymphatic organ or site ($III_E$) or spleen ($III_s$) or both ($III_{se}$) |
| Stage IV | Diffuse or disseminated involvement of one or more extralymphatic organs with or without associated lymph node involvement. The organ(s) involved should be identified by a symbol:<br>A = Asymptomatic<br>B = Fever, sweats, weight loss > 10% of body weight |

Devita VT Jr, Hellman S, Rosenberg SA, eds. Cancer: principles and practice of oncology. 3rd ed. Philadelphia; JB Lippincott, 1989.

disease with other histologic types is treated with radiation and combination chemotherapy.

The standard mantle field for midline mediastinal radiation to doses of 4000 rads results in fetal exposure to a greater-than-acceptable degree. It has been recommended that the fetus in the first trimester of pregnancy should not be exposed to more than 10 rads (0.1 cGy). Internal radiation scatter from standard mantle fields cannot be shielded and would result in a greater exposure rate to the fetus than the dose recommended for continuation of the pregnancy. Patients with pelvic disease or disease localized to the inguinal or abdominal region should undergo therapeutic abortion prior to radiation therapy. Similar disease first recognized in the third trimester would be treated with localized radiation therapy once fetal maturity was achieved and the infant delivered. Patients found to have rapidly progressing disease routinely receive chemotherapy, with the decision for initiating treatment based on the trimester of pregnancy and the patient's desires.

Advanced (stage III and stage IV) Hodgkin's disease has been successfully treated with the MOPP regimen—Mustargen (nitrogen mustard), Oncovin (vincristine), procarbazine, and prednisone. The role for chemotherapy in the management of Hodgkin's disease in the first trimester of pregnancy is only beginning to become defined. Patients who must be treated in the first trimester because of infradiaphragmatic disease that is difficult to follow, systemic symptoms, visceral involvement, or disease progression could receive vinblastine during the first trimester with "minimal risk" to the fetus. When the patient enters into the second trimester, a modified mantle radiation field and vinblastine or a change to a combination chemotherapy if disease progresses is possible. Therapeutic abortion should be offered to those patients in the first half of pregnancy who are unwilling to accept an increase in risk of adverse fetal outcome potentially attributable to treatment.

## NON-HODGKIN'S LYMPHOMA

Fewer than 50 cases of non-Hodgkin's lymphomas during pregnancy have been published. The mean age of patients with non-Hodgkin's lymphoma is 42 years, suggesting that most patients are past their childbearing years or are in a subfertile period of their reproductive life. The most important prognostic features for non-Hodgkin's lymphoma are the histologic type and the stage of disease. Histologically, the nodular type is more indolent; untreated, it has a survival period of approximately 4 years. The diffuse type is more virulent and has a life expectancy measured in months.

## ACUTE LEUKEMIA

Acute leukemia rarely complicates pregnancy, the incidence being less than 1 case in 75,000 pregnancies. The disease is usually first recognized in the second or third trimester. Presenting symptoms are easy fatigability, bleeding diathesis, or recurrent infections that reflect bone marrow failure. Specific physical findings associated with acute leukemia include sternal tenderness, skin pallor, petechiae, ecchymoses, and hepatosplenomegaly. Patients with acute lymphocytic, myelocytic, or monocytic leukemia usually have normocytic, normochromic anemia, mild to marked thrombocytopenia, and leukocytosis. Acute myeloblastic leukemia may be differentiated from acute lymphoblastic leukemias by the presence of Auer rods in the cytoplasm of myeloblasts. High serum and urine lysozyme levels are associated with acute monoblastic leukemias. The clinical impression is confirmed by bone marrow aspiration studies.

Pregnancy does not influence the natural history of acute leukemia. Substantial improvement in the survival of women with acute leukemia in pregnancy has occurred with the use of chemotherapy, radiation therapy, and supportive care, including blood products, antibiotics, and autologous bone marrow transplantation.

Anthracycline antibiotics have been used in pregnancy as single agents or in combination therapy without evidence of fetal malformation. *Vinca* alkaloids have been used for treating acute leukemia in pregnancy. Long-term follow-up of 26 children born to 23 women with leukemia in pregnancy suggests no long-term sequelae from the chemotherapy. Unfortunately, although remission may be achieved in 50% to 80% of treated patients, the median survival is less than 1 year.

## CHRONIC MYELOCYTIC LEUKEMIA

Chronic myelocytic leukemia makes up 90% of the chronic leukemias complicating pregnancy. Pregnancy does not adversely affect the natural history of chronic myelocytic leukemia. Treatment is palliative.

The most useful drugs in the management of this disease are busulfan, hydroxyurea, dibromomannitol, and cyclophosphamide. Approximately 96% of pregnant women with chronic myelocytic leukemia survive to delivery. Fetal survival throughout the gestation is 84%.

## MELANOMA

Pregnancy frequently induces a darkening in the appearance of pigmented nevi, but a bluish or slightly gray appearance to a nevus requires immediate excisional biopsy. Indeed, pigmented nevi that have become darker or irregular in outline and elevated should always be promptly excised in pregnancy under local anesthesia. Pregnancy does not change the natural history of melanoma.

Most patients with malignant melanoma present with stage I disease, disease limited to a primary cutaneous lesion. Stage I disease is pathologically staged according to the Clark's level of deepest anatomic invasion or the Breslow system, which places patients with disease invading to a maximum depth of less than 0.76 mm at a low risk, those with invasion of 0.76 to 1.5 mm at an intermediate risk, and those with invasion of greater than 1.5 mm at a high risk. Stage II disease represents patients with metastases to regional lymph nodes or disease in lymphatic channels leading to those regional nodes. Stage III disease involves distant, blood-borne metastases. Stage I lesions are usually treated with wide local excisions. Stage II lesions are treated surgically with complete regional lymph node dissections. Stage III disease is treated with systemic chemotherapy, including agents such as dimethyltriazenoimidazole-carboxamide (DTIC) or nitrosoureas such as chloroethylcyclohexyl nitrosourea (CCNU). Response rates are low (20% to 25%), and the median duration of remission is only 8 to 10 months. Surgery should be performed promptly in patients with stage I and stage II disease, whereas patients with stage III disease can only be palliated. Early delivery of the fetus in the third trimester once fetal lung maturation has been achieved should be routinely considered for stage III patients.

Placental or fetal metastases have only been reported 16 times, with four fetal deaths due to transplacental metastases of malignant melanoma. Although malignant melanoma is the most common malignancy to metastasize to the placenta and fetus, this is such a rare event as to preclude the recommendation of pregnancy termination for the management of the disease to avoid transplacental carcinogenesis or to induce a remission.

## GASTROINTESTINAL CANCER

### COLORECTAL CANCERS

Cancers of the gastrointestinal tract rarely complicate pregnancy. There is no evidence that pregnancy changes the natural history of colorectal cancer, the most common of these neoplasms. Most pregnant patients with gastrointestinal cancers have rectal carcinomas. Approximately 20% of patients have carcinoma presenting in the sigmoid colon. Unfortunately, diagnosis is frequently difficult in pregnancy, and there is a considerable delay in diagnosis. Typical presenting symptoms include severe constipation, abdominal distention, and rectal bleeding. Delay in diagnoses can be associated with intussusception, obstruction, or perforation. Carcinoembryonic antigen (CEA) is routinely elevated in pregnancy and is of little use in diagnosing colorectal cancers in the gravid state. The diagnosis may be established through the use of digital rectal examination, examination of the stool for occult blood, and proctoscopy or flexible sigmoidoscopy.

Early-stage colorectal cancers diagnosed in the first and second trimester should be treated with prompt surgery, and the pregnancy should be allowed to go to term. Patients with large colorectal lesions with metastases suspected or present have been allowed to carry the pregnancy until fetal maturity and then have undergone a cesarean section and bowel resection, provided they remained relatively asymptomatic. Most colorectal cancer patients are delivered by cesarean section, since labor may result in dystocia or hemorrhage. Lesions identified initially in the third trimester usually are not treated until fetal maturity is achieved. Standard therapy for curable lesions is definitive surgery, including standard bowel resections, low anterior resections, or abdominal perineal resections.

## PANCREATIC TUMORS

Pancreatic carcinoma rarely complicates pregnancy and is difficult to diagnose in the presence of pancreatitis. The most common presenting symptoms are abdominal pain and gastrointestinal symptoms. The most effective way to make the diagnosis is by endoscopic retrograde pancreatography with cytologic examination of pancreatic secretions. Eight cases of insulinoma have been reported in pregnancy. Each was recognized in the first trimester as a result of hypoglycemic episodes.

## STOMACH TUMORS

Gastrinomas rarely complicate pregnancy. They may present with a severe ulcer diathesis postpartum. Gastrinomas are associated with elevated serum gastrin, peptic ulceration, and secretion of gastric acid. Their management is surgical.

Gastric cancers rarely complicate pregnancy, and their symptoms are similar to those normally experienced in pregnancy, including gastrointestinal discomfort, nausea, and vomiting. Diagnosis may be made by gastroscopy, which avoids diagnostic radiation exposure. Only one-half of reported cases of gastric carcinomas are resectable in women who are not pregnant. The remainder are invariably fatal.

## LIVER TUMORS

Hepatocellular carcinomas are rare in women and usually present in postmenopausal women.

## SOFT TISSUE SARCOMA

Soft tissue sarcomas rarely complicate pregnancy. The overall prognosis is poor. Osteogenic sarcoma is the most frequent sarcoma reported in pregnancy. No survival differences were noted in 18 cases of osteogenic sarcoma managed in pregnancy when they were matched with nonpregnant women for skeletal tumor location, histologic appearance, and age. Therapeutic abortion has been recommended in the first trimester for patients exposed to intense cytotoxic chemotherapy. However, it is usually recommended that patients diagnosed in the third trimester undergo early delivery once fetal maturity has been established.

## ENDOCRINE TUMORS

### THYROID CANCER

The thyroid is an infrequent site for cancer to develop in pregnancy. Patients at high risk for thyroid cancer include women exposed to radiation therapy to the head, neck, or chest during childhood. Most cancers of the thyroid present as solitary nodules. Pregnancy changes should not result in the misdiagnosis of thyroid cancer. Most thyroid nodules appear in the first and third trimester of pregnancy and are benign.

The most common type of thyroid cancer to be diagnosed in pregnancy is the papillary carcinoma or mixed papillary follicular carcinoma. These carcinomas usually present as solitary nodules, but on careful sectioning of the tissue, 30% to 40% of patients will have multifocal disease.

Fine-needle aspiration biopsies are used to diagnose thyroid cancer in pregnancy. Radionuclide scans are contraindicated in pregnancy because of the theoretical risk of destroying the fetal thyroid. Fine-needle aspiration biopsy is associated with a false-negative rate of only 6%.

Since the overwhelming number of thyroid cancers presenting in pregnancy are histologically well differentiated, there is no reason to terminate pregnancy or avoid future pregnancies. Pregnancy does not appear to influence the course of thyroid cancer. Thyroid suppression therapy may be administered until delivery, regardless of the trimester in which the cancer was diagnosed. Patients should undergo prompt surgery if metastases develop in regional lymph nodes during suppression therapy or if the tumor is fixed to surrounding tissue and enlarges during suppression therapy.

## ADRENAL TUMORS

Pheochromocytoma is the most common tumor rising in the adrenal gland in pregnancy. Computed tomography scans and arteriography have been replaced by magnetic resonance imaging (MRI) for studying pregnant patients suspected of having a pheochromocytoma, because MRI does not result in fetal exposure to ionizing radiation. Magnetic resonance imaging may be used to confirm the presence, laterality, and location of the tumor. Further laboratory confirmation of the diagnosis of pheochromocytoma can be achieved by confirming elevated 24-hour urine collection levels of catecholamines, vanillylmandelic acid (VMA), and metanephrines.

The management of pheochromocytoma has been surgical in the first two trimesters and delivery by cesarean section followed by tumor resection in the third trimester. Medical management of the disease includes preoperative alpha-adrenergic blockade with oral phenoxybenzamine to lower the blood pressure, and propranolol to reduce the heart rate and prevent arrhythmias through the beta-adrenergic receptor blockade.

## URINARY TRACT MALIGNANCIES

### KIDNEY TUMORS

Renal cell carcinoma is the most common malignancy rising in the urinary tract in pregnancy. Twenty-two of 37 cases of renal tumors reported in one series were renal cell carcinoma. Hematuria is the most common presenting symptom. Nephrectomy with or without radiation therapy is standard treatment.

## BLADDER CANCERS

Bladder cancers have only infrequently been reported in pregnancy. The histologic distribution is similar to that in the nonpregnant state, with an overwhelming majority being transitional cell carcinoma followed by squamous cell and adenocarcinomas. Standard treatment of superficial, well-differentiated bladder cancers is fulguration. Management of deeply invasive cancer requires radiation therapy followed by partial or complete cystectomy. The diagnosis of a bladder cancer in early pregnancy requires therapeutic abortion if radiation therapy is necessary. Patients diagnosed late in pregnancy may delay treatment until fetal viability is achieved.

## CENTRAL NERVOUS SYSTEM TUMORS

Central nervous system tumors rarely complicate pregnancy. Patients present with headaches and visual disturbances. Magnetic resonance imaging allows for rapid evaluation without radiation exposure. Patients with infratentorial lesions have a particularly poor prognosis. The overall maternal mortality for patients with central nervous system tumors is 60%. Therapeutic abortions have been recommended for patients diagnosed in the first trimester to have malignant brain tumors because of the rapid course of such tumors. Elevated cerebrospinal fluid pressure requires surgical decompression, and steroids are given to reduce cerebral edema. Spinal cord tumors presenting in pregnancy may be diagnosed through magnetic resonance imaging, and decompression procedures should be promptly performed.

# PART XI. MEDICAL AND SOCIAL CONSIDERATIONS IN PREGNANCY

# 53.  IMPORTANT PSYCHIATRIC PROBLEMS DURING PREGNANCY AND THE POSTPARTUM PERIOD

## PSYCHIATRIC DISORDERS DURING PREGNANCY

### MANAGEMENT OF PSYCHOTIC DISORDERS

The woman with a history of psychotic disorder who intends to become pregnant should consult in advance with both an obstetrician and a psychiatrist to evaluate (1) whether she should remain on medication during pregnancy and (2) the indications for prophylaxis against postpartum psychosis, a condition for which she is at increased risk. She should remain under the care of both an obstetrician and a psychiatrist for the duration of the pregnancy and for at least the first 3 months postpartum.

Patients with a history of schizophrenia and schizophrenia-like disorders will most likely have been treated with, and sometimes maintained on, either oral phenothiazine (e.g., chlorpromazine, haloperidol, trifluoperazine) or IM injection of depot long-acting phenothiazine (e.g., fluphenazine) or thioxanthenes (e.g., flupentixol).

When clinically possible, any neuroleptics and medications for side effects should be withdrawn. If there is a history of recurrent episodes or chronic residual symptoms, then it may be necessary to continue a neuroleptic, at the minimal possible dosage, throughout the pregnancy. Choice of the specific neuroleptic must be made carefully, based on the patient's history of response and the likelihood of side effects.

Because of the known physical and behavioral teratogenic effects of the medications commonly used to treat neuroleptic side effects (anticholinergics and diphenhydramine) it is advisable to withdraw any anticholinergic or antihistamine for the first 12 to 16 weeks of pregnancy and to readminister it only if necessary.

A woman who has recovered from a single episode of mania will usually be taking a neuroleptic, as described earlier, and/or lithium carbonate, either for continued control of manic symptoms or for prophylaxis. If she has had only one episode of mania, then it is reasonable to discontinue the lithium and the neuroleptic prior to conception. However, if she has had more than one episode or if the risk of relapse seems high, then maintenance of a neuroleptic during pregnancy may be indicated.

The use of lithium is usually contraindicated during pregnancy. Lithium is teratogenic in the first trimester and is associated with an increased occurrence of cardiac defects, especially Ebstein's anomaly.

Therefore, lithium should ideally be withdrawn at least 1 month before conception or immediately after the patient is found to be pregnant. If lithium is necessary to help control otherwise unmanageable manic symptoms, it can be administered beginning in the second trimester. Shifts in fluid balance during pregnancy often require doubling of the lithium dose to achieve therapeutic blood levels. At delivery, however, renal clearance is reduced. To avoid toxicity to both mother and infant, the lithium dose should be decreased by 50% or more in the week prior to the anticipated delivery date or, if the risk of relapse is too high, when labor begins.*

A woman who has had a single episode of depression with psychosis is most likely to have been treated with tricyclic antidepressants, in conjunction with a neuroleptic, or with electroconvulsive (ECT) therapy. If she has had only one episode and is currently symptom-free, a trial off medications throughout the pregnancy should be considered. If there is a history of recurrent episodes or

---

*With their consent, women taking lithium during pregnancy or lactation should be registered with the American Register of Lithium Babies Registry, Langley Porter Neuropsychiatric Institute, 401 Parnassus Avenue, San Francisco, CA 94122.

chronic residual symptoms, it may be necessary to maintain her on medication during the pregnancy.

In this circumstance, the most conservative course of action is to maintain the patient on a phenothiazine alone through the first trimester, adding tricyclic antidepressant only if the phenothiazine does not provide adequate symptom control. It is prudent to reduce the tricyclic antidepressant to a minimum maintenance dose throughout the pregnancy and to withdraw it gradually before delivery even if it must be restarted soon afterward.

Monoamine oxidase inhibitors should not be used during pregnancy because of increased rates of fetal malformation. So little is known about the teratogenic effects of the newer agents that they should not be used except under special circumstances and with consultation.

Drug-induced psychoses (organic hallucinosis-delusional syndrome) are usually self-limited. The patient with a history of such an episode is unlikely to be maintained on medication unless she has an additional underlying disorder such as schizophrenia. The history of a drug-induced psychosis, particularly if recent and with an addictive drug such as cocaine, should alert the obstetrician to possible continuing drug use. Pregnant women with positive toxicology studies require careful education by the physician and staff as to the adverse effects of continued drug exposure on both mother and baby. Every effort should be made to admit these women to drug rehabilitation programs while they are pregnant.

### Management of Psychotic Episodes

The patient who suffers the onset of a psychotic episode while pregnant requires hospital admission to obtain skilled psychiatric nursing care, the careful observation needed for differential diagnosis, and a thorough workup for organic factors that might contribute to the illness. Such a workup is most efficiently accomplished on a psychiatric unit that is part of a general hospital. Since pregnancy per se is not associated with an increased risk of mental disorder, it cannot be assumed to be the etiologic agent. Drug use is probably the most likely organic factor contributing to a psychotic episode during pregnancy, but such conditions as cerebral embolism, pulmonary embolism with hypoxia, autoimmune disorders, and infections of the central nervous system must also be considered.

## MANAGEMENT OF NONPSYCHOTIC DISORDERS

### Depressive Episodes

A woman who has recovered from a single major depressive episode (without psychosis) but is still on antidepressants (e.g., tricyclics, monoamine oxidase inhibitors) should be advised to withdraw from these antidepressants before conception. If there is a substantial risk of relapse based on multiple past episodes, it may be necessary to continue an antidepressant during pregnancy. This should be a tricyclic on which there is some information as to potential risks (e.g., amitriptyline or imipramine).

### Anxiety, Panic Attacks, and Obsessive Disorders

A more common obstetric problem is the woman who comes for preconception counseling or early in pregnancy and reports that she has been taking a benzodiazepine (such as diazepam, alprazolam, lorazepam) for generalized anxiety symptoms. Benzodiazepines have been associated with an increased incidence of fetal malformations, especially cleft lip or palate. Although the evidence is controversial, it is probably best to avoid benzodiazepines during the first trimester.

### Substance Abuse

Women with chronic uncontrolled substance abuse often do not present until they go into labor, whereas women who use drugs only occasionally and heroin-addicted women who are engaged in methadone-maintenance programs are more likely to present for prenatal care. Any woman giving a history of drug abuse or with a positive urine toxicology should be counseled regarding the risks to her and her infant of continued drug use during the pregnancy. Women with addictions to alcohol, heroin, tranquilizers, and pain killers can be referred to established drug detoxification programs with adjunctive use of self-help groups like Alcoholics Anonymous and Pills Anonymous. Although no drug has yet been found that reliably blocks cocaine cravings, and drug rehabilitation programs are presently hard to find for cocaine addicts, every effort should be made to refer pregnant women for the treatment available. The physician should inform himself or herself of the laws requiring reporting of positive urine toxicology results to authorities, since in some states women with positive urine toxicology at time of delivery are not allowed to take their babies home and it is the physician's legal responsibility to report the situation.

### Eating Disorders

Anorexia nervosa and bulimia nervosa are eating disorders with important consequences for weight and reproductive function. Anorexia nervosa is a syndrome characterized by persistent concerns about eating and weight as well as dieting in the face of subaverage weight (85% of expected weight for height). Amenorrhea of at least 3 months duration is required for the diagnosis. Bulimia nervosa is a syndrome characterized by repeated binge eating and attempts at counteracting weight gain through severe dieting or compulsive laxative use or self-induced vomiting. Oligomenorrhea or amenorrhea are common in bulimia nervosa but are not required for the diagnosis. Anorexia nervosa and bulimia nervosa may be concurrent. Intermediate syndromes are currently called atypical eating disorders.

Women with active anorexia have higher rates of prematurity and low birth weight, attributed to the relationship between low maternal weight and infant weight. Although women with bulimia may experience improvement in their symptoms as pregnancy progresses, most have a return of symptoms in the first postpartum year.

## PSYCHIATRIC DISORDERS DURING THE POSTPARTUM PERIOD

It is important to be aware of the differing symptom patterns of the rare but serious disorders (postpartum psychosis and nonpsychotic major depression) and the common but less disabling disorders (initial maternal indifference and the maternity blues) (Table 53-1).[†]

† The Marce Society, a scientific society to promote study and the exchange of information on postpartum psychosis, was established in 1982. Information about the society is available from Dr. Beth Alder, Queen Margaret College, Clerwood Terrace, Edinburgh, UK EHIZ 8TS.

**TABLE 53-1.** Psychiatric Problems During the Postpartum Period

| | Initial Maternal Indifference | Postpartum "Blues" | Postpartum Psychosis |
|---|---|---|---|
| Prevalance | 40% (among primiparas) | 50% to 70% | 0.1% to 0.3% |
| Major risk factors | Obstetric (amniotomy and/or unusually painful labor) | Not known | Primiparous, previous postpartum psychosis, history of bipolar affective disorder |
| Typical onset | Day 1 | Day 3 to 1 month | Day 3 to 1 month |
| Typical duration | 3 days | Less than 10 days | 6–8 weeks (longer without treatment) |
| Potential for suicide or infanticide | Rare | Rare | Significant |
| Management | Education by physician, support from family | Education by physician, support from family | Hospitalization, medication, social support, psychotherapy |
| Prognosis with treatment | Good | Good | Variable, at risk for recurrence |

The vast majority of postpartum psychoses are affective (i.e., manic or depressive psychoses). A minority are schizophrenia-like conditions, distinguished from schizophrenia by the shorter duration of illness. It is very rare for true schizophrenia to begin during the postpartum period. Most episodes of postpartum psychosis start very abruptly between day 3 and day 14 of the postpartum period. These psychotic episodes are some of the most severe to be observed in psychiatry and usually present as a mixture of delirium and psychosis, with perplexity, confusion, and prominent delusions and hallucinations. Within a few days of treatment the confusional symptoms lessen, and a picture consistent with depressive, manic, or, less commonly, schizophrenia-like psychosis emerges. The onset of symptoms soon after delivery and the prominent features of delirium suggest an organic, most likely hormonal, factor, but this has yet to be conclusively determined.

Women with postpartum psychosis require skilled psychiatric nursing care within a hospital setting and should be admitted with their babies whenever possible. Manic illness often responds very quickly to treatment within 2 weeks, sometimes within days.

## BREAST-FEEDING

Extreme caution is warranted in breast-feeding an infant while the mother is taking any psychotropic medication. The deleterious effects of lithium and benzodiazepines are the best established, whereas the evidence for tricyclics and neuroleptics is more equivocal. The safest approach is to recommend that mothers on any form of psychotropic medication substitute bottle-feeding for breast-feeding.

# 54. MULTIFETAL PREGNANCY REDUCTION

Complications or improper use of fertility drugs such as human menopausal gonadotrophin (Pergonal) or newer agents such as Metrodin, and associated reproductive technologies such as in vitro fertilization (IVF) or gamete intrafallopian transfer (GIFT) have created one of the ultimate ironies in medical care. Usually reserved as the last resort for couples with very significant infertility problems, the overdosage of such drugs or transfer of multiple embryos has led to situations in which women previously infertile now bear more fetuses than they can possibly carry to viability. Spectacular reports, both in the medical literature and in the lay media, have detailed successes such as the Dionne quintuplets of the 1930s, but they have also described equally infamous tragedies, such as the Frustaci septuplets in California in 1985 (see also Fig. 54-1). Although the successes have touched the public's heart, the reality is that the tragedies of prematurity, with its associated high risks of fetal demise and significant impairment for survivors, have more generally been the rule.

Advances in prenatal care and intensive neonatal care have reduced the mortality of multifetal pregnancies. However, neonatal advances have not been equally successful on morbidity. Even in the best hands, the obstetric outcome for three or more fetuses is significantly worse than that for singleton or even twin pregnancies. The ability to carry quadruplets or more is, by any reasonable definition, significantly compromised, and in grand multiple cases such as sextuplets or more, it has hardly ever been seen.

When faced with such potentially tragic circumstances, couples have had to choose among several unnerving options. One option is termination of the entire pregnancy with the intent to conceive again. However, because conception is not guaranteed, particularly since most of these patients are infertility cases, this option has generally been very unpalatable. The second option is to continue with all the fetuses. In cases of quadruplets or even quintuplets, survival of some or all is certainly a possibility, but there is significant risk of long-term morbidity. With six or more fetuses, the chance of survival is extremely low, and, for example, in cases of octuplets that we encountered, the chance was certainly zero.

Over the course of the past few years the multifetal pregnancy reduction has become a realistic option in the face of perinatal tragedy from multiple fetuses. In the literature several terms have been used to describe the procedures discussed in this chapter. A consensus has been reached to use *selective termination* for a procedure performed because of an abnormality diagnosed in one fetus and *multifetal pregnancy reduction* (MFPR) when the indication is solely fetal number without demonstrable fetal defects.

## SELECTION OF PATIENTS AND TECHNIQUES

Three different technical procedures have been reported: transcervical, transvaginal, and transabdominal. A technique involving transcervical suction to remove

E. Albert Reece, John C. Hobbins, Maurice, J. Mahoney and Roy H. Petrie (Eds). *Handbook of Medicine of the Fetus & Mother.* Copyright © 1995 by J.B. Lippincott Company

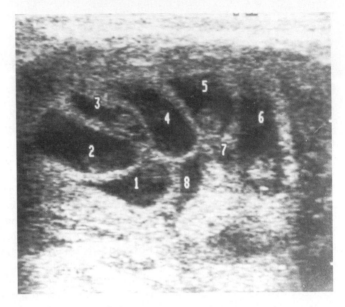

**FIGURE 54-1.** Ultrasound at 8 weeks showing an octuplet gestation. A ninth sac was empty. (Reprinted with permission from Obstet Gynecol 1988;71:290.)

embryos at 8 to 11 weeks was reported in 1986. Another method that has been tried successfully is a transvaginal aspiration of the early embryo, usually at about 6 to 7 weeks. This technique is analogous in many respects to oocyte aspiration for in vitro fertilization and may be particularly useful when the attempt is made very early in gestation. Proponents of transvaginal techniques now believe that delaying the procedure to at least 9 to 10 weeks is desirable to permit at least a rudimentary fetal visualization to look for worrisome signs such as, for example, nuchal folds.

The technique that is generally technologically most feasible involves the transabdominal insertion under ultrasound guidance of a spinal needle (usually 22-gauge). The needle is maneuvered into the thorax of the fetus, and a small dose of potassium chloride is injected (Fig. 54-2). This injection (about 0.5 to 1.0 mL) results in cardiac standstill, usually within 1 to 2 minutes of the injection, with ultimate reabsorption of the sac (Fig. 54-3). On occasion, cardiac motion will continue for a longer time, but a definite slowing, which appears "preterminal," will be apparent.

The decision of which embryo to choose has been strictly a technical issue of which embryos are easiest to reach. Anecdotal experience suggests that it is better not to choose the embryo closest to the cervix, since vaginal discharge is likely and devitalization of tissue near the cervix might predispose to ascending infection and increased risk of fetal loss. Also, there is concern about removal of amniotic fluid, because a sudden decrease in uterine size might induce contractions.

Composite data suggest success (defined as the ultimate live birth of babies) in approximately 75% of cases. In the vast majority of cases, the procedure is technically not very difficult for physicians experienced in performing ultrasound-guided needle procedures.

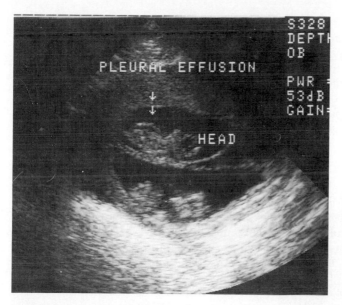

**FIGURE 54-2.** Pleural effusion in thorax of a fetus at 11 weeks following injection of 0.7 mL KCl. Cardiac standstill was confirmed within 30 seconds.

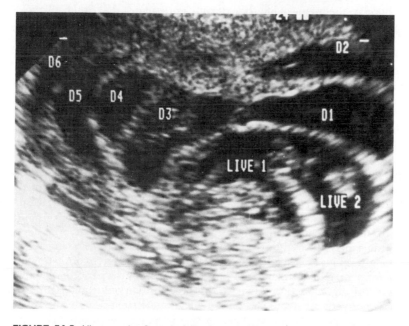

**FIGURE 54-3.** Ultrasound at 9 weeks following selective termination of three embryos at 8 weeks and three more at 9 weeks (D-1 through D-6). Twins were left (live 1 and live 2), who went 35 weeks and were then delivered—two boys who were healthy at 18 months of age. (Reprinted with permission from Evans MI, Fletcher JL, Zador IE, et al. Selective first trimester termination in octuplet and quadruplet pregnancies: clinical and ethical issues. Obstet Gynecol 1988;71:290.)

## TIMING

Most of the transabdominal cases reported to date have been performed at 10 to 12 weeks of pregnancy. Although there are few data, it would seem that transabdominal attempts prior to 8 weeks would be technically more difficult, and the transvaginal approach will probably be best at very early gestational ages. However, the chance at this time of a "natural" spontaneous loss of the remaining embryos is still a considerable possibility and therefore poses a risk of losing the only remaining embryo(s). Consequently, even some transvaginal advocates now wait until about 10 weeks.

## HOW MANY?

From the beginning our bias, based on existing obstetrical data, has been to believe that twins are the best place to stop. Not surprisingly, therefore, the decisions of both the patient and physician have almost always been to leave twins. We felt that by leaving twins there is still some "margin for error." Although the obstetric outcome for twins is not quite as good as that of singleton pregnancies, it is considerably better than that for triplets or more.

In some cases triplets have been left. Obstetrically, the outcome of triplets can be satisfactory, but the risks of prematurity and morbidity are certainly increased above those for twins. Such risks can be justified if the couple understands the high likelihood of alterations of life-style during a pregnancy that could still yield an unsatisfactory outcome.

We have believed that leaving only one would generally be a poor medical decision because of the risk of losing the pregnancy if there is a problem with the only remaining embryo. Exceptions to this conclusion would include a woman with diethylstilbestrol-induced uterine malformations or very significant medical disease such as cardiac failure, for which the added burden of multiple gestation might be the difference between a viable pregnancy and one that is not. The ethics of how many to leave are intertwined with the medical realities of obstetric outcome. Ethics evolve with technology. We have argued in several publications that since the obstetric management of twins is well known to all obstetricians and should not generally present major difficulties, reducing the number of fetuses below two does not generally seem justified. Others have not necessarily agreed, and some routinely have reduced pregnancies to singletons. The data have led us to reevaluate our position. Unlike most problems in which more data clear up problems, in this case the situation has only become more complex.

Overall, the experience of the world's largest groups suggests a 6% short-term and 12% long-term loss rate with MFPR. However, the loss rates correlate with initial fetal number, and therefore with number of procedures performed (Table 54-1). Not surprising, reduction of five to two is riskier than reduction of three to two. What is not yet settled and is certainly a legitimate subject of debate is the relative merits of the reduction of three to two versus three to one. The one survivor in the latter may have a lower morbidity, but that must be balanced against the certain mortality of the second fetus. With further experience it should be possible to define more accurately the risks both of performing and of not performing selective termination. Only with such data will it be possible to

**TABLE 54-1.** Results of Multifetal Pregnancy Reduction

| Initial No. Fetuses | No. Performed | Average Final No. Fetuses | Early Loss | Late Loss | Total Loss |
|---|---|---|---|---|---|
| 9 | 1 | 2.00 | 0.00% | 0.00% | 0.00% |
| 8 | 2 | 2.00 | 0.00% | 0.00% | 0.00% |
| 7 | 10 | 2.20 | 10.00% | 22.20% | 30.00% |
| 6 | 13 | 2.15 | 15.38% | 22.73% | 34.60% |
| 5 | 29 | 2.00 | 13.79% | 20.00% | 31.03% |
| 4 | 130 | 2.00 | 5.38% | 16.14% | 21.15% |
| 3 | 106 | 1.89 | 6.60% | 12.63% | 18.40% |
| 2 | 19 | 1.00 | 0.00% | 0.00% | 0.00% |
| | 310 | 1.905 | 0.06 | 0.12 | 0.17 |

determine the exact risks and benefits of the procedure and whether twins are the ideal end point for the procedure.

## TREATMENT OF INFERTILITY AND MULTIPLE PREGNANCY

The vast majority of cases of quadruplets or more are iatrogenic. Many of these have been associated with suboptimal Pergonal use or in vitro fertilization and embryo transfer of large numbers of embryos. With the development of cryopreservation, the incidence of IVF multiple gestations has been decreasing. With malpractice litigation initiated by patients who had poorly controlled Pergonal cycles, such cases may also diminish. However, it is absolutely clear that, with about 20,000 patients in the United States receiving Pergonal or its equivalent annually, multifetal pregnancies can and will happen even occasionally to women in the care of excellent physicians using the best of equipment and intent. Furthermore, there are some patients for whom there is a very narrow margin of Pergonal use between no response and hyperstimulation. The availability of selective termination should allow physicians to take "calculated" risks for patients who otherwise would probably not become pregnant.

## MANAGEMENT OF PREGNANCIES AFTER MFPR

Our experiences and those of other groups involved in these procedures raise concern for the possibility of midtrimester pregnancy loss. Since a noticeable proportion of the late losses we have seen have had confounding factors, it is not possible to delineate exact components of risk. Data on the natural history in the early and midtrimester of multifetal pregnancies for risks are poor and hinder evaluation of selective termination assessment. The risks of congenital malformations should be no different, and invasive studies such as amniocentesis should be considered as otherwise indicated. Chorionic villus sampling seems ill-advised, since excessive manipulation of the uterine contents around the time of the procedure might increase the risks of fetal loss. Once past the middle trimester, there is no reason to believe that late pregnancy management should be any different from that with any other twins.

## PREVENTION

Two approaches to prevention of iatrogenic causes of multifetal pregnancy are possible. First, one can draw the moral line before any technological intervention for infertility. The 1987 Vatican statement held that technologies like IVF or artificial insemination are inherently immoral because the unitive and procreative functions of human sexuality are wrongly separated. Another opinion is that any infertility treatment is improper for a psychosocial reason. The anxiety that brings women into fertility treatment is caused by "dehumanizing socialization" in which "having a child is the ultimate need and in which infertility is seen as personal failure and a sign of worthlessness." In this view, if they had only come to terms with these (supposed) feelings, they would have never found themselves in this situation.

"Dehumanizing socialization" is not the basic cause of the despair of most infertile couples. Straightforward biological causes of infertility can sometimes be remedied by a number of methods, including IVF. The position just cited creates passive resignation in the face of a remediable problem. Infertility is a significant form of human suffering, and if something can be done about it, there is a strong moral obligation to do it. However, one is not ethically permitted simply to do "anything" to achieve or preserve pregnancy, as we hope the discussion has shown.

How should the human need for a child be evaluated on ethical grounds? Is there a moral duty to have a child of one's own? Is there a "right" to have a child? We believe that no moral or legal right exists to have children in a positive or enabling sense. Society is not obliged to grant each person an "entitlement" to a child in the same sense that it gives rights to life, freedom and speech, and protection from enemies. On the other hand, there is a negative duty not to restrain or prevent women from childbearing. In our society, such a right should be guarded by the legal right to privacy.

Once they have obtained medical help in becoming pregnant, women deserve further help to achieve their aim, as long as the means used are proportionate to the ends sought and as long as the consequences of the intervention meet the tests of ethical principles widely accepted in society. Among all the principles involved, the primary one to be used in multifetal pregnancies is proportionality. A proportionate relationship between means and ends entails two criteria. First, there must be no other way to achieve the end—in this instance, the end of preserving a viable and desired pregnancy. Second, the way chosen must be the one that results in least harm and most good for all involved. We have studied the ethical attitudes of physicians, ethicists, and clergy likely to encounter these situations. Overall there is considerable support for couples to have choices in these decisions and against legislated morality over such complex issues.

The second way to ensure prevention is better medicine. Most cases of multiple pregnancy are iatrogenic and avoidable by more diligent use of fertility drugs and better patient management. Selective termination should be viewed as a provisional approach only—until improved fertility treatment obviates its use. Research with spare embryos is also needed to help improve the efficacy and efficiency of in vitro fertilization, thereby also diminishing the requirements for multiple embryos to achieve a high likelihood of pregnancy.

# 55. PREGNANCY BEFORE AGE 20 AND AFTER AGE 35

Although it may at first seem incongruous to combine early and delayed child-bearing in the same chapter, they share many similarities:

1. Each has been poorly defined.
2. Each occurs at times of instability of the hypothalamic-pituitary-ovarian-uterine axis.
3. Each has been associated with increased complications of pregnancy and poorer obstetric outcome.
4. Each requires specialized evaluation, counseling, and care.
5. Numerous myths and expectations may obscure true risks.
6. Their outcome has complex socioeconomic situations.

Advances in medical-care systems and changes in demography and attitudes have changed our concept of "old" and "young" that have led to the application of numerous judgmental definitions and stigmata. Chronologic age alone may not adequately reflect biological age or the physiological, psychological, or socio-logical environment surrounding the pregnancy. For a more thorough discussion of this topic, please see Chapter 83 in Reece EA, Hobbins JC, Mahoney MJ, and Petrie RH, eds. Medicine of the fetus & mother. J.B. Lippincott, 1992.

## PREGNANCY BEFORE AGE 20

### EPIDEMIOLOGY

In the United States about 1 million teenagers, or 5% to 8% of the teenage population, become pregnant each year. Teenage pregnancies represent about one-eighth of all live births and one half of all births to unmarried women. Half of teenage pregnancies proceed to delivery, with about 20% of the babies being placed for adoption. The teenage pregnancy rate in the United States is one of the highest among industrialized nations.

### Ectopic Pregnancy

Diagnosing ectopic pregnancy is more difficult in adolescents because of inherent irregularity of menses, increased incidence of dysmenorrhea, difficulty in obtaining a reliable sexual history, and fear of parental anger. The rate of ectopic pregnancy in women age 15 to 24 is 13.9 per 1000 pregnancies compared to 19.5 per 1000 for older women. Mortality rates are higher in younger women (16.8 deaths per 1000 ectopic pregnancies in the 15- to 19-year-old age group versus 8.7 per 1000 in the 25- to 34-year-old age group).

E. Albert Reece, John C. Hobbins, Maurice, J. Mahoney and Roy H. Petrie (Eds).
*Handbook of Medicine of the Fetus & Mother.* Copyright © 1995 by J.B. Lippincott Company

## Gestational Trophoblastic Disease

In one study, the incidence of hydatidiform mole was two times greater for women younger than 15 than for all other ages. Malignant sequelae were less common (37.5%), although the figure was not statistically significant. Treatment was 100% successful in the adolescents. A study of adolescents undergoing elective abortion showed a high incidence (1 in 500) of unsuspected hydatidiform mole.

## MEDICAL COMPLICATIONS OF PREGNANCY

### Pregnancy-Induced Hypertension

In a controlled study of 471 patients under age 15, the incidence of pregnancy-induced hypertension was 34.2% (compared with an overall rate of 25.3%). Forty percent of 222 teenage patients in a Memphis study were toxemic during pregnancy. Essential hypertension and other preexisting factors may be more important in the risk of pregnancy-induced hypertension than age alone.

### Infectious Diseases

Adolescent women tend to have infection patterns different from those of their older counterparts. Pregnant teenagers are more likely to have otitis media, varicella, mumps, pertussis, and other childhood illnesses. Adolescent pregnant women have a lower relative risk for urinary tract infections, chorioamnionitis, and postpartum endometritis and a higher relative risk for STDs.

### Nutrition

According to the American Dietetic Association in 1989, pregnant adolescents are nutritionally at risk and require nutrition intervention early in and throughout pregnancy. Teenage pregnancy is inseparably linked with early sexual maturation. Thus, the pregnant teenager is smaller in stature and weight than her older counterpart. One-fourth of all pregnant teenagers have a diet deficient in calcium, protein, vitamins, and iron. A weight gain considered adequate to support pregnancy is a 20% weight increase above the 50th percentile for height, along with a protein intake of 1.5 to 1.7 g/kg/day. A diet containing 20% protein, 30% to 35% fat, and 45% to 50% carbohydrates should provide adequate energy and structural needs.

## PERINATAL OUTCOME

### Delivery Method

A study from a comprehensive clinic in New York found a fourfold increase from the 1960s to the 1980s in the rate of cesarean section among adolescents. Another study, which matched 471 patients with an older, similar control group, showed a significant increase in the rate of cephalopelvic disproportion (8.7% versus 4.9%) but an insignificant increase in the cesarean section and midforceps rates.

## OUTCOME OF PREGNANCY

### Birth Weight

The general incidence of small-for-gestational-age infants is closely related to the obstetric history and to the trimester during which prenatal care began. When corrections are made for race, socioeconomic status, and gravidity, birth weights of infants of adolescents—even the youngest teenagers—are similar to those of young adults. Adolescents with prior births show the highest frequency of low-birth-weight infants, and an adolescent smoker is three times more likely to have a small-for-gestational-age infant than is a nonsmoker.

### Maternal Mortality

Older studies showed a significant mortality risk for adolescent pregnancies, but current information does not substantiate this concern. The Maternal Mortality Collaborative reported an overall rate of 14.1 deaths per 100,000 live births in 1980 to 1985. A woman over 30 was 3.2 times more likely to die from pregnancy than a woman in her 20s. The risk of death from abortion in women age 15 to 19 was 1.2 per 100,000.

### Congenital Anomaly

In Great Britain, the rate of perinatal death from complications of congenital abnormalities is higher in the offspring of women under 20; central nervous system malformations are the most frequent anomaly.

### Childhood Morbidity and Mortality

Infant mortality is only slightly higher in older white teenagers (28 per 1000) than in 20- to 24-year-olds (22 per 1000). Teenagers younger than 15 have a significantly increased risk (48 per 1000).

## HEALTH CARE OF THE PREGNANT TEENAGER

Teenagers often cite physicians as the most credible and preferred source of information, but more uniformly teenagers seek counsel about pregnancy alternatives from their mother, partner, or best girlfriend. There are many barriers to effective communication between teenagers and physicians. The obstetrician may deal with low reading levels, language barriers, and erratic attendance by even the most mature and dedicated adolescents.

Adult underestimations of the intensity of teen attitudes might explain the physicians' observations of casual, nonchalant, or disinterested demeanors in the teenagers. Such postures might actually camouflage concerns, and further exploration of these differences is needed to enhance communication.

It is incorrect to assume that teenage pregnancy is always unplanned or unwanted. Pregnancy may be an attempt to enhance self-image or societal position. It also may be part of normal psychosocial development. The prenatal health information needs of adolescents seem to be related to matters of self-esteem and good use of health care.

### Prenatal Care

Ten percent of adolescents delay prenatal care until the third trimester or receive none at all, a proportion two to three times higher than among adults. Adolescents with a repeat pregnancy tend to seek prenatal care later, even though they are older and presumably more aware of the availability and advantages of the health-care system.

The most successful programs for adolescent care use a team approach to ensure that the patient's concerns and needs are not overlooked. A team of physicians, nurses, public-health personnel, social workers, psychologists, educators, nurse-midwives, dietitians, and community resource people can provide a comfortable environment for the adolescent; all involved share an interest in the well-being of both mother and child. In a successful program, patients are valued as individuals and cared for nonjudgmentally.

Prenatal counseling should include an open discussion of reproductive biology, physiological changes of pregnancy, warning signs and symptoms of disease, nutrition, childbirth and anesthesia, child care, and lactation. The program should not ignore the individual needs and character of the adolescent and should provide mechanisms to involve the adolescent and her support people in all aspects of pregnancy care.

## PREGNANCY AFTER AGE 35

### EPIDEMIOLOGY

The baby boomers (born between 1947 and 1965) who delayed childbearing to realize other life objectives have initiated the new baby boom of the 1980s and 1990s. This has created an older population of women reproducing and wanting to reproduce. Since the early 1970s, the rate of women age 25 to 39 having their first child has increased steadily. The most dramatic increase has been in women age 30 to 34 (from 7.3 per 1000 in 1970 to 14.6 per 1000 in 1982).

#### Fertility and Infertility

It is clear from the studies that advancing maternal age correlates with decreased fecundity, but it is less clear how this relates to the fertility of the individual patient. If 50% of women age 40 or 41 are fertile, it does not imply that an individual 40-year-old is 50% fertile. Population statistics should be applied only to populations, not to individuals.

### MEDICAL COMPLICATIONS OF PREGNANCY

#### Hypertension

Actuarial studies confirm that with age, systolic and diastolic blood pressures gradually rise. Most reports also indicate an increased incidence of pregnancy-induced hypertension with age. In a study of data from several centers on a total of 36,482 deliveries, women age 25 to 29 had a 2.5% incidence of toxemia, those age 35 to 39 had an incidence of 4.0%, and those over age 40 a 4.6% incidence.

It remains unclear whether the patient or her age is the most important factor. Essential hypertension should be controlled before initiation of pregnancy. Routine monitoring for hypertension (blood pressure, patient weight, and urine protein determination with physical examination) should be performed at each visit. Pregnancy-induced hypertension should be managed using the same guidelines regardless of age.

## Diabetes Mellitus

Diabetes, like hypertension, is a systemic disease that shows an age-related increase. It is debatable if this can be translated into a pregnancy-related increase, although most published reports support this relationship.

## Anatomical Changes of the Uterus

The reported incidence of leiomyomata patients is 3% to 6% in patients over age 40. Possible complications are the same as in younger patients. One study found an overall occiput anterior presentation in 81.8% of 22,264 patients and in 68.9% of women age 40 to 44. The increase found in all types of malpresentation was thought to be due to an increased incidence of uterine fibroids. The incidence of breech presentation may be slightly increased, with varying reports of 1% to 6%. An earlier study using x-ray pelvimetry found that pelvic types unfavorable for vaginal delivery occurred four times more often in primigravidas over age 35 than in those under age 25.

Aging may cause sclerotic changes of vessels, resulting in inadequate vascular perfusion of the maternal-fetal unit. Uteroplacental underperfusion may be a unifying etiology of placental infarcts, placental growth retardation, and placental abruption, as well as a sequela of pregnancy-induced hypertension and diabetes. When parity is controlled, there is no increased risk of previa.

## OBSTETRIC COMPLICATIONS

### Maternal Fever/Chorioamnionitis

One study showed an increase in chorioamnionitis in older women, but this effect disappeared when socioeconomic bias was eliminated.

### Premature Labor

A report showing increased incidence in premature labor among older nulliparous patients was not substantiated. As the etiology and mechanisms of premature labor become better defined, perhaps so will its relationship to age.

### Induction of Labor

In a large Dublin study, the induction of labor rate of 25.5% in women over age 40 was more than twice that of women less than 40. Another study, on primigravidas over age 35, reported an induction rate of 19%, an average induction interval of 17.5 hours, and a failure rate of 38%; hypertension was involved in the decision for induction in 71% of cases.

### Abnormalities of the Labor Curve

Most studies report a significantly higher cesarean section rate for older patients. Although this association is clearly confirmed, most studies contain too many variables to make the results meaningful. If the covariables of meconium-stained amniotic fluid, fetal distress, induction of labor, and epidural anesthesia are removed, the rate is still increased in both primigravidas and multigravidas.

## OUTCOME OF PREGNANCY

### Birth Weight

Several studies have reported increased birth weights among older women, but other studies found that when other covariates were excluded, maternal age was not predictive of birth weight.

### Maternal Mortality

One study reviewed death certificates collected by the Centers for Disease Control from 1974 to 1978 on women age 35 and older. Maternal mortality rates for women age 35 to 39 were 50.9 per 100,000; age 40 to 44, 86.1 per 100,000; and over age 45, 198.8 per 100,000. In 1982, the mortality rate for women over age 34 had fallen to 24.2 per 100,000. This decrease was thought to be due to a high number of women in the under-40 age group and an overall trend toward lower parity.

### Perinatal Mortality and Morbidity

Analysis of 44,386 pregnancies (1959 to 1966) in 12 hospitals as part of the Collaborative Perinatal Project found that the combined mortality rate rose from 25 per 1000 for women age 17 to 19 to 69 per 1000 for those age 40 or older.

An investigation of the total singleton birth population of New York City from 1976 to 1978 (320,726 births) stratified by age, parity, race, and socioeconomic status showed that the adjusted fetal death rate rose at about 9% per year of age from the late 20s to the early 40s (5.4 deaths per 1000 births in the 25- to 29-year-old group versus 22.3 per 1000 over age 40). Prior fetal loss had a strong and consistent association with antepartum and intrapartum stillbirths and neonatal deaths, whereas age had no association with intrapartum fetal death.

The risk of spontaneous abortion increases with gravidity irrespective of age and with age irrespective of gravidity.

There is incontrovertible evidence that the incidence of genetic defects, especially the autosomal trisomies, increases with maternal age. Age increases the rate of all autosomal trisomies, but only trisomy 13, 18, and 21 are compatible with life. This collection of acrocentric chromosomes may be particularly prone to the consequences of prolonged meiotic arrest. Although trisomies account for less than 20% of abortions in women under age 25, they are responsible for 67% of abortions in women over 40. A significant inverse relationship was found with 45 XO cases. Paternal age did not appear to have a significant effect. Although maternal serum alpha fetoprotein screening provides an additional benefit in screening for trisomy 21, it adds little to the detection of other trisomic disorders. No age-specific difference in maternal alpha fetoprotein levels has been found.

### Gestational Trophoblastic Disease

A significant increase in trophoblastic disease has been seen in women over age 40. The highest risk of malignancy was in women over 50.

## PSYCHOLOGICAL CONSIDERATIONS

One study found that older women were less troubled by pregnancy and reported fewer symptoms in the first trimester. Although the level of anxiety increased as the pregnancy progressed, older patients were typically better adjusted as they entered the last trimester. Overall, older mothers may differ psychologically, but show no differences in their adaptability.

## HOW OLD IS TOO OLD?

Although there are scattered reports of pregnancy after age 50, pregnancy in women over age 45 is exceedingly uncommon. Overall, older patients may show little difference from their younger counterparts except in their decreased fecundity. Although there may be an increased rate of specific pregnancy complications, resulting in increased maternal morbidity and higher health-care costs, a child born to an otherwise healthy private patient in a tertiary-care facility has no increased risk of an adverse neonatal outcome. This is usually the single most important factor to the woman contemplating a pregnancy after age 35.

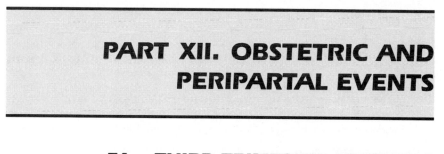

# PART XII. OBSTETRIC AND PERIPARTAL EVENTS

# 56. THIRD TRIMESTER BLEEDING

Bleeding in the third trimester is a major cause of perinatal morbidity and mortality. Its exact incidence is unclear because of a lack of comprehensive reporting, but community-based studies suggest frequency rates of 3% to 4.8%. In 30% of cases definite features of placental abruption exist; placenta previa is responsible for 20% of cases. In about half of these women, no clear reason for the bleeding can be identified, and it is presumed to be from either local lesions in the birth canal, marginal separation, or trauma.

## PLACENTAL ABRUPTION

Placental abruption, defined as premature detachment of a normally implanted placenta, recognizably occurs in 1% of pregnancies. Commonly associated with preterm labor and delivery, it accounts for 15% to 25% of all perinatal mortality. Symptoms of abruption include visible maternal hemorrhage in 65% to 80% of patients before delivery; a tense, irritable uterus; fetal distress; and coagulopathy in the most severe situations. More commonly, however, painful vaginal bleeding is the hallmark. This variability of clinical presentation necessitates a high index of suspicion for the diagnosis.

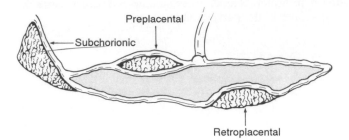

**FIGURE 56-1.** Sites of periplacental hemorrhage that have been described sonographically. Subchorionic hemorrhage may be remote from the placenta but is thought to arise from marginal abruptions. The term *preplacental hemorrhage* has been chosen to describe both subamniotic hematoma and massive subchorial thrombosis. Intraplacental hemorrhages (intervillous thrombi) also may be identified but are difficult to distinguish from placental lakes or other intraplacental sonolucencies.

The clinical classification of placental abruption is based on the observation of bleeding at three principal sites (Fig. 56-1). Nyberg and associates (1987) described bleeding seen by ultrasound at the following locations:*

1. Subchorionic: between the myometrium and the placental membranes
2. Retroplacental: between the myometrium and the placenta
3. Preplacental: between the placenta and amniotic fluid.

The sonographic characteristics of placental hemorrhage change with time. Initially hemorrhage appears to be either hyperechoic or isoechoic with the placenta; after a week the appearance is hypoechoic, and by the end of the second week it is likely to be sonolucent. These factors act as confounding variables when the sensitivity of ultrasound to identify the presence or absence of placental abruption is in question.

Page and coworkers (1954), using a constellation of maternal and fetal signs, devised a classification system based on the degree of morbidity (Table 56-1). The classification, which uses four grades, continues to have practical significance.

Ultrasound visualization of a clot occurs in only about 25% of clinically suspected cases; as a result, the absence of ultrasound findings should not preclude the diagnosis. Irrespective of the ultrasound appearance or progression of the clot, the clinical, hemodynamic, and hematologic parameters are most important.

Some investigators have suggested that when a clot is visible, its size may be clinically significant. This can be assessed by using Sauerbrei and Pham's method: the volume of the hemorrhage is estimated by multiplying the three perpendicular diameters by 0.52, using the formula for an ellipsoid.

Abruptions may occur throughout gestation. It has been demonstrated that 18% occur before 32 weeks and 42% occur after 37 weeks.

*Nyberg D, Cyr D, Mack LA, et al. Sonographic spectrum of placental abruption. AJR 1987;148:161.

**TABLE 56-1.** Classification of Placental Abruption According to Maternal and Fetal Signs

| Grade* | Concealed Hemorrhage | Uterine Tenderness | Maternal Hypotension | Coagulopathy | Fetal Distress |
|--------|----------------------|--------------------|----------------------|--------------|----------------|
| 0 | no | no | no | no | no |
| 1 | no | no | no | no | no |
| 2 | yes | yes | no | rare | yes |
| 3 | yes | yes | yes | often | death |

* Grade 0 is a retrospective diagnosis from inspection of the placenta. Grade 1 includes "marginal sinus" separation or other limited processes of abruptio placentae. Grades 2 and 3 imply significant hemorrhage requiring immediate therapy with the possibility of maternal complications.
From Page EW, King EB, Merrill JA. Abruptio placenta: dangers of delay in delivery. Obstet Gynecol 1954;3:385.

## CLINICAL ASSOCIATIONS

Placental abruption is associated with increasing parity, abdominal trauma, sudden decompression of polyhydramnios, and external cephalic version. The relationship with hypertension is unclear. In assessing a woman with placental abruption, the possibility of physical abuse or cocaine usage must not be overlooked.

## MANAGEMENT PRINCIPLES

The important features of the pregnancy assessment are summarized in Table 56-2.

### Mild Abruption

Mild abruption may spontaneously resolve or preterm labor may begin. If the fetus is remote from term and appears healthy, the obstetrician should consider arresting labor. The use of tocolysis in this clinical situation is controversial because theoretically it may promote further bleeding; however, evidence to support this position is lacking. The link between abruption and preterm labor is thought to be due either to the presence of extravasated blood in the myometrium, which triggers uterine activity, or to a fetal response to a hostile intrauterine environment.

**TABLE 56-2.** Important Features of the Pregnancy Assessment

| Fetal | Maternal |
|-------|----------|
| • Fetal distress | • Hypovolemia |
| • Fetal demise | • Coagulation status |
| • Gestational age/size | • Uterine activity and tone |
| • Size of placental abruption | • Pain |
| | • RH status |

## Moderate to Severe Abruption

In moderate to severe abruption, maternal resuscitation is the priority. The degree of hypovolemia is often underestimated because of the following:

1. The hemorrhage may be concealed.
2. It may have occurred outside of the hospital.
3. An increase in maternal peripheral resistance may occur, giving rise to false reassurance regarding her blood pressure.

Moderate to severe abruption requires aggressive volume replacement. Clotting defects should be sought with a high index of suspicion. A prolonged bedside clotting time serves as a useful marker of the degree of placental separation and coagulopathy.

When assessing the fetus, the obstetrician should remember that in 81% of cases the estimated fetal weight is below the mean for gestational age. Signs of fetal distress, including fetal tachycardia and severe variable or late decelerations, may also be present. If fetal demise has occurred, there will be significant alterations in maternal cardiovascular and coagulation status.

Clinical management decisions in moderate to severe placental abruption must be individualized, and aggressive plans should be made for delivery if there is evidence of hemodynamic or coagulation instability. The state of the cervix is another important variable: in the presence of an otherwise healthy fetus, it may allow vaginal delivery. Caution should, however, be exercised when a prolonged interval from abruption to delivery is expected. Further placental separation and worsening of the coagulopathy may occur without warning. Rh-immune prophylaxis is recommended in Rh-negative women who do not have antibodies.

## PLACENTA PREVIA

In two large series, placenta previa occurred in the third trimester in 0.4% to 0.9% of patients. It is a much more common ultrasound diagnosis in the second trimester of pregnancy, with an incidence then of 5.3%. At least 90% of these cases convert by term to a normal placental location, giving rise to the concept of placental migration.

Multiparity, advanced maternal age, multiple pregnancy, and previous cesarean section have been noted in association with placenta previa. A twofold increase in the rate of placenta previa has been seen after a previous section; the risk is greatest in the pregnancy immediately after the section.

## DIAGNOSIS

Using transabdominal ultrasound with a full maternal urinary bladder, the accuracy of this diagnosis ranges from 93% to 97%. Diagnostic errors are due to several factors. Overdistention of the urinary bladder, resulting in apposition of the anterior and posterior walls of the lower uterine segment, is common. Normally the uterine wall is convex toward the bladder; this relationship is reversed when bladder overdistention occurs (Fig. 56-2). Other causes for diagnostic errors include myometrial contractions, fibroids, blood clots, late placental migration, and

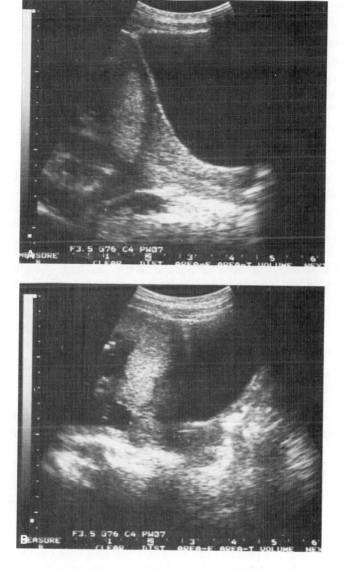

**FIGURE 56-2. (A)** An anteriorly located placenta with a full maternal urinary bladder. A false impression of placenta previa is created. **(B)** The urinary bladder in the same patient has been partially emptied. The placenta is now clear of the cervix.

a posterior placental location, with the calcified fetal head obscuring the exact placental edge.

Some have championed the use of endovaginal sonography to clarify placental location. Closely approximating the probe tip to the site of interest allows the use of a higher-frequency probe, and a higher-resolution image is obtained. It appears that the procedure can be conducted safely with no risk of bleeding. Others have demonstrated that anterior wall placentas are more likely to convert than posteriorly positioned ones.

## MANAGEMENT

Management options in the third trimester are based on the existing clinical possibilities and fetal health. These situations may be summarized as follows:

1. The patient has never bled.
2. Heavy bleeding is occurring.
3. Bleeding has stopped in a preterm patient.
4. The fetus is 37 weeks or older.

All third trimester patients with ultrasound confirmation of complete previa should be admitted to the hospital. For women who have never bled, it is important to note that in over 50% of patients with placenta previa, the first episode of bleeding may occur after 31 weeks. Repeat ultrasound at 2- to 3-week intervals for placental localization may indicate if migration has occurred.

If heavy bleeding is occurring, emergency measures to rapidly stabilize the mother's cardiovascular system are indicated, and delivery should be performed by cesarean section. Prophylactic Rh immunoglobulin is recommended for all women who are Rh negative without antibodies. For women whose bleeding has stopped, Macafee's expectant approach continues to be the standard. There is general agreement that there is no place for expectant management in the term patient with placenta previa. An elective cesarean section should be performed if the diagnosis is confirmed.

## PLACENTA ACCRETA WITH PLACENTA PREVIA

Placenta accreta, the abnormal adherence of the placenta to the uterine wall, is due to an underdeveloped decidua basalis. Conditions thought to predispose women to placenta accreta include previous dilatation and curettage, uterine scarring due to cesarean section or myomectomy, and manual removal of the placenta. Of these, the most common association of placenta accreta is placenta previa in the presence of a previous cesarean section scar.

Under normal prenatal conditions a thin hypoechoic zone is present between the myometrium and the placenta. This zone is on average 9.5 mm thick, and after 18 weeks gestation it should be seen in all cases throughout the entire placental implantation site. When this hypoechoic zone is breached in whole or in part and is not apparent, placenta accreta, increta, or percreta may be present. The sensitivity and specificity of these observations have not yet been established.

Management principles are no different from those for patients with placenta previa, except that massive blood transfusions and hysterectomy are quite common because of the profound hemorrhagic shock that may occur. Uterine inversion in the postpartum period may be the first sign of placenta accreta.

## OTHER CAUSES OF THIRD TRIMESTER BLEEDING

### CIRCUMVALLATE PLACENTA

This finding occurs in 1% to 2% of pregnancies and may be associated with bleeding and placental abruption.

## MARGINAL SINUS BLEEDING

Bleeding in this situation occurs at the placental margin, and some clinicians contend that this is a form of placental abruption.

## VASA PREVIA

Bleeding from vasa previa is a fetal obstetric emergency. It is primarily associated with velamentous insertion of the umbilical cord or vessels to a succenturiate lobe of the placenta. The hemorrhage in this situation is relatively small by adult standards and usually occurs after spontaneous rupture of the fetal membranes. The sudden fetal heart rate changes that occur with this fetal hemorrhage must raise a high index of suspicion. There is not always time to confirm the presence of fetal red cells by the Apt test, because prompt delivery is the only management option available.

## TRAUMA

Direct trauma to the pregnant uterus may occur from accidents (e.g., motor vehicle or fall) and physical abuse. Quite commonly massive placental bleeding is concealed, and even though the clear priority is the assessment and maintenance of maternal health, the fetus and the integrity of the uteroplacental environment should not be ignored. At a minimum, fetal evaluation should include the assessment of fetal-maternal bleeding by the Kleihauer-Betke test and external fetal heart rate monitoring for several hours.

Physical abuse occurs in about 8% of pregnant women. The literature indicates that 25% to 63% of battered women report battering during pregnancy; in some cases, the first episode of abuse occurred during pregnancy.

## CERVICAL AND VAGINAL LESIONS

Nine percent of all cases of antepartum hemorrhage may be due to lower genital tract causes. It is important to exclude local lesions (e.g., polyps, erosions); this is done by direct visualization of the cervix and genital tract by speculum examination.

## CONCLUSION

Bleeding in the third trimester, however slight, requires prompt attention and complete evaluation. It is unwise to attempt pelvic examination in a location that is not equipped to manage profuse bleeding.

# 57. NORMAL AND ABNORMAL LABOR

To a large extent, obstetric decision making about labor aberrations is a process of estimating the probability of a safe vaginal delivery. All the clinical information used in reaching decisions about obstetric interventions (use of oxytocin, conduction anesthesia, cesarean or instrumental delivery) should be viewed from this perspective.

## NORMAL CERVICAL DILATATION

The relationship between cervical dilatation and time during labor is described by a sigmoid curve (Fig. 57-1). Dilatation is divided into a latent phase and an active-phase. These constitute the first stage of labor. The second stage then encompasses the time between complete cervical dilatation and delivery of the fetus. The *latent phase* extends from the onset of labor until the upward inflection of the dilatation curve and is associated with little or no incremental change in dilatation. The *active-phase* follows, during which most of the cervical dilatation occurs. During the terminal portion of the active-phase, dilatation appears to slow, but this is more apparent than real and relates to the fact that the cervix is now pulled around the edges of the presenting part and is moving in a cephalad rather than a coronal direction. Parity has a major effect on the duration and pattern of labor. In general, the labors of multiparas are shorter than those of nulliparas, with shorter latent phase and more rapid rates of dilatation and descent in the active-phase and second stage. The labors of multiparous women who have had all previous babies by cesarean section should be judged by labor criteria established for nulliparas.

## LATENT PHASE

During the *latent phase*, preparation of the cervix occurs for the more rapid dilatation that will occur subsequently. Biochemical and physical changes in the cervix evolve that result in the process of maturation or "ripening." These alterations involve palpable softening, effacement, and anterior rotation, and sometimes a small degree of dilatation of the cervix.

The cervix may dilate slowly (maximally 0.5 cm/hr) or not at all during the latent phase. This phase tends to be shorter in multiparas then in nulliparas, a consequence, at least in part, of the fact that multiparas tend to begin with labor with more cervical dilatation than do nulliparas.

## ACTIVE-PHASE

Except for the relatively brief acceleration and deceleration portions of the active-phase, cervical dilatation is linear. Clinical labor assessment takes advantage of this fact by measuring the speed at which the cervix dilates during the active

E. Albert Reece, John C. Hobbins, Maurice, J. Mahoney and Roy H. Petrie (Eds). *Handbook of Medicine of the Fetus & Mother.* Copyright © 1995 by J.B. Lippincott Company

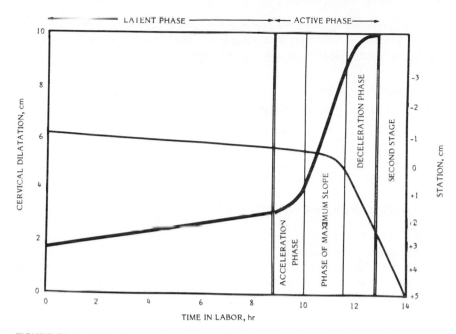

**FIGURE 57-1.** Composite of normal cervical dilatation and fetal descent curves showing their interrelations and components. (From Cohen WR, Friedman EA, eds. Management of labor. Aspen Publishers, 1983.)

phase to determine normality. Two observations of cervical dilatation are necessary to calculate the slope of the dilatation line. Once established, this rate tends to be constant for each individual (i.e., if the labor is normal dilatation will continue at the same rate until the deceleration phase is reached). Abnormalities of the activephase are defined by deviation from this projected rate of dilatation. Full cervical dilatation is diagnosed when the cervix has retracted to the widest portion of the presenting part.

## NORMAL DESCENT

As the cervix dilates in late active-phase, the resistance to fetal descent decreases and the force of uterine contractions, coupled after complete dilatation with the mother's active bearing-down efforts, begins the expulsion of the fetus from the uterus and birth canal. By the time complete cervical dilatation has been reached, descent has usually become linear and during the second stage normally proceeds in this manner until the presenting part encounters the pelvic floor. The normality of the descent mechanism can be judged from the rate of descent. It is apparent that descent also has a latent phase during which little change in station occurs under most circumstances (see Fig. 57-1). The degree of descent that has occurred before the onset of labor influences the length of the latent phase and has prognostic importance for the probability of vaginal delivery. The overall risk of cesarean section for presumed cephalopelvic disproportion when the fetal presenting part is unengaged in nulliparas at the onset of labor may be as high as 30%. Of most importance in this regard is that lack of fetal descent prior to active-phase labor is not prima facie evidence of a labor aberration or of fetopelvic disproportion.

## ABNORMAL LABOR

### LATENT-PHASE DYSFUNCTION

One abnormality of the latent phase is identifiable. *Prolonged latent phase* (Fig. 57-2, Table 57-1) is diagnosed when the latent phase exceeds 20 hours in nulliparas or 14 hours in multiparas. It is particularly likely to occur when labor begins with the cervix minimally effaced and dilated. Prolonged latent phase does not appear in and of itself to be associated with an increased need for operative delivery and is not a predictor of the more serious labor disorders of the active-phase, which have a strong association with cephalopelvic disproportion.

Treatment of a prolonged latent phase may consist of active efforts to stimulate uterine contractility or of heavy maternal sedation. Oxytocin stimulation is effective in 85% of cases in converting latent to active-phase. A similar proportion of patients respond favorably to narcotic sedation. After a dose of morphine sulfate the patient often sleeps for several hours and awakens in active-phase labor. Oxytocin stimulation is still necessary for the approximately 10% of women who persist in a desultory latent phase after the effects of the narcotic have abated. About 5% of women have their contractions cease and are presumed to have been in false labor.

The choice between uterine stimulation and therapeutic rest depends on the clinical situation. Whenever a fetal or maternal condition exists that could be jeopardized by prolonging the labor, active intervention should be used unless there is a clear contraindication to the administration of oxytocin. Similarly, when there is a reason to minimize the duration of labor, it is reasonable to intervene in

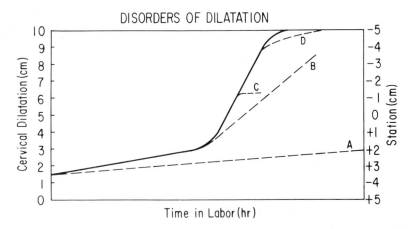

**FIGURE 57-2.** Schematic showing disorders of dilatation. (A, prolonged latest phase; B, protracted active-phase dilatation; C, arrest of dilatation; D, prolonged deceleration phase, a form of arrest disorder.)

**TABLE 57-1.** Patterns of Abnormal Labor

| Pattern | Diagnostic Criterion |
|---|---|
| **Disorders of Dilatation** | |
| Prolonged latent phase | |
| Nulliparas | Latent phase duration >20 hours |
| Multiparas | Latent phase duration ≥14 hours |
| Protracted active phase | |
| Nulliparas | Maximum slope of dilatation ≤1.2 cm/hr |
| Multiparas | Maximum slope of dilatation ≤1.5 cm/hr |
| Arrest of Dilatation | Cessation of active-phase progress for 2 hours |
| **Disorders of Descent** | |
| Failure of descent | No descent by full cervical dilatation |
| Protracted descent | |
| Nulliparous | Maximum slope of descent ≤ 1.0 cm/hr |
| Multiparas | Maximum slope of descent ≤ 2.0 cm/hr |
| Arrest of descent | Cessation of descent for 1 hour |

Modified from Friedman EA. Labor: clinical evaluation and management. 2nd ed. New York: Appleton-Century-Crofts, 1978.

the latent phase even before it reaches the limit of normal. The presence of prolonged rupture of membranes, preeclampsia, early intrauterine infection, or certain acute maternal illnesses would thus favor an approach of active stimulation of labor.

## ACTIVE-PHASE DYSFUNCTION

There are two abnormalities of active-phase dilatation (Fig. 57-2, Table 57-1). A *protracted active-phase* is diagnosed when cervical dilatation progresses linearly after commencement of active-phase, but at a rate below the established limits of normal. *Arrest of dilatation* occurs when cervical dilatation ceases for 2 hours during the active-phase. The designation of *prolonged deceleration phase* may be used to describe protracted or arrested labor during the terminal portions of cervical dilatation. The limits for the duration of the deceleration phase are 3 hours in nulliparas and 1 hour in multiparas.

The obstetric conditions associated with protraction and arrest disorders are similar, but the therapeutic approaches to the abnormalities differ. Both dysfunctions occur commonly in association with cephalopelvic disproportion, minor malpositions or abnormal attitudes, excessive sedation or anesthesia, and chorioamnionitis. Myometrial dysfunction, which may be primary or may be a consequence of the preceding factors, also contributes to active-phase dysfunction. The same clinical associations, diagnostic assessments, and treatment options exist for the analogous protraction, arrest, and failure disorders of descent to be described subsequently.

In the evaluation of protracted active-phase or arrest of dilatation, thorough examination of the patient to identify any associated predisposing conditions is necessary. Careful cephalopelvimetry is useful to ascertain the likelihood of disproportion. The Müller-Hillis maneuver (vaginal examination during the peak of a contraction with gentle fundal pressure applied) provides a useful assessment of the degree of descent, rotational tendencies, and attitudinal changes likely to occur with subsequent contractions. If cephalopelvic disproportion seems unlikely and the position of the fetal head is normal, then assessment of uterine contractility, a search for infection, and evaluation of medications that have been administered are necessary. The risk of dysfunctional active-phase labor is increased in older mothers, but diagnosis and therapy should not be influenced by maternal age.

Whether to use oxytocin in the presence of protraction abnormalities is controversial. The best available evidence suggests that when these disorders arise de novo (i.e., not provoked by infection, medication, etc.) they are not amenable to correction by stimulating uterine contractions. Enhancing uterine contractile force in such circumstances probably does not alter the rate of dilatation or descent appreciably. If, however, the protraction disorder appears to have resulted from inhibitory influences, oxytocin may overcome it.

Protraction disorders are sensitive to many inhibitory factors and may be exacerbated or even converted to arrest disorders under some circumstances. An excessively large dose of conduction anesthesia may do this. Rupture of the fetal membranes as a treatment for protraction disorders has not proved to be of benefit and may sometimes worsen the situation by precipitating the development of an arrest of dilatation.

Arrest of dilatation may evolve during a protracted active-phase or one that has been progressing normally. Arrest disorders are more commonly associated with cephalopelvic disproportion than are protraction disorders. Also, therapeutic considerations differ because arrest disorders have the potential to respond to augmentation of uterine activity by oxytocin. In the presence of an arrest abnormality, the cephalopelvic relationships must be evaluated carefully and a judgment made about the probability of disproportion. Major degrees of bony disproportion occur in at least 40% of women with arrest disorders. If the evidence for fetopelvic disproportion is considerable, it may be appropriate to move directly to cesarean section. If the pelvis is adequate or seems probably adequate, stimulation of uterine activity is reasonable, especially if uterine activity appears normal.

Three outcomes are possible when oxytocin is administered in arrest disorders: absence of further change in dilatation or descent, progress that is as good as or better than that prior to the arrest, or progress at a rate lower than the prearrest rate. Of those women who respond to oxytocin, about 85% will have done so by the end of 3 hours. Under most circumstances, if there has been no respond to oxytocin stimulation after about 3 hours, cesarean section is necessary. If oxytocin stimulation results in dilatation that is at least as rapid as that prior to the arrest, the likelihood of eventual vaginal delivery is high; but if dilatation resumes at a rate slower than existed prior to the arrest, disproportion or an insurmountable problem with uterine contractility is likely.

The potential benefit of artificial rupture of membranes in the management of labor is controversial. Although there is no doubt that rupture of the membranes can induce labor in many individuals, its influence on labor already established is less certain. Some studies have shown a modest shortening of active-phase labor in response to rupture of membranes, and one randomized trial on a very small sample of mixed parity demonstrated a shortening of the first stage by about 2 hours. Although amniotomy may increase uterine work, its salutary effect on dysfunctional labor has not been proved. It is nevertheless reasonable to rupture membranes when an arrest disorder has been identified. Those few patients who respond will do so promptly.

## THE SECOND STAGE OF LABOR

### DISORDERS OF DESCENT

During the second stage of labor, the focus of interest changes from that of cervical dilatation to fetal descent. The rate at which active descent occurs is influenced by several factors, including uterine contractile force, voluntary maternal expulsive efforts, fetal size, position, and attitude, the deformability of the fetal head, pelvic architecture, and the characteristics of the pelvic floor. Three kinds of descent disorders can be identified, *protracted descent, arrest of descent*, and *failure of descent* (Fig. 57-1, 57-3). All three descent abnormalities are similar in terms of their associated obstetric conditions, and in many respects they are analogous to the protraction and arrest disorders of dilatation. In a protracted descent pattern, the presenting part descends progressively, but at a rate below 1 cm/hr in nulliparas or 2 cm/hr in multiparas. This may continue until delivery, or may convert to an arrest of descent (which may also occur when the preceding rate of descent was normal), diagnosed when there has been no change in fetal station for 1 hour during the second stage. A failure of descent is identified when there has been no descent during labor at the time complete cervical dilatation has been reached. This is a relatively uncommon but, nevertheless, frequently overlooked labor abnormality with a very high associated likelihood of the need for cesarean delivery.

Careful cephalopelvimetry as well as evaluation for other associated obstetric problems (the same as those that occur with active-phase dilatation abnormalities) is necessary when descent disorders are diagnosed. Oxytocin stimulation of uterine activity is generally not beneficial in the presence of protracted descent,

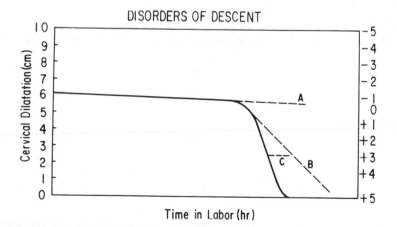

**FIGURE 57-3.** Schematic showing disorders of descent. (A, failure of descent; B, protracted descent; C, arrest of descent.)

except insofar as it is used to overcome inhibitory effects on contractility. An arrest or failure of descent is more likely to respond to uterotonic drugs.

## CEPHALOPELVIMETRY

The elegant work of Caldwell and Moloy (1933, 1938) formalized obstetric thinking with regard to the relationship between variations in human pelvic structure and the mechanism of labor.* The knowledge of pelvic architecture and its relation to labor should be used as a complementary technique to the analysis of labor curves. This allows one to explain the observed mechanism of labor, to judge the effects of labor on the fetal skull, and to assess the probability of the need for operative intervention. The value of a keen interpretation of cephalopelvic relationships along with the evaluation of the labor curves cannot be overestimated as a means of providing intelligent and safe conduct of dysfunctional labor. Neither kind of information can be used optimally without the other. Decisions concerning management and intervention in the second stage must be based on careful evaluation of maternal and fetal condition and of the progress of descent. Under some circumstances a fetus may descent at a normal rate and still take more than 2 hours to encounter the pelvic floor. To subject such patients to potentially traumatic operative procedures merely because they have not delivered within 2 hours after the second stage has begun carries little benefit and considerable risk.

## SHOULDER DYSTOCIA

After the descending head extends under the pubic symphysis and crosses perineum, there is occasionally an obstruction to further descent caused by shoulder dystocia. Management of this complication of the second stage of labor includes assessment of each patient in labor for risk factors for shoulder dystocia.

If gentle downward traction on the head at delivery fails to release the shoulders, a vaginal examination should be performed to assess the position of the bisacromial diameter and the degree of descent of the posterior shoulder. If the shoulders are in the anteroposterior diameter of the pelvis, they should be shifted to an oblique dimension. Sometimes this results in the anterior shoulder stemming under the pubic symphysis. If the anterior shoulder does not descend, the mother's thighs may be flexed against her abdomen—the McRobert's maneuver. If no success follows, the Woods corkscrew maneuver should be applied. This involves rotating the posterior shoulder 180° to the anterior position, at which point it generally moves under the symphysis and can be delivered. After or instead of the Woods maneuver, one may attempt to deliver the posterior fetal arm by drawing it across the fetal chest. Should this be unsuccessful, the remaining options are to fracture the fetal clavicle intentionally or to perform the Zavenelli

---

* Caldwell WE, Moloy HC. Anatomical variations in the female pelvis and their effect in labor with a suggested classification. AM J Obstet Gynecol 1933;26:479. Caldwell WE, Moloy HC, D'Esopo DA. Studies on pelvic arrests. AM J Obstet Gynecol 1938;36:928.

maneuver, which involves pushing the fetal head back into the vagina and delivering by cesarean section.

## EPISIOTOMY

Episiotomy for vaginal delivery has been a common part of obstetric care in North America for the last half century. However, recent trends away from operative deliveries and an enlightened attitude toward childbirth have shown that episiotomy is not always necessary. In general, one may view the decision to use episiotomy as a matter of obstetric judgment, a procedure to be performed when the alternative risks of spontaneous laceration or delay in delivery would be more hazardous than the operative incision.

## CODA

The obstetrician cannot guarantee a good outcome of every childbirth, but through the application of the principles expressed in this chapter, he or she can promise to seek the best outcome possible for a mother and fetus with the maximal obtainable safety. This can occur in the context of a birth experience that is emotionally enriching for the parturient and her family and treats the laboring mother with the requisite gentleness, dignity, and compassion demanded by the process of giving birth.

# 58. NORMAL AND OPERATIVE DELIVERIES

## PREPARATION FOR DELIVERY

Delivery of the infant is a continuation of the cardinal movements of the fetal head through the mother's pelvis. In primiparous and multiparous women, it is not unusual (in fact, it is normal) for engagement to take place during the second stage. The head usually is flexed, and then goes through the following cardinal movements: descent, internal rotation, extension, and external rotation. Delivery occurs during the third movement, when the head extends itself as it moves under the symphysis pubis.

When delivery is imminent the ACOG guidelines are:

1. The patient should not be left unattended.
2. No attempt to delay the birth with restraint or anesthesia should be made.
3. Maternal and fetal monitoring during the second stage of labor should be maintained (fetal heart by electronic means or every 5 minutes by auscultation; maternal pulse and blood pressure every 15 minutes).

## NORMAL VAGINAL DELIVERY

The usual technique of a normal vaginal delivery consists of the following: as the vertex of the fetal head appears at the vaginal introitus, the patient is placed in the lithotomy position.

Some patients may prefer to deliver from a squatting position, and physiologically this is a reasonable alternative. The uterus of the patient in the supine position compresses the great vessels.

Once the patient has been draped and continues to push with contractions, the perineum is allowed to distend gradually. With slow delivery, the mother is less likely to lacerate her perineum. *Crowning* occurs as the largest diameters of the head are passing through the introitus. Too rapid birth and sudden expansion of the cranial bones may lead to laceration of the dural sinuses and development of a subdural hematoma.

Although some may advocate episiotomy as a routine procedure, more recent studies have advocated selective use of this procedure. With malpresentations or larger infants, an episiotomy is necessary to create more room for the delivery. In some cases, especially during a case of shoulder dystocia, a mediolateral episiotomy may be necessary usually on the right side. With previous vaginal surgery, an episiotomy may be performed to prevent extensive lacerations.

After the head has delivered, the obstetrician assesses whether the umbilical cord is wrapped around it. If it is, it should be passed over the head. If the cord is too tight, it can be doubly clamped and cut prior to the birth of the infant's body. Note that if monoamniotic twins are being delivered vaginally, a nuchal cord around the first baby may be the cord of the second infant.

At this point, the oropharynx and nasopharynx are suctioned. If meconium is present, a flexible catheter is passed into the fetal stomach to empty it, in addition to aspirating meconium from the mouth and nose. After the head has delivered, the obstetrician assesses whether the shoulders will deliver easily or whether dystocia is likely. If dystocia is suspected, an attempt is made to deliver the anterior shoulder before complete external rotation (restitution) occurs. As the normal delivery progresses, the clinician pulls down on the fetal head toward the floor to deliver the anterior shoulder. The head is then lifted to deliver the posterior shoulder and the rest of the body is then delivered. The mouth and nose are once again suctioned as necessary. The blood gases at the time of birth are an indicator of the acid-base status of the infant and reflect recent trends just prior to the delivery.

## FETAL AND NEONATAL EFFECTS OF VAGINAL DELIVERY

The vast majority of women have a short second stage. The median time for the nulliparous patient is 23 minutes and that for the multiparous patient is 9 minutes. However, the 95th percentile for the nulliparous patient is 2.5 hours, and that for the multiparous patient is 70 minutes. Nonocciput anterior positions and patients with epidural anesthesia can prolong the second stage.

As the length of the second stage increases, the pH decreases and the umbilical artery lactate levels increase. During the second stage the patient may have scalp samples obtained as part of monitoring in the delivery room. Fetal distress is usually defined as a pH below 7.2. However, brief periods of bradycardias during the last moments of the second stage of labor may cause the cord pH to decrease below 7.2 without necessarily representing fetal distress.

The heart rate of the infant varies considerably during the end of labor and immediately following the delivery. In one study, there was a tachycardia of 180 bpm associated with the first cry that lasted approximately 10 minutes after the delivery in all infants. Then the heart rate slowed to the predelivery average of 140. By the next day, the heart rate of the infants was 120 bpm.

Immediately after the delivery, the flow of blood in the umbilical cord can markedly alter the blood volume in the infant. If there is a delay in cord clamping, blood will flow from the placenta to the infant by as much as 90 mL/kg. If the infant is held above the mother, the placental transfer can be completely eliminated.

## COMPLICATIONS OF VAGINAL DELIVERY

Some of the problems after a vaginal delivery include maternal trauma and infant trauma, meconium aspiration and postpartum hemorrhage.

## EPISIOTOMY

This procedure is not without complications. The patient usually loses about 200 mL of blood. There may be an extension through the rectal sphincter and possibly through the rectum itself. The perineal defect may occasionally rupture in the postpartum period. If the rupture occurs because of infection, a primary repair with clindamycin for 5 days may be done.

## LACERATIONS

If the cervix is lacerated, it should be repaired immediately with absorbable suture. The primary cautions to the physician are to inspect the vagina and cervix if increased bleeding is present or if extensions of the episiotomy are seen. It is helpful to palpate the anus and rectum after episiotomy repair before the patient leaves the delivery room to ensure that the mucosa is intact, the sphincter is present, and sutures are not palpated in the rectum.

## INFANT TRAUMA

Infant trauma may occur after either spontaneous or operative vaginal delivery. Risk factors include: weight greater than 3500 g, second stage of labor more than 1 hour, shoulder dystocia, and forceps delivery.

## SHOULDER DYSTOCIA

Physical injury may occur when the obstetrician exerts force on the infant's head and neck while trying to deliver the anterior shoulder. If shoulder dystocia occurs, calls for assistance, including the help of an anesthesiologist and a pediatrician. Fundal pressure is not advised.

The management of shoulder dystocia is described in more detail in Chapter 57.

## FRACTURED CLAVICLE

This will often occur in cases of shoulder dystocia. It is not quite as common (about 2 in 1000 births) as brachial plexus injury, which occurs in 2.6 in 1000 births. It may also occur without the presence of shoulder dystocia. Most of these fractures resolve without disabilities.

## INTRAVENTRICULAR HEMORRHAGE

This may be associated with operative vaginal delivery, but it is more commonly associated with low birth weight, low 5-minute Apgar score, cord pH <7.2, and severe respiratory distress syndrome.

## MECONIUM ASPIRATION

Meconium aspiration is a potentially dangerous complication in the newborn. It can cause pneumonitis or pneumonia, persistent fetal circulation, respiratory distress, and long-term complications.

When meconium is present at the time of birth, it must be suctioned from the infant's mouth and nose immediately. Surprisingly, the method of suctioning (bulb versus deLee) probably does not make much difference. Regardless of the methodology, the obstetrician and pediatrician in the delivery room must be experienced in the resuscitation of the newborn when meconium is present.

## POSTPARTUM HEMORRHAGE

Postpartum hemorrhage may be caused by uterine atony, unrecognized pelvic injury, retained placenta or accreta, uterine rupture, or uterine inversion. First, the patient should have at least one large-bore intravenous line in place and enough physiologic solutions infused to prevent hypovolemia. The patient is moved to the delivery room if she is not already there. A careful and complete pelvic exam should attempt to identify the source of the bleeding. If there is uterine atony, uterine massage is done and additional oxytocin is added to the intravenous solution. Ergot alkaloids or prostaglandins may also be used. The uterus is explored and curetted for additional portions of the placenta. If there is an accreta, or a rupture that cannot be repaired, a hysterectomy may be necessary. If the uterus is inverted, laparotomy is usually not necessary for its replacement if tocolytics are used.

## BREECH AND OTHER MALPRESENTATIONS

Most presentations other than the cephalic are breech presentations. More of the breech presentations are premature. As the body catches up in size late in the pregnancy, the heavier head then moves toward the pelvis. The placement of the placenta may influence the fetal position at or near term. The breech fetus and placenta weigh less than their nonbreech counterpart. There is a higher rate of congenital abnormalities, and the perinatal mortality and morbidity rates are higher. Complications in labor that are increased in the breech infant compared to the nonbreech infant include abruptio placentae, placenta previa, and prolapsed cord. A nuchal cord is less common in the breech infant than in the nonbreech infant.

The most common position is the frank breech, when the buttocks are in the pelvis, the hips are flexed, and the knees are extended, placing the legs up against the chest. If the fetus is sitting "cross-legged" with both the hips and knees flexed, this is the complete breech presentation. If the buttocks are higher in the pelvis and one or both of the feet are the presenting part, this is the footling or double-footling presentation. With exceptions, footling breech presentation is usually delivered by cesarean since the cervix does not dilate as well with only small parts in the pelvis. The exceptions are a nonviable infant, stillbirth, or a precipitous delivery.

A vaginal delivery is done in the delivery room with at least one assistant present in case an emergency cesarean needs to be performed. If the fetus is preterm, the delivery may be less traumatic if the membranes are not ruptured until the entire infant has delivered.

Macrosomic breech infants greater than 4500 g are usually delivered by cesarean. The position of the neck and head may also be evaluated by ultrasound or flat plate of the abdomen, and a cesarean is performed if the head is extended. Finally, clinical pelvimetry is performed to assess the size of the pelvis.

As much of the delivery as possible is allowed to progress spontaneously. Once the body has delivered to the umbilical cord, the pulse may be palpated directly to assess the status of the infant. The legs and buttocks will deliver simultaneously. If the mother is unable to push out the legs after the breech has delivered, the operator pushes the thigh away from the midline to flex the knee and bring the foot down.

As the infant is delivering, an assistant palpates the fetal head through the abdominal wall and maintains pressure to keep it flexed to prevent its entrapment by extension. If rapid traction is applied to the body, this increases the likelihood that one or both of the arms may become trapped behind the neck. The body can be rotated to try to dislodge the nuchal arm. If the arms are not nuchal, the operator can reach for the upper arm and sweep it across the chest to deliver it.

The head is delivered by flexing it through the pelvis promptly to prevent the cervix from closing on the neck. Although an assistant applies suprapubic pressure, the obstetrician delivers the head with the Mauriceau maneuver. This is performed by laying the infant's body on the upturned palm of one hand and arm. The fingers of that hand are placed over the fetal maxillae to help flex the head. The fingers of the other hand then grasp the shoulder, and traction is gently applied as the head is flexed. If the head fails to deliver, Piper forceps may be applied to the head to deliver it (Fig. 58-1). These are inserted from below the infant while an assistant holds the body. In the unlikely event that the cervix has closed on the neck and all attempts to deliver the head have failed, Dührssen incisions can be performed by incising the cervix with a scissors at 10 o'clock and 2 o'clock.

Today a majority of breech infants are delivered by cesarean, at least in part out of fear of medical malpractice suits.

## BIRTHS OF MULTIPLE INFANTS

Procedures for delivering multiple infants are somewhat different. First, there must be additional pediatricians, nurses, and equipment. Second, an anesthetic

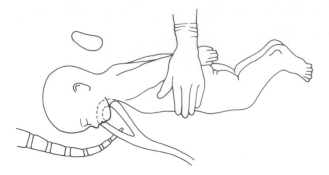

**FIGURE 58-1.** The Piper's forceps are inserted from beneath the infant while an assistant holds the body.

support is desirable. An ultrasound machine may help determine the position of the additional fetus(es).

If the first fetus is not vertex, some obstetricians will perform a cesarean. There is the possibility of interlocking heads, where the head of a second fetus descends into the pelvis before the head of the fetus that is being delivered. If this occurs, a vaginal delivery without injury or death of one or both infants is virtually impossible.

In the delivery room, all fetuses are monitored until they are delivered. If possible, fetal monitors with different ultrasound frequencies may be used. Transducers with the same frequency may interfere with each other and produce strange sounds and readings on both monitors. If two different transducers are not available, the first fetus can be connected to an internal ECG lead and the second fetus can be monitored with the ultrasound transducer. The literature has not demonstrated differences in neonatal outcome between those delivered vaginally and by cesarean, regardless of the effect of labor.

There is no compelling reason to deliver the next infant in a hurry if both the mother and fetus(es) are in good condition. Morbidity-mortality of the second nonvertex infant following elective breech extraction, external version, or immediate cesarean has been studied. In at least one study there were no differences.

## OPERATIVE VAGINAL DELIVERY

Today appropriate indications for operative vaginal delivery may include inability of the mother to push in the presence of an adequate pelvis and normal-size fetus; relative contraindication to pushing, such as cardiac disease or cerebral vascular problem; or development of fetal distress with the fetus at a low station and with an adequate pelvis.

Both vacuum and forceps apply traction to the fetal head, but the vacuum applies its force to the scalp whereas the forceps pulls against the bony parts of the head. The modern Silastic version is not traumatic by itself when it is placed. However, when the vacuum is applied, an increasing amount of force is applied to the fetus. After the delivery, the primary complication that occurs is a cephalohematoma of the scalp. This is potentially dangerous because a layer of blood 1 cm thick beneath the surface of the scalp over the entire surface of the head, although it may look innocuous, may represent one-half of the infant's blood volume.

If an operative vaginal delivery is performed, a number of guides to making this decision should be present. The cervix must be completely dilated and the membranes ruptured. In addition, the mother should be in the delivery room and an anesthesiologist should be available. The bladder is drained just prior to the delivery. The position of the fetal head is identified. The shape of the maternal pelvis is evaluated or known. Finally, the obstetrician should be experienced in the type of delivery to be performed.

If a vacuum delivery is performed, the cup is applied between contractions. However, vacuum and traction are applied only with contractions.

There are four types of forceps deliveries. An outlet forceps delivery is done when the scalp is at the introitus without separating the labia, the fetal skull has reached the pelvic floor, the sagittal suture is in the anterior-posterior diameter or in the right or left occiput anterior or posterior position, and the fetal head is at or on the perineum. A rotation of the fetal head cannot exceed 45° in an outlet forceps delivery. A low forceps delivery is done when the leading position of the skull is at +2 station or more. A midforceps delivery is done when the fetal head is engaged but is above +2 station.

In the presence of molding, a Simpson's forceps or equivalent with its 18-cm blades can be used. If there is no molding, an Elliot or Tucker-McLane, with its 15-cm blades, is the more usual choice.

In the occiput anterior position, the left branch of the forceps is inserted first (Fig. 58-2). The second and third fingers of the right hand are used to guide the blade along the scalp and inside the cervix while the thumb helps push the blade in. If insertion does not go easily, the forceps may be at the wrong angle. It is adjusted if necessary (Fig. 58-3). Then the right branch of the forceps is inserted. Once both blades are in, the position is checked for the correct application prior to applying traction.

Traction is then applied in the axis of the vagina. The descent of the fetus may be

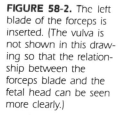

**FIGURE 58-2.** The left blade of the forceps is inserted. (The vulva is not shown in this drawing so that the relationship between the forceps blade and the fetal head can be seen more clearly.)

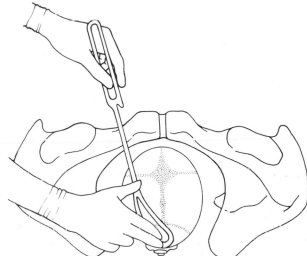

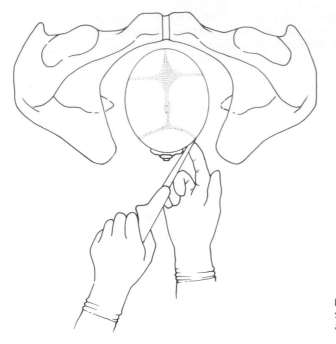

**FIGURE 58-3.** The position of the forceps is adjusted, if necessary.

more effective if traction is applied during a contraction. The blades may be left on until the head is completely outside of the vagina, or they may be removed just as the head starts to deliver. If the blades are left on, the combination of the head and blades may cause more trauma to the perineum.

## CESAREAN DELIVERY

When the scalp pH is less than 7.2 or there is a severe prolonged bradycardia before the cervix is completely dilated, or for other reasons, a cesarean delivery may be indicated. In preparation for the delivery, a patient who has fetal distress may benefit from an intravenous tocolytic to relax the uterus.

If the cesarean delivery is an emergency, a vertical incision may be made in the skin to facilitate a more rapid delivery. If speed is not essential, a Pfannenstiehl incision can be made. If more room may be necessary for a large infant or one with a large malformation, a Maylard muscle-cutting incision may be considered. If the lower uterine segment is well developed, a low transverse incision is recommended, because the potential complications in future pregnancies are lessened with this type of incision. If the lower uterine segment is not well developed or if there is a malpresentation, especially in a premature infant, a vertical incision may be made in the uterus.

If there is chorioamnionitis, both aerobic and anaerobic cultures are obtained at the time of cesarean. If antibiotic prophylaxis is utilized, there is no evidence that any regimen from the newer cephalosporins is any better than ampicillin or a first-generation cephalosporin. If intraexamination infection is evident early in the intrapartum period, antibiotics may be used without adverse neonatal outcome.

## CONCLUSION

For a healthy infant, the most important points in the care of the mother are the careful monitoring of the patient and her fetus. In the case of a difficult delivery, an experienced obstetrician and an anesthesiologist may be required. A pediatrician is needed in the delivery room to care for a premature or depressed infant.

---

# 59. PREMATURE LABOR

---

## EPIDEMIOLOGY AND DEMOGRAPHY

Definitions of preterm birth differ. According to the World Health Organization, a preterm birth is any birth, regardless of birth weight, that occurs before 37 menstrual weeks gestation. The current classification of low birth weight (LBW) is summarized in Table 59-1.

Preterm birth is one of the most important issues in reproductive medicine. It is directly responsible for 75% to 90% of all neonatal deaths not due to lethal congenital malformations. Preterm birth also accounts for a large proportion of perinatal mortality and short- and long-term neonatal morbidity. The major diseases of the preterm infant are due to organ immaturity; therefore, their incidence is inversely related to gestational age. These conditions include respiratory distress syndrome, bronchopulmonary dysplasia, patent ductus arteriosus, necrotizing enterocolitis, hyperbilirubinemia, apnea of prematurity, intraventricular hemorrhage, retinopathy of prematurity, and neonatal sepsis. In the past, if preterm infants survived at all, they faced a high risk of significant handicap (blindness, deafness, cerebral palsy, or mental retardation). For more background on topics relating to preterm birth, please see Chapter 87 in Reece EA, Hobbins JC, Mahoney MJ, and Petrie RH, eds. Medicine of the fetus & mother, J.B. Lippincott, 1992.)

Preterm birth and LBW differ in their pathogenesis but share many predisposing factors (Table 59-2). Although the rate of LBW in the United States declined by 11% from 1975 to 1985 (most of the decline occurred before 1980), the rate of very LBW increased by 4%, all of it after 1980. From 1985 to 1987, the rates of moderately LBW and very LBW increased by 2.2% and 2.5%, respectively.

The incidence of preterm birth is 18.3% in blacks and 8.5% in whites. Reasons for these demographic differences are complex and relate to socioeconomic and biological differences between the races.

Many epidemiologic risk factors are not etiologic per se, but instead are simply markers identifying patients at increased risk. Table 59-3 lists the identifiable causes most proximate to preterm birth. Most preterm births do not belong to the

**TABLE 59-1.** Birthweight Categories

| Category | Grams |
|---|---|
| Low birth weight (LBW) | <2500 |
| Very low birth weight (VLBW) | <1500 |
| Extremely low birth weight (ELBW) | |
| or | |
| Very very low birth weight (VVLBW) | ≤1000 |
| Incredibly low birth weight (ILBW) | ≤750 |

From Amon E. Limits of fetal viability: obstetric considerations regarding the management and delivery of the extremely premature baby. Obstet Gynecol Clin North Am 1988;15:321, with permission.

idiopathic category; only after known or suspected causes are eliminated should patients be diagnosed with idiopathic preterm labor. Recent studies have shown that clinically evident membrane rupture, medical or obstetric maternal complications, or fetal complications account for about 70% of preterm births.

## PATHOPHYSIOLOGY

The pathophysiology of preterm labor is unknown. This is not surprising, since the mechanisms that initiate parturition spontaneously at term are also unknown.

**TABLE 59-2.** Categories of Risk For LBW

Economic
  Poverty
  Unemployment
  Maternal father's poor socioeconomic
    status
  Uninsured, underinsured
  Poor access to prenatal care
  Poor access to food
Cultural-Behavioral
  Low educational status
  Poor health-care attitudes
  No or inadequate prenatal care
  Cigarette, alcohol, drug abuse
  Age <16 or >35 yr
  Unmarried
  Short interpregnancy interval
  Lack of support group (husband, family,
    church)
  Stress (physical, psychological)
  Poor weight gain during pregnancy
  Black race*

Biological-Genetic-Medical
  Previous LBW infant
  Low maternal weight at her birth
  Black race*
  Low weight for height
  Short stature
  Poor nutrition
  Chronic medical illnesses
  Inbreeding (autosomal recessive?)
  Intergenerational effects
Reproductive
  Multiple gestation
  Premature rupture of membranes
  Infections (systemic, amniotic, extraamniotic, cervical)
  Preeclampsia/eclampsia
  Uterine bleeding (abruptio placentae, placenta previa)
  Parity (0 or >5)
  Uterine-cervical anomalies
  Fetal disease
  Anemia or high hemoglobin
  Idiopathic premature labor
  Iatrogenic prematurity

* Black race is a risk factor for both growth retardation and premature birth. The risk is twice that for whites and remains present when confounding social and economic variables are controlled. Classification of risks for blacks as cultural and biological is due to the uncertainty of the role of these variables.
From Kliegman RM, Rottman CJ, Behrman RE. Strategies for the prevention of low birth weight. Am J Obstet Gynecol 162:1073, with permission.

**TABLE 59-3.** Proximate Causes of Preterm Birth

Iatrogenic Preterm Delivery
  Physician error
Maternal Causes
  Significant systemic medical illness
  Significant nonobstetric abdominal pathology
  Illicit drug abuse
  Severe preeclampsia/eclampsia
  Trauma
Uterine Causes
  Malformation
  Acute overdistention
  Large myomata
  Deciduitis
  Idiopathic uterine activity
Placental Causes
  Abruptio placentae
  Placenta previa
  Marginal placental bleeding
  Large chorioangioma
Amniotic Fluid Causes
  Oligohydramnios with intact membranes
  Preterm rupture of chorioamniotic membranes
  Polyhydramnios
  Subclinical Intra-amniotic infection
  Clinical chorioamnionitis
Fetal Causes
  Fetal malformation
  Multifetal gestation
  Fetal hydrops
  Fetal growth retardation
  Fetal distress
  Fetal demise
Cervical Causes
  Cervical incompetence
  Acute cervicitis/vaginitis

However, there is extensive literature on the biomolecular processes closely involved with labor.

## PROGESTERONE WITHDRAWAL

Progesterone withdrawal is not an accepted theory in humans, especially when viewed from a classical endocrine aspect. However, the concept of progesterone withdrawal as a quintessential biological phenomenon cannot be easily abandoned. First, such a mechanism is dominant in the mammalian world. Second, during the normal menstrual cycle, physiological progesterone withdrawal occurs after ovulation and before menses. Third, corpus luteectomy before 8 weeks gestation is followed by spontaneous abortion.

## OXYTOCIN

The second theory of parturition is the oxytocin theory. Infusions of oxytocin can induce labor near or at term, but there is little evidence that levels of oxytocin in maternal serum are increased before or during labor. Increases in plasma oxytocin occur primarily during the second stage of labor and postpartum. However, oxytocin does not appear to cause myometrial contraction in the absence of gap junction formation between myometrial cells. Oxytocin is not the primary agent in the initiation of labor, but simply a facilitator of myometrial forces.

## ORGAN COMMUNICATION

The third hypothesis is that of organ communication. During labor, many substances accumulate in the amniotic fluid (including free arachidonic acid, prostaglandins, platelet-activating factors, and cytokines), allowing investigators to view with unusual clarity an exciting repository of biomolecular processes relating to parturition. Decidual cells have properties that resemble those of macrophages in many ways. Activation of these cells relates to the initiation of labor.

The anatomical site of the organ communication system is the interface between the chorion and the decidua, which is also where maternal and fetal tissues meet. Lysosomal release of various enzymes may trigger prostaglandin biosynthesis and activate cervical collagenase. The amnion, chorion, and decidua have the biochemicals necessary for the propagation of labor.

The choriodecidual interface is a unique anatomical structure that provides the core for both immunologic and paracrine interactions. These may ultimately be the keys to understanding the physiology of term labor and the pathophysiology of preterm labor.

## CLINICAL USE OF RISK FACTORS

Many risk factors antedate the diagnosis of preterm labor, but unfortunately these factors are not very specific. This lack of specificity is further compounded by the inability to diagnose true preterm labor, let alone subclinical preterm labor, accurately in the early stage.

Various risk-scoring systems have been developed to identify women at above-average risk for preterm birth. These scores subject empirically collected data to various statistical analyses. However, these scores often do not make clear to what extent the predicted preterm birth relates to a treatable entity. Assuming that spontaneous preterm labor with intact membranes is treatable with tocolytic agents, there are many other proximate causes of preterm birth (see Table 59-3) for which tocolysis is absolutely contraindicated (e.g., antepartum stillbirth, significant maternal hemorrhage, chorioamnionitis, lethal congenital abnormalities, eclampsia).

Although risk-scoring systems (Table 59-4) may identify a subset of patients at increased risk for preterm birth, most patients who actually deliver preterm cannot be identified with these methods. The false-positive rate is very high in those identified as high risk. As a rule, the positive predictive value of a high-risk score is less than 30%. There are significant costs and problems associated with

**TABLE 59-4.** Major and Minor Risk Factors of the Modified
Scoring System for Spontaneous Preterm Labor

| Major Factors* | Minor Factor† |
|---|---|
| Multiple gestation | Febrile illness during pregnancy |
| Previous preterm delivery | Bleeding after 12 weeks |
| Previous preterm labor, term delivery | History of pyelonephritis |
| Abdominal surgery during pregnancy | Cigarette smoking (> 10 per day) |
| Diethylstilbestrol exposure | One second trimester abortion |
| Hydramnios | More than two first trimester abortions |
| Uterine anomaly | |
| History of cone biopsy | |
| Uterine irritability (admission to rule out preterm labor) | |
| More than one second-trimester abortion | |
| Cervical dilation (>1 cm) at 32 weeks | |
| Cervical effacement (<1 cm) length at 32 weeks | |

*Presence of one or more indicates high risk.
†Presence of two or more indicates high risk.
From Holbrook RH, Laros RK, Creasy RK. Evaluation of a risk scoring system for prediction of preterm labor. Am J Perinatol 1989;6:62, with permission.

initiating and maintaining surveillance and therapy in identified high-risk patients. These concerns are important because the low positive predictive value of risk scoring implies that most women so identified will nonetheless deliver at term, regardless of treatment. Needless treatments and interventions may cause unnecessary anxiety and stress, and limited resources may be allocated to populations where they are needed the least. If uterine activity per se becomes a significant factor for initiating therapy, then in some series up to 50% of all pregnancies would be subject to tocolytic therapy.

## EARLY CLINICAL DIAGNOSIS
### CHIEF COMPLAINT

A host of complaints may herald preterm labor (Table 59-5). Many of these symptoms are common in normal pregnancy and are often dismissed by many prenatal care providers.

Vague constitutional symptoms may also presage preterm labor. A not uncommon set of complaints relates to painless uterine activity, described as "balling up" or tightening of the uterus. Some complaints are misinterpreted and consequently mis-reported by the patient, thus misleading both physician and patient. These include gas pains, constipation, and an increase in fetal movements and may represent undiagnosed actual increases in rhythmic uterine activity. It is generally a good idea to instruct patients, especially those at increased risk, about the vague signs and symptoms of preterm labor. Patients experiencing these should be encouraged to contact the physician as soon as possible.

**TABLE 59-5.** Chief Symptoms of Preterm Labor

---

Abdominal pain
Back pain
Pelvic pain
Menstrual-like cramps
Vaginal bleeding
Pinkish staining
Increased vaginal discharge
Pelvic pressure
Urinary frequency
Diarrhea

---

## CERVICAL DILATATION

Asymptomatic cervical dilatation may represent silent preterm labor, cervical incompetence, or a normal anatomical variation. In a general obstetric population, the frequency of preterm asymptomatic cervical dilatation increases as gestation advances. The frequency was evaluated in a large study by Papiernik and associates in 1986 (Table 59-6).

Some investigators have argued that some change in management is useful when a pregnant patient is found to have asymptomatic cervical dilatation at cervical examination. These options include monitoring uterine activity, performing more frequent surveillance, restricting activity, administering tocolytic agents, and obtaining endocervical cultures. Although these options appear logical to the clinician, there is little published data to support them. These options appear more reasonable if the patient has been previously identified as high risk.

Although these services may be useful in a few circumstances, to date they are not considered to be the standard of care and are not fully endorsed by the American College of Obstetricians and Gynecologists.

The hallmark of threatened preterm labor is uterine activity. The diagnosis of threatened preterm labor is applied to the patient with uterine activity but no evidence of cervical changes. About 85% of patients with threatened preterm labor will deliver at term. In the past, many of these patients may have been diagnosed as having painful Braxton-Hicks contractions. The change in terminol-

**TABLE 59-6.** Percentage of General Obstetric Patients with Cervical Dilation of the Internal Os 1 cm

| Weeks Gestation | Percent | Total | % Preterm Birth |
|---|---|---|---|
| 19–24 | 2.4 | 2124 | 17.3 |
| 25–28 | 4.4 | 2415 | 23.4 |
| 29–31 | 10.6 | 1750 | 21.6 |
| 32–34 | 12.4 | 2967 | 17.4 |
| 35–36 | 22.5 | 1921 | 11.1 |
| 37–38 | 32.8 | 2693 | — |

ogy is clinically important. The recurrence rate of threatened preterm labor in the current pregnancy is about 30%; of these women, about half will deliver preterm.

Documenting cervical change requires serial documentation of cervical status, ideally by the same examiner. One method of determining cervical change is by noting changes in the Bishop score. Dilatation of the internal cervical os or effacement of cervical length is most significant; other measures of change, such as consistency and position, seem to be inadequate for accurate diagnosis.

Fetal station, although not part of the diagnostic criteria for actual preterm labor, has prognostic value: the lower the station, the greater the risk of spontaneous preterm delivery. A patient who experiences a lower frequency of documented uterine contractions and who is known to have a high degree of cervical compliance based on the Bishop scoring criteria (e.g., Bishop score > 6) is at increased risk for premature delivery.

Many practitioners believe that for tocolytic therapy to be most successful, it should be started before serial cervical change is documented. Thus, many practitioners initiate tocolytic therapy as early as possible.

## MANAGING PRETERM LABOR

Once the diagnosis of preterm labor is made, appropriate evaluations and initial management plans are instituted. The diagnostic evaluation has two major parts. In the first, the need for tocolytic therapy is assessed, with attention focused on the specific nature of the agents to be used. The second part is an etiologic diagnostic workup.

During evaluation, the physician seeks contraindications to actively prolonging pregnancy. Absolute contraindications include fetal demise, lethal fetal anomaly, severe preeclampsia/eclampsia, severe hemorrhage, and chorioamnionitis. Relative contraindications include fetal heart-rate monitor abnormalities, fetal growth retardation, mild preeclampsia, relatively stable late second trimester and third trimester bleeding, progressive structural but nonlethal fetal anomalies, significant maternal medical disease, and cervical dilatation of 5 cm or more. The fundamental issue is whether the risk of delivery outweighs the risk of prolonging the pregnancy.

The lower limit for initiating tocolysis in a favorable candidate is about 17 to 20 weeks gestation. As for the upper limits of fetal age and weight, different opinions exist for appropriate tocolytic therapy. In "uncomplicated" patients, some physicians initiate tocolytic therapy at 36 weeks gestation and continue oral treatment until 37 to 38 weeks.

Once therapy is determined, the choice of tocolytic agent is the next major decision. The physician must consider the mother's adrenergic state and the presence of diabetes mellitus, heart disease, hypertension, renal disease, neuromuscular disease, or gastrointestinal disease. These factors are discussed in greater detail later under the specific tocolytic agents. The physician must seek contraindications to beta-sympathomimetic agents, including situations in which beta-receptor stimulation is undesirable (e.g., New York Heart Association functional class 2 or higher cardiac disease, cardiac arrhythmias, severe hypertension, thyrotoxicosis, asymmetric septal hypertrophy, uncontrolled diabetes mellitus, neurologic thromboembolic phenomenon). Contraindications to magnesium sulfate include myasthenia gravis, some cardiac rhythm disturbances, myocardial damage, and severe renal disease.

During the initial evaluation period, some authors recommend performing microbiological cultures, urine toxicology, and baseline maternal cardiac, hematologic, and electrolyte evaluations. While these test results are pending and the mother and fetus are deemed stable, a thorough ultrasound examination is done to complete the evaluation. Factors to be assessed are listed in Table 59-7. Many of these factors have a tremendous influence on clinical management.

## FETAL AGE, WEIGHT, AND GROWTH STATUS

One of the most important determinations that must be made is that of gestational age. This usually has already been determined during prenatal care. Of course, gestational age is not one true number but rather a range of numbers based on the best obstetric estimate. Sonography is often used to confirm optimal menstrual age or to be consistent with suboptimal menstrual age within a given number of days. At best, sonographic fetal age based on biometry is an estimate determined by the mean for a population of normally grown and uncomplicated fetuses.

Routine fetal biometric measurements should be taken, including the biparietal diameter (BPD), head circumference (HC), cephalic index (CI), abdominal circumference (AC), and femur length (FL). After the gestational age is determined or confirmed, fetal weight should be estimated. For practical purposes, I recommend using fetal weight tables based on the calculations of the Shepard formulae

**TABLE 59-7.** Fetal and Maternal Assessment via Sonography

---

Fetal Evaluation
    Fetal age, weight, and growth status
    Fetal life and fetal number
    Fetal lie, presentation, position
    Fetal well-being
    Fetal behavior
    Fetal anatomy and gender
    Fetal blood sampling (funicentesis) for rapid karyotype, blood gases, disease-specific hematologic profiles
Amniotic Fluid Evaluation
    Polyhydramnios
    Oligohydramnios
    Amniocentesis for infection, fetal pulmonary maturation, fetal hemolysis
Placental and Funic Evaluation
    Previa
    Abruption
    Marginal bleed with membrane separation
    Location, internal anatomy, contour, thickness, and grade
    Umbilical cord insertion sites
    Funic presentation
Uterine Evaluation
    Defective uterine scar
    Uterine septum
    Weak lower uterine segment
    Myomatous uterus

---

(1982).* As in gestational age, estimating fetal weight by sonography carries with it inherent error. But unlike gestational age, postdelivery birth weight is a reproducible number without a significant range of error: this unequivocal number is the cornerstone of immediate neonatal prognosis, particularly for infants <1000 g. Therefore, determining fetal weight is useful for predelivery counseling regarding prognosis.

After age and weight are determined, intrauterine growth status should be assessed. Several investigators have suggested that fetal growth retardation is more common than expected in the setting of preterm labor.

The clinical relevance of finding fetal growth retardation is again of great importance to management at the lower limits of fetal viability (i.e., 22 to 26 weeks). In these situations sonographic measurements may erroneously underestimate fetal age secondary to suboptimal growth, and the infant may be erroneously declared previable. At the other end of the prematurity spectrum (32 to 36 weeks), it is not uncommon to find fetal pulmonary maturity when performing transabdominal amniocentesis. One explanation for the presumably "accelerated" pulmonary phospholipid determinations may be that suboptimal fetal growth manifests as preterm labor.

## FETAL DEMISE

In patients with inadequate prenatal care, fetal demise and multiple gestation not uncommonly present as preterm labor. These entities are reliably ruled in or out with the use of ultrasound. Tocolytic therapy is contraindicated in fetal demise; labor is either allowed to proceed or augmented.

## FETAL NUMBER

In patients with multiple gestation, extreme care must be used when administering parenteral tocolytic therapy. When using either beta-agonists or magnesium sulfate combined with fluid therapy, the risk of pulmonary edema is higher in multiple gestation than in singleton pregnancies. To prevent pulmonary edema, total fluid intake should be restricted to 2500 mL per 24 hours of salt-free or salt-poor solutions. Multiple gestation results in preterm labor at least 12 times more commonly than in singleton pregnancies. Moreover, multiple gestation carries with it a higher incidence of many other maternal and fetal complications that strongly influence management of preterm labor and delivery. Not uncommonly, multiple gestation is complicated by fetal malformation, polyhydramnios, or nonimmune hydrops. The overall likelihood that a multiple gestation will be delivered before 37 weeks is about 40%.

## MALPRESENTATION

Fetal malpresentation is common in patients with preterm labor and delivery. The incidence of malpresentation is inversely related to gestational age. It is possible

*Shepard MJ, Richards VA, Berkowitz RL, et al. An evaluation of two equations for predicting fetal weight by ultrasound. AM J Obstet Gynecol 1982;142:47.

with sonography to detect an associated uterine malformation, placental abnormality, polyhydramnios, oligohydramnios, or fetal abnormality. One's index of suspicion for a fetal malformation or genetic syndrome must be raised because there is a higher incidence of fetal malformation in the preterm breech infant: Nisell and associates (1981) reported an incidence of 13.6% in Sweden in all breech infants born after 28 weeks gestation and weighing less than 2500 g at birth.[†]

Ordinarily, I recommend performing a cesarean section for infants estimated to weigh 750 to 1500 g with a gestational age of 26 to 32 weeks. Below 750 g or less than 26 weeks gestation, inherent fetal biology is thought to be a better predictor of survival than the delivery mode. Above 1500 g, there is little information demonstrating any significant advantage of cesarean section for the breech-presenting fetus.

A less popular but increasingly common option to manage the breech-presenting fetus is the careful, selective performance of external cephalic version under ultrasound guidance.

## FETAL WELL-BEING

Since the contraction stress test is strongly contraindicated in the presence of preterm labor, the test of choice for further fetal evaluation is the biophysical profile. Fetal tone, movement, amniotic fluid volume, and fetal breathing movements (FBM) all become normally manifest weeks before classical fetal heart reactivity. Fetal oxygenation is sufficient if these four parameters are present, regardless of reactivity.

## FETAL BREATHING MOVEMENTS

Although many factors influence the presence of FBM in the nonlabor state, there seems to be a significant decrease in FBM during true labor. Several investigators have observed that the presence or absence of FBM may distinguish between the patient in preterm labor destined to deliver within 48 or 56 hours and the patient destined to deliver within a week of diagnosis. This prediction is most accurate in uncomplicated preterm labor without membrane rupture, antepartum hemorrhage, or multiple gestation, and prior to tocolytic therapy. How FBM can be applied to the management of preterm labor remains unclear, but this is an exciting area of clinically pertinent investigation.

## FETAL MALFORMATION

There is an increased incidence of fetal malformation in patients with preterm labor. Often these patients have advanced preterm labor, spontaneous rupture of membranes, or vaginal bleeding.

It is important to perform a complete fetal malformation screen in preterm labor and delivery. If sonographic evidence suggests aneuploidy, a fetal karyotype may be useful for optimal medical and obstetric management of labor, mode of deliv-

---

[†] Nisell H, Bistoletti P, Palme C. Preterm breech delivery: early and late complications. Acta Obstet Gynecol Scand 1981;60:363.

ery, place of delivery, and neonatal resuscitation. The rapidity of a karyotypic determination depends on the clinical exigencies; time is one factor influencing the decision to use amniocentesis versus funicentesis. If a virtually lethal chromosomal constitution is discovered, then management should focus on the mother's safety, and nonaggressive management for the fetus or newborn should be used. Tocolytic therapy should be discontinued.

## POLYHYDRAMNIOS

Polyhydramnios is an uncommon but important cause of preterm labor due to uterine overdistention. It has been defined as an amniotic fluid volume of greater than 2000 mL. The diagnosis is suspected when uterine enlargement is greater than expected for gestational age. There is usually difficulty in palpating fetal parts. Occasionally, the uterine wall is exceedingly tense and tender. Respiratory compromise and postrenal obstruction may result from massive uterine overdistention. As many as 40% of patients with polyhydramnios experience preterm labor and delivery.

Maternal causes include diabetes mellitus and red cell alloimmunization (anti-D, anti-Kell, etc.). These entities are readily excluded by laboratory tests. Fetal etiologies include complicated multiple gestation, nonimmune hydrops, and structural congenital malformations. Up to 75% of singleton pregnancies with nonimmune hydrops have associated polyhydramnios. Fetal congenital malformations occur in up to 50% of cases with polyhydramnios. Fetal malformations were found in 75% of cases with severe polyhydramnios, compared to a 29% rate of fetal abnormality in mild cases.

One placental cause of polyhydramnios is a large chorioangioma, a benign vascular malformation that acts like an arteriovenous shunt. Tumors large enough to produce polyhydramnios and preterm labor are rare. They are usually circumscribed, solid or complex masses protruding from the fetal surface of the placenta and are larger than 5 cm when associated with fetal hydrops.

## OLIGOHYDRAMNIOS

Oligohydramnios is diagnosed easily with ultrasound as a significant reduction in amniotic fluid volume. In the setting of preterm labor this may be due to premature rupture of the membranes, severe intrauterine growth retardation, or a genitourinary malformation in which fetal urination into the amniotic cavity is absent. Serial sonography and invasive procedures allow for differentiation among the etiologies.

The diagnosis of lethal renal diseases is important, since many of these cases may present with fetal distress or malpresentation during preterm labor. About 60% of patients with Potter's syndrome develop preterm labor, and 40% to 60% are in the breech presentation. In these situations, cesarean section is performed solely for maternal indications. However, unless studied serially, it may be impossible to differentiate from severe growth retardation.

## FETAL GENDER

Female fetuses have been found to benefit from the use of antenatal dexamethasone to reduce the incidence of respiratory distress syndrome. By regression analysis, Fleisher and coworkers (1985) found that the L/S ratio in females reached 2:1 at 33.7 weeks, 1.4 weeks earlier than in males.[‡] Phosphatidylglycerol first appeared at 34 weeks for females and at 35 weeks for males. The female infant has a significant survival advantage, particularly if her birth weight is 1000 g or more.

## AMNIOCENTESIS AND NEONATAL OUTCOME

Amniocentesis in experienced hands carries minimal risk in the late second trimester or third trimester. There is no scientific evidence that it stimulates labor.

The appropriate management of patients with positive intra-amniotic cultures remains controversial. Some regimens include antibiotics and immediate delivery, but in others the fetus is delivered only when there is frank clinical evidence of infection, particularly if the fetus is 28 weeks or younger. If there is no evidence of intra-amniotic infection, there is documented significant immaturity (i.e., L/S < 1.5), and there is a significant risk of delivery between 24 hours and 1 week, then it is reasonable to give a course of betamethasone 12 mg intramuscularly twice, 24 hours apart. In these situations aggressive tocolytic therapy is reasonable if the fetus is less than 35 weeks gestation. In contrast, if the L/S is 2:1 or higher, phosphatidylglycerol is present, or if there is a positive shake test, some authors are not as aggressive because the benefit of tocolysis does not seem to outweigh the risk.

We recently analyzed neonatal morbidity in infants born with mature amniotic fluid tests. The mothers presented with spontaneous preterm labor and were potential candidates for tocolytic therapy. In view of the pulmonary maturity, tocolytic agents were discontinued in many patients. Entry criteria were singleton gestation, transabdominal amniocentesis, uncontaminated amniotic fluid, delivery within 72 hours of amniocentesis, and absence of antenatal steroids, diabetes mellitus, and significant malformations. We found that despite "pulmonary maturity," respiratory distress and other morbidities still occurred as an inverse function of gestational age. Hence, prolongation of pregnancy should still be attempted even in the presence of mature amniotic fluid indices. It should be noted that none of the infants had significant respiratory distress at 34 weeks or more. Two recent studies of neonatal morbidity have found an inverse relationship between neonatal morbidity and gestational age (Tables 59-8, 59-9).

## UTERINE MALFORMATION

In one study of uterine anomalies the complete septate uterus had the best fetal survival rate (86%), and the complete bicornuate uteri (50%) and unicornuate (40%) the worst. The patients with complete bicornuate uteri had the highest incidence of preterm labor (66%). Didelphia and all varieties of bicornuate uteri were associated with an incidence of preterm labor that was above 20%. Preterm labor occurred in 10.3% to 37.5% of patients with unicornuate uteri. In cases of uterine anomalies, associated cervical incompetence, malpresentation, and pre-

---

[‡]Fleisher B, Kulovich MV, Hallman M, et al. Lung profile: sex differences in normal pregnancies. Obstet Gynecol 1985; 66:327.

**TABLE 59-8.** Neonatal Morbidity in Infants Born with Mature Amniotic Fluid Tests

| | Weeks Gestation | | | |
|---|---|---|---|---|
| | <33 (n = 15) | 33 (n = 13) | 34 (n = 19) | 35–36 (n = 35) |
| Respiratory distress | 7 (47%) | 2 (15%) | 0 | 0 |
| Air leak | 2 (13%) | 1 (8%) | 0 | 0 |
| NEC | 1 (7%) | 3 (23%) | 0 | 0 |
| IVH | 4 (27%) | 1 (8%) | 2 (11%) | 0 |
| Sepsis | 7 (47%) | 2 (15%) | 0 | 0 |
| Blood transfusion | 8 (53%) | 4 (31%) | 2 (11%) | 1 (3%) |
| TPN | 8 (53%) | 5 (39%) | 1 (5%) | 1 (3%) |
| BWT (mean ± SD) | 1563 ± 489 | 1925 ± 283 | 2177 ± 259 | 2442 ± 333 |

From Amon E, Leventhal S, Allen GS, et al. Neonatal outcome following spontaneous preterm labor after demonstrated lung maturity by amniocentesis. Society for Gynecologic Investigation, 37th annual meeting, St. Louis, Missouri, #169, with permission.

term labor are not uncommon; therefore, uterine malformation may be suspected when associated obstetric problems arise. Likewise, in cases of known uterine anomalies, one must have a high index of suspicion for the development of associated problems. Unfortunately, uterine anomalies are often not recognized until patients have obstetric or gynecologic problems.

## MANAGEMENT DECISIONS AT THE LOWER END OF VIABILITY

Managing preterm delivery at the lower limits of viability—currently 22 to 24 weeks gestation—is a vexing problem. The a priori determination of viability for a severely preterm yet normally formed fetus requiring delivery remains a statisti-

**TABLE 59-9.** Morbidity Rates per Gestational Age at Birth

| | Gestational Age (Wk) | | | | | |
|---|---|---|---|---|---|---|
| Complication | 26–27 (n = 16) | 28–29 (n = 32) | 30–31 (n = 33) | 32–33 (n = 44) | 34 (n = 40) | 35 (n = 36) |
| Intensive-care nursery | 16 (100) | 32 (100) | 31 (94) | 40 (91) | 29 (73) | 8 (22) |
| Respiratory distress syndrome | 13 (81) | 19 (59) | 10 (30) | 13 (30) | 9 (23) | 1 (3) |
| Patent ductus arteriosus | 8 (50) | 16 (50) | 7 (21) | 6 (14) | 5 (13) | — |
| Sepsis | 5 (31) | 8 (25) | 5 (15) | 3 (7) | 2 (5) | 2 (6) |
| Intraventricular hemorrhage | 5 (31) | 4 (13) | 1 (3) | — | — | — |
| Necrotizing enterocolitis | 4 (25) | 2 (6) | 2 (6) | 1 (2) | — | — |

Percentages (in parentheses) are rounded to nearest percent.
From Konte, et al. Short-term neonatal morbidity. Am J Perinatol 1986;3:285, with permission.

cal, not an absolute, concept. Biological and clinical variables associated with obstetric and neonatal management that favorably influence neonatal outcome have been reviewed. It is optimal for delivery in such cases to occur in immediate proximity to a neonatal intensive-care center.

A highly individualized, thoughtful, thorough, and compassionate approach to the patient is required. Survival rates as a function of gestational age and birth weight are shown in Table 59-10.

Because there are inherent inaccuracies in estimating fetal age and weight, consideration on behalf of the fetus between 22 to 23 weeks gestation and 450 to 600 g should be made. Since the likelihood for survival in these instances is dismal (i.e., < 5% to 10%), cesarean section for fetal indications is best avoided.

## TOCOLYTIC AGENTS

### BETA-SYMPATHOMIMETIC AGENTS

Beta$_1$ receptors predominate in the heart, small intestine, and adipose tissue, beta$_2$ receptors in the uterus, blood vessels, bronchioles, and liver. Some of these agents (for example, ritodrine) have been publicized as having selective beta$_2$ activity. Beta$_2$-selective sympathomimetic amines are structurally related to catecholamines and stimulate all beta receptors throughout the entire body. With continued use, tachyphylaxis is noted.

The side effects of these agents represent an exaggeration of their physiological effects. In the cardiovascular system, there is a decrease in diastolic blood pressure, tachycardia, an increase in cardiac output, and a tendency toward arrhythmogenesis. Chest pain not uncommonly occurs with parenteral administration. Since these drugs increase oxygen demand and decrease coronary artery perfusion, it is reasonable to assume that they may cause myocardial ischemia. There may be transient ST segment depression that resolves with discontinuation of

**TABLE 59-10.** Survival Rates (%) of Extremely Low Birth Weight Infants

| Birth Weight (g) | Yu et al. Melbourne, 1977–83 (n = 220)* | Amon et al. Memphis, 1983–85 (n = 263)† | Amon‡ St. Louis, 1985–86 (n = 197)† |
|---|---|---|---|
| 500–599 | 11 | 9 | 9 |
| 600–699 | 27 | 29 | 29 |
| 700–799 | 44 | 43 | 36 |
| 800–899 | 59 | 66 | 62 |
| 900–1000 | 64 | 64 | 69 |

* Includes those with birth defects; survival as of 1 year.
† Survival = discharge home alive.
‡ Previously unpublished data.
Other reports describing survival in 100-g increments may include outborn infants, may exclude delivery room deaths, may define survival only up to 27 days of postnatal life, or may consolidate data from multiple institutions and thus make comparisons less meaningful.
From Amon E. Limits of fetal viability: obstetric considerations regarding the management and delivery of the extremely premature baby. Obstet Gynecol Clin North Am 1988;15:321, with permission.

drug therapy. These clinical and EKG findings may relate directly to drug therapy or indirectly to electrolyte disturbance per se rather than to ischemia.

Pulmonary edema may occur in a small percentage of patients treated with parenteral beta-sympathomimetic agents. This life-threatening complication has several predisposing factors: multiple gestation, a positive fluid balance, blood transfusion, anemia, infection, associated hypertension, polyhydramnios, and underlying cardiac disease.

Metabolic complications, such as hypokalemia due to increases in glucose and insulin, hyperglycemia due to glucagon stimulation and glycogenolysis, and an increase in free fatty acids due to lipolysis, are common with intravenous therapy. Less common is lactic acidosis and ketosis. Occasionally there have been cases of diabetic ketoacidosis.

### Ritodrine

Ritodrine infusions should be given according to the guidelines in the manufacturer's package insert, or based on Caritis's method. Attention should be paid to contraindications, maternal tachycardia, diabetic status, and fluid balance. Some physicians give ritodrine intramuscularly in the belief that this route may lead to fewer side effects and require less fluid hydration. The technique has been described by Gonik and associates.[§]

### Terbutaline

Terbutaline is commonly used in the initial management of preterm labor. Initially, its efficacy was thought to be quite significant, but subsequent studies have found that it has only limited efficacy. Terbutaline has significant, potentially life-threatening side effects similar to those of ritodrine, especially when given intravenously.

An alternative route is subcutaneous administration: the drug effect is rapid and apparently has fewer side effects. The ease of administration and the avoidance of intravenous hydration makes subcutaneous use a reasonable alternative. In a commonly used regimen, 0.25 mg is given subcutaneously every 20 to 60 minutes until contractions have subsided. Close attention is paid to the maternal heart rate and symptoms to prevent serious complications. Oral administration of terbutaline results in widely varying serum concentrations. The common daily dose ranges from 10 to 20 mg; the maximum daily dose is about 40 mg.

## PROSTAGLANDIN SYNTHETASE INHIBITORS

Prostaglandin synthetase inhibitors are among the most effective drugs known for inhibiting preterm labor.

Of all the tocolytic agents available, indomethacin is likely to have the greatest efficacy.

Maternal side effects are minimal and include primarily gastrointestinal upset, which may require the use of Maalox. Indomethacin is contraindicated in patients

---

[§] Gonik B, Benedetti T, Creasy RK, et al. Intramuscular versus intravernous ritrodine hydrochloride for preterm labor management. Am J Obstet Gynecol 1988;159:323.

with hematologic dysfunction, peptic ulcer disease, and known allergy. Indomethacin does not significantly affect uteroplacental perfusion or Apgar scores.

The most significant potential complications in the fetus relate to the premature closure of the ductus arteriosus, right-sided heart failure, and fetal death. In the neonate the most feared complication is persistent pulmonary hypertension. Fetal and neonatal oliguria is not uncommon; in fact, idiopathic polyhydramnios may be treated effectively with indomethacin. Sonographic surveillance for oligohydramnios is indicated when indomethacin is used for more than 72 hours. There are case reports of bowel perforation. Hyperbilirubinemia may occur because indomethacin may displace bilirubin from the binding sites of albumin.

Nevertheless, a growing database suggests that the selective use of indomethacin before 34 weeks gestation causes no substantial side effects to the fetus or neonate. Since prostaglandin synthetase inhibitors are effective, easily administered, and tolerated well by the mother, these agents may be used with proper precautions to minimize fetal and neonatal effects. These include very short courses (24 to 48 hours) in patients less than 34 weeks gestation.

## MAGNESIUM SULFATE

The clinical use of magnesium sulfate has several advantages. American obstetricians have extensive experience with it in patients with preeclampsia/eclampsia. Properly used, magnesium sulfate for both tocolysis and seizure prophylaxis is safe.

### Pharmacology

The mechanism by which hypermagnesemia exerts its relaxant effects on smooth muscle differs from that of skeletal muscle. Smooth muscle undergoes pharmacomechanical coupling mediated by various agonists rather than the electromechanical coupling characteristic of skeletal muscle. Excess magnesium depresses the peripheral neuromuscular system in three ways: the inhibition of acetylcholine release, the reduction of sensitivity of the motor endplate, and the reduction of the amplitude of the motor endplate potential. Acetylcholine is unnecessary for spontaneous contractility of smooth muscle.

The exact mechanism by which magnesium diminishes or abolishes uterine activity remains unclear. Experimental data support the view that extracellular magnesium ion concentration affects the uptake, binding, and distribution of intracellular calcium in vascular smooth muscle. Similar mechanisms may operate in gravid uterine smooth muscle.

### Maternal Side Effects

Table 59-11 summarizes the major maternal clinical side effects of maternal hypermagnesemia.

One of the most important side effects encountered during standard tocolytic therapy with magnesium sulfate is chest pain, possibly due to myocardial ischemia. This rarely occurs due to magnesium sulfate therapy alone; more often there are additional factors. Some have reported an increased rate of chest pain with and without EKG changes in patients receiving initial therapy with ritodrine and magnesium sulfate simultaneously compared to ritodrine alone. This finding is

**TABLE 59-11.** Potential Maternal Effects of Hypermagnesemia

Common Side Effects
  Loss of deep tendon reflexes
  Warmth during infusion
  Mild central hypothermic effect
  Increase in skin temperature
  Cutaneous vasodilatation
  Transient peripheral arterial vasodilatation
  Nausea, possible emesis
Not Uncommon Side Effects (seen with moderately elevated serum levels)
  Somnolence, lethargy, lightheadedness
  Visual blurring, diplopia
  Dysarthria
  Nystagmus
  Constipation and dyspepsia
Uncommon Side Effects
  Potentiation of other neuromuscular blockers
  Lengthening of the P-R and QRS interval
  Controversial effect on the T wave
  Chest pain
  Pulmonary edema
Effects Seen at Very High Serum Concentrations
  Respiratory depression
  Cardiac arrest
  Profound muscular paralysis
  Amnesia
  Decreased rate of impulse formation of the S-A node
Rare Side Effects
  Profound hypotension
  Maternal tetany
  Hypersensitivity urticarial reaction
  Paralytic ileus

not entirely unexpected, based on the known cardiovascular effects of both agents. The results of this study emphasize that such combined tocolytic treatment is potentially life-threatening.

The other potentially lethal side effect encountered during magnesium sulfate tocolytic therapy is pulmonary edema. Its incidence is about 1%, compared to 5% in patients receiving beta-sympathomimetics. Generally, these cases are complicated by other factors associated with pulmonary edema: multiple gestation, polyhydramnios, preeclampsia, anemia, blood transfusion, chorioamnionitis, positive fluid balance, operative delivery, dual-agent therapy, and prolonged therapy. With proper patient selection, judicious use of therapy, and close monitoring, the risk of pulmonary edema can be minimized.

### Perinatal Side Effects
Neonatal and fetal effects are summarized in Table 59-12. None of the neonatal effects appear to be due to magnesium alone, since they may be related to confounding variables such as maternal illness, fetal growth retardation, and prematurity. Magnesium sulfate is an effective tocolytic agent that has minimal

**TABLE 59-12.** Potential Fetal/Neonatal Effects of Hypermagnesemia

1. Controversial effects on fetal heart rate variability
2. Lack of significant effect on fetal umbilical Doppler studies
3. Fetal breathing movements decrease
4. Mean baseline fetal heart rate decreases
5. Flaccidity, hyporeflexia
6. Need for assisted ventilation
7. Weak or absent cry
8. Transient decreased active tone of neck extensors
9. Possible transient radiographic bony changes

adverse effects in patients at risk for preterm delivery and is as effective as intravenous beta-sympathomimetic agents and is safer than beta-mimetic agents. Dual-agent intravenous therapy with magnesium sulfate and a beta-sympathomimetic agent carries with it the potential for extremely serious effects compared to single-agent therapy and thus cannot be recommended.

### Long-Term Therapy
The most important problem arising from prolonged therapy appears to be emotional depression and anxiety of the patient and family due to prolonged bedrest and hospitalization.

### Recommended Clinical Protocol
Most reports in the literature have used a loading dose of 4 g intravenous magnesium sulfate followed by 2 g per hour, but some have advocated 6-g loading doses. The clinical protocol allows for fine-tuning of infusion rates without the potential for fluid overload and is well tolerated by most patients. Of course, this assumes that contraindications to magnesium therapy are respected (myasthenia gravis, heart block, recent myocardial infarction, and severe renal disease). Paying careful attention to fluid intake and output diminishes the risk of pulmonary edema and magnesium toxicity. Although solutions containing some salt are used, continuous isotonic crystalloid infusion is restricted to patients undergoing the final labor and delivery process.

### NIFEDIPINE

The calcium-channel blockers are better called "calcium antagonists" since they do not completely block calcium influx into the cell. Calcium antagonists are divided into three classes: phenylalkylamines, 1,4-dihydropyridines, and benzothiazepines. The respective prototypes are verapamil, nifedipine, and diltiazem.

The mechanism of action of nifedipine appears limited to the inhibition of the slow voltage-dependent channels regulating calcium influx. Adverse pharmacologic effects include vasodilation, negative inotropism, and S-A or A-V node conduction disturbances. Because it is a potent vasodilator, nifedipine may cause dizziness, lightheadedness, flushing, headache, and peripheral edema. Although the overall incidence of side effects is 17%, severe effects necessitating discontinuation of therapy occur in 2% to 5% of patients. The negative inotropic and dromotropic (affecting cardiac nodal conduction) effects of nifedipine are minimal. This is due in large part to the heart's baroreflex response to peripheral vasodilation. Idiosyncratic reactions to nifedipine is rare.

Nifedipine is rapidly and almost completely absorbed from the gastrointestinal tract. Absorption after sublingual administration is rapid but less complete, with levels being measurable in the plasma within 5 minutes. The rate of absorption of oral and sublingual capsules varies widely among patients.

### Clinical Experience

One study reported on 58 women in preterm labor who were randomized to receive oral nifedipine or intravenous ritodrine. It found that nifedipine was as effective as ritodrine and had significantly fewer side effects. Nifedipine, when clinically used as a tocolytic agent, does not have the untoward cardiovascular and metabolic effects reported with ritodrine tocolysis.

## PROGESTATIONAL AGENTS

Progestational agents have been widely used to prolong pregnancy in women who are judged to be at increased risk of miscarriage or preterm birth. The most commonly used agent is 17-α-hydroxyprogesterone caproate. In several controlled trials this drug was primarily given weekly in doses of 250 to 1000 mg. Therapy was often started at the initiation of prenatal care or in the third trimester. This drug seems to be more useful for prophylaxis than for inhibiting active preterm labor.

## ANTENATAL GLUCOCORTICOIDS

Data from 12 controlled trials involving over 3000 participants demonstrated that corticosteroids could reduce the incidence of respiratory distress syndrome in each subgroup examined. Reductions in respiratory morbidity were also associated with reductions in intraventricular hemorrhage, necrotizing enterocolitis, and neonatal death. Fortunately, these beneficial effects occurred in the absence of strong evidence for adverse effects of corticosteroids.

Nonrandomized trials have supported the use of corticosteroids in very preterm gestations. A survey of maternal-fetal specialists shows that this therapy, even at 24 weeks gestation, is not unreasonable.

## ADJUNCTIVE THERAPY

Adjunctive therapy to optimize the perinatal outcome of impending preterm delivery is threefold:

1. Administering antenatal steroids to prevent respiratory distress syndrome with thyroxine or thyrotropin-releasing hormone
2. Preventing intraventricular hemorrhage by medical therapies such as the antenatal administration of phenobarbital and vitamin K and operative interventions such as prophylactic forceps and prophylactic cesarean section

3. Administering antenatal antibiotics beyond the accepted standard treatment to prolong "subclinically" infected pregnancies and to prevent neonatal sepsis

None of these therapies have gained widespread acceptance. Further research regarding their safety and efficacy is warranted before their use can be recommended outside of a research protocol.

## PREVENTING PRETERM BIRTH

Preventing preterm birth is a major undertaking, but success would lead to a major improvement in health and welfare. It is difficult to imagine how such a multifaceted problem could be solved by simple interventions, especially when we lack an essential understanding of the mechanisms that give rise to the multitudinous proximate causes of preterm birth (Table 59-3).

Regardless of the medical component of these programs, it is clear that socioeconomic variables, such as educational status, income, nutrition, housing, child care, and sociologic and psychological stress, place a substantial burden on those experiencing preterm delivery. Many investigators believe that the greatest potential impact will not come from the medical component per se; rather, reduction of preterm delivery will come from social, educational, and economic changes.

# 60. PREMATURE RUPTURE OF THE MEMBRANES

In most women, the chorioamniotic membranes remain intact during pregnancy and rupture spontaneously during active labor. Rupture before the onset of labor is called "premature rupture of the fetal membranes" (PROM). The word *premature* is often used in obstetrics to refer to preterm gestation, and PROM can also occur in the full-term gestation. (For a more thorough discussion of this topic, please see Chapter 88 in Reece EA, Hobbins JC, Mahoney MJ, and Petrie RH, eds. *Medicine of the fetus & mother*. J.B. Lippincott, 1992.)

There is no agreement on how long the interval between rupture of membranes and onset of labor should be before the diagnosis of PROM can be made. The latency period has ranged from 1 to 12 hours in different reports. Generally, clinical decision-making issues arise when spontaneous labor does not occur within several hours after the membranes rupture. Some authors have suggested the phrase *prolonged PROM* to define a latency period of more than 24 hours.

## RELEVANCE AND FREQUENCY

The incidence of PROM is about 10% after 37 weeks and 2% to 3.5% before 37 weeks gestation. Despite this apparently low prevalence in preterm gestation, 30% to 40% of preterm neonates are born to women with PROM, making PROM the leading identifiable cause of preterm delivery. Although most cases of preterm PROM occur after 32 weeks gestation, the major contribution to perinatal mortality is attributable to PROM at less than 32 weeks. The main maternal risks associated with PROM are chorioamnionitis and puerperal infection. The risk of maternal death has decreased from about 0.2% in 1958–1959 to 0.03% (1 in 3400) in 1982. The greatest number of women with spontaneous rupture of membranes as a function of cervical dilatation have rupture of membranes at the end of the first stage of labor.

## NORMAL HISTOLOGY

The fetal membranes are formed by the apposition of amnion and chorion. The amnion is derived from the cytotrophoblast and consists of an epithelium, which faces the amniotic cavity; a compact layer, which is responsible for most of the strength of the amnion; and a spongy layer interposed between amnion and chorion. The spongy layer allows the amnion some freedom to slide over the fixed chorion. The chorion contains several collagen layers, the outermost of which is closely attached to and often indistinguishable from the decidua capsularis.

## HISTOLOGIC FINDINGS

A comparison of histologic findings in membranes of patients with term PROM with those of patients with uncomplicated pregnancies suggests that inflammation (and probably infection) is in many cases the cause, and not only a consequence, of preterm PROM.

## BIOPHYSICAL STUDIES

Two groups of investigators have shown that membranes that rupture before labor have decreased elasticity. It has been suggested that a localized defect in the amnion may be responsible for PROM.

## BIOCHEMICAL DATA

Since infection has been associated with PROM, the mechanisms by which microbial invasion of the membranes may lead to membrane rupture have been a subject of intensive investigation. Microorganisms are a source of proteases or phospholipases that could predispose to membrane rupture. Indeed, incubating bacteria with chorioamniotic membranes in vitro reduces the bursting pressure of these tissues. Another host mechanism that may be involved in membrane rupture is the peroxidase-hydrogen peroxide-halide system. Recently, cytokines have also been implicated in PROM.

## CLINICAL RISK FACTORS

Many risk factors have been implicated in PROM, some on the basis of small and often uncontrolled studies. Since many risk factors can coexist in the same patient, multivariate statistical analysis is the best way to distinguish primary factors from confounding variables.

Harger and coworkers (1990) compared demographic factors and medical, obstetric, gynecologic, and sexual histories of 341 women with preterm PROM (20 to 36 weeks) and 253 controls matched for maternal age, gestational age, parity, type of care (private versus clinic), and previous vaginal or cesarean delivery. When multiple logistic regression analysis was conducted, only three factors remained significant: previous preterm delivery, vaginal bleeding during the index pregnancy, and cigarette smoking. Table 60-1 shows the odds ratio and the 95% confidence limits for these risk factors.

## PREVIOUS PRETERM PROM

Naeye examined the outcome of two successive singleton pregnancies in 5230 women (1982). The recurrence rate of preterm delivery after PROM was 21%; that after term PROM was 26% (Table 60-2). Asrat and associates reported a 32% recurrence risk in 121 patients with previous preterm PROM (1991).

## VAGINAL BLEEDING

The mechanisms by which vaginal bleeding may lead to preterm PROM are unknown. One possibility is that decidual bleeding with clot formation may impair the nutritional support of the membranes; subsequent stretching of the weakened area would lead to rupture. An alternative explanation is that an ascending infection may cause deciduitis manifested by vaginal bleeding.

## SMOKING

The study, previously cited, by Harger and colleagues (1990) also found that smoking throughout pregnancy doubled the risk of preterm PROM (odds ratio = 2.08; 95% confidence limits: 1.37 to 3.13). It is of interest that patients who smoked but stopped during pregnancy did not have a higher risk of PROM than women who never smoked.

**TABLE 60-1.** Clinical Risk Factors for Preterm PROM Multivariate Analysis*

| Risk Factor | Odds Ratio | 95% Confidence Limits |
|---|---|---|
| Previous preterm delivery | 2.84 | 1.40–2.48 |
| Cigarette smoking | 2.08 | 1.37–3.13 |
| Bleeding during pregnancy: | | |
|   Never | 1.00 | — |
|   During first trimester | 2.38 | 1.47–3.86 |
|   During second trimester | 4.42 | 1.62–12.03 |
|   During third trimester | 6.44 | 1.81–22.91 |
|   More than one trimester | 7.43 | 2.16–25.60 |

* Adjusted for income and race.
Adapted from Harger JH, Hsing AW, Tuomala RE, et al. Risk factors for preterm premature rupture of fetal membranes: a multicenter case-control study. Am J Obstet Gynecol 1990;163:130.

**TABLE 60-2.** Risk Factor: Previous Preterm Delivery

| First Pregnancy | Second Pregnancy | |
| --- | --- | --- |
| | Preterm PROM (%) | Full-Term PROM (%) |
| Preterm, PROM | 21 | 17 |
| Preterm, no PROM | 10 | 13 |
| Term, PROM | 7 | 26 |
| Term, no PROM | 4 | 17 |

Naeye RL. Factors that predispose to premature rupture of the fetal membranes. Obstet Gynecol 1982;60:93.

## SEXUAL INTERCOURSE

There is little evidence to implicate coitus during pregnancy in the etiology of PROM.

## CONNECTIVE TISSUE DISORDERS

It is now apparent that Ehlers-Danlos syndrome comprises a group of at least eight inheritable connective tissue disorders. Type I, or gravis type, is inherited with an autosomal dominant pattern; it seems to be associated with preterm PROM and preterm birth.

## PREVIOUS OPERATIONS ON THE GENITAL TRACT

Harlap and Davies (1975), using stepwise regression analysis, found that the rate of PROM was not higher in patients with one or more previous abortions than in patients without abortions.*

## COLONIZATION OF THE LOWER GENITAL TRACT WITH SELECTIVE MICROORGANISMS

In view of the proposed role of ascending infection in the etiology of PROM, cervicovaginal flora in PROM has been investigated in several studies. There is good evidence to support an association between infection with *Chlamydia trachomatis* (CT) and *Neisseria gonorrhoeae* (NG) and PROM. Similarly, an association between colonization with group B streptococcus (GBS) and PROM has been reported.

## MICROBIAL INVASION OF THE AMNIOTIC CAVITY

### PREVALENCE

The overall prevalence of positive amniotic fluid cultures is 28.5%, but this figure probably underestimates the true prevalence of microbial invasion of the amniotic

---

*Harlap S, Davies AM. Late sequelae of induced abortion: complications and outcome of pregnancy and labor. Am J Epidemiol 1975;102:217.

cavity. Retrieval of amniotic fluid by amniocentesis is extremely difficult in women with preterm PROM and severely reduced amniotic fluid volume.

## MICROBIOLOGY

In general, the microorganisms isolated from the amniotic fluid of women with PROM are similar to those normally found in the lower genital tract. The most common microorganisms isolated from women with term PROM were *Ureaplasma urealyticum*, *Peptostreptococcus*, *Lactobacillus*, *Bacteroides* species, and *Fusobacterium*.

## RELATIONSHIP BETWEEN LABOR AND MICROBIAL INVASION

The onset of labor in the setting of PROM has traditionally been considered an early sign of intrauterine infection.

Are there differences in the type of microorganisms and inoculum size between women in labor and not in labor with preterm PROM? The only study examining this issue published to date reported that patients with preterm PROM in active labor on admission had a higher inoculum size than women not in labor on admission.[†] No gross differences in qualitative microbiology could be detected between women with and without active labor on admission. Microbial invasion limited to *Mycoplasma* was found in only 8% of patients in labor versus 20% of those not in labor.

## CONSEQUENCES

Patients with microbial invasion of the amniotic cavity are more likely to develop chorioamnionitis, endometritis, and neonatal sepsis than patients with a negative amniotic fluid culture on admission. The microorganisms isolated from septic newborns are similar to those found in the amniotic fluid.

## MICROBIAL INVASION: CAUSE OR CONSEQUENCE OF PROM?

A growing body of evidence suggests that PROM may be the result of subclinical infection and inflammation. Patients with PROM for 1 to 4 hours before the onset of labor had a higher prevalence of histologic chorioamnionitis than patients who delivered preterm without PROM (Table 60-3). Since it is unlikely that inflammation of the chorioamniotic membranes develops in 4 hours, these data suggest that in these cases histologic chorioamnionitis precedes rather than follows PROM.

Microbial invasion of the amniotic cavity can also be the consequence of PROM. The frequency of positive amniotic fluid cultures increases with time. Indeed, 75% of patients who were quiescent on admission and subsequently went into labor had a positive amniotic fluid culture; however, only 25% of these patients had a

---

[†] Romero R, Quintero R, Oyarzun E, et al. Intra-amniotic infection and the onset of labor in preterm rupture of the membranes. Am J Obstet Gynecol 1988;159:661.

**TABLE 60-3.** Duration of PROM and Frequency of Chorioamnionitis

| | Weeks of Gestation | | |
|---|---|---|---|
| | 20–28 | 29–32 | 33–37 |
| PROM after onset of labor | 23% | 15% | 11% |
| PROM 1–4 hours before onset of labor | 48% | 29% | 32% |

Modified from Naeye RL, Peters EC. Causes and consequences of premature rupture of fetal membranes. Lancet 1980;1:192.

positive culture on admission, and the remaining 50% became positive during the latency period.

## ABRUPTIO PLACENTAE

Abruptio placentae occurs more frequently in patients with preterm PROM than in the general obstetric population (5.5% versus 0.8%). The mechanisms responsible for separation of the placenta in preterm PROM have not been determined. Some have proposed that leakage of fluid after PROM may lead to a disproportion between the placental and uterine surfaces that in turn would favor placental separation.

An alternative etiopathogenetic hypothesis postulates that a disorder of decidual hemostasis leads to separation of the membranes from the decidua, with subsequent compromise of their nutritive support. Weakening of the membranes eventually may lead to rupture. Secondary infection of the decidua could cause inflammation and facilitate premature placental detachment. An association between histologic chorioamnionitis and abruptio placentae has been reported.

## DIAGNOSIS

The diagnosis of membrane rupture must be considered in patients who complain of watery vaginal discharge or a sudden gush of fluid from the vagina. The diagnosis may also be made incidentally in patients admitted in preterm labor, in patients with ultrasound-demonstrated oligohydramnios, or during pelvic examinations done for other indications. The woman should be carefully questioned as to the time of the initial loss of vaginal fluid, the color and consistency of the discharge, and any odor noted. These questions may help to differentiate PROM from loss of the mucous plug in prodromal labor, vaginal discharge associated with infection, normal leukorrhea of pregnancy, and urinary incontinence (sometimes present in pregnancy), and also to determine the presence of blood, meconium, or vernix particles.

Evaluation of the patient begins with a sterile speculum examination. Visualization of a vaginal pool or obvious leakage of fluid from the cervix into the posterior fornix is strong evidence supporting the diagnosis of ruptured membranes. A sterile swab of fluid should be obtained from the posterior fornix and placed on a clean glass slide and on a piece of nitrazine paper. Amniotic fluid, when put on a slide and allowed to dry, will show arborization ("ferning") under the microscope at low magnification. This method has an overall accuracy of 96%. Rare false-positive ferning results have been described in association with fingerprints on the slide or contamination with semen and cervical mucus. False negatives (5% to 10%) may be caused by dry swabs or by contamination with blood. The slide should be evaluated after at least 10 minutes of drying to decrease the false-negative rate.

Nitrazine paper turns from yellow to blue when exposed to any alkaline fluid (i.e., pH of 7.0 or more); the normal gestational pH of the vagina is 4.5 to 5.5, and that of the amniotic fluid is 7.0 to 7.5. This method has an overall accuracy of 93.3%. False-positive results range from 1% to 17% and can result from alkaline urine, blood, semen, vaginal discharge in cases of bacterial vaginosis, or *Trichomonas* infection. False negatives may occur in up to 10% of cases.

If no fluid is present in the posterior fornix, the patient can be reexamined after rest in the supine position for several hours to allow for accumulation of further fluid in the posterior fornix. Additionally, a speculum examination allows for collection of vaginal and cervical cultures, and of amniotic fluid from the pooling in the posterior fornix for fetal lung maturity studies (see below).

Ultrasound visualization of decreased amniotic fluid volume can help confirm the diagnosis of PROM when other findings are ambiguous. However, the diagnostic value of sonographic assessment of amniotic fluid volume has not been rigorously examined to date. Other causes of oligohydramnios such as severe fetal growth retardation or fetal urinary-tract anomalies must be carefully ruled out. Conversely, a normal amount of amniotic fluid does not exclude the diagnosis of PROM.

In rare instances more invasive techniques are needed, such as transabdominal injection of dye (indigo carmine, Evans blue, fluorescein) into the amniotic cavity. Methylene blue should not be used because it may cause fetal methemoglobinemia. A tampon in the vagina can document subsequent leakage in cases of PROM. These invasive methods can be justified, since the diagnosis of PROM requires special maternal and fetal surveillance; in cases of very preterm gestation, the mother must be transferred to a tertiary-care center.

Whether a digital examination should be performed is a commonly asked question in the setting of PROM. The only justification for performing a digital examination is to determine cervical status. This information can be adequately obtained by sterile speculum examination and visual examination of the cervix. Digital vaginal examinations significantly shorten latency periods at each gestational age.

## INITIAL MANAGEMENT

Any patient with an established diagnosis of PROM should be assessed for gestational age, fetal well-being, signs and symptoms of chorioamnionitis, and preterm labor. Antepartum surveillance has been undertaken in patients with PROM with the nonstress test (NST) or biophysical profile (BPP); the oxytocin stress test and the nipple stimulation test have been avoided in these patients because of the risk of initiating labor. Although these tests were originally developed to detect uteroplacental insufficiency, their primary use in PROM is to diagnose impending infection.

## NONSTRESS TEST

Lack of reactivity should not be ascribed to prematurity without further testing. Isolated fetal heart rate decelerations seems to be related to the amniotic fluid volume, since the amniotic fluid index is lower in patients with decelerations than in patients without them.

Table 60-4 shows the diagnostic indices of a nonreactive NST in the prediction of total infectious morbidity (i.e., proven or suspected neonatal sepsis, and maternal chorioamnionitis), of culture-documented neonatal sepsis, and of microbial invasion of the amniotic cavity. Since the false-positive rate of a nonreactive NST is around 35%, it would be inappropriate to make a management decision solely on the results of this test.

## AMNIOTIC FLUID VOLUME

The amniotic fluid index (AFI) in patients with preterm PROM remains stable after the membranes rupture. Patients with a vertical amniotic fluid pocket less than 1 cm have a shorter latency period and a higher incidence of chorioamnionitis and neonatal sepsis than patients with a vertical pocket greater than 2 cm. A reduction in amniotic fluid volume is also associated with an increased incidence of microbial invasion of the amniotic cavity. Table 60-5 shows the diagnostic indices of a vertical pocket less than 1 cm.

## FETAL BREATHING MOVEMENTS

Preterm PROM is associated with a significant and prolonged reduction of fetal breathing movements lasting about 2 weeks. This phenomenon seems to be related to rupture of membranes per se, rather than to infection, hypoxia, or intrauterine growth retardation (Table 60-6).

The best approach to monitoring the patient with preterm PROM is probably a combination of ultrasound and amniocentesis. Patients may be monitored with

**TABLE 60-4.** Diagnostic Indices of Nonreactive NST in the Prediction of Infectious Outcome

|  | Chorioamnionitis, Possible Neonatal Sepsis, Documented Neonatal Sepsis* | Documented Neonatal Sepsis* | Positive Amniotic Fluid Culture† |
| --- | --- | --- | --- |
| Sensitivity | 94% (15/16) | 100% (7/7) | 88% (23/26) |
| Specificity | 70% (26/37) | 59% (27/46) | 75% (45/60) |
| Positive predictive value | 58% (15/26) | 27% (7/26) | 60% (23/38) |
| Negative predictive value | 96% (26/27) | 100% (27/27) | 94% (45/48) |
| Prevalence | 30% (16/53) | 13% (7/53) | 30% (26/86) |

* From Vintzileos AM, Campbell WA, Nochimson DJ, et al. The fetal biophysical profile in patients with premature rupture of the membranes: an early predictor of infection. Am J Obstet Gynecol 1985;152:510.
† From Romero R. Unpublished observations.

**TABLE 60-5.** Diagnostic Indices of Amniotic Fluid Volume (<1 cm) in the Prediction of Infectious Outcome

| | Chorioamnionitis, Possible Neonatal Sepsis, Documented Neonatal Sepsis* | Documented Neonatal Sepsis* | Positive Amniotic Fluid Culture† |
|---|---|---|---|
| Sensitivity | 56% (9/16) | 71% (5/7) | 77% (21/27) |
| Specificity | 89% (33/37) | 83% (38/46) | 66% (39/59) |
| Positive predictive value | 69% (9/13) | 38% (5/13) | 51% (21/41) |
| Negative predictive value | 82% (33/40) | 95% (38/40) | 87% (39/45) |
| Prevalence | 30% (16/53) | 13% (7/53) | 31% (27/86) |

* From Vintzileos AM, Campbell WA, Nochimson DJ, et al. The fetal biophysical profile in patients with premature rupture of the membranes: an early predictor of infection. Am J Obstet Gynecol 1985;152:510.
† From Romero R. Unpublished observations.

either the BPP or total body activity. If a patient has a BPP score above 6 (original Manning score) or a total activity more than 3 minutes (10% in a 30-minute period) (Table 60-7), the likelihood of a positive amniotic fluid culture or neonatal sepsis is extraordinarily low. These patients can be followed with serial ultrasound examinations. On the other hand, if a patient has a BPP of less than 6 or a total activity lower than 10%, amniocentesis can be performed to determine if there is microbial invasion of the amniotic cavity.

## CHORIOAMNIONITIS

Conservative management of the preterm PROM pregnancy enjoys widespread but not universal acceptance. The greatest concern arising from this noninterventional strategy is the development of infection. The classical signs of chorioam-

**TABLE 60-6.** Diagnostic Indices of Fetal Breathing Movements (<30 Sec Duration in 30-Min Observation) in the Prediction of Infectious Outcome

| | Chorioamnionitis, Possible Neonatal Sepsis, Documented Neonatal Sepsis* | Documented Neonatal Sepsis* | Positive Amniotic Fluid Culture† |
|---|---|---|---|
| Sensitivity | 100% (16/16) | 100% (7/7) | 92% (23/25) |
| Specificity | 73% (27/37) | 59% (27/46) | 49% (19/39) |
| Positive predictive value | 61% (16/26) | 27% (7/26) | 53% (23/43) |
| Negative predictive value | 100% (27/27) | 100% (27/27) | 90% (19/21) |
| Prevalence | 30% (16/53) | 13% (7/53) | 39% (25/64) |

From Vintzileos AM, Campbell WA, Nochimson DJ, et al. The fetal biophysical profile in patients with premature rupture of the membranes: an early predictor of infection. Am J Obstet Gynecol 1985;152:510.
† From Roberts AB, Goldstein I, Romero R, et al. Comparison of total fetal activity measurement with the biophysical profile in predicting intra-amniotic infection in preterm premature rupture of membranes. Ultrasound Obstet Gynecol 1991;1:36.

**TABLE 60-7.** Prediction of Positive Amniotic Fluid
Cultures: Biophysical Profile vs Total Fetal Activity

|  | Biophysical Profile | Total Fetal Activity (10%) |
|---|---|---|
| Sensitivity | 92% (23/25) | 96% (24/25) |
| Specificity | 59% (23/39)* | 82% (32/39) |
| Positive predictive value | 59% (23/39) | 77% (24/31) |
| Negative predictive value | 92% (23/25) | 97% (32/33) |

* Significant difference between specificities, $p < .05$.
From Roberts AB, Goldstein I, Romero R, et al. Comparison of total fetal activity measurement with the biophysical profile in predicting intra-amniotic infection in preterm premature rupture of membranes. Ultrasound Obstet Gynecol 1991;1:36.

nionitis include fever, maternal and fetal tachycardia, foul-smelling amniotic fluid, and maternal leukocytosis with a left shift in the differential. These signs are insensitive, however, and will detect only about 12% of patients with positive amniotic fluid cultures.

Several studies have examined the value of C-reactive protein (CRP) in monitoring the patient with preterm PROM. The emerging picture is that a normal maternal serum CRP has a high negative predictive value for clinical and histologic chorioamnionitis. On the other hand, the positive predictive value of CRP is limited but can be improved by serial testing. A steady rise in serum CRP is associated with impending chorioamnionitis. Several studies have demonstrated that CRP is an earlier and more accurate laboratory parameter than the white blood cell count and differential in the diagnosis of chorioamnionitis.

## TERM PROM

The traditional management of patients with term PROM has been induction of labor to prevent maternal and neonatal infection. However, no scientific evidence has ever been presented to support the contention that inducing labor will decrease perinatal mortality and maternal morbidity.

Four randomized clinical trials have compared expectant management versus induction of labor with oxytocin in the context of term PROM within the last 10 years. Meta-analysis of these trials indicates that induction of labor is associated with a higher incidence of cesarean section (Table 60-8) and maternal infectious morbidity, while failing to reduce the incidence of neonatal sepsis (Table 60-9).

These trials have compared expectant management versus induction by oxytocin infusion alone. However, other methods of induction (i.e., prostaglandin administration) may be more effective than oxytocin infusion. Five randomized clinical trials compared induction with prostaglandin $E_2$ administration versus oxytocin infusion in the setting of term PROM. Their meta-analysis indicates that induction with prostaglandins is associated with a lower incidence of cesarean section (Table 60-10).

From the preceding analysis, we conclude that there is insufficient evidence to favor any of the alternatives to manage term PROM. The apparently worse results obtained with induction of labor may be attributed to the method of induction and the definition of failed induction rather than to induction per se. Studies in which

**TABLE 60-8.** Effect of Induction of Labor on the Cesarean Section Rate in Term PROM

| Study | Expectant | Induction | Odds Ratio Induction/Expectant (95% CL) |
|---|---|---|---|
| Duff et al. (1984)* | 7% (5/75) | 20% (12/59) | 3.57 (1.07–12.56) |
| Morales et al. (1986)† | 7% (11/167) | 21% (31/150) | 3.69 (1.70–8.18) |
| Tamsen et al. (1990)‡ | 8% (4/50) | 0% (0/43) | 0.15 (0.02–1.76) |
| Van der Walt et al. (1989)§ | 0% (0/20) | 30% (6/20) | 3.35 (0.17–34.44) |
| Typical odds ratio | | | 2.75 (1.64–4.61) |

*Duff P, Huff RW, Gibbs RS. Management of premature rupture of membranes and unfavorable cervix in term pregnancy. Obstet Gynecol 1984;63:697.
†Morales WJ, Lazar AJ. Expectant management of rupture of membranes at term. South Med J 1986;79:995.
‡Tamsen L, Lyrenas S, Cnattingius S. Premature rupture of the membranes: intervention or not. Gynecol Obstet Invest 1990;29:128.
§Van der Walt D, Venter PF. Management of term pregnancy with premature rupture of the membranes and unfavourable cervix. S Afr Med J 1989;75:54.

patients have been managed expectantly indicate that labor will spontaneously begin by 12 hours in 50%, by 24 hours in 70%, by 48 hours in 85%, and by 72 hours in 95% of cases.

Given that PROM could be a risk factor for chorioamnionitis, puerperal endometritis, and neonatal sepsis, it is a relevant issue whether patients with term PROM should receive prophylactic antibiotics. This has been addressed by one double-blind randomized trial in which women with PROM were randomized to receive dimethylchlortetracycline or placebo. The administration of antibiotics significantly reduced the rate of endometritis but did not decrease the perinatal mortality or the incidence of infectious neonatal complications. No contemporary study has addressed this issue. Tetracycline is certainly not the drug of choice for this indication, given the fetal risks.

**TABLE 60-9.** Effect of Induction of Labor on the Incidence of Neonatal Infection in Term PROM

| Study | Expectant | Induction | Odds Ratio Induction/Expectant (95% CL) |
|---|---|---|---|
| Duff et al. (1984)* | 0% (0/75) | 2% (1/59) | 9.69 (0.19–502) |
| Morales et al. (1986)† | 0% (0/167) | 0% (0/150) | N.C. |
| Tamsen et al. (1990)‡ | 4% (2/50) | 0% (0/43) | 0.15 (0.01–2.49) |
| Van der Walt et al. (1989)§ | 0% (0/20) | 5% (1/20) | 7.39 (0.15–372) |
| Typical odds ratio | | | 1.15 (0.16–8.23) |

N.C., not computable.
*Duff P, Huff RW, Gibbs RS. Management of premature rupture of membranes and unfavorable cervix in term pregnancy. Obstet Gynecol 1984;63:697.
†Morales WJ, Lazar AJ. Expectant management of rupture of membranes at term. South Med J 1986;79:995.
‡Tamsen L, Lyrenas S, Cnattingius S. Premature rupture of the membranes: intervention or not. Gynecol Obstet Invest 1990;29:128.
§Van der Walt D, Venter PF. Management of term pregnancy with premature rupture of the membranes and unfavourable cervix. S Afr Med J 1989;75:54.

**TABLE 60-10.** Effect of Induction of Labor with $PGE_2$ or Oxytocin on the Cesarean Section Rate in Term PROM

| Study | C/S with $PGE_2$ | C/S with Oxytocin | Odds Ratio $PGE_2$/Oxytocin (95% CL) |
|---|---|---|---|
| Ekman-Ordeberg et al. (1985)* | 0% (0/10) | 40% (4/10) | 0.09 (0.01–1.36) |
| Westergaard et al. (1983)† | 5.5% (6/109) | 4.8% (4/84) | 1.16 (0.28–5.11) |
| Hauth et al. (1977)‡ | 14% (7/50) | 22% (11/50) | 0.58 (0.18–1.82) |
| Lange et al. (1981)§ | 0% (0/99) | 2.9% (3/102) | 0.14 (0.01–2.30) |
| Van der Walt et al. (1989)# | 0% (0/20) | 30% (6/20) | 0.10 (0.02–0.79) |
| Typical odds ratio | | | 0.40 (0.21–0.78) |

\* Ekman-Ordeberg G, Uldbjerg N, Ulmsten U. Comparison of intravenous oxytocin and vaginal prostaglandin $F_2$ gel in women with unripe cervixes and premature rupture of the membranes. Obstet Gynecol 1985;66:307.
† Westergaard JG, Lange AP, Pedersen GT, Secher NJ. Use of oral oxytocics for stimulation of labor in cases of premature rupture of the membranes at term: a randomized comparative study of prostaglandin $E_2$ tablets and demoxytocin resoriblets. Acta Obstet Gynecol Scand 1983;62:111.
‡ Hauth JC, Cunningham FG, Walley PJ. Early labor initiation with oral $PGE_2$ after premature rupture of the membranes at term. Obstet Gynecol 1977;49:523.
§ Lange AP, Secher NJ, Nielsen FH, Pedersen GT. Stimulation of labor in cases of premature rupture of the membranes at or near term: a consecutive randomized study of prostaglandin $E_2$-tablets and intravenous oxytocin. Acta Obstet Gynecol Scand 1981;60:207.
# Van der Walt D, Venter PF. Management of term pregnancy with premature rupture of the membranes and unfavourable cervix. S Afr Med J 1989;75:54.

## PRETERM PROM

## MANAGEMENT ISSUES

There are several issues in the management of preterm PROM that play no part in term PROM:

1. Should tocolysis be started, and if so when (prophylaxis prolong versus therapeutically)?
2. Will antibiotic prophylaxis prolong the latency period and reduce the incidence of chorioamnionitis and neonatal sepsis?
3. Should steroids be given to enhance fetal lung surfactant production?
4. What are the best methods of antenatal fetal surveillance?

### Tocolysis

Since two of three randomized clinical trials of intravenous tocolysis have suggested that treatment results in some prolongation of pregnancy, it is relevant to determine whether enough time could be gained to complete steroid administration and reduce the incidence of RDS. Meta-analysis of the two trials that provided adequate information indicates that tocolysis does not result in prolongation of pregnancy of more than 48 hours (Table 60-11). Thus, there is insufficient evidence to justify the use of tocolytic agents in patients with PROM for this specific reason.

### Antibiotics

Several investigators have conducted randomized clinical trials to examine the potential benefits of antibiotic administration. Meta-analysis of three contempor-

**TABLE 60-11.** Effect of Tocolysis on Prolongation of Pregnancy > 48° in Preterm PROM

| Study | Expectant | Tocolysis | Odds Ratio Tocolysis/Expectant (95% CL) |
|---|---|---|---|
| Garite et al. (1987) | 75.0% (30/40) | 65.2% (15/23) | 0.87 (0.61–1.23) |
| Weiner et al. (1988) | 76.1% (32/42) | 87.9% (29/33) | 1.15 (0.93–1.42) |
| Typical odds ratio | | | 1.07 (0.89–1.28) |

Data from Garite TJ, Keegan KA, Freeman RK, Nageotte MP. A randomized trial of ritodrine tocolysis versus expectant management in patients with premature rupture of membranes at 25 to 30 weeks of gestation. Am J Obstet Gynecol 1987;157:388, and Weiner CP, Renk K, Klugman M. The therapeutic efficacy and cost-effectiveness of aggressive tocolysis for premature labor associated with premature rupture of the membranes. Am J Obstet Gynecol 1988;159:216.

ary trials indicates that antibiotic administration is associated with a reduction in the incidence of chorioamnionitis and documented (culture-proven) neonatal sepsis (Tables 60-12 and 60-13).

## Steroid Administration
The use of steroids in patients with preterm PROM is an issue of clinical relevance because RDS is the major cause of neonatal morbidity and mortality. Meta-analysis of randomized trials has been conducted, and two out of three meta-analyses have shown that steroid administration results in a significant reduction in the incidence of RDS.

## Amniocentesis
Only one small randomized clinical trial has examined the value of amniocentesis in the setting of preterm PROM. Neonates born to women who had amniocenteses had a lower incidence of fetal distress during labor (as judged by fetal heart rate tracing) and a shorter hospital stay than those born to women randomized not to have amniocenteses. No difference in the rate of neonatal sepsis, maternal chorioamnionitis, or endometritis was noted between the two groups. This study had very limited power to detect differences in neonatal morbidity.

**TABLE 60-12.** Effect of Antibiotic on the Incidence of Chorioamnionitis in Preterm PROM

| Study | Placebo | Antibiotic | Odds Ratio (95% CL) |
|---|---|---|---|
| Amon et al. (1988)* | 10% (4/39) | 16% (7/43) | 0.66 (0.21–2.12) |
| Morales et al. (1989)† | 26% (22/84) | 4% (3/81) | 5.81 (1.80–18.76) |
| Johnston et al. (1990)‡ | 36% (16/45) | 7.5% (3/40) | 3.76 (1.17–12.1) |
| Typical odds ratio | | | 2.42 (1.23–4.74) |

*Amon E, Lewis SV, Sibai BM, Villar MA, Arheart KL. Ampicillin prophylaxis in preterm premature rupture of the membranes: a prospective randomized study. Am J Obstet Gynecol 1988;159:539.
†Morales WJ, Lazar AJ. Expectant management of rupture of membranes at term. South Med J 1986;79:995.
‡Johnston MM, Sanchez-Ramos L, Vaughn AJ, Todd MW, Benrubi GI. Antibiotic therapy in preterm premature rupture of membranes: a randomized, prospective, double-blind trial. Am J Obstet Gynecol 1990;163:743.

**TABLE 60-13.** Effect of antibiotic on the Incidence of Neonatal Sepsis in Preterm PROM

| Study | Placebo | Antibiotic | Odds Ratio Antibiotic/ Placebo (95% CL) |
|---|---|---|---|
| Amon et al. (1988)* | 16.7% (6/36) | 2.4% (1/42) | 0.12 (0.02–1.12) |
| Morales et al. (1989)† | 9.5% (8/84) | 4.9% (4/81) | 0.49 (0.12–1.91) |
| Johnston et al. (1990)‡ | 4.4% (2/45) | 0.0% (0/40) | 0.15 (0.01–2.41) |
| Typical odds ratio | | | 0.32 (0.13–0.77) |

*Amon E, Lewis SV, Sibai BM, Villar MA, Arheart KL. Ampicillin prophylaxis in preterm premature rupture of the membranes: a prospective randomized study. Am J Obstet Gynecol 1988;159:539
†Morales WJ, Lazar AJ. Expectant management of rupture of membranes at term. South Med J 1986;79:995.
‡Johnston MM, Sanchez-Ramos L, Vaughn AJ, Todd MW, Benrubi GI. Antibiotic therapy in preterm premature rupture of membranes: a randomized, prospective, double-blind trial. Am J Obstet Gynecol 1990;163:743

## Assessing Pulmonic Maturity

In addition to clinical studies, data generated from experimental observations provide further support for the lack of effect of vaginal contamination on the L/S ratio results. The available evidence indicates that fetal lung maturity studies can be performed on amniotic fluid obtained from the vagina and that a mature L/S ratio or the presence of PG is associated with a very low risk of RDS. Moreover, this noninvasive, low-risk approach allows for serial L/S and PG determinations.

## Mature Phospholipid Studies

A mature phospholipid study has been demonstrated in about 50% of patients with preterm PROM with gestational ages below 34 weeks. The incidence of RDS in neonates with immature L/S was 33% (5 in 15). In patients with a mature phospholipid profile, there is no evidence that active intervention is beneficial to the neonate.

## Amnioinfusion During Labor

Oligohydramnios is a risk factor for the development of severely abnormal fetal heart rate patterns during labor. In one study patients with preterm PROM had a higher incidence of cesarean section for fetal distress than patients with preterm labor and intact membranes.

The available evidence indicates that prophylactic amnioinfusion during labor may reduce the prevalence of abnormal fetal heart patterns and therefore may decrease the need for fetal scalp sampling. Further studies are required to determine if this treatment decreases the prevalence of biochemically confirmed fetal distress and the cesarean section rate for this indication.

## SECOND TRIMESTER PROM

Until recently, the management of patients with ruptured membranes before 26 weeks gestation often consisted of pregnancy termination.

Recent studies have provided data with which to counsel patients with this complication. Four studies have examined the outcome of 310 patients with preterm PROM before 26 weeks. The overall survival rate in this collected series was 40%; among the deaths, 29% occurred in utero and the remainder post-natally. Respiratory insufficiency and intraventricular hemorrhage were the most common neonatal complications. Clinical neonatal sepsis was reported in 25%.

Three of the four studies have follow-up data in some newborns; the length of follow-up ranges from 3 months to 6 years. Fifty-seven percent of infants were normal at follow-up. Long-term sequelae included chronic lung disease, developmental and neurologic abnormalities, hydrocephalus, and cerebral palsy.

Preterm delivery occurred in 57% of patients within 1 week, 60% and 79% within 1 month after PROM. An inverse relationship between gestational age at rupture of membranes and interval to delivery was noted in two of the four studies.

The main maternal complication associated with PROM before 26 weeks is chorioamnionitis, which occurred in 46% in this collected series. Leakage of amniotic fluid after second trimester amniocentesis should be considered separately. It occurs with an incidence of 1.2% and is usually transient in nature. The risk of delayed PROM in these cases is no different than in the general population.

## PULMONARY HYPOPLASIA

The frequency of pulmonary hypoplasia is related to the gestational age at the time of membrane rupture.

One study has used logistic regression analysis to determine the risk factors for the development of pulmonary hypoplasia. Gestational age at the time of PROM, but not the duration of the latency period or the severity of oligohydramnios, was associated with pulmonary hypoplasia.

Less clear is the role of the duration of rupture of membranes in the development of pulmonary hypoplasia. More clinical data are required to settle this issue. Studies of experimental oligohydramnios in the guinea pig suggest that the duration of PROM plays a role in the genesis of pulmonary hypoplasia, although the magnitude of this effect is smaller than the time of rupture.

Fetal breathing movements are considered important for normal lung development. Although some have reported absent fetal breathing in fetuses that subsequently died with pulmonary hypoplasia, others have found no difference between fetuses with and without pulmonary hypoplasia in the time spent breathing.

# 61. POSTTERM PREGNANCY

The definition of *postterm* implies a gestation that has progressed to 42 completed weeks from the first day of the last menstrual period. Many authors refer to the precise number of days, with 294 days being equivalent to 42 completed weeks. In some recent reports, patients are included in postterm studies when 287 days of gestation have passed. The terms *postdate, prolonged,* and *postterm pregnancy* are often used interchangeably. The term *postmature* is often misused when a pregnancy has merely gone a specified number of days beyond the expected date of confinement (EDC). This latter term should be reserved for postterm pregnancies that have resulted in the birth of a dysmature infant.

The postterm pregnancy is a complication of pregnancy considered to be associated with significant morbidity for both the fetus and mother. Earlier reports demonstrated a significant increase in perinatal mortality. More recent reports continue to confirm increased perinatal morbidity, but they have not shown an increased perinatal mortality (PNM) rate compared to term. This change is likely due to the development of antepartum surveillance, intrapartum monitoring, and improved neonatal care.

## INCIDENCE

The incidence of postterm gestation ranges from 3% to 12%. The postterm pregnancy is often further categorized as poor dates versus good dates, referring to accuracy of dating.

Many reports define postterm pregnancy by the following criteria:

- Positive pregnancy test by 6 weeks from the first day of the LMP
- Bimanual exam in the first trimester that confirms gestational age (GA)
- Fetal heart tones (FHT) heard by DeLee stethoscope at 20 weeks GA or 22 weeks or more of auscultated FHTs
- Confirmatory ultrasound prior to 26 weeks

An ultrasound should be performed in the patient who is unsure of her LMP, has irregular menstrual cycles, has recently discontinued oral contraceptives, or has evidence of a size-date discrepancy. This is most valuable when done prior to 20 weeks GA and more accurate when done early in gestation. A crown-rump length obtained between 6 and 12 weeks has an accuracy of ±3 to 5 days, and biparietal diameter and/or femur length between 14 and 20 weeks should be ±1 week. If the estimated GA by these early measurements differs from that calculated based on LMP by more than 10 to 12 days, the GA should be corrected to that based on ultrasound. After 20 weeks GA, the accuracy of ultrasound-based GA is substantially reduced, being ±3 weeks (in the third trimester), and therefore is not useful in redating a pregnancy.

E. Albert Reece, John C. Hobbins, Maurice, J. Mahoney and Roy H. Petrie (Eds).
*Handbook of Medicine of the Fetus & Mother.* Copyright © 1995 by J.B. Lippincott Company

## COMPLICATIONS

### MACROSOMIA

Numerous reports have described an increase in the frequency of macrosomic infants in the postterm population. Macrosomic infants at any GA experience increased birth trauma shoulder dystocia, and have more cesarean section births.

### OLIGOHYDRAMNIOS

Oligohydramnios is noted more commonly in the postterm gestation. Ultrasound descriptions of oligohydramnios have been based on subjective impressions, measurement of the deepest vertical fluid pocket, and determination of what is termed the amniotic fluid index (AFI). The AFI is a semiquantitative assessment of amniotic fluid volume. It is accomplished by dividing the maternal abdomen into four quadrants, using the umbilicus and the linea nigra. The ultrasound transducer is placed along the patient's long axis and directed perpendicular to the floor. The deepest vertical pocket is measured in each quadrant. The AFI is the sum of the measurements in centimeters from four quadrants. Using the AFI, amniotic fluid volume increases until around 30 weeks GA and plateaus at 12 cm until term. After 40 weeks, the AFI decreases, with as much as a 30% decrease between 40 and 42 weeks.

### MECONIUM

Various reports have described an increased incidence of meconium passage in the postterm pregnancy. The mere presence of meconium in the amniotic fluid is not considered a sensitive or specific indicator of intrauterine fetal distress. Meconium passage may simply reflect the maturing fetal vagal system and be provoked by fetal stress. Even when meconium passage is not secondary to fetal stress, it may pose the threat of meconium aspiration. This problem is further complicated with oligohydramnios, since the mixture of meconium and AF will be thicker. Recognition of meconium in the amniotic fluid requires active oropharyngeal suctioning at delivery to minimize meconium aspiration morbidity. Even so, this will not eliminate the meconium aspiration syndrome (MAS), because aspiration may have occurred in utero. MAS is most often encountered in high-risk gestations exhibiting abnormal fetal heart findings.

### POSTMATURITY

An infrequent but significant morbidity associated with the postterm gestation is the occurrence of the postmaturity syndrome. Associated synonyms for this finding include *placental dysfunction* and *dysmaturity syndrome*. The latter term is preferable, because this syndrome may also occur in the term infant. Dysmaturity probably results from subacute placental dysfunction-insufficiency that results in nutritional deprivation and fetal wasting. Features of dysmaturity include failure of fetal growth; loss of subcutaneous tissue; dry, wrinkled skin; and a high incidence of meconium staining. The incidence of dysmaturity findings is 3% at term compared to 10% to 20% in the postterm infant. Postnatally, such infants often manifest hypothermia or hypoglycemia, perhaps due to decreased fat and glycogen stores. Additionally, hyperviscosity and polycythemia are not uncommon and probably reflect a chronic hypoxemic fetal environment.

## MANAGEMENT

There is little disagreement that the postterm pregnancy presents as a high-risk situation with an increased potential for both maternal and fetal morbidity.

### ROUTINE INDUCTION

Neither routine induction nor expectant management should be instituted as a general rule. Individualization is currently often the chosen clinical approach, although there may be variances of detail in each management scheme. Currently, acceptable expectant management approaches propose selective induction of those postterm patients with inducible cervixes or with any medical or obstetrical complication.

The definition of an inducible cervix was systematized by Bishop's scoring system of 1964. The Bishop score evaluated five characteristics of the cervical-pelvic exam that he found useful in predicting the success of elective induction. These included cervical position, consistency, dilation, effacement, and station of the presenting part. The Bishop score could range from 0 to 13. Bishop noted that, given a score of 9 or greater, the average duration of labor, following amniotomy and oxytocin, was 4 hours or less, with no failed inductions.

The other subpopulation of postterm patients that should undergo induction are those that demonstrate any evidence of medical or additional obstetrical complications. This includes patients with hypertensive disorders, either pregnancy-related or preexisting; diabetes mellitus; and renal, cardiac, or collagen-vascular diseases. Obstetrical conditions warranting intervention include abnormal fetal lie, suspected macrosomia, or fetal dysmaturity. Historical factors such as prior stillbirth should also be taken into consideration.

### ANTEPARTUM SURVEILLANCE

Current information in the literature supports the concept of selective induction, with expectant management of those postterm patients with unfavorable cervices, if careful antepartum surveillance is conducted. The next question that arises is which antepartum test, if any, is superior and at what interval the test results should be obtained. Various tests have been applied to the postterm population and include the contraction stress test (CST), nonstress test (NST), biophysical profile, and ultrasound assessment of amniotic fluid volume.

The CST is useful in following the postterm patient but has the disadvantage of a large number of equivocal results that require repeat testing. Other limitations of the CST approach are the time consumed, cost, inconvenience, and skill necessary to interpret the test. Given the limitations of the CST, other means of surveillance have been examined. The NST is generally thought to be very reliable in predicting fetal well-being.

The biophysical profile test, first described by Manning in 1980, includes five variables: fetal movement, fetal muscular tone, fetal breathing, amniotic fluid volume (normal ≥ 1-cm pocket), and an NST. The total score possible is 10, with two points given for each parameter found to be normal and nothing given if abnormal.

Although original reports used a weekly test interval, more recent work supports twice-weekly surveillance. Given the high-risk nature of the postterm patient, it is prudent to maintain a high level of suspicion and to be willing to intervene when any suggestion of fetal compromise exists. The presence of FHR decelerations or evidence of oligohydramnios is especially disconcerting and usually warrants delivery.

## INTRAPARTUM MANAGEMENT

### INDUCTION

When expectant management is used in the postterm patient, in addition to antepartum surveillance, one must often consider how to effect delivery for either medical or obstetrical indications. In the setting of an inducible cervix, the standard approach of amniotomy and oxytocin achieves a high degree of success. The patient with an uninducible cervix presents the classic obstetrical dilemma. If the concern for fetal well-being is extreme, one may proceed directly to cesarean section, especially when adequate fetal evaluation is not feasible (e.g., fetal scalp pH assessment). In those cases where the indication for delivery is less emergent, an effective means of induction must deal with the unfavorable cervix. Current options include using oxytocin alone or using prostaglandin to ripen the cervix prior to oxytocin. Prostaglandin has been used to ripen the unfavorable cervix in a variety of clinical situations at different gestational ages.

As with any treatment, one must weigh overall benefits against the risks. With regard to the use of $PGE_2$ for ripening of the cervix, the benefits appear limited to initiation of labor in a large number of patients, and possibly a reduction in the length of labor, without adversely increasing the rate of cesarean births. Given the known potential effects on the fetus, $PGE_2$ should be used only with caution in those situations when induction is initiated for concerns of fetal well-being. In such cases, fetal heart rate monitoring must be continuously used following placement of the $PGE_2$. Relative contraindications to $PGE_2$ usage may include evidence of oligohydramnios, the presence of maternal diseases adversely affected by prostaglandins (e.g., asthma), and (because of the risk of uterine hypertonia) the presence of a uterine scar.

If $PGE_2$ is being electively used for cervical ripening and the fetus appears well, fetal heart rate should be monitored for 2 to 4 hours. If labor has not begun and FHR is reassuring, the patient may be discharged home, to return for subsequent oxytocin induction.

### FETAL MONITORING

Regardless of whether labor is spontaneous or induced for favorable Bishop score or because of fetal or maternal indications, the postterm fetus should have continuous evaluation at the onset and throughout labor. Initial assessment should include ultrasound evaluation of amniotic fluid volume and of estimated fetal

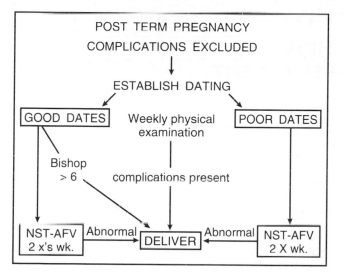

FIGURE 61-1. Management of the postterm pregnancy. (AFI, amniotic fluid index.)

weight. Although a firm rule cannot be made regarding at what weight a cesarean section should be performed, the risks of macrosomia and attendant birth trauma should be strongly considered when the estimated fetal weight is greater than 4500 g. The decision to proceed with a trial of labor in fetuses estimated to weigh between 4000 and 4500 g should be based on a number of factors, including prior obstetrical history, maternal size, presence of diabetes, and maternal consent. Additional specific intrapartum concerns include the increased incidence of meconium passage with risk of aspiration, oligohydramnios with associated umbilical cord vulnerability, and uteroplacental insufficiency.

Oligohydramnios is another risk for the postterm fetus. Saline amnioinfusion has been useful, given variable decelerations when oligohydramnios is confirmed.

## RECOMMENDATIONS

Initially, accuracy of the postterm diagnosis should be confirmed and followed by a search for any medical (e.g., hypertension) or obstetrical (e.g., growth retardation, abnormal fetal lie, spontaneous rupture of membranes) complications warranting delivery. (Fig. 61-1 illustrates management of the postterm pregnancy.) For those patients lacking accurate dating criteria (i.e., poor dates), expectant management should be initiated, with twice-weekly NST and AFV assessment. Any plan to induce a patient with unsure dates electively necessitates verification of fetal lung maturity. In those patients diagnosed postterm by good dating criteria, cervical inducibility should be evaluated and, if present (Bishop score >6), labor induction should be considered. The remaining postterm patients with unfavorable cervices can be assessed by ultrasound. Delivery should be considered when the fetal weight is estimated at >4000 g or oligohydramnios (AFI < 5) is present. If the ultrasound suggests neither of these, expectant management can be undertaken with twice-weekly NST and amniotic fluid volume measurement. The patient should have weekly exams to evaluate cervical inducibility, development of medical complications, or obstetrical factors indicating delivery.

# 62. ANESTHESIA IN THE HIGH-RISK PATIENT

Anesthetic management of the high-risk parturient aims at maintenance of maternal cardiovascular function and oxygenation; and maintenance, and possibly improvement, of the uteroplacental blood flow.

## CARDIOVASCULAR DISEASES

### PREECLAMPSIA–ECLAMPSIA

Although preeclampsia is accompanied by exaggerated retention of water and sodium, the shift of fluid and proteins from the intravascular into the extravascular compartment may result in hypovolemia, hypoproteinemia, and hemoconcentration. This phenomenon may be further aggravated by proteinuria. The mean plasma volume in women with preeclampsia has been found to be 9% below normal, and in those with severe disease, it was as much as 30% to 40% below normal. Prior to the start of therapy these patients usually have a low cardiac index, low pulmonary capillary wedge pressure, and high systemic vascular resistance. Thrombocytopenia and elevation in the serum concentration of fibrin-fibrinogen degradation products are not uncommon in severe cases. In addition, a significant proportion of patients with preeclampsia develop an acquired defect in platelet function (impaired thromboxane $B_2$ biosynthesis), resulting in prolongation of bleeding time. HELLP syndrome, a variant of severe preeclampsia, may develop either antepartum or postpartum. It is characterized by hemolysis, elevated liver enzymes, and a low platelet count. Maternal and fetal prognoses are poor.

### General Management

The mainstay of anticonvulsant therapy in this country is magnesium sulfate; though its efficacy in preventing seizures has been well substantiated, its mechanism of action remains controversial. Magnesium potentiates the duration and intensity of action of both depolarizing and nondepolarizing muscle relaxants.

The aim of fluid therapy is to raise the CVP and pulmonary capillary wedge pressure to the normal range (4 to 6 cm $H_2O$ and 5 to 10 mmHg, respectively) and to raise the urine output to 1 mL/kg/h. This has been shown to improve the cardiac index and to prevent abrupt, often precipitous drops in blood pressure associated with vasodilator therapy.

Hydralazine (Apresoline) is the most commonly used vasodilator in preeclampsia, since it has been shown to increase both uteroplacental and renal blood flows. Sodium nitroprusside (Nipride), a potent vasodilator of resistance and capacitance vessels with an immediate but evanescent action, is useful in preventing dangerous elevations in systemic and pulmonary blood pressure during laryngoscopy and intubation. Infusion rates of sodium nitroprusside below 5 to

E. Albert Reece, John C. Hobbins, Maurice, J. Mahoney and Roy H. Petrie (Eds). *Handbook of Medicine of the Fetus & Mother.* Copyright © 1995 by J.B. Lippincott Company

10 μg/kg/min, depending on the length of administration, can be maintained without undue risk of cyanide toxicity in the mother and fetus. Trimethaphan (Arfonad), a ganglionic blocking agent, is particularly useful in hypertensive emergencies, since it will not cause vasodilation in the brain. Other agents include alphamethyldopa and clonidine, as well as nitroglycerin, ketanserin (a serotonin receptor antagonist), atenolol (a beta-adrenoreceptor antagonist), and labetalol (a nonselective beta blocker with some alpha$_1$-blocking effects).

### Anesthetic Management
Epidural anesthesia for labor and delivery should no longer be considered contraindicated in preeclampsia, providing there is no clotting abnormality or plasma volume deficit. In volume-repleted patients positioned with left uterine displacement, epidural anesthesia leads to a significant improvement in placental perfusion.

For cesarean section, the level of regional anesthesia must extend to T3–T4, making adequate fluid therapy and left uterine displacement even more vital. Should hypotension occur, its correction will require a reduced dose of ephedrine in view of the increased sensitivity to vasopressors.

General anesthesia in preeclamptic patients has its particular hazards. The rapid-sequence induction and intubation necessary to avoid aspiration are occasionally difficult because of upper-airway edema. Marked rises in systemic and pulmonary arterial pressure occurring at intubation and extubation enhance the risk of cerebral hemorrhage and pulmonary edema. An appropriate antihypertensive therapy, such as administration of trimethaphan or nitroprusside infusion, will minimize these hemodynamic changes. Ketamine and ergot alkaloids should be avoided. Relaxants should be administered with caution (using a nerve stimulator) to avoid overdosage.

## HEART DISEASE

Heart disease during pregnancy remains the leading nonobstetric cause of maternal mortality. Cardiac decompensation and death occur most commonly at the time of maximum hemodynamic stress (i.e., in the third trimester of pregnancy, during labor and delivery, and in the immediate postpartum period).

### Rheumatic Heart Disease
Mitral stenosis is the most frequent valvular lesion in parturients with rheumatic heart disease. Other valvular diseases—namely, mitral regurgitation and aortic stenosis or regurgitation—are found much less frequently. Together they amount to between 10% and 35% of all cases.

### Congenital Heart Diseases
Patent ductus arteriosus, atrial septal defect, and ventricular septal defect are the more common congenital cardiovascular abnormalities. Pulmonary hypertension may develop late in the natural history of these diseases, causing a reversal of the shunt (Eisenmenger's syndrome). During pregnancy, the decrease in systemic vascular resistance, in the presence of fionary vascular resistance, results in a significant increase in the right-to-left shunt.

Tetralogy of Fallot is the most common cyanotic congenital heart disease seen during pregnancy.

### Anesthetic Management

Continuous epidural block not only eliminates pain and tachycardia throughout labor and delivery, but also prevents the progressive increase in cardiac output and stroke volume normally occurring during parturition. It also abolishes the bearing-down reflex. In view of these advantages, continuous lumbar epidural analgesia is recommended for most pregnant women with rheumatic valvular diseases except for those with severe, symptomatic aortic stenosis, in whom even transient episodes of hypotension may result in serious coronary hypoperfusion, arrhythmias, and even cardiac arrest. Intrathecal narcotics have been used to provide obstetric analgesia without the risk of hypotension. Morphine (0.5 to 1.5 mg) or fentanyl (37.5 to 50 μg) is usually effective in relieving the pain of uterine contractions, but pudendal block is required for delivery. If general anesthesia is required for cesarean section, the standard thiopental-nitrous oxide-halogenated anesthetic-muscle relaxant technique is recommended. In cases of severe mitral stenosis, etomidate (0.2 to 0.3 mg/kg) or a slow induction with halothane or intravenous fentanyl is preferred.

## DIABETES MELLITUS

Insulin-dependent diabetes mellitus is one of the most common medical complications encountered in pregnancy, occurring in about 0.1% to 0.5% of all pregnant women.

## GENERAL MANAGEMENT

Close control of diabetes is equally important in the intrapartum period. Several techniques may be used to maintain glucose levels during labor. A continuous intravenous infusion of both insulin and glucose is common. Ten units of regular insulin added to a 1000-mL solution of 5% dextrose, given at the rate of 100 mL/h by constant infusion pump, will result in glucose levels below 100 mg/dL. An alternative is to give the patient one-third of the prepregnancy dose of intermediate-acting insulin on the morning of delivery. Capillary glucose measurements should be determined every 1 to 2 hours, and regular insulin supplements should be given if necessary. In the immediate postpartum period the patient's insulin requirements are usually lower than those before pregnancy, so that for 48 hours insulin should be given only as needed. If cesarean section is anticipated, the morning insulin dose should be omitted, the procedure planned for early in the day, and a 5% dextrose solution infused, with hourly blood glucose determinations.

## ANESTHETIC MANAGEMENT

One of the most specific changes that affects anesthetic management of diabetic parturients is the decrease in uteroplacental blood flow, which may be decreased by as much as 35% to 45% in the last trimester.

## Labor

Lumbar epidural block can provide excellent pain relief for both labor and delivery, if necessary. Avoidance, or immediate treatment, of maternal hypotension is extremely important for the reasons stated earlier. Rapid infusion of a dextrose-free solution should be administered via a second intravenous catheter, and ephedrine 10 to 30 mg IV can be given promptly if there is an episode of hypotension despite careful precautions.

## Cesarean Section

For cesarean section regional anesthesia is useful, since it enables the anesthesiologist to evaluate the mental status of the patient and to detect potential hypoglycemia. Care should be taken to avoid hypotension by adequate left uterine displacement and administration of dextrose-free solutions. Ringer's lactate, because of the high lactate content, is not ideal, and Normosol-R is preferable for plasma volume expansion. General anesthesia is not contraindicated, as long as there is adequate care in avoiding hypoglycemia.

# NEUROLOGIC DISEASES

Only those more commonly seen will be discussed here: epilepsy, myasthenia gravis, multiple sclerosis, paraplegia, and muscular dystrophy. Subarachnoid hemorrhage, caused by rupture of an aneurysm or arteriovenous angioma, is rare but very important because of the high mortality associated with it.

# EPILEPSY

Idiopathic epilepsy is fairly frequent in our society (incidence approximately 0.5%) and is most commonly seen first in the child or young adult. Many anticonvulsant drugs are in common use, such as phenobarbital, phenytoin, and primidone.

## Anesthetic Management

Local anesthetic techniques may be useful in labor and delivery, since no greater sensitivity to these drugs has been shown than that in normal patients. Where general anesthesia is used for cesarean section, drugs with convulsive potential should be avoided (e.g., enflurane, ketamine, and methohexital), as should wide variations in $pCO_2$. Narcotic-diazepam combinations are useful after delivery.

Status epilepticus requires rapid intervention, with control of seizures and ventilation, and monitoring of vital signs and acid—base status, as well as fetal heart rate. Diazepam infusion to blood concentrations of 0.2 to 0.4 $\mu$/mL is usually sufficient, but general endotracheal anesthesia, with the use of nondepolarizing muscle relaxants, may be necessary.

# MYASTHENIA GRAVIS

Myasthenia gravis is an autoimmune disorder that is characterized by excessive muscle fatigue with exercise, affecting the ocular, laryngeal, facial, and respiratory muscles. Partial recovery follows rest and treatment with anticholinesterase drugs.

Remission is common in pregnancy, but muscle weakness has also been known to increase.

Facilities for intensive respiratory care should be available at the time of delivery. For pain relief, the most useful, if feasible, is lumbar epidural anesthesia, which affords the flexibility of allowing rest in the first stage of labor and adequate analgesia for elective outlet forceps delivery (often undertaken to shorten the second stage); it can also be extended for cesarean section. Large doses of ester-type local anesthetics, such as 2-chloroprocaine (Nesacaine), because of their hydrolysis by cholinesterase, carry a potential for greater toxicity in patients on anticholinesterase drugs.

## MULTIPLE SCLEROSIS

Multiple sclerosis (MS) is a demyelinating disease characterized by remissions and exacerbations, with progressive deterioration of the central nervous system. The relapse rate during the first 3 months postpartum is several times higher than that in the pregnant state, and the exacerbation rate is lower during pregnancy. Evidence relating any form of anesthesia to the progress of MS has been lacking, and many argue that patients should not be denied regional anesthesia for pain relief during labor and delivery.

## PARAPLEGIA

Paraplegia may result from trauma or from spinal cord tumors or poliomyelitis. Patients are particularly vulnerable to impaired respiratory function, decubitus ulcers, fractures due to osteoporosis, impaired temperature regulation, and urinary tract infections. The phenomenon known as "autonomic hyperreflexia" occurs in almost half of patients with lesions above T7. It consists of sweating, facial flushing, pilomotor erection, headache, bradycardia, and severe hypertension in response to stimulation of skin, or distention or contraction of hollow organs, such as bladder, uterus, or gut below the level of the lesion. Cesarean section is not more common than in uncomplicated pregnancy, but weak expulsive efforts may necessitate the use of forceps to shorten the second stage of labor.

### Anesthesia

From 1 week following a spinal injury, or in neuromuscular diseases where there are denervated or degenerating muscles (e.g., muscular dystrophies, multiple sclerosis), potassium leaks from the muscle cell in response to succinylcholine. Thus, administration of succinylcholine can lead to hyperkalemia, which may cause severe arrhythmias, even ventricular fibrillation. Regional anesthesia is therefore safer for the parturient with paraplegia. Little actual analgesia is required, but the continuous epidural or spinal technique can be very valuable in controlling hyperreflexia during labor. Epidural narcotic may prove to be a useful alternative, with less effect on blood pressure and heart rate.

## MUSCULAR DYSTROPHY

Muscular dystrophy is an inherited disorder characterized by progressive loss of muscular function. There are several major categories, but patients generally have muscle weakness leading to contractions and deformities such as scoliosis and lordosis, and bones are readily fractured. Myocardial myopathy may be present, and respiratory failure is an ever-present hazard. Swallowing may be compromised, and aspiration of secretions leads to pneumonitis. Administration of succinylcholine causes hyperkalemia, hyperthermia, and elevated enzymes, such as creatinine phosphokinase (CPK). These increases may mimic, but do not always indicate, the potentially lethal malignant hyperthermia (MH).

### Anesthesia

Because of delayed gastric emptying and weak intestinal mobility, there is a special disposition to aspiration. A histamine receptor antagonist such as ranitidine (150 mg orally the night before, and 50 mg IV 1 to 2 hours before surgery) or cimetidine (300 mg orally the night before, and 300 mg IM an hour before surgery) can be given. Sodium citrate (30 mL) is also administered orally prior to induction. As is standard with all obstetric patients, cricoid pressure is applied until the larynx is intubated and the cuff is inflated. Succinylcholine should not be used, since it may produce a contracture, without fasciculations, which makes ventilation difficult. Small doses of nondepolarizing muscle relaxants may be used.

### SUBARACHNOID HEMORRHAGE

The incidence of subarachnoid hemorrhage is about 1 in 10,000 pregnancies. Conservative management is associated with a maternal mortality as high as 50% in the few weeks following hemorrhage, whereas surgery gives the best prognosis for mother and baby. There are several reports of cesarean section followed directly by aneurysm clipping at the same procedure; usually, however, pregnancy is allowed to continue after surgery until the occurrence of labor and vaginal delivery at term. Successful fetal outcome following both maternal hypothermia and induced hypotension have been reported. Trimetaphan (Arfonad) may be the safer drug with which to induce hypotension, since it is rapidly hydrolyzed and has a high molecular weight, but sodium nitroprusside has been used without incident. Where possible, the fetal heart rate should be monitored throughout. Transient bradycardia, with rapid return to normal after the end of hypotension, is the rule. In the case of recent bleeding, the goals during induction of anesthesia are to control hypertension and avoid fluctuations in blood pressure during laryngoscopy and endotracheal intubation. Smooth induction is followed by reduction of intracranial pressure and induced hypotension.

During labor the parturient requires sufficient pain relief in the first stage of labor to avoid marked changes in blood pressure and increases in cardiac output. This is best provided by lumbar epidural analgesia, which is also useful in preventing the Valsalva maneuver in the second stage. Forceps may be applied to shorten this stage and avoid bearing down. For cesarean section also, epidural anesthesia is the method of choice. If general anesthesia is necessary because of fetal distress, antihypertensive drugs may be used to prevent the response to endotracheal intubation.

### DRUG ABUSE DURING PREGNANCY

Illicit drug use for recreational purposes has reached epidemic proportions. In contrast to earlier years, when depressants or hypnotics like marijuana or methaqualone were popular, the present wave involves stimulants such as cocaine and methamphetamine. These exert their effect by modulating the sympathetic nervous system to a degree that may result in physiologic alterations affecting anesthetic and obstetric management.

For the fetus, maternal cocaine use is particularly hazardous. Numerous studies have identified an increased incidence of fetal wastage, low fetal weight, and premature labor and delivery, as well as low Apgar scores, placental abruption, and intrauterine death following cocaine abuse.

Maternal medical complications are also common. These include acute myocardial infarction, myocarditis, lethal ventricular arrhythmias, asystole, and rupture of the ascending aorta or intracranial aneurysm. With large doses, generalized convulsions, coma, cerebrovascular accident, or subarachnoid hemorrhage are not uncommon. Smoking, or "free-basing," the drug may result in bronchospasm, pulmonary edema, or adult respiratory distress syndrome.

It is not unusual for the perinatal care team to be presented with an acutely ill mother and a fetus in need of urgent obstetric intervention. Seizures should be quickly terminated with intravenous injection of thiopental (50 to 100 mg) or diazepam (5 to 10 mg), the airway protected, and adequacy of ventilation and oxygenation ensured. Hypertension may be exacerbated by unopposed alpha stimulation following the use of a beta-adrenergic receptor blocker. Therefore, a combined alpha and beta receptor antagonist, such as labetalol, may be preferable.

Nitroprusside is currently the favored drug for management of hypertensive crisis. The calcium channel antagonist verapamil can prevent ventricular fibrillation induced by cocaine, which is due to enhanced calcium influx into myocardial cells.

Ketamine should be avoided, since it has potent sympathomimetic actions of its own. Thiopental remains the standard induction agent. Agents sensitizing the myocardium to the arrhythmogenic effects of catecholamines, such as halothane, should be avoided.

Regional anesthesia (spinal or epidural) may be used in more elective cesarean sections. For labor and vaginal delivery, intravenous narcotics may be used to provide pain relief, but administration must be titrated carefully, since their effects may be potentiated by cocaine. Epidural analgesia provides more complete pain relief.

Anesthetic considerations in managing the parturient abusing amphetamines are similar to those for cocaine.

## THIRD TRIMESTER BLEEDING

The two most common conditions resulting in antepartum hemorrhage are placenta previa and abruption. In severe cases, the mother may require rapid intravascular volume replacement with a crystalloid solution and/or blood products. Thus, placement of large-bore intravenous cannulae (14- or 16-gauge) is strongly recommended. Blood-component therapy with fresh-frozen plasma, cryoprecipitate, and platelet concentrate may be necessary to treat dilutional or disseminated intravascular coagulopathy. Invasive monitoring of arterial and central venous pressures may be warranted. Emergency cesarean section is often necessary and is usually performed under general anesthesia because of time constraints and uncorrected hypovolemia. Patients with placenta previa and prior cesarean sections have an increased incidence of placenta accreta and greater potential for severe hemorrhage.

## OBESITY

Obesity enhances the risks of obstetric and anesthetic interventions, and recent data suggest that it is a leading contributor to maternal morbidity and mortality. A patient is considered to be obese when her weight is more than 20% above ideal body weight.

Additional demands imposed by pregnancy can result in cardiac decompensation. Associated with obesity are hypertension, coronary artery disease, and diabetes mellitus, which further limit cardiac reserve during the stresses of labor and delivery. Changes in the respiratory system predispose to development of hypoxemia. The most serious consequences of obesity are manifested in the "obesity hypoventilation (Pickwickian) syndrome," characterized by chronic hypoxemia, hypercarbia, right-sided cardiac failure, and somnolence. Obesity is associated with higher volumes and more acidic gastric juices, thus enhancing the risk of aspiration pneumonitis.

## ANESTHETIC CONSIDERATIONS

Analgesia blunts increases in cardiac output and ventilation associated with pain of labor and vaginal delivery. Intravenous narcotics, however, must be used cautiously so as to avoid airway obstruction and hypoventilation. Epidural analgesia, being more effective in providing complete pain relief, is preferable, but not without risk, such as unintended intravascular or intrathecal injection of local anesthetic.

For cesarean section, regional anesthesia should be used whenever possible, thus avoiding potentially difficult laryngoscopy and endotracheal intubation. Where general anesthesia cannot be avoided, prophylaxis against aspiration of gastric contents and careful evaluation of the airway should be performed. Awake laryngoscopy and endotracheal intubation under topical anesthesia may be preferred prior to induction. Since postoperative pulmonary complications are common, chest physical therapy, incentive spirometry, and early ambulation are to be encouraged.

## PRETERM LABOR AND DELIVERY

Although preterm deliveries occur in 8% to 10% of all births, they contribute to approximately 80% of early neonatal deaths. Several maternal complications of tocolysis have been reported, such as hypotension, hypokalemia, hyperglycemia, myocardial ischemia, pulmonary edema, and death. General anesthesia may be risky in the presence of preexisting tachycardia, hypotension, and hypokalemia. Delaying anesthesia by at least 3 hours from the cessation of tocolysis, if possible, will allow beta-mimetic effects to dissipate. Potassium supplementation is not necessary.

## FETAL SURGERY

Recent improvements in invasive as well as noninvasive technology have made it possible to diagnose and, in some cases, treat fetal anomalies.

The fetus has the ability to react to noxious stimuli and thus requires analgesia/anesthesia for painful procedures. Direct fetal injection of nondepolarizing muscle relaxants can provide immobilization for relatively simple procedures that do not require major anesthesia, such as fetal blood transfusion. Administration of d-tubocurarine (1.5 mg/kg estimated fetal weight) or pancuronium (0.3 mg/kg) into the fetal buttock (with the use of ultrasound, if need be) has resulted in the onset of paralysis within 5 minutes, lasting 4 and 7 hours, respectively. When feasible, continuous fetal heart rate monitoring, in conjunction with acid-base measurements, appears to be adequate for determination of fetal well-being. Postoperative administration of tocolytic agents is recommended.

---

# 63.  THE PUERPERIUM AND LACTATION

---

The puerperium operationally defines a period of 6 weeks following delivery in which a number of changes in the anatomy and physiology of reproduction occur, such as the menstrual cycle, systemic changes, and lactation.

## THE REPRODUCTIVE SYSTEM

### THE CERVIX

Ultrasonography of both the nongravid and puerperal uterus reveals the variation in normal uterine size. The normal pregravid weight of the uterus is 50 to 100 g, depending on parity. The uterus achieves a term weight of 1000 to 2000 g and is composed of 83% water. The uterine length also changes appreciably during pregnancy, from 6 to 8 cm in the nonpregnant state to 40 cm or more at term.

Following parturition, the cervix is very distensible, thin, and flabby, even in the presence of a well-contracted uterus with little or no bleeding. There may or may not be multiple tears along the cervical margin. This laxity in the cervix results in a dilated state of about 2 to 3 cm for the first few days following delivery. By the end of the first week, the cervix will return to a state resembling nonpregnancy, but dilated to about 1 cm. This state will persist for up to 6 weeks, or occasionally up to 3 months.

### THE UTERUS

Immediately after expulsion of the placenta, strong uterine contractions decrease uterine size. Within 24 hours the uterine size approximates the size at 20 weeks gestation. By 48 hours, the uterine size approaches 14 weeks gestation. Within 2 weeks postpartum, the uterus decreases further in size, descending into the pelvic cavity and eventually below the pubic symphysis. The nonpregnant uterine size will be achieved within 4 weeks postpartum. Pathologic estimates of these changes indicate that immediately following delivery the contracted uterus weighs approximately 1 kg; 1 week later, about 500 g; and 2 weeks later, about 300 g. Uterine weights of less than 100 g can be observed as soon as 3 weeks postpartum.

Within 24 to 36 hours, patients will begin to pass blood-tinged discharge with particulate matter (lochia) through the vagina. The lochia contains the superficial necrotic layer of the pregnant endometrium (the decidual). Microscopically, the lochia consists of red blood cells, pieces of decidual epithelial cells, and bacteria. The nonpregnant endometrium is regenerated by the endometrial gland and the connective tissue. Within 10 days, a new endometrium regenerates rapidly throughout most of the endometrial surface. Regeneration at the placental implantation site takes longer, since such a process awaits sloughing from necrotic cells, followed by repair of these epithelial structures. A delay in involution at the placental site over a protracted period may result in postpartum hemorrhage. Sloughing of the placental site, resulting in infarction and necrosis, is believed to occur secondary to constriction and thrombosis of vessels supplying the placental site.

## THE VAGINA

Following parturition, the vagina is hyperemic, swollen, and smooth. The normally present rugae are often absent but reappear within 3 weeks postpartum. The edema and swelling usually resolve by 6 weeks postpartum.

## THE MENSTRUAL CYCLE

Return of the menstrual cycle following delivery occurs at variable time periods, and the menstrual flow may be in variable quantities. Some patients may present with intermittent spotting after delivery, or with a normal menstrual flow as early as 5 weeks postpartum. The average time for return of the menses for nonlactating women is about 8 to 10 weeks, with a range of up to 17 to 18 weeks postpartum. Histologic evidence of secretory endometrium demonstrates that ovulation may occur in nonlactating women as early as 27 days or 36 days after delivery. Earlier studies had reported that ovulation occurred later. Delayed return of menses is usually seen in lactating women. Infant suckling intensity and frequency, coupled with the timing of introduction of supplementary foods to the infant, determine the duration of anovulation and amenorrhea in well-nourished women.

## SYSTEMIC CHANGES

Cardiovascular status, which alters significantly during pregnancy, returns to a nonpregnant state shortly after delivery. For example, the blood volume decreases by about 20% with 72 hours postpartum. This decrease in blood volume may be secondary to the blood loss that occurs during parturition, as well as the postpartum diuresis. Other cardiovascular changes, such as increased heart rate and cardiac output, return to baseline within the first 2 weeks postpartum.

## THE URINARY SYSTEM

Pregnancy induces both functional and structural changes in the urinary system. The functional changes seem to remit promptly after delivery; however, the structural changes may persist for several months. Renal blood flow in nonlactating women returns to nonpregnant levels by 6 weeks postpartum. A puerperal diuresis usually occurs within the first 3 days postpartum, and this enhances the return of blood volume to normal.

Dilation of the bladder ureters and renal pelvis may persist for 3 or more months postpartum. The puerperal bladder with an increased capacity is somewhat refractory to increased intravesicular pressure; hence, overdistention and incomplete emptying may result. In fact, about 20% of postpartum women will experience incomplete emptying.

## THE LIVER

During pregnancy, plasma proteins—such as coagulation factors, immunoglobulins, transport and binding proteins, cholesterol, triglyceride, and lipoproteins—increase. The blood levels of these proteins fall precipitously within 24 to 48 hours postpartum, and by 2 to 3 weeks after delivery their levels return to baseline. Liver function test values remain normal during pregnancy and elevated values should be considered abnormal.

## LACTATION

### STAGES OF LACTATION

The cycle of human lactation consists of four separate stages: mammogenesis (mammary growth), lactogenesis (the initiation of milk secretion), galactopoiesis (the maintenance of lactation), and finally involution (the cessation of lactation).

### Lactogenesis (Secretory Phase)

The hormonal environment of the mother changes abruptly at parturition. Two factors, the loss of progesterone-induced inhibition and prolactin-induced stimulation, are thought to trigger lactogenesis, the initiation of secretion of a copious milk supply. The release of inhibition linked to the decrease of progesterone is thought to be the active factor responsible.

### HORMONAL CONTROL OF LACTATION

#### Endocrine Control

The minimal hormonal requirements for the maintenance of normal lactation are prolactin, insulin, and hydrocortisone. In response to suckling, prolactin surges to an apex at 30 minutes and returns to basal levels after 2.5 to 3 hours from the end of the first to approximately the 12th week postpartum. An adequate prolactin response may also be needed to establish necessary levels of prolactin receptors on the mammary epithelial cells and thus appears critical to the establishment of successful lactation. By the third month postpartum, serum prolactin levels approach prepregnancy values and do not respond to suckling. Nevertheless, adequate milk production can still continue.

Suckling also stimulates the release of oxytocin from the posterior pituitary. Auditory, olfactory, or emotional cues also lead to the release of oxytocin. Oxytocin produces a contraction of the myoepithelial cells, releasing milk from the alveoli and small ducts into the larger ducts and sinuses. Oxytocin release and the subsequent serum peak of prolactin are not related.

## COMPOSITION AND QUANTITY OF HUMAN MILK

Human milk contains more lactose and nonprotein nitrogen and less protein nitrogen than bovine milk (Table 63-1). For human milk the figures are averages that change as lactation progresses through each of the stages described earlier. Moreover, each sample from an individual at a particular time can differ in content and composition from each previous sample or from those of women otherwise matched for time, age, diet, and so on.

The mammary gland produces colostral milk for the first 3 days postpartum. This milk contains a higher protein and lower fat, calorie, and lactose content than milk produced later. Colostrum appears yellow when it contains high levels of carotene. Colostrum is rich in immunoglobulins that may provide protection against gastrointestinal infections.

By 2 weeks postpartum, the mammary gland produces a stable and mature milk, although compositional differences are still seen. Once widening starts, mammary gland function deteriorates and milk composition again changes.

## EFFECT OF MATERNAL DIET ON MILK COMPOSITION AND PRODUCTION

Maternal dietary intake has little effect on human milk macronutrient content and is not affected significantly by maternal dietary intake, whereas milk fatty acid composition reflects maternal dietary fat intake. Maternal fat-soluble vitamin intake can affect milk composition, but the effect of dietary intake of water-soluble vitamins varies and depends on the specific vitamin transport system involved. Little evidence exists that links moderate maternal caloric deprivation with decreased milk production.

**TABLE 63-1.** General Composition of Human and Bovine Milks

| Species | Protein (%) | Casein (% Protein) | Fat (%) | Lactose (%) | Ash (%) | Kilocalories (per 100 mL) |
|---------|---------|---------|---------|---------|---------|---------|
| Human | | | | | | |
| Mature, 36 d | 1.0 | 40 | 3.9 | 6.8 | 0.2 | 63 |
| Colostrum, 3 d | 2.3 | — | 3.0 | 5.5 | — | 58 |
| Bovine | 3.4 | 82 | 3.7 | 4.8 | 0.7 | 75 |

From Jensen RG, et al. Nutrition today 1988: (Nov/Dec): 20. with permission. Adapted from Blanc B. World Rev Nutr Diet 1981;36:1. Harzer G, et al. Z Ernah 1986;25:77.

## PRENATAL AND PERINATAL PRACTICES THAT AFFECT BREAST-FEEDING

### PRENATAL EXAMINATION

Several abnormalities can be detected and treated during the prenatal period. Among these are treatable conditions such as inverted nipples, conditions that will require special counseling but that should not preclude nursing (e.g., silicone breast implantation and unilateral mastectomy), and conditions that preclude adequate lactation (e.g., insufficient glandular development and breast reduction procedures that have severed nerve endings to the areola and nipple). Even when the physical exam yields no apparent problem, the clinician should take a detailed lactation history early in the pregnancy, since the problems multiparous women have with lactation with one child repeat with later children.

### Maternal Health Problems

Few maternal conditions preclude lactation. Failure to lactate may occur secondary to Sheehan's syndrome (postpartum pituitary necrosis), to destructive diseases of the hypothalamic-pituitary system, and to hypophysectomy. Alternative feeding for the infant is necessary when the composition of the milk is deleterious, when necessary maternal drug therapy would be detrimental to the infant, or when the milk contains a transmittable substance such as a virus, as in human immunodeficiency virus (HIV), or an environmental contaminant. The infant with galactosemia, a rare occurrence of 1 in 60,000 births, must be maintained on a lactose-free diet. Since lactose is the major carbohydrate in human milk, its use is obviously precluded.

**Substance Abuse.** Most abused substances clearly enter the milk and can cause harm to the infant.

*Smoking of Cigarettes.* If the mother smokes cigarettes, nicotine and its major derivative, cotinine, derived from tobacco use, are found in the serum and urine of infants in direct proportion to the amount of exposure from breast milk and/or passive exposure. If the mother must smoke while nursing, the clinician should caution her to allow an interval of at least 1.5 hours between smoking a cigarette and nursing the infant. This may be difficult, since most infants do not feed on a schedule that would allow such planning in early lactation. Also, to avoid the addition of passive exposure of tobacco derivatives to that already obtained from the milk, mothers must be cautioned not to "light up" when they nurse.

*Caffeine.* Caffeine freely crosses the human alveolar cell into the milk and is detectable within 15 minutes after oral ingestion. Levels of caffeine in breast milk are approximately 1% of the maternal dose. Accumulation of low doses of caffeine is possible, especially in breast-fed infants, since caffeine elimination is delayed and adult clearance levels are not achieved until 3 to 4 months of age.

*Alcohol.* Ethanol and many other substances in alcoholic beverages are transferred into the milk. Maximal blood concentration after a standard dose has occurred between 30 and 60 minutes after ingestion in a ratio of 0.9 in milk to maternal plasma. Once the ethanol is in the milk, it does not break down readily to acetaldehyde, which is thought to be the toxic compound in alcohol metabolism.

Large amounts of alcohol would have to be consumed by the mother before there would be an obvious clinical effect on the infant. At toxic levels, however, the effects can be significant. Foremost, of course, is the concern about the drunken mother's ability to care for the infant. Large amounts of alcohol also interfere with breast-feeding, first by hindrance of the milk-ejection reflex through inhibition of oxytocin release and second through the depressant effect on the infant, which causes less vigorous suckling.

**Other Recreational Drugs.** All known recreational drugs are excreted into breast milk, and pharmacokinetic data for humans are not available for most of them. Some, like marijuana and phencyclidine (PCP), are known after exposure to be in higher concentrations in the milk than in the maternal serum. The appearance of addictive drugs in breast milk, therefore, often precludes the continuance of breast-feeding.

## Pre-Existing Maternal Health Problems

**Maternal Phenylketonuria.** Limited data indicate that a phenylketonuric mother under strict dietary control should be allowed to breast-feed. No data are available on the potential problems encountered by a mother with uncontrolled phenylketonuria.

**Thyroid Disease.** Because conditions of hypothyroidism are often associated with infertility in females, they occur only rarely with lactation. When they do occur, breast-feeding can continue uninterrupted, since the therapy is usually full replacement with desiccated thyroid.

## Infectious Diseases Acquired Postpartum

**Human Immunodeficiency Virus (HIV).** Almost all infants who are positive for human immunodeficiency virus (HIV) in the early postpartum period contracted the disease during gestation. However, HIV has been isolated in breast milk, and although a minor transmission route for the disease, it appears that an infant may contract the syndrome through exposure to breast milk.

In developing countries, given the poor mortality prognosis of all infants who acquire AIDS or AIDS-related complex prenatally, breast-feeding should not necessarily be discouraged for that group, since the mortality risk from other infections, diarrhea, and dehydration from bottle-feeding may be greater than the increased mortality associated with HIV exposure. In developed countries, where safe feeding alternatives are available, bottle-feeding may be a safer course.

**Other Infectious Diseases.** Other retroviruses—such as human T-cell leukemia (HTLV-1) and cytomegalovirus (CMV), herpes simplex virus (HSV), rubella, and hepatitis B virus—have been isolated in breast milk. Breast-feeding may be the major mother-infant transmission route for HTLV-1. The Centers for Disease Control recommends that for all the viruses mentioned earlier, except HTLV-1, breast-feeding should not be discouraged. For HTLV-1, guidelines similar to those for HIV exposure should be followed.

## Contaminants

**Drug Therapy.** Most medications are found in human milk at 1% of maternal circulation. The rate of passage from maternal circulation to the milk depends on the molecular weight of the drug, the percentage that is protein-bound, pH, and water and lipid solubility. No unnecessary medications should be given to a nursing mother, since data are lacking on most drugs. The potential effects on the infant are largely unknown. Some drugs are clearly contraindicated during breast-feeding. Drug dosage, peak appearance, and the feeding schedule need to be coordinated. Usually the best time to give a drug is immediately after a feed.

## SUPPORT STRATEGY FOR MOTHER AND INFANT

With reduced time in the hospital after delivery, health professionals have little time to prepare the mother for nursing. Therefore, it is imperative that mothers receive sufficient preparation for lactation during the prenatal period and that both an emotional and educational support system be established for after delivery.

## PERINATAL CARE

### LABOR AND DELIVERY

#### Method of Delivery
Labor and delivery practices that encourage early mother-infant contact, reduced medication, and vaginal delivery extend the duration of lactation.

#### Mother-Infant Contact
Early mother-infant contact promotes frequent and early feeds and thus leads to lactation success. Frequent feeds may encourage increased milk intake and production through the suckling stimulation of the lactogenic hormone, prolactin. Increased nursing frequency also empties the breasts more often, and breast emptying may signal milk synthesis as well. Length of time at breast may have little or no independent effect on milk intake, although severely restricting the length of the feed may promote early involution and breast engorgement.

#### Maternal Fatigue and Stress
Maternal physical and emotional stress may inhibit prolactin and oxytocin release, which in turn limits milk production and letdown. If letdown is delayed because of anxiety or stress, then the relaxation can be coupled with the judicious use of synthetic oxytocin delivered nasally to promote letdown. Factors that promote successful lactation are listed in Table 63-2.

## COMMON PROBLEMS IN POSTPARTUM CARE

### INADEQUATE MILK SUPPLY

In the first 2 weeks of lactation, many women also express concern that they are not producing enough milk for their infant. If the baby is given formula supple-

**TABLE 63-2.** Practices That Promote Successful Lactation

---

Early maternal-infant contact
  Frequent and early feeds
    Complete breast emptying
Reduced medication
Vaginal delivery
Reduced maternal fatigue and stress
Reduced use of formula supplementation

---

mentation to assuage the mother's concerns, the infant will need less milk and the total time at the breast will be reduced, as will total milk production, thus aggravating the problem. When a substitute food is used in place of breast milk, the infant intakes of these two energy sources will be related inversely. The infant's appetite will regulate total caloric intake so that changes in consumption of one food will be offset by complementary changes in intake of the other food. Once lactation has been established, use of supplementary feeds may not reduce total milk production.

## MASTITIS

Mastitis is an inflammation of the mammary gland from some infectious process. Breast-feeding is contraindicated only if the abscess ruptures into a duct and contaminates the milk. If rupturing occurs, the breasts should be pumped so that gland involution will not take place.

## CONTRACEPTION

Since ovulation and menstruation can occur within the first 6 weeks for the woman who chooses to bottle-feed or partially breast-feed her infant, women who are sexually active should be counseled on contraception options during the early puerperal period. For women who choose to breast-feed exclusively, barrier methods or progestin-only oral contraceptives are the preferred methods. Combined estrogen and progestin pills, even of the low-dosage variety, appear to affect milk production and the duration of lactation.

# INDEX

Numbers followed by an f indicate a figure; t following a page number indicates tabular material

Abdominal anomalies, ultrasound diagnosis of, 211, 211f
Abdominal cancer, fetal, 206
Abdominal circumference
  indicative of IUGR, 244–245, 249t
  normal values for, 246t
Abdominal wall, defects of, 166–168
Abnormal labor
  active-phase dysfunction, 593–595
  disorders of descent, 595–597
  latent-phase dysfunction, 592–593
  patterns of, 593t
ABO hemolytic disease, 505
Abortion
  lupus erythematosus and, 539–540
  saline, 465
  septic, 339–340, 465
  spontaneous, 16–23, 397
Abruptio placentae, 333, 583–584
  causing DIC, 464
  clinical associations of, 585
  management of, 585–586
  in PROM, 629
  sites of, 584t
Abstinence syndrome, 64–65
Acetaminophen, pregnancy use risk, 71t, 532
Acetone, impact on fetus, 74t
Acetylcholinesterase (AChE) testing, 224
  to diagnose neural tube defects, 227
Achondrogenesis, 192–193
Achondroplasia, 193
Acid-base status, fetal, 289t, 290t, 292–295
Acrania, 210f
Acromelia, 179, 180t
Acute fatty liver of pregnancy, 437, 438f
Acute leukemia, 561–562
Acute renal failure, 444–445
  causes of, 444t
Acute urethral syndrome, 525
Adams-Oliver syndrome, 197
Adenocarcinoma, endometrial, 564
Adnexa, pregnancy-related changes in, 308
Adrenal gland
  cancers of, 565
  changes in pregnancy, 412

fetal, 413
  function of, 411–412
  hypersecretion disorders of, 413–415
  hyposecretion disorders of, 415–416
  laboratory testing of, 412–413, 414t
Adrenal hyperplasia, congenital, 416
Adrenal insufficiency, 415
Adult polycystic kidney disease, 172–174
Adult respiratory distress syndrome. See ARDS
AFAFP screening, 225f
  to diagnose neural tube defects, 226–227
  false measurements in, 226–227, 234
African sleeping sickness, in fetus, 114
Agenesis of the corpus callosum, 136–137
Aglossia-adactylia syndrome, 196
AIDS, 65
  malignancies associated with, 518t
  opportunistic infections in, 517t
  pneumonia in, 378
Air embolism, venous, 379–380
Alcohol
  adverse effects of, 320, 324–325
  mother's milk contaminated by, 656–657
  pregnancy use risk, 72t
  teratogenic capability of, 59–60, 61–63
Alloimmune thrombocytopenia, fetal, 471–472
Alpha fetoprotein (AFP), 224
  biology of, 223–236
  abnormal transport of, 234–236
  normal transport of, 233–234
  screening of. See AFAFP screening; MSAFP screening
Alpha thalassemia, 125
Amebiasis, in fetus, 115
American sleeping sickness, in fetus, 114
Amikacin, pregnancy use risk, 71t
Aminoglycosides, obstetric use of, 121
Aminophylline, pregnancy use risk, 72t
Aminopterin, pregnancy use risk, 55t, 73t
Amitriptyline, pregnancy use risk, 72t
Amniocentesis
  complications of, 219
  in first trimester, 214, 220

etiology and definition of, 238–240
management of, 46
prevention of, 44
risk factors of, 239t
ultrasound data in, 273
Intravascular fetal transfusion (IVT), 493
advantages and disadvantages of, 500
blood for, 494
delivery following, 501
in hydrops fetalis, 498–499
patient selection for, 494
risks of, 499–500, 500t
success rate of, 499, 499t
technique of, 496–498
Intraventricular hemorrhage, 600
Iodides
pregnancy use risk, 73t, 405
teratogenic capability of, 58t
Iodine deficiency, teratogenic capability
of, 58t
Ipsilateral oophorectomy, 32
Iron, requirements in pregnancy, 476,
477t
Iron deficiency anemia, 481
Isoimmunization, Doppler ultrasound
findings in, 257
Isoniazid, pregnancy use risk, 71t
Isotretinoin, teratogenic capability of, 57t

Jejunoileal bypass, 426
Jeune syndrome, 195
Juvenile respiratory papillomatosis, 92–93

Kala-azar, in fetus, 115
Karyotyping, fetal, 220
Kernicterus, 488–489
Ketoacidosis, diabetic, 394–396
Kidney. See also Renal entries
defects of, 170–174
dialysis in pregnancy, 447
postpartum changes in, 654
pregnancy-related changes in, 313
transplantation of, 447
Killed-virus vaccines, pregnancy use risk,
71t
Kniest syndrome, 195
Kyphosis, 181

Labor, 590–592
abnormal, 592–597. See also Abnormal
labor
induction of
in postmature pregnancy, 641, 642
in PROM, 633–635, 634t
preterm, 397, 606–624
Lactation
endocrine control of, 654–655
factors influencing, 658
inadequate, 658–659

milk composition and production, 655
promotion of, 658t
stages of, 654
Laparoscopic salpingostomy, 35
Laparoscopy, in diagnosis of ectopic preg-
nancy, 25
Late deceleration, 291–292
Lead, impact on fetus, 74t
Lecithin/sphingomyelin ratio (L/S), 12, 14,
14f
Leg length, fetal, 183t
Leiomyoma, degenerating, causing DIC,
466
Leishmaniasis, in fetus, 115
Leptospirosis, in fetus, 112
Lethal multiple pterygium syndrome, 18
Leukemia, 562
Lindane, obstetric use of, 123
Lipid metabolism, in pregnancy, 388
Listeriosis, in fetus, 108–109
Lithium carbonate, pregnancy use risk,
56t, 72t, 567
Live-virus vaccines, pregnancy use risk,
71t
Liver
postpartum changes in, 654
pregnancy-related changes in, 315, 316t
rupture of, 334–335
Liver diseases
cancer, 439, 564
differential diagnosis of, 434t
effects on pregnancy, 439–440
exacerbated by pregnancy, 438–439
unique to pregnancy, 433–437
Liver fluke, treatment during pregnancy,
513t
Long bone length, gestational age from,
248t
Low back pain, effects on pregnancy, 536
Low-birth-weight (LBW) infants
MSAFP diagnosis of, 235
risk factors for, 322
survival rates for, 618
Lung
pregnancy-related changes in, 312–313
scanning of, 456
Lupoid chronic active hepatitis, 440
Lupus anticoagulant, 21–23
Lupus erythematosus. See Systemic lupus
erythematosus (SLE)
Lupus obstetric syndrome, Doppler ultra-
sound findings in, 257
Luteal phase defects, 20
Lyme disease, 453, 514
in fetus, 111–112
Lymphocytes, disorders of, 127
Lymphocytic hypophysitis, 403
Lymphoma, non-Hodgkin's, 561